The Nutrition Bible

Also by Jean Anderson

The Doubleday Cookbook★ (with Elaine Hanna)

The Family Circle Cookbook (with the Food Editors of *Family Circle*)

The Grass Roots Cookbook

Jean Anderson's Processor Cooking

Half a Can of Tomato Paste & Other Culinary Dilemmas† (with Ruth Buchan)

Jean Anderson Cooks

The New Doubleday Cookbook (with Elaine Hanna)

The Food of Portugal‡

Micro Ways (with Elaine Hanna)

Jean Anderson's Sin-Free Desserts

The New German Cookbook (with Hedy Würz)

Also by Barbara Deskins

Everyone's Guide to Better Food and Nutrition

★Winner of the R. T. French Tastemaker Award, Best Basic Cookbook of the Year (1975), and Best Cookbook of the Year, Overall (1975).

†Winner of the R. T. French Tastemaker Award, Best Specialty Cookbook of the Year (1980).

‡Winner of the Seagram/International Association of Cooking Professionals Award, Best Foreign Cookbook of the Year (1986).

The Nutrition Bible

•

A Comprehensive, No-Nonsense Guide to Foods,
Nutrients, Additives, Preservatives, Pollutants
and Everything Else We Eat and Drink

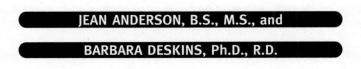

JEAN ANDERSON, B.S., M.S., and

BARBARA DESKINS, Ph.D., R.D.

Quill
William Morrow
NEW YORK

LIBRARY OF CONGRESS CATALOGING-IN-PUBLICATION DATA

Anderson, Jean
    The nutrition bible : a comprehensive, no-nonsense guide
to foods, nutrients, additives, preservatives, pollutants and
everything else we eat and drink / Jean Anderson, Barbara Deskins.
      p.   cm.
    Includes index.
    ISBN 0–688–15559–6
    1. Nutrition—Dictionaries.   I. Deskins, Barbara B.   II. Title.
RA784.A533   1995
613.2'03—dc20
                                        94–38080
                                          CIP

PRINTED IN THE UNITED STATES OF AMERICA

First Quill Edition

    3   4   5   6   7   8   9   10

BOOK DESIGN BY VERTIGO DESIGN

EDITORIAL ASSISTANCE PROVIDED BY K&N BOOKWORKS

Introduction

In this age of fitness, arcane words and terms come at us from every quarter. They glare at us from television screens, confront us in newspapers and magazines, lurk on supermarket shelves, even surface in our refrigerators, freezers and cupboards.

These are the mind-deadening, polysyllabic words of *nutri-speak*. The language of diet, fitness and health.

If the 1980s were the decade of culinary excess, the 1990s are the decade of eating right and keeping fit, of questioning (if not altogether abandoning) the old nutritional myths, of understanding the true relationship between good diet and good health.

Since the beginning of time, man has used food to prevent or cure disease, although early on he had no knowledge of nutrition. Just as Jewish mothers now administer chicken soup to thwart colds and flu, shamans once brewed broths of evergreen branches (in each case, the fragrant steam opens the respiratory passages). Nutritionists now know so many of the killer and metabolic diseases of generations past (beriberi, pellagra, rickets, scurvy) to be nothing more than acute vitamin deficiencies (of thiamin, niacin, vitamin D and vitamin C, respectively). These are diseases that proper diets would have prevented.

Even in the high-tech times of today, the old adage "You are what you eat" still applies. Most of us now know that too much fat, too much sugar, too much salt—the staples of junk food—are bad and that fresh fruits and vegetables are good. The nutritionally aware among us are scaling back on portions, choosing whole grains and flours over those that are refined and using monounsaturated vegetable oils instead of saturated fats, which are known to increase the risk of coronary heart disease. But now there are even newer concerns.

With bacteria such as salmonella invading many of America's henhouses and *Escherichia coli* cropping up in our hamburgers, we worry about the safety of our food. We fret about water pollution, about toxic fallout both industrial and agricultural. We're afraid of additives, stymied by shifting theories about vitamins and exasperated by conflicting reports about what we should and shouldn't eat. Finally, we're frustrated by the language of nutrition (not least the nutri-babble of package labels).

Our minds are muddled with such terms as HDL ("good" cholesterol) and LDL ("bad" cholesterol), with antioxidants, trans fatty acids and genetic engineering. And what do we really know about carbohydrates, proteins, fats, vitamins and minerals? About those exciting new nonnutrients called functional foods, phytochemicals or nutraceuticals, which hold such promise in preventing (or thwarting) a variety of diseases, including cancer? What do we really know about the effects of food irradiation? Antioxidants? Anorexia? Herbal teas and folk remedies?

With America's interest in nutrition intensifying, with those who barely knew a vitamin from a virus suddenly getting into fitness and becoming concerned about what they put into their mouths, we felt it was time for a comprehensive, commonsense nutrition decoder. A nononsense dictionary that defines in lay language all the baffling words and phrases of nutri-speak. A "good book" written by nutritionists with postgraduate degrees who tell it like it is, separating fact from fiction.

We've spent years on the project, consulted with scientific experts, done untold time in library stacks, plowed through every reputable source we could find. It has been arduous, this labor of love. But we were determined that the truth be told.

So we begin with A, VITAMIN, and proceed right through ZWIEBACK, discussing foods and health foods; nutrients, additives and pollutants; enzymes and hormones; food-related diseases and deficiencies. We take them up one by one, translating the terms into plain English and presenting the latest nutritional findings.

We have included nutrient counts for all the major foods and beverages (and some of the minor ones) because we believe it's important to learn which foods are high (or low) in fat or saturated fat, in calories or cholesterol. To know, too, which vitamins and minerals they supply in abundance, which they contain in moderate amounts and which they lack altogether. We're aware that figures vary somewhat from source to source—but not enough to seriously misrepresent nutrient content overall. Our figures, for the most part, are taken from the U.S. Department of Agriculture's *Composition of Foods: Raw, Processed, Prepared, Parts 1 through 21* (we list supplementary sources for nu-

trient counts in the Bibliography). Thus you can compare the amount of protein or vitamin C, for example, in a portion of any food with your Recommended Dietary Allowance.

Although *The Nutrition Bible* is designed to answer questions about nutrition and health, it is in no way intended to replace a visit to the doctor, a registered dietitian or another health-care provider.

Its purpose, quite simply, is to unscramble all the nutri-jabber that surrounds us and to present, in as readable and reliable a fashion as possible, all the latest food and nutrition information available. *The Nutrition Bible* was written for the millions of Americans genuinely concerned about eating right and staying fit (as well as for those who may "get nutrition" one day soon). May they find it as essential as *Webster's*.

—JEAN ANDERSON, B.S., M.S., *New York*
—BARBARA DESKINS, Ph.D., R.D.,
    Associate Professor, Clinical Dietetics
    and Nutrition Department,
    University of Pittsburgh

Abbreviations Used in This Book

α-TE = alpha-tocopherol equivalent (the unit of measure used for vitamin E)

CDC = Centers for Disease Control

EPA = Environmental Protection Agency

ESADDI = Estimated Safe and Adequate Daily Dietary Intake

FDA = U.S. Food and Drug Administration

g = gram

GRAS = Generally Recognized as Safe, by the FDA (applied to food additives)

IU = international unit, the unit of measurement for such fat-soluble vitamins as D and E

mcg = microgram

mg = milligram

NA = nutrient count not available

NE = niacin equivalent

RDA = Recommended Dietary Allowance (daily; of vitamins, minerals and protein)

RE = retinol equivalent (the unit of measure used for vitamin A)

USDA = U.S. Department of Agriculture

Notes

Cross-references are indicated by small capital letters; "see ALGINATES," for example. Boldface type is used to indicate alternate terms as well as subcategories within entries.

•

The Recommended Dietary Allowances (RDAs) given for all vitamins and minerals, and also for protein, are adapted from *Recommended Dietary Allowances,* Tenth Edition, by the Food and Nutrition Board of the National Research Council (Washington, D.C.: National Academy Press, 1989). Because RDAs are updated only every five to ten years, these figures are the most current ones available.

•

About recipe nutrient counts: All nutrient counts are based strictly upon recipe ingredients, not upon suggested accompaniments. If a recipe suggests alternative or optional ingredients, the nutrient counts for these are not included unless otherwise stated.

In these nutrient counts (both for individual foods and for recipes), the first figure represents total fat content; the second the amount of the total that is saturated. For example: *7 g fat, 2 saturated* means that there are 7 total grams of fat and that 2 of those 7 grams are saturated.

The Nutrition Bible

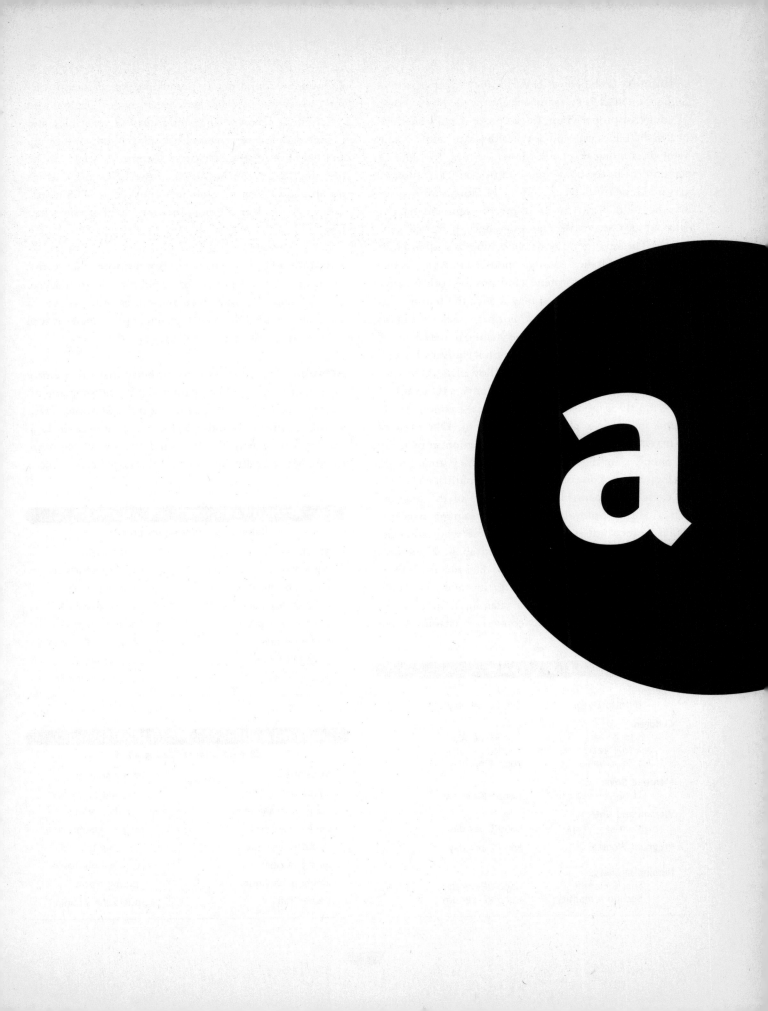

A, Vitamin: Absolutely essential for the proper growth of children, vitamin A or **retinol** is also needed by children *and* adults for proper vision (it can prevent and sometimes cure night blindness) and for healthy skin and mucous membranes lining the body's inner cavities. In addition, vitamin A helps the body fight infection and, according to Harvard University's recent Nurses' Health Study, may reduce the risk of breast cancer. Its precursor present in many plants, BETA-CAROTENE, may also reduce the risk of some cancers. The latest good news, according to a Johns Hopkins School of Medicine study conducted in Africa, is that vitamin A and beta-carotene (and possibly other carotenoid vitamin A precursors) may reduce the transmission of AIDS from mother to infant. Formerly measured in international units (IU), which some vitamin bottle labels still list, vitamin A is now measured in retinol equivalents (RE). The latest Recommended Dietary Allowance (RDA) lists RE only, so that's what we use. To convert IU to RE: 1 RE = 3.3 IU if food source is an animal (retinol), 10 IU if food source is a plant (beta-carotene). **DEFICIENCY SYMPTOMS:** Lowered resistance to infection; rough, dry and pimply skin; digestive problems; kidney stones; night blindness and eye disease, including xerophthalmia, which can cause permanent blindness. Results of the ongoing Nurses' Health Study (an eight-year program involving 89,000 women nurses) suggest that those who didn't get enough beta-carotene and retinol had about 25 percent more breast cancers than those whose diets met the RDAs. **GOOD SOURCES:** Liver, eggs, margarines and whole milk and low-fat milks fortified with vitamin A. In addition, beta-carotene, which the body converts to vitamin A, can be found in abundance in pumpkins, winter squash, carrots, sweet red peppers, apricots, mangoes, papayas and other bright yellow/orange/red fruits and vegetables, also in such dark leafy greens as chard, spinach, mustard, turnip and beet tops. **PRECAUTIONS:** Vitamin A is fat soluble, meaning that it can be stored in the body and that it's possible to OD on high-dosage supplements. The worst-case scenario: blurred vision, increased skull pressure, hair loss.

Accutane: The brand name for **isotretinoin,** a derivative of vitamin A that's prescribed in pill form to treat severe cases of acne. Because Accutane causes birth defects, it should be avoided by women planning pregnancies as well as by women who are already pregnant.

Acerola: A Caribbean cherry or berry that is extremely high in vitamin C. Most vitamin C pills and supplements labeled "natural" are made from acerola. **SEASON:** Fresh acerola is difficult to find at any season of the year in U.S. markets although in the West Indies it's available year-round. Many health-food stores sell bottled acerola juice.

RDA FOR VITAMIN A	
Babies:	
Birth to 1 year	375 RE per day
Children:	
1 to 3 years	400 RE per day
4 to 6 years	500 RE per day
7 to 10 years	700 RE per day
Men and Boys:	
11 to 51+ years	1,000 RE per day
Women and Girls:	
11 to 51+ years	800 RE per day
Pregnant Women:	800 RE per day
Nursing Mothers:	
First 6 months	1,300 RE per day
Second 6 months	1,200 RE per day

NUTRIENT CONTENT OF 1 CUP RAW ACEROLA	
(about 3½ ounces; 98 grams)	
31 calories	7 mg sodium
0 g protein	143 mg potassium
0 g fat, 0 saturated	0 g dietary fiber
0 mg cholesterol	75 RE vitamin A
8 g carbohydrate	0.02 mg thiamin
12 mg calcium	0.05 mg riboflavin
9 mg phosphorus	0.3 mg niacin
0.2 mg iron	1,644 mg vitamin C

NUTRIENT CONTENT OF 1 CUP FRESH ACEROLA JUICE	
(8 fluid ounces; 242 grams)	
51 calories	7 mg sodium
1 g protein	235 mg potassium
0.7 g fat, 0 saturated	1 g dietary fiber
0 mg cholesterol	123 RE vitamin A
12 g carbohydrate	0.05 mg thiamin
24 mg calcium	0.15 mg riboflavin
22 mg phosphorus	1.0 mg niacin
1.2 mg iron	3,872 mg vitamin C

Acesulfame-K (additive; artificial sweetener): Sold as Sweet One and Sunette, this newest noncaloric, non-nutritive sweetener (200 times sweeter than sugar and okay for baking) was FDA-approved in 1988. It's still under scrutiny, however, because its chemical structure closely resembles that of saccharin, a weak carcinogen. Although more than ninety studies have shown acesulfame-K, a potassium salt that supposedly passes through the body unchanged, to be safe, some tests suggest otherwise. The findings: A group of rats fed acesulfame-K developed more tumors than those not fed it; also, acesulfame-K raised the blood cholesterol levels of diabetic rats. Consumer watchdogs want further testing. GRAS.

Acetaminophen: Although the painkiller acetaminophen does not cause gastrointestinal bleeding (as aspirin sometimes does), it can, on rare occasions, bring on anemia or jaundice or significantly lower the white blood cell count. It's best to take acetaminophen products, such as Tylenol, with food and to avoid alcohol while using it. Indeed, one liver expert, testifying recently before an FDA panel, warned that if you down more than two alcoholic drinks a day, you should halve the maximum recommended daily dosage of acetaminophen. As a result, the FDA panel recommended that serious drinkers be warned: Taking large doses of acetaminophen while continuing to drink can mean severe liver damage.

Acetic Acid (additive): The acid in vinegar (4 to 6 percent) and an ancient food additive. It is used to flavor fruit beverages, cheeses, pickles, relishes, ketchup, baked goods, also to control their acidity. GRAS.

Acetone Peroxide (additive): A bleach and conditioner used in milling flour. Although the FDA considers it safe, it's due further testing. GRAS.

Achiote: See ANNATTO.

Acid: A chemical compound that has the power to neutralize alkalies such as lye. The strength of acids is measured on the pH scale (*pH* stands for "potential hydrogen," because acids release hydrogen ions into water solutions). Anything with a pH of 7 is considered neutral, but the lower the pH number—6, 5, 4, 3 and so forth—the stronger the acid. Most foods are slightly acidic and those that are highly acid—lemon juice and vinegar, to name two—are distinctly sour.

Acidophilus Milk: A tart and creamy milk made by injecting a culture of *Lactobacillus acidophilus*. It's often prescribed for people who can't properly digest LACTOSE (milk sugar), usually because their digestive tracts lack the necessary enzyme LACTASE. It is also recommended to those who've been taking antibiotics and need to have "benign" or beneficial bacteria reintroduced into their digestive tracts. The nutritive value of acidophilus milk is the same as the milk from which it's made. Before 1970 most people hated acidophilus milk because it was so sour. What's sold today throughout America is "sweet" acidophilus milk, a highly palatable but no less effective form made possible through improved methods. To capsulize, *Lactobacillus acidophilus* bacteria are introduced into sweet milk *after* it's pasteurized, then the milk's kept refrigerated so they can't proliferate and sour the milk.

Acid Reflux: This painful form of heartburn is now better known as reflux ESOPHAGITIS.

Acne (diet and): In the old days, dermatologists and dietitians fingered chocolate, french fries, potato chips, nuts, colas (all the junk foods teenagers adore) as the culprits behind "bumps" or "zits." Now they're more inclined to blame heredity, androgens (hormones that kick into overdrive when children, especially boys, reach puberty), stress, oily cosmetics and shampoos. Still, vitamin A and/or zinc deficiency may play a role. For acute cases, ACCUTANE is prescribed; also ointments or liquids containing RETIN-A (a vitamin A derivative). Many nutritionists aren't closing the book on diet and acne, however, and suggest avoiding any foods that seem to trigger outbreaks.

Acorn Squash: See SQUASH.

Acrolein: A volatile mucous membrane-damaging aldehyde formed when fats reach the smoke point. This chemical breakdown (specifically the dehydration of glycerol) is most apt to happen when meats are broiled or grilled too close to the flame or when foods are sautéed or deep-fat-fried at intense heat.

Additives: To some, all additives are bad. In truth, many of them are not only *not hazardous to our health; they are essential to the preservation of our health.* Broadly speaking, additives can be classified according to function. There are flavorings and flavor enhancers; colorings; nutritional supplements (usually vitamins and minerals added to flours and cereals to replace nutrients lost during milling and refining); antioxidants (to prevent rancidity); preservatives (to retard spoilage); emulsifiers, stabilizers and texturizers (to keep creamy foods creamy); thickeners; humectants (to keep foods moist); anticaking agents (for free-flowing flours and salts); leavening agents; bleaches; dough conditioners; and sweeteners. Of the nearly 3,000 "chemicals" U.S. processors intentionally add to food, 98 percent are nothing more than sugar, corn syrup, salt, pepper, citric acid (found naturally in citrus fruits), baking soda, mustard and vegetable colors. Then there are the unintentional additives that make their way into our food supply on its long journey from farm to dinner table. These include residuals of drugs given to animals, of pesticides and herbicides, even of chemicals that migrate into food from plastic packaging and metal cookware.

The FDA is mandated by law to regulate the food industry and ensure the safety of our food supply. Not always with complete success, as consumer watchdogs are quick to point out. Anyone scanning a food label will be bewildered (frightened, perhaps) by the number of additives. It's impossible to cover them all, but we do discuss the most commonly used and controversial ones elsewhere in this book. They're listed alphabetically.

Adipic Acid (additive): Used to impart tartness to fruit-flavored gelatins and soft drinks. GRAS.

Adipose Tissue: Fatty tissue or deposits formed when the body stores unused calories in the form of fat. Contrary to popular opinion, fat—or at least moderate amounts of it—is necessary to cushion such organs as the kidneys, also to help insulate the body and keep it at a constant temperature.

Adult-Onset Diabetes: See DIABETES.

Adzuki Beans: See BEANS, DRIED.

Aflatoxin: A poison produced when a specific mold (ASPERGILLUS FLAUUS) grows on contaminated peanuts, corn and other grains. Aflatoxin has been linked to liver tumors, which are common in parts of Africa where peanuts are a staple. In the United States, susceptible foods are carefully screened for aflatoxin and the mold that produces it. The FDA sets the tolerance level for aflatoxin at 5 parts per billion (ppb) for milk and 20 ppb for other foods. Many scientists would like to see these limits lowered to ensure that our food supply is even safer. Because of America's growing awareness of aflatoxin and parental concern about its presence in peanut butter, Consumers Union recently tested three top brands—Jif, Peter Pan and Skippy—for aflatoxin and found no more than a trace in any of them. Not so supermarket "generics," which averaged five times as much aflatoxin as the brand names. Worst of all, with ten times the aflatoxin of brand-name peanut butters, were the freshly ground, health-food "natural" peanut butters.

Agar (additive): A clear, flavorless form of seaweed sold in bars, leaves and flakes, usually in Asian grocery stores, that's used to thicken foods much the way gelatin does. Vegetarians depend on agar because true gelatin is made from calves' feet. Many commercial ice cream manufacturers also rely on agar to give their ice creams and sherbets a rich, butter-smooth consistency. As an additive, agar is rated GRAS.

Aging (diet and): Do your nutritional needs change after you pass the big Five-O? Certainly the RDAs set by the National Academy of Sciences treat all adults more or less the same regardless of age. Many scientists, however, now believe that nutritional needs do indeed change with age. Body processes slow, nutrients are less efficiently metabolized, immune systems break down, medications interfere with digestion and assimilation of nutrients and some of them stress vital organs and accelerate bone loss. To counteract, or at least temper, the effects of aging, some nutritionists recommend boosting intake of the B vitamins B_6, B_{12} and folic acid; of vitamins C, D and E; and of beta-carotene and calcium. They deplore the lack of research on geriatric nutrition and call for studies to pinpoint how dietary needs change with age. Meanwhile, they don't advocate megadoses of vitamins. On the contrary, they suggest eating fewer high-calorie, high-fat, high-cholesterol foods, more whole grains, fresh fruits and vegetables. They also recommend more exercise and perhaps, if needed, a daily multivitamin tablet.

AIDS (acquired immune deficiency syndrome) (diet and):

AIDS is a viral disease that impairs the immune system of the human body, leaving the victim open to various infections. Because AIDS manifests itself in so many ways (infections, malignancies, neurologic disease), dietary management must be individually tailored to the needs of the patient. Many patients suffer from PEM (protein-energy malnutrition), some from mouth sores that make eating difficult, others from diarrhea. Many also show reduced blood levels of vitamin A and its precursor beta-carotene, as well as selenium, which is believed to trigger the formation of immune-system-bolstering T-cells. Will bulking up on these nutrients (especially the nontoxic beta-carotene) slow the progress of AIDS? No medical researcher is willing to climb out on that limb. Yet. However, promising results are just in from an African study conducted by the Johns Hopkins School of Medicine in Baltimore. It suggests that mothers deficient in vitamin A, beta-carotene and/or other carotenoids are more likely to pass the AIDS virus along to their newborns than mothers with "healthy" blood levels of these nutrients. Before AIDS reaches the terminal stage, it's important for patients to eat a well-balanced diet each and every day, avoiding, perhaps, raw fruits and vegetables and undercooked meats, fish and poultry that might be contaminated with disease-causing bacteria. Each AIDS patient must be monitored and reevaluated by physicians and dietitians as the disease progresses.

Airplane Food:

One frequent international flier never eats airline food east or south of Rome because catering kitchens overseas are not as carefully monitored for sanitation and safe handling of food as they are in this country. Another always orders the children's plate on foreign carriers, knowing it will be given special attention. And a third packs fruit, bread and cheese, then picnics aloft. Although food poisoning is a distinct possibility with airline food (savvy travelers avoid aspics, creamed foods, seafood, gelatin salads and desserts), the FDA, through the U.S. Public Health Service Act, makes every effort to watchdog domestic airline caterers, both on the ground and in the air,

to assure travelers of safe food and drink. Many airlines cater to those on restricted diets, because of either health or religious taboos, but require at least twenty-four hours' notice for a special menu (low-calorie, low-fat, kosher, etc.).

Aji-no-moto:

You'll see bottles of this white powder in Asian grocery stores, also in upscale supermarkets. It's nothing more than MONOSODIUM GLUTAMATE sold under its Japanese brand name.

Alanine:

One of the nonessential AMINO ACIDS.

Alar:

The trade name for **daminozide,** a chemical used by apple growers to ripen their crops all at once, reduce premature windfalls, firm and redden apples and prolong their storage life. A few years back, Alar was reported to cause cancer, especially in children, and the public outcry was so heated apple growers voluntarily stopped using Alar and the manufacturer withdrew it from the market. Apples grown in the United States have been Alar-free since 1989 and Alar is no longer registered for use on any food crops.

Albacore:

The "white meat" yellowfin tuna, which Americans prefer to either light or dark meat tuna. Albacore isn't really white, however, but ivory-hued or pink. When canned, albacore is labeled "white meat tuna" and is packed in either vegetable oil or water. For the nutrient content, see TUNA.

Albumins:

Proteins found in food (**ovalbumin** is the protein in egg white, **lactalbumin** one of those found in milk). Albumin is also present in blood serum; indeed, its blood serum value is used in nutrition assessment. If, for example, the blood serum value is low, it may mean malnutrition or liver disease.

Alcohol, Alcoholic Beverages:

Few people consider alcohol food, yet it's loaded with calories and can pack on the pounds. Researchers at the Beltsville Human Nutrition Research Center in Maryland have recently proved that the body doesn't burn "alcohol calories" any faster or more efficiently than it does those from fat or carbohydrate. Alcohol weighs in at 7 calories per gram, versus 9 for fat, 4 for carbohydrate and protein—something to bear in mind when you want a second martini or can of beer. Alcohol (or **ethyl** alcohol, to be technically correct) is produced as yeasts metabolize certain sugars. **Gin** (from grain with juniper for flavor) and **vodka** (from potatoes or grain) are the purest forms of alcohol. **Scotch whisky** comes from barley; **bourbon** from corn; **rye** from rye; **rum** from sugarcane; **tequila** from cactus; **wine** from grapes; and **beer, ale** and **stout** from hops. The higher a beverage's proof (alcohol content) and the sweeter it is, the more the calories. For example:

1 oz light beer = 7 to 9 calories

1 oz beer, ale or stout = 11 to 14 calories

1 oz table wine = 17 to 29 calories
(depending on sweetness and alcoholic content)

1 oz sparkling wine = 21 to 42 calories
(depending on sweetness and alcoholic content)

1 oz dessert (fortified) wine = 35 to 52 calories (depending on sweetness and alcoholic content)

1 oz 80-proof whiskey = 65 calories

1 oz 86-proof whiskey = 70 calories

1 oz 90-proof whiskey = 74 calories

1 oz 94-proof whiskey = 77 calories

1 oz 100-proof whiskey = 83 calories

1 oz liqueur = 82 to 116 calories
(depending on proof and added sweeteners)

According to a recent ten-year study conducted on 130,000 adults by the Kaiser Permanente Medical Center in Oakland, California, moderate drinking lowers your risk of dying of heart disease by 30 percent. It may also mean 65 percent fewer colds—provided you don't smoke (or so a new English/American study of 400 healthy men and women suggests). By *moderate drinking,* researchers mean 12 ounces of beer per day *or* 5 ounces of wine *or* 1½ ounces of whiskey for women and twice that for men. The flip side is that moderate drinking may increase a woman's chance of breast cancer by about 10 percent. Pregnant women who drink—even a glass of beer or wine a day— risk having babies with FETAL ALCOHOL SYNDROME. A major problem with alcohol is that few people can limit themselves to one or two drinks a day. Although beers and wines do contain some carbohydrate and minerals, whiskey offers nothing but calories and, when downed in quantity, depletes the body's supply of vitamin B₁ (thiamin) and magnesium (see ALCOHOLISM). It should be noted, how-

ever, that when wine and spirits are used in cooking, much of the alcohol quickly evaporates, leaving only their flavors behind. See also WINES.

Alcoholism (diet and): Alcoholism is as much a disease as, say, cancer, and it can be equally deadly. Both chronic and progressive, it is characterized by a physical dependency on alcohol, which can savage the liver. Eating poorly and obtaining 50 to 60 percent of their calories from drink, most alcoholics are malnourished. They are particularly deficient in protein, thiamin and other vitamins of the B-complex, which are squandered in the oxidation of alcohol, a process that takes place in—and ultimately damages—the liver. In addition to cirrhosis, alcoholics often suffer from high blood pressure, gastritis, pancreatitis, kidney disease and dementia. Rehab involves team efforts by physicians, psychiatrists and dietitians, who prescribe liquids at the start, then balanced menus of solid food plus supplements to boost the body's supply of B vitamins.

Aldicarb: A highly toxic pesticide, still in use, that's showing up in well water. It has been a particular problem on Long Island, New York, where, after years of use in the potato fields, it has begun leaching into the aquifer. Among the aware, there's a movement to ban aldicarb.

Ale: Like beer, ale is a fermented malt beverage made from hops. But because it is brewed in a slightly different way, ale tastes much "hoppier" than beer. **Stout** is a popular strong, coffee-dark ale, brewed for the most part in Ireland.

NUTRIENT CONTENT OF 1 CUP ALE	
(8 fluid ounces; 267 grams)	
98 calories	17 mg sodium
1 g protein	8 mg potassium
0 g fat, 0 saturated	0 g dietary fiber
0 mg cholesterol	0 RE vitamin A
9 g carbohydrate	0.10 mg thiamin
12 mg calcium	0.70 mg riboflavin
72 mg phosphorus	1.4 mg niacin
0 mg iron	0 mg vitamin C

Aleurone: The layer of cells just beneath the bran in grains, especially in kernels of wheat and barley. Aleurone is rich in nutrients but is removed when wheat is milled into white flour.

Alfalfa Sprouts: The tiny silvery shoots of germinating alfalfa seeds. Mild and tender, they're a salad-bar staple and can now be bought at many supermarkets in little plastic boxes. According to some food professionals, however, they can be toxic if eaten in large quantities. Certainly, they are a gassy food, capable of inducing heartburn and bloating. Alfalfa sprouts are very low in calories but contain small amounts of vitamins A and C, thiamin, riboflavin and niacin. **SEASON:** Year-round.

NUTRIENT CONTENT OF 1 CUP ALFALFA SPROUTS	
(about 1¼ ounces; 33 grams)	
10 calories	2 mg sodium
1 g protein	26 mg potassium
0 g fat, 0 saturated	1 g dietary fiber
0 mg cholesterol	5 RE vitamin A
1 g carbohydrate	0.03 mg thiamin
10 mg calcium	0.04 mg riboflavin
23 mg phosphorus	0.2 mg niacin
0.3 mg iron	3 mg vitamin C

Alfalfa Tea: Although this herbal tea (made from the same legume that's grown for silage) has its champions, its saponins (toxic sugar derivatives) can wreck the digestion, even interfere with breathing.

Algae: Pond scum and seaweed are among the aquatic plants called algae. Some of them are adored by the Japanese. In this country, health-food stores push SPIRULINA (a blue-green alga) powder, tablets and liquid (all expensive), multibilling them as energy powerhouses, pound melters, magical sources of active vitamin B_{12}, even as miracle cures for Alzheimer's disease. In truth, spirulina isn't very nutritious. Ten capsules don't even supply 3 percent of the RDA of protein—most of this in the form of PHENYLALANINE, an amino acid that's toxic to those with PHENYLKETONURIA (PKU) because they can't metabolize it. All alga add fiber to the diet, some vitamin A and an unusable form of B_{12}. Some forms of spirulina, which the FDA promptly seized, were found to contain a poisonous alga. And here are more facts about this so-called superfood: Some people taking spirulina have suffered severe gastrointestinal upsets; there have even been cases of suffocation. Still, algae are being touted as the foods of tomorrow. And in their quest for energy, celebrities and athletes are already scarfing down freeze-dried algae.

Alginates (additives): **Ammonium alginate, calcium alginate** and **potassium alginate** are gelatinous substances obtained from seaweeds used to keep ice creams creamy and breads, cakes, cookies and candies moist. They are also used to remove mineral particles from cheeses, cheese products, sugar-free jams and jellies. GRAS.

Alimentary Canal: The digestive tract or gastrointestinal tract.

Alitame: An artificial sweetener, said to be 2,000 times sweeter than sugar, which can be used for baking. The FDA has yet to approve it.

Alkali, Alkaline: The opposite of acids, alkalies are also called **bases.** They neutralize acids in a water solution, the reaction that baking powder uses in the process of leavening (the gas released when acids and alkalies collide, bubble through batters and doughs, causing cakes, quick breads and cookies to rise). Most alkaline substances (baking powder among them) taste bitter, almost soapy. Very few foods are alkaline.

Alkaloids: These odorless, intensely bitter, nitrogen-based compounds occur naturally in certain plants and can affect animals profoundly. Certain alkaloids—**strychnine** and **cocaine,** to name two—are among the most powerful poisons and narcotics known to man. Even CAFFEINE, an alkaloid/stimulant present in chocolate, coffee, tea and cola nuts, packs a wallop.

Allergy: Anyone who's exploded into a sneezing fit or spent days suffering from a dripping nose and red, running eyes knows what an allergy is. By definition, an allergy is an immune reaction to a foreign substance (pollen, to name one) that causes the body to manufacture antibodies. What are often passed off as allergies are actually food intolerances—the inability to digest **lactose** (milk sugar), for example, because the body doesn't produce enough of the proper enzyme (**lactase**). The foods most apt to cause grief (both allergies and intolerances) are nuts, eggs, milk, soybeans, wheat, peanuts, chicken, fish and shellfish. Although many people say they're allergic to the sodium bisulfites used in food preparation, processing and preservation, this is less a true allergy than a sensitivity (see SULFITES). Those with any serious reactions to food should consult a physician whose specialty is allergies.

Allicin: Down through the ages, garlic has been prized for its medicinal properties, and with good reason. Today food scientists are zeroing in on allicin, a sulfur compound present in garlic that may be a powerful anticarcinogen.

Almond Paste: See MARZIPAN.

Almonds: Two types of these nuts grow throughout the world: **bitter almonds** (illegal in the United States because of their prussic acid content), from which oil and flavorings are extracted; and **sweet almonds,** the nuts we love to nibble and our main concern here. **NUTRITIVE VALUE:** Although loaded with fat and calories, almonds contain no cholesterol and their fat is at least unsaturated. Almonds are also a moderate source of protein, dietary fiber, iron, potassium and riboflavin. If unsalted, they are low in sodium.

NUTRIENT CONTENT OF 1 OUNCE (28 GRAMS) BLANCHED UNSALTED ALMONDS

170 calories	1 mg sodium
5 g protein	219 mg potassium
15 g fat, 1 saturated	3 g dietary fiber
0 mg cholesterol	0 RE vitamin A
6 g carbohydrate	0.05 mg thiamin
66 mg calcium	0.26 mg riboflavin
143 mg phosphorus	0.9 mg niacin
1.3 mg iron	0 mg vitamin C

NUTRIENT CONTENT OF 1 OUNCE (28 GRAMS) DRY-ROASTED UNSALTED ALMONDS

150 calories	5 mg sodium
7 g protein	90 mg potassium
14 g fat, 1 saturated	3 g dietary fiber
0 mg cholesterol	0 RE vitamin A
5 g carbohydrate	0.04 mg thiamin
100 mg calcium	0.17 mg riboflavin
150 mg phosphorus	0.8 mg niacin
1.1 mg iron	0 mg vitamin C

NUTRIENT CONTENT OF 1 OUNCE (28 GRAMS) ROASTED, SALTED ALMONDS

178 calories	218 mg sodium
5 g protein	219 mg potassium
16 g fat, 2 saturated	2 g dietary fiber
0 mg cholesterol	0 RE vitamin A
6 g carbohydrate	0.04 mg thiamin
67 mg calcium	0.26 mg riboflavin
143 mg phosphorus	1.0 mg niacin
1.3 mg iron	0 mg vitamin C

Alpha-tocopherol, Vitamin E (additive): When used as an additive, alpha-tocopherol helps to keep fats and oils from turning rancid. See also E, VITAMIN. GRAS.

Aluminum, Aluminum Cookware: Although there's no known function for aluminum in the body at present, our bodies contain between 50 and 150 milligrams of it and most Americans swallow from 10 to 100 milligrams more of it every day (plant and animal foods both contain aluminum and so may drinking water). Does aluminum cause Alzheimer's disease? One controversial epidemiological survey reported that the risk of Alzheimer's was 1½ times greater in areas where the water supply contained high levels of aluminum than in areas where it was low. And autopsies have shown that there are high concentrations of aluminum in the brains of those who have died of Alzheimer's. *Still, most scientists believe that this is probably the result of the disease, not the cause.* And what about cooking in aluminum pots and pans? Is it dangerous? Not really. Very little aluminum leaches into the food although a recent French study suggests that if the food is acidic (tomatoes, for example) the absorption of aluminum may be somewhat higher. Still, other items up our aluminum intake far more—baking powders, for example, and antacids made with aluminum hydroxide.

Aluminum Sulfate, Cake Alum, Patent Alum (additive): Usually called just **alum** and so sour it will turn your mouth inside out, this white compound is used by commercial and home canners to keep pickles crisp and firm. GRAS.

Alzheimer's Disease (diet and): This cruel, irreversible degeneration of the brain, which now afflicts four million Americans (and nearly four times as many people worldwide), causes premature and progressive senility. The brains of Alzheimer's victims contain abnormally high levels of aluminum. And according to recent experiments conducted at Massachusetts General Hospital in Boston (a

Harvard affiliate), there also appears to be a link between zinc and Alzheimer's. Test-tube studies suggest that zinc may cause certain proteins to become insoluble and clump in the brain, destroying gray matter. A buildup of this "brain plaque" is common in Alzheimer's patients. Is dietary zinc to blame? The Boston researchers doubt it, but they do warn against taking megadoses of this trace element. A major problem with Alzheimer's patients is that they often forget to eat or eat poorly. Many seem almost addicted to sweets and, if given the chance, will eat huge quantities of them, sometimes to the exclusion of other food. Some Alzheimer's patients pace constantly and need up to 1,600 extra calories a day for energy.

Amaranth: Once a staple of the Aztecs, this ancient South American plant is being rediscovered. Its grain, which can be ground into flour or cooked like rice, is a source of high-quality protein, fiber and iron. And its green leaves, best boiled like kale, are powerhouses of potassium and vitamin A. **SEASON:** Spring and summer for the leaves, year-round for the grain.

Amberjack: A deep-sea, warm-water fish, firm and light of flesh, that can weigh as much as 175 pounds. These monsters are often riddled with parasites and may also contain ciguatoxin, which can lay you low for weeks, even months, with severe flulike symptoms (see CIGUATERA POISONING). Small jacks (less than 5 pounds) are the best— and safest—to eat. Brown-skinned, with glints of amber and lavender, amberjack is particularly popular in the Caribbean and Gulf of Mexico as a chowder fish (it toughens and dries when broiled, fried, grilled or baked). In the United States, amberjacks are often dismissed as "trash fish," although in Florida smoked amberjack is considered a special delicacy. For approximate nutrient counts, see FISH, LEAN WHITE.

American Cheese: Originally a sharp, natural CHEDDAR, American cheese is, to most Americans, the butter-smooth processed variety, a blend of Cheddar and Colby. It's lower in protein than unprocessed Cheddar, higher in sodium. It comes as sandwich slices, in bricks both solid and soft. The soft ones have had considerable water added and are classified as cheese food or cheese spread, as are many dips and spreads.

NUTRIENT CONTENT OF ½ CUP AMARANTH GRAIN
(about 3½ ounces; 98 grams)

364 calories	21 mg sodium
14 g protein	356 mg potassium
6 g fat, 1 saturated	27 g dietary fiber
0 mg cholesterol	0 RE vitamin A
65 g carbohydrate	0.08 mg thiamin
148 mg calcium	0.20 mg riboflavin
443 mg phosphorus	1.3 mg niacin
7.4 mg iron	4 mg vitamin C

NUTRIENT CONTENT OF ½ CUP BOILED AMARANTH LEAVES
(about 2½ ounces; 66 grams)

14 calories	14 mg sodium
1 g protein	423 mg potassium
0 g fat, 0 saturated	1 g dietary fiber
0 mg cholesterol	183 RE vitamin A
3 g carbohydrate	0.01 mg thiamin
138 mg calcium	0.09 mg riboflavin
47 mg phosphorus	0.4 mg niacin
1.5 mg iron	27 mg vitamin C

NUTRIENT CONTENT OF 1 OUNCE (28 GRAMS) AMERICAN CHEESE

106 calories	405 mg sodium
6 g protein	46 mg potassium
9 g fat, 6 saturated	0 g dietary fiber
27 mg cholesterol	82 RE vitamin A
0 g carbohydrate	0.01 mg thiamin
174 mg calcium	0.10 mg riboflavin
211 mg phosphorus	0.02 mg niacin
0.1 mg iron	0 mg vitamin C

NUTRIENT CONTENT OF 1 OUNCE (28 GRAMS) AMERICAN CHEESE FOOD

94 calories	274 mg sodium
6 g protein	103 mg potassium
7 g fat, 4 saturated	0 g dietary fiber
18 mg cholesterol	57 RE vitamin A
2 g carbohydrate	0.01 mg thiamin
140 mg calcium	0.13 mg riboflavin
113 mg phosphorus	0 mg niacin
0.2 mg iron	0 mg vitamin C

NUTRIENT CONTENT OF 1 OUNCE (28 GRAMS) AMERICAN CHEESE SPREAD

82 calories	380 mg sodium
5 g protein	69 mg potassium
6 g fat, 4 saturated	0 g dietary fiber
16 mg cholesterol	54 RE vitamin A
2 g carbohydrate	0.01 mg thiamin
159 mg calcium	0.12 mg riboflavin
201 mg phosphorus	0 mg niacin
0.1 mg iron	0 mg vitamin C

Amino Acids: The chemical components or building blocks of protein, which the body requires for growth, maintenance, repair and the manufacture of various hormones, antibodies and enzymes. There are twenty-one amino acids in all, nine of them essential, meaning that the body cannot synthesize them in sufficient quantities to satisfy the nutritional requirements for good health and that they must be included in the diet. The nine **essential amino acids** are HISTIDINE, ISOLEUCINE, LEUCINE, LYSINE, METHIONINE, PHENYLALANINE, THREONINE, TRYPTOPHAN and VALINE; their best sources are meat, fish, fowl, eggs and dairy products. In addition, CYSTEINE (cystine) and TYROSINE, sometimes classified as nonessential amino acids, are now considered **semiessential** because if the diet contains them (meat, milk, fish, poultry and legumes are good sources), the body can use them in place of two essential amino acids—methionine and phenylalanine—to make protein. The **nonessential amino acids?** Alanine, ARGININE, asparagine, aspartic acid, GLUTAMIC ACID, GLUTAMINE, glycine, proline, serine and TAURINE.

What about taking amino acid supplements? Some athletes use tyrosine to build physical strength, combat fatigue and increase mental alertness. And insomniacs swallow tryptophan supplements as so-called natural sleeping pills. Because indiscriminate use of tryptophan has both crippled and killed, the FDA wants amino acid supplements reclassified as medicines and made available by prescription only. See also LIMITING AMINO ACIDS.

Ammoniated Glycyrrhizin (additive): A supersweet licorice flavoring used in candies, root beer and items that taste of wintergreen. Though considered safe by the FDA, it can raise blood pressure, cause headaches, edema and fatigue. There is now talk of label warnings for foods containing this additive.

Ammonium Alginate (additive): See ALGINATES.

Ammonium Bicarbonate (additive): An alkali used in leavening quick breads, cakes, cookies, confections and cocoa products. GRAS.

Ammonium Chloride (additive): Used in baking to provide food for yeast and to condition doughs. It can acidify urine, act as an expectorant and, in 0.5- to 1-gram doses, induce nausea. GRAS.

Ammonium Phosphate (Monobasic, Dibasic), Ammonium Sulfate (additives): Buffers, leaveners and acidifiers used in baking and brewing. GRAS.

Ammonium Sulfide (additive): An artificial spice flavoring used in baking. Because it is used in such minute quantities, it need not be listed on package labels (and rarely is). GRAS.

Amoebic Dysentery: An infection of the gastrointestinal tract caused by a waterborne amoeba. The most likely victims are world travelers who aren't careful about what they eat and drink. Symptoms of amoebic dysentery are severe diarrhea, dangerous because of dehydration and subsequent loss of minerals and water-soluble B and C vitamins. **BEST PREVENTIVES:** Eating well-cooked vegetables only (no salads or sliced tomatoes); eating no raw fruits other than thick-skinned ones you peel yourself; drinking nothing more than boiled coffee or tea, beer, wine or carbonated bottled water or soft drinks (without ice); taking all alcoholic drinks "straight up"; carrying your own disposable plastic glasses; brushing your teeth with mouthwash (don't rinse the brush under the tap); and not letting a drop of tap water pass your lips.

Amphetamine: A chemical compound, also known as **speed**, that stimulates the central nervous system. Though it is sometimes prescribed by doctors to help those struggling to lose weight, it's addicting and dangerous over time. Besides, amphetamines kill the appetite for only a week or two. When it returns, more speed is needed to stay hunger pangs and unless dosages are increased, the dieter regains all the lost weight. And then some.

Amylopectin: One of the components of starch (the other is AMYLOSE). Amylopectin remains clear when heated in water and doesn't gel. It's commonly used in commercially frozen sauces and gravies because it won't break down and weep (ooze water) after it's thawed. Foods rich in amylopectin include potatoes and tapioca.

Amylose: The second component of starch (the first is AMYLOPECTIN). Amylose forms a gel when heated in liquid. Wheat flour contains it in abundance, and so do arrowroot and cornstarch.

Anaheim Peppers: See HOT PEPPERS under PEPPERS, CAPSICUMS.

Analogue: A meat look- and taste-alike made out of vegetable protein, usually soy. Analogues are actually higher in protein than true meat (50 percent versus 20 to 30 percent) but contain only a third as much fat and, better still, zero cholesterol. Meat analogues are usually sold in health-food stores and are suitable for vegetarians.

Anchos: See HOT PEPPERS under PEPPERS, CAPSICUMS.

Anchovies: Tiny, oily, strong-flavored fish that are most at home in the Mediterranean, offshore waters of Portugal and the Bay of Biscay. The anchovy, writes Alan Davidson in *North Atlantic Seafood*, "is unique among the important food fishes in that it is not normally eaten fresh." The most popular market forms are fillets canned in oil and anchovy paste, although anchovies are also salted, smoked and dried. Their pungent brininess is what gives three classic salads— green goddess, Caesar and Niçoise—their distinctive flavors, also *vitello tonnato* (cold sliced veal in tuna sauce). And, of course, they're a popular topping for pizza and its Provençal equivalent, *pissaladière*.

Anemia: Not only a low hemoglobin count in red blood cells but also any condition in which there are too few mature red blood cells or cells large enough to carry sufficient oxygen to body tissues. Hemoglobin, which contains iron, is what distributes oxygen to cells throughout the body, enabling them to burn food as energy. The most common type of anemia is iron-deficiency anemia, but nutritional anemias can also be caused by a lack of copper, vitamin B_{12} and folic acid. The major symptoms of anemia include a pale, washed-out look, headaches and fatigue. In children, anemia may cause behavioral or learning problems.

Angel Food Cakes: Although these featherweight, high-rising cakes have a reputation of being the very devil to make, they are the dieter's best friend because they're low in calories and fat and contain no cholesterol. The principal ingredients are stiffly beaten egg whites (which leaven the cake), sugar, flour and flavorings (usually vanilla, almond and/or lemon).

NUTRIENT CONTENT OF ONE (2½-INCH) SLICE ANGEL FOOD CAKE

(about 2 ounces; 53 grams)

137 calories	77 mg sodium
3 g protein	32 mg potassium
0 g fat, 0 saturated	0 g dietary fiber
0 mg cholesterol	0 RE vitamin A
32 g carbohydrate	0 mg thiamin
50 mg calcium	0 mg riboflavin
63 mg phosphorus	0.1 mg niacin
0.2 mg iron	0 mg vitamin C

NUTRIENT CONTENT OF 10 WELL-DRAINED CANNED ANCHOVIES

(about 1½ ounces; 40 grams)

84 calories	1,466 mg sodium
12 g protein	216 mg potassium
4 g fat, 1 saturated	0 g dietary fiber
0 mg cholesterol	8 RE vitamin A
0 g carbohydrate	0.03 mg thiamin
93 mg calcium	0.15 mg riboflavin
101 mg phosphorus	8.0 mg niacin
1.9 mg iron	0 mg vitamin C

Annatto (additive, coloring): Also called **achiote,** these small, dark-red seeds from the annatto tree are used throughout Mexico, the Caribbean and Latin America to color and flavor meat and fish. They are exceptionally hard and must be boiled about 5 minutes, then soaked several hours before they can be ground into paste or powder. The flavor of annatto is somewhat earthy and musty, definitely an acquired taste. The pigment of annatto is used by the dairy industry to give cheeses and butters their sunny orange and yellow colors.

Annona: See CHERIMOYA.

Anorexia: A medical term meaning "lack of appetite."

Anorexia Nervosa: A grave eating disorder that most often afflicts teenage girls. Because of social pressures, fear of obesity and distorted images of their own bodies, anorexics suffer a psychological loss of appetite, may lose 25 percent of their body weight and, sometimes, quite literally starve themselves to death. See also BULIMIA.

Antacids: Medications taken to neutralize stomach acids. Those containing magnesium or aluminum block the absorption of calcium in the body. For that reason, antacids made with calcium carbonate are a better choice for osteoporosis sufferers (and others) who need to boost their calcium intake. Indeed, calcium carbonate antacids actually do double duty. They ease the symptoms of acid indigestion *and* supply the body with the most usable form of calcium available.

Anthocyanins: The red, purple and blue pigments present in such fruits and vegetables as red cabbage, beets, raspberries, red and blue plums. Anthocyanin is an indicator, meaning that it, like litmus paper, changes color depending upon whether it's in the presence of an acid or an alkali. Clever cooks long ago learned to capitalize on the chameleon nature of anthocyanin. For example, by adding vinegar to beets or by cooking red cabbage in the company of cranberries, they could turn these foods a dazzling ruby red that did not fade on standing.

Anthoxanthins: The white pigments of such vegetables and grains as onions, cauliflower, potatoes, rice and flour, which change to creamy white, or even bright yellow, in the presence of an alkaline solution. Adding a pinch of cream of tartar to the cooking water will keep them white and bright.

Antibiotics: These, quite literally, are substances, natural or synthetic, that have the power to destroy or thwart the growth of microorganisms. **Penicillin,** derived from a mold, is one well-known antibiotic. Modern medicine relies on a large arsenal of antibiotics to treat a variety of infectious diseases. Some antibiotics must be taken with meals, so it's important to follow your doctor's or pharmacist's directions. **Tetracycline,** for example, decreases the absorption of calcium, so it should not be taken with milk or other dairy foods. The effectiveness of **penicillin G** and **erythromycin** can be destroyed by fruit juices or other acidic beverages, so they should be taken on an empty stomach. Antibiotics also kill "friendly" intestinal bacteria, which can lead to nausea and vomiting. They can also destroy the bacteria that manufacture vitamin K, so those taking antibiotics should eat plenty of vitamin K-rich foods—broccoli, snap beans, peas and dark leafy greens. It pays to read the fine print; also to ask your doctor, pharmacist or nutritionist about the effect of a particular antibiotic on nutrition. And what about the antibiotics now being routinely mixed into cattle and poultry feed? How much remains in the meat and are these residual antibiotics harmful? Dangerous? Food faddists would have you think so. Here are the facts: Anyone raising cattle, sheep, hogs or poultry for the table must withdraw all antibiotics early enough for the animal tissues to show no discernible traces of them. Unfortunately, not all farmers follow the rules. The U.S. Food and Safety Inspection Service, in a late-1980s survey, found antibiotic residues in 5.3 percent of the carcasses tested, most of them pork. And another turned up residues of **sulfamethazine,** a known carcinogen, in milk (this antibiotic was never approved for use in the dairy industry and the discovery of it has led to closer surveillance). As for antibiotic residues in meat, thorough cooking renders them inactive. Still, people with allergies may be at risk. And others, over time, may develop a resistance to the antibiotics.

Antioxidants: Chemicals that keep other substances from being oxidized (turning brown or rancid, etc.). **Vitamin E** is a natural antioxidant present in vegetable oils. **Vitamin C** is another natural antioxidant, and it's added to fresh, frozen and canned fruits such as apples, peaches and pears to keep them from darkening. Every time we sprinkle a cut avocado with **lemon** or **lime juice,** we're preventing—or at least retarding—oxidation. In commercial food processing such artificial antioxidants as **butylated**

hydroxyanisole (see BHA) and **butylated hydroxytoluene** (BHT) are added to keep fats from turning rancid. There is now intense interest in the role of antioxidants in the body because they may destroy free radicals, which some scientists believe may not only accelerate aging but also contribute to the formation of cancers and cataracts. In addition, antioxidants, and vitamin E especially, keep "bad" cholesterol (LDL) from being oxidized. It's *oxidized* LDL, biomedical researchers now believe, that's the true culprit behind arterial plaque buildup and thus a major cause of heart disease. **Beta-carotene** (a precursor of vitamin A) and vitamins C and E are all effective antioxidants, but taking megadoses of vitamin C may be harmful. As for vitamin E, no one knows for certain whether large doses help or harm. A recent, controversial Finnish study of male long-term smokers to the contrary, many scientists still believe that diets rich in antioxidants (even antioxidant vitamin supplements) may decrease the onset and severity of many chronic diseases, among them cancer.

Antivitamins, Vitamin Antagonists: There exist certain substances—mostly in medications—that render specific vitamins useless (or, at best, less useful to the human body). One of the agents of chemotherapy, for example, deactivates **pyridoxine** (one of the B-complex) and another, used to treat leukemia, is antagonistic to **folacin** (another of the B-complex). The coumarin blood thinners depower **vitamin K.** Raw egg whites contain an antivitamin of another sort called AVIDIN, which bonds with **biotin** (another B vitamin), forming a compound the body can't metabolize. Though the chemistry of such interractions isn't fully understood, it's important to be aware of them.

Appetize: The brand name of a new high-tech shortening from Source Food Technology that's synthesized from polyunsaturated vegetable oils plus butter, beef tallow and lard that have been stripped of their CHOLESTEROL. Like conventional fats, Appetize contains 9 calories per gram. But unlike margarine, shortening and other hydrogenated vegetable oils, it contains no TRANS FATTY ACIDS. It's also lower in cholesterol than natural animal fats. The food technologists who developed Appetize say that it fries and deep-fries like a dream, that it makes feathery cakes and flaky pastries and that it's full of old-fashioned flavor. It's packaged like shortening. Look for it.

Apple Cider, Apple Juice: The juice pressed from apples, either fresh or bottled. With most of the fiber left behind in the press, apple cider and juice are not particularly nutritious (it's best to buy those fortified with vitamin C). Many cooks now keeping an eye on their calories will boil apple cider or juice down to a thick syrup that can be brushed over open-face fruit tarts in place of the more caloric jams or jellies usually used. It can also be used to sweeten fresh berries and other fruits.

NUTRITIVE CONTENT OF 1 CUP BOTTLED APPLE CIDER OR JUICE

(8 fluid ounces; 248 grams)

117 calories	2 mg sodium
0 g protein	250 mg potassium
0 g fat, 0 saturated	0 g dietary fiber
0 mg cholesterol	0 RE vitamin A
30 g carbohydrate	0.05 mg thiamin
15 mg calcium	0.04 mg riboflavin
22 mg phosphorus	0.2 mg niacin
1 mg iron	2 mg vitamin C

Apples: What Adam and Eve ate in the Garden of Eden, historians suspect, was a pomegranate, not an apple. The fact is, apples probably originated in the colder climes of northern Europe and weren't known in the New World until the Pilgrims and Virginia settlers introduced them. Today the United States has emerged as the world's top apple grower. The best-seller is the Delicious, of which American essayist A. J. Liebling once wrote, "People who don't like food have made a triumph of the Delicious apple because it doesn't taste like an apple, and of the Golden Delicious because it doesn't taste like anything." Nutri-

NUTRIENT CONTENT OF 1 MEDIUM-SIZE APPLE WITH SKIN

(about 5 ounces; 138 grams)

81 calories	0 mg sodium
0 g protein	157 mg potassium
1 g fat, 0 saturated	3 g dietary fiber
0 mg cholesterol	7 RE vitamin A
21 g carbohydrate	0.02 mg thiamin
10 mg calcium	0.02 mg riboflavin
10 mg phosphorus	0.1 mg niacin
0.3 mg iron	8 mg vitamin C

tionally speaking, the size of the apple has more to do with its nutrient content than the variety. Although an apple a day may not keep the doctor away, it does provide plenty of dietary fiber, small amounts of vitamin C, zero cholesterol and sodium. **SEASON:** Year-round, but at their peak in autumn.

NUTRIENT CONTENT OF 1 CUP APPLESAUCE
(about 8¾ ounces; 244 grams)

117 calories	2 mg sodium
0 g protein	250 mg potassium
0 g fat, 0 saturated	4 g dietary fiber
0 mg cholesterol	7 RE vitamin A
30 g carbohydrate	0.02 mg thiamin
15 mg calcium	0.04 mg riboflavin
22 mg phosphorus	0.2 mg niacin
1.5 mg iron	2 mg vitamin C

Apricots: These small, buttery fruits surfaced in the wilds of China thousands of years ago, grew in the Hanging Gardens of Babylon and were considered a delicacy by the Romans. Today, the world's best apricots grow in the Loire Valley of France, but bumper crops come from California. Though apricots look like small peaches, their flavor is part apple, part lemon, thanks to their MALIC ACID and CITRIC ACID content. They contain impressive amounts of vitamin A, some vitamin C and potassium but few calories (except syrup-canned or dried apricots). **SEASON:** Summer, early fall.

NUTRIENT CONTENT OF 3 MEDIUM-SIZE PITTED FRESH APRICOTS
(about 3¾ ounces; 106 grams)

55 calories	1 mg sodium
1 g protein	313 mg potassium
0 g fat, 0 saturated	2 g dietary fiber
0 mg cholesterol	277 RE vitamin A
12 g carbohydrate	0.03 mg thiamin
15 mg calcium	0.04 mg riboflavin
20 mg phosphorus	0.6 mg niacin
0.6 mg iron	11 mg vitamin C

NUTRIENT CONTENT OF 1 CUP DRAINED CANNED APRICOT HALVES (HEAVY-SYRUP PACK)
(about 9¼ ounces; 258 grams)

222 calories	3 mg sodium
2 g protein	604 mg potassium
0 g fat, 0 saturated	3 g dietary fiber
0 mg cholesterol	317 RE vitamin A
57 g carbohydrate	0.05 mg thiamin
28 mg calcium	0.05 mg riboflavin
39 mg phosphorus	1.0 mg niacin
0.8 mg iron	10 mg vitamin C

NUTRIENT CONTENT OF 1 CUP DRIED SULFURED APRICOT HALVES (UNCOOKED)
(about 4½ ounces; 130 grams)

338 calories	34 mg sodium
7 g protein	1,273 mg potassium
1 g fat, 0 saturated	10 g dietary fiber
0 mg cholesterol	941 RE vitamin A
87 g carbohydrate	0.01 mg thiamin
87 mg calcium	0.21 mg riboflavin
140 mg phosphorus	4.3 mg niacin
7.2 mg iron	16 mg vitamin C

NUTRIENT CONTENT OF 1 CUP APRICOT NECTAR
(8 fluid ounces; 251 grams)

140 calories	8 mg sodium
1 g protein	286 mg potassium
0 g fat, 0 saturated	2 g dietary fiber
0 mg cholesterol	331 RE vitamin A
36 g carbohydrate	0.02 mg thiamin
18 mg calcium	0.04 mg riboflavin
23 mg phosphorus	0.7 mg niacin
1.0 mg iron	2* mg vitamin C

*If the apricot nectar is fortified with vitamin C, the vitamin C content per cup zooms to 136 milligrams.

Aquaculture: The raising of fish, shellfish and aquatic plants in controlled-environment fish farms both offshore and on. What Americans know best are farm-raised Mississippi catfish (which account for 50 percent of the aquaculture business) and farm-raised Maine mussels. A handful of government agencies regulate America's infant aquaculture industry, among them the USDA, FDA, EPA, National Oceanic and Atmospheric Administration and Fish and Wildlife Service. Other than complaints that farm-raised fish lack flavor, the biggest problems are the fish farmers' dependence on disinfectants to kill bacteria, herbicides to reduce plant growth in ponds and antibiotics to fight diseases and parasites. So far the FDA has approved the use of only five chemicals, but fish farmers are begging for more.

Arachidonic Acid: This was once thought to be one of the essential fatty acids (see FAT). But because the body can, in a pinch, manufacture arachidonic acid from linoleic acid, it is not essential in the diet. Arachidonic acid is found in meat and milk. It's also added to infant formulas. Some food researchers are now linking psoriasis to diet and specifically to the inability, in some people, to metabolize arachidonic acid normally. Stay tuned.

Arginine: Although arginine is considered one of the nonessential AMINO ACIDS, children can't synthesize enough of it to support growth, so must get plenty of it in their diet (good sources: beef, milk, soybeans).

Arrowroot: A fine, odorless, powdery white starch used to thicken puddings, sauces and glazes. True arrowroot comes from the rootstock of a plant grown on Bermuda, Jamaica and other Caribbean islands. The roots are peeled, beaten to a milky pulp, then allowed to stand until the starch settles. The starch is dried in the sun—or more recently in drying houses—then bottled for sale. Arrowroot has about twice the thickening power of flour. There's an added advantage, too. Once thickened, arrowroot sauces are crystal clear, making them the perfect choice for glazing open-face fruit tarts.

NUTRIENT CONTENT OF 1 TABLESPOON ARROWROOT
(about ⅓ ounce; 8 grams)

29 calories	0 mg sodium
0 g protein	1 mg potassium
0 g fat, 0 saturated	0 g dietary fiber
0 mg cholesterol	0 RE vitamin A
7 g carbohydrate	0 mg thiamin
3 mg calcium	0 mg riboflavin
0 mg phosphorus	0 mg niacin
0 mg iron	0 mg vitamin C

Arsenic: Arsenic trioxide, a powerful but poisonous and possibly carcinogenic insecticide, has been widely used by farmers and citrus growers. And arsenic, a toxic metal, frequently shows up in shellfish. Repeated exposure to arsenic can damage the kidneys, impair brain function, even, some researchers believe, cause cancer. Yet this deadly poison is now considered a trace mineral essential to the metabolism of methionine but it is needed only in minute quantities (see AMINO ACIDS).

Arthritis (diet and): Hucksters constantly push miracle arthritis-cure diets upon the elderly and infirm, the most likely candidates for this painful inflammation of the joints. For example, one popular claim is that by eliminating members of the nightshade family—eggplant, potatoes, tomatoes—you can ease the pain. The truth is that none of these claims is known to prevent, cure or even relieve the symptoms of this debilitating disease. What *is* generally agreed: Keeping weight down will help because it reduces the load on weight-bearing joints, and eating a well-balanced diet low in saturated fats but high in eicosapentaenoic acid (see EPA), a fatty acid found in fish, may ease some of the inflammation. On the other hand, about a third of those afflicted with rheumatoid arthritis swear that certain foods—milk, in particular—exacerbate the pain and swelling in their joints. Researchers, who've so far failed to prove that food can aggravate rheumatoid arthritis, are listening nonetheless. From Massachusetts now comes word of a new dietary study that shows great promise as a treatment for rheumatoid arthritis. A physician at Boston's Beth Israel Hospital mixed liquid chicken collagen with orange juice, served it every breakfast to twenty-eight arthritis sufferers and discovered that all had improved significantly after three months; indeed, four patients seemed to have gone into remission. Further studies are planned.

Artichokes, Globe or French: Probably native to Sicily or North Africa, artichokes are the buds of a Mediterranean thistle. When artichokes are large, only the heart and fleshy bases of the leaves are eaten. But anyone who has traveled in France or Italy also knows the small tender varieties that are bounced in and out of a skillet and eaten, prickles and all. Catherine de Médicis, it's said, introduced artichokes to France in the sixteenth century when she married Henry II. In those days, artichokes were considered an aphrodisiac but in truth they are neither aphrodisiacal nor very nutritious (except for some vitamin A and C and assorted minerals). In a freshly picked artichoke, the carbohydrate exists in the form of INULIN, a starch the body can't digest. In storage, however, inulin turns to sugar, so the calorie content of artichokes varies widely. For example, a just-picked, boiled-right-away artichoke may contain only 9 calories, whereas that same artichoke, after weeks in storage, may contain six times that. Still hardly high calorie. **SEASON:** Fresh artichokes are in season from October through June but at their best in April and May.

NUTRIENT CONTENT OF 1 MEDIUM-SIZE BOILED/STEAMED ARTICHOKE	
(about 4⅓ ounces; 120 grams)	
60* calories	114 mg sodium
4 g protein	424 mg potassium
0 g fat, 0 saturated	6 g dietary fiber
0 mg cholesterol	22 RE vitamin A
13 g carbohydrate	0.08 mg thiamin
54 mg calcium	0.08 mg riboflavin
103 mg phosphorus	1.2 mg niacin
1.6 mg iron	12 mg vitamin C

*The fresher the artichoke, the lower the calories.

Artichokes, Jerusalem; Sunchokes:

Jerusalem artichokes aren't artichokes and they aren't from Jerusalem. They're the tubers of a sunflower native to North America and their name is thought to be a corruption of *girasole,* the Italian word for "sunflower." The *artichoke* part is easy to explain: These fleshy tubers taste like globe artichokes. Like them, too, their starch is at first present in the form of inulin, which the body can't metabolize (inulin is used to manufacture a pasta that health-food stores tout as being safe for diabetics; the truth is, regular pasta is also safe for

NUTRIENT CONTENT OF 1 CUP SLICED RAW JERUSALEM ARTICHOKE	
(about 5½ ounces; 150 grams)	
114 calories	6 mg sodium
3 g protein	644 mg potassium
0 g fat, 0 saturated	2 g dietary fiber
0 mg cholesterol	3 RE vitamin A
26 g carbohydrate	0.30 mg thiamin
21 mg calcium	0.09 mg riboflavin
117 mg phosphorus	2.0 mg niacin
5.1 mg iron	6 mg vitamin C

diabetics). Jerusalem artichokes are surprisingly nutritious, providing generous amounts of iron, potassium, thiamin and niacin. They add welcome crunch when sliced raw into salads. They can also be boiled and mashed like potatoes. **SEASON:** October through March.

Artificial Sweeteners: Indispensable to diabetics and dieters, these sugar substitutes, some scientists believe, may actually heighten your craving for sweets. Some artificial sweeteners have been banned as carcinogenic (CYCLAMATE); others (ASPARTAME, ACESULFAME-K and SACCHARIN), though under ongoing scrutiny, are used to sweeten everything from soft drinks to diet desserts. Until the jury is in, all should be used in moderation. See also SORBITOL; SUCRALOSE.

Arugula, Arugola, Rugola: Also known as **rocket,** this pungent green beloved by Italians is related to the radish, which may explain its bite. In recent years arugula has spread beyond America's Little Italys and now appears with some regularity in supermarkets across the country. Home gardeners dote on it, too, and have no difficulty raising bumper crops. The emerald, tongue-shaped leaves of arugula are superb in salads, adding welcome piquancy and upping the nutritional content. **SEASON:** Year-round.

NUTRIENT CONTENT OF 1 CUP ARUGULA (LEAVES AND STEMS)	
(about ¾ ounce; 20 grams)	
4 calories	6 mg sodium
0 g protein	74 mg potassium
0 g fat, 0 saturated	NA g dietary fiber
0 mg cholesterol	48 RE vitamin A
1 g carbohydrate	0.10 mg thiamin
32 mg calcium	0.20 mg riboflavin
10 mg phosphorus	0 mg niacin
NA mg iron	NA mg vitamin C

Ascorbic Acid, Vitamin C (additive): Used in canning, pickling and preserving to keep fruits and vegetables from darkening. Safe. See also C, VITAMIN.

Asiago: A hard, bacteria-ripened, Parmesan-like grating cheese made of partially skimmed cow's milk that comes from Vicenza, Italy.

NUTRIENT CONTENT OF 1 OUNCE (28 GRAMS) ASIAGO

106 calories	74 mg sodium
8 g protein	32 mg potassium
8 g fat, 5 saturated	0 g dietary fiber
26 mg cholesterol	72 RE vitamin A
1 g carbohydrate	0.01 mg thiamin
271 mg calcium	0.10 mg riboflavin
171 mg phosphorus	0 mg niacin
0 mg iron	0 mg vitamin C

Asian Pears: They look a little like apples, taste a little like pears and, writes Elizabeth Schneider in her benchmark *Uncommon Fruits & Vegetables: A Common Guide,* are all "crunch and juice, so crisp-firm they can be cut paper-thin, their nectar welling up and pouring off each slice." Asian pears are moderately good sources of vitamin C, niacin and fiber, but they aren't very sweet or flavorful. Twenty-five different varieties of Asian pear grow in the United States, so the ones that land in your supermarket may be shiny or russeted, yellow-green or brown, big or little (small ones weigh in at about 4 ounces apiece, medium-size ones 8 ounces and whoppers ¾ pound). Asian pears can be sliced and eaten out of hand or cooked like apples and pears. Cooking intensifies their flavor but does nothing to soften their texture. **SEASON:** Late summer until winter.

NUTRIENT CONTENT OF 1 MEDIUM-SIZE ASIAN PEAR (WITHOUT SKIN)

(about 8 ounces; 227 grams)

95 calories	0 mg sodium
1 g protein	275 mg potassium
0 g fat, 0 saturated	3 g dietary fiber
0 mg cholesterol	0 RE vitamin A
24 g carbohydrate	0.06 mg thiamin
9 mg calcium	0.16 mg riboflavin
25 mg phosphorus	2.5 mg niacin
0.4 mg iron	9 mg vitamin C

Asparagine: One of the nonessential AMINO ACIDS.

Asparagus: Unlike many foods, which have fallen in and out of favor over the centuries, asparagus has always been popular—*except* with children who turn up their noses at the "sparrow grass" on their plates. Asparagus, as we now know it, was developed from a spindly wild grass by the Romans, who lavished so much time on their asparagus beds some stalks weighed 3 pounds apiece. The French, equally keen on asparagus, developed the only variety Europeans consider worth eating: White asparagus—in truth, nothing more than green asparagus grown underground. The stalks, deprived of sunlight, remain as pale as ivory. White asparagus is milder than the green, softer, too. All asparagus is low in calories. **SEASON:** In many areas, year-round, but the best asparagus come to market between early March and June.

NUTRIENT CONTENT OF 4 LARGE COOKED GREEN ASPARAGUS SPEARS

(about 2 ounces; 60 grams)

20 calories	1 mg sodium
2 g protein	183 mg potassium
0 g fat, 0 saturated	1 g dietary fiber
0 mg cholesterol	32 RE vitamin A
4 g carbohydrate	0.16 mg thiamin
21 mg calcium	0.18 mg riboflavin
50 mg phosphorus	1.4 mg niacin
0.6 mg iron	26 mg vitamin C

Aspartame (artificial sweetener): Sold under the brand names Equal and NutraSweet—and, now that original manufacturer's patent has expired, as the cheaper Natra-Taste—aspartame is synthesized out of two amino acids: aspartic acid and phenylalanine. After years of both private and FDA testing, it's still controversial. Complaints have been filed with the FDA claiming such adverse reactions as headaches, dizziness and nausea; however, careful research casts doubts on whether aspartame causes headaches. It is definitely unsafe for those with phenylketonuria (PKU), a congenital condition that makes it impossible for the body to metabolize phenylalanine. Toxic compounds build up in the body and cause abnormal nerve or brain function (even mental retardation), mild seizures, skin rashes and reduced pigmentation (meaning blond hair and pale skin). **CALORIES:** 4 per 0.04-ounce (1-gram) packet.

Aspartic Acid: One of the nonessential AMINO ACIDS.

Aspergillus: A widespread genus of molds. The one that concerns us here is *Aspergillus flavus,* a common mold that can ruin whole bins of stored grain or nuts (particularly peanuts) by producing a hazardous mycotoxin (see AFLA-TOXIN). The FDA routinely tests grains and nuts for *A. flavus* and aflatoxin and withdraws all contaminated lots from the market. This is not to suggest that our food supply is entirely free of *A. flavus.* The cost of eliminating it entirely would be prohibitive. Most researchers agree, however, that the small amounts present in grains and nuts do not pose health risks. Still, it's advisable to reject all grains or nuts that look shriveled, discolored or moldy. There are, by the way, beneficial strains of *Aspergillus.* Food processors capitalize on the fermentative powers of *Aspergillus niger* to facilitate the extraction of CITRIC ACID, an additive, from beet molasses. Citric acid is one of the safest, most widely used food additives in the United States. Finally, *A. niger* is used to make Beano, an antiflatulent sold in health-food and drugstores.

Aspirin, Acetylsalicylic Acid (diet and): One of the first painkillers, aspirin is not without its side effects, some of them serious. It can cause stomach bleeding (and subsequent iron-deficiency anemia). It can decrease the absorption of amino acids and it depletes the body's supply of vitamins C and K, thiamin, folic acid and potassium. Thus anyone taking large and/or prolonged doses of aspirin (as arthritis sufferers often do) may need to supplement the lost vitamins and minerals. A daily multivitamin/mineral tablet may be all that's necessary. Ask your doctor or, better yet, a registered dietitian (R.D.).

Asthma (diet and): Among the foods suspected of triggering asthma attacks (wheezing and extreme difficulty in breathing) in children are chocolate, colas, eggs, fish, nuts, milk and dairy products. SULFITES, too, can touch off violent fits of coughing and wheezing in persons of all ages. Indeed, so many people are acutely or fatally sensitive to sulfites that in 1986 the FDA revoked the GRAS status for sulfites used on fresh vegetables and fruits. With one exception: potatoes used by restaurants. But the FDA may soon extend its sulfites ban to include spuds, too. Sulfites are the antioxidants chefs used to keep potatoes, onions and other foods from discoloring, also to keep such salad-bar staples as lettuce and tomatoes fresh and moist (safer

antioxidants are now used). Sulfites are still used by vintners; fortunately, labels on all domestic and some foreign wines containing sulfites now state this fact.

Atemoya: Now being grown in Florida, this custardy tropical fruit is a cherimoya-sugar apple hybrid. It's sweet, bland, ivory-fleshed and best when chilled well and eaten raw, either out of hand or diced into fruit salads. As for nutrient content, atemoyas are a good source of dietary fiber, potassium, vitamins C and K. They are also low in sodium. **SEASON:** August through November. **NOTE:** Specific nutrient counts unavailable.

Atherosclerosis: A buildup of fatty deposits in the arteries, including those surrounding the heart, which can eventually lead to heart attacks. The current medical/nutritional thinking is that a diet low in saturated fat and cholesterol will delay the onset of atherosclerosis.

Athletes: See SPORTS NUTRITION.

Atkins Diet: See FAD DIETS under DIETS.

Attention Deficit Hyperactivity Disorder (ADHD), Attention Deficit Disorder (ADD): The modern term for **hyperactivity** or **hyperkinesis**, which may afflict as many as 20 percent of American children, most of them boys. Such children are disruptive at home and in school; they find it impossible to concentrate and seem to be in perpetual motion. Though some parents believe that diet—specifically artificial food colors and flavorings, sugar, the sugar substitute ASPARTAME, indeed sweets in general—causes or at least exacerbates ADHD, a series of nutritional studies conducted over the years (notably one at the Yale University School of Medicine and another at Vanderbilt University) have shown that sugar has little effect on children's behavior. Now there's an update: The latest answer to the "Does sugar turn little angels into little devils?" question seems to be "Maybe." Or "Sometimes." Pediatric researchers at Yale's School of Medicine have discovered that if children are fed a lot of sugar on empty stomachs, their adrenaline levels soar. As a result, they may tremble, become agitated and lose the ability to concentrate. Not so adults put through the same tests or, for that matter, children given sweets at the end of a proper meal.

The Yale researchers insist, however, that their findings are preliminary (more tests are to come) and do not prove that sugar causes hyperactivity in children. What they do suggest is that children would be wiser to snack on peanut butter crackers or cheese than on sweets. Whether sugar hops children up remains to be seen. There's no denying, however, that it fills them up, leaving little room—or appetite—for nutritious food. See also FEINGOLD DIET.

Avidin: A protein antivitamin (see ANTIVITAMINS) found in raw egg whites that can bind biotin, a B-complex vitamin, and keep the body from absorbing it. Fortunately, cooking destroys avidin.

Avocado Oil: The green-gold oil of the avocado, now bottled and sold like olive oil in upscale food markets. It has a faintly fruity-nutty flavor and is best used to dress salads. Buy in small quantities; avocado oil quickly turns rancid. **NOTE:** Like other oils, avocado oil will weigh in at 120 calories per tablespoon and 14 grams fat (in this case most of it is monounsaturated).

Avocados: These "alligator pears" are native to Mexico. Yet they weren't grown to any extent north of the border until the turn of the century. Most of the U.S. crop now comes from Florida (big, smooth-skinned, bright green avocados) and California, where the smaller, wartier green **Fuerte** and black **Hass** varieties are grown. For flavor, connoisseurs insist on Hass and won't use anything else for guacamole. What's remarkable about the avocado is its high fat content (British schooners sailing the Caribbean routinely took avocados aboard to be used as "midshipman's butter"). Although caloric, avocados contain substantial amounts of potassium, vitamins A and C and niacin. They are low in sodium and contain zero cholesterol. **SEASON:** Florida avocados come to market in late summer/early fall and the Californias in midwinter.

NUTRIENT CONTENT OF 1 LARGE AVOCADO (NOT PEELED OR PITTED)	
(about 10 ounces; 280 grams)	
369 calories	9 mg sodium
5 g protein	1,303 mg potassium
37 g fat, 6 saturated	8 g dietary fiber
0 mg cholesterol	171 RE vitamin A
13 g carbohydrate	0.24 mg thiamin
22 mg calcium	0.43 mg riboflavin
91 mg phosphorus	3.5 mg niacin
1.3 mg iron	30 mg vitamin C

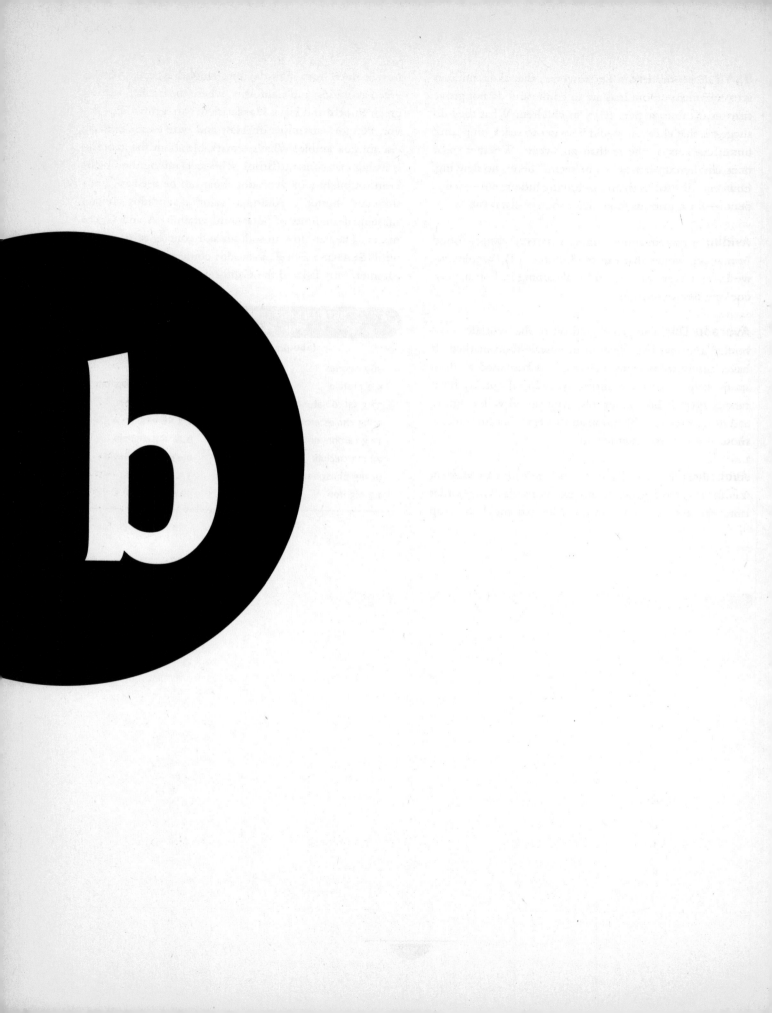

B₁, Vitamin; Thiamin: The chief function of this vitamin is to cooperate with other members of the B-COMPLEX in converting glucose to energy, which fuels the body. It is also important for a healthy nervous system. For years doctors blamed beriberi, a devastating nerve disease that once rampaged through Asia, on something harmful *in* food. Only with the turn of the twentieth century did scientists discover that rice bran, removed to create the polished white rice Asians preferred, contained something that prevented beriberi. And only in 1926 were crystals of this "beriberi vitamine" used to cure beriberi in people. Today we know this substance as thiamin or vitamin B_1 and it is one of the nutrients added to grains and flours during the enrichment process. **DEFICIENCY SYMPTOMS:** Depression, irritability, attention deficit, muscular weakness. Severe thiamin deficiency can cause beriberi with symptoms including edema, paralysis and heart failure. Those most apt to be lacking in thiamin are alcoholics and those who constantly junk out on soft drinks, candy, pretzels, chips and other high-carb foods made with unenriched flours. **GOOD SOURCES:** Brewer's yeast, meats (especially pork and liver), peas and beans, both fresh and dried, whole or enriched grains and breads. **PRECAUTIONS:** Being water soluble, thiamin tends to leach out in the cooking water. It is also destroyed by heat. Indeed, as much as 30 percent of the thiamin can be lost as a loaf of bread bakes and another 10 to 30 percent as a slice of it toasts. Alcohol impairs the body's ability to absorb thiamin, as does tea, if drunk in prodigious quantities.

B₂, Vitamin; Riboflavin: Like thiamin, riboflavin helps the body metabolize carbohydrates. But it also aids in the metabolism of fats and proteins. In addition, it's essential to the proper function of three other B vitamins (B_6, folacin and niacin), to the making of red blood cells and maintenance of body tissues, especially those of the skin and eyes. **DEFICIENCY SYMPTOMS:** Dry and scaly facial skin, cracks at the corners of the mouth, oral inflammation. **PRECAUTIONS:** Riboflavin is water soluble, so some of it will be lost in cooking. In alkaline solutions it's quickly destroyed by heat (a strong argument against adding a pinch of baking soda to the cooking water), but it is fairly stable if cooked in an acid medium or by dry heat. A greater danger is light. The sun's ultraviolet rays are particularly ruinous. In the old days when milk was delivered door-to-door, bottles left on a sunny stoop for two hours would have lost half their riboflavin. As with thiamin, milling removes much of the riboflavin in grains, but enrichment puts it back. Riboflavin is also lost when rice is polished, but here, alas, it is not replaced (all the more reason to eat brown rice). **GOOD SOURCES:** Meats, liver, eggs, milk, yogurt, cheese, whole and enriched grains and such dark green vegetables as beet greens, spinach and broccoli.

RDA FOR VITAMIN B₁ (THIAMIN)	
Babies:	
Birth to 6 months	0.3 mg per day
6 months to 1 year	0.4 mg per day
Children:	
1 to 3 years	0.7 mg per day
4 to 6 years	0.9 mg per day
7 to 10 years	1 mg per day
Men and Boys:	
11 to 14 years	1.3 mg per day
15 to 50 years	1.5 mg per day
51+ years	1.2 mg per day
Women and Girls:	
11 to 50 years	1.1 mg per day
51+ years	1 mg per day
Pregnant Women:	1.5 mg per day
Nursing Mothers:	
First 6 months	1.6 mg per day
Second 6 months	1.6 mg per day

RDA FOR VITAMIN B₂ (RIBOFLAVIN)	
Babies:	
Birth to 6 months	0.4 mg per day
6 months to 1 year	0.5 mg per day
Children:	
1 to 3 years	0.8 mg per day
4 to 6 years	1.1 mg per day
7 to 10 years	1.2 mg per day
Men and Boys:	
11 to 14 years	1.5 mg per day
15 to 18 years	1.8 mg per day
19 to 50 years	1.7 mg per day
51+ years	1.4 mg per day
Women and Girls:	
11 to 50 years	1.3 mg per day
51+ years	1.2 mg per day
Pregnant Women:	1.6 mg per day
Nursing Mothers:	
First 6 months	1.8 mg per day
Second 6 months	1.7 mg per day

B₆, Vitamin; Pyridoxine: Necessary for the metabolism of protein, pyridoxine also converts glycogen (a complex carbohydrate) into glucose (a sugar), which can be utilized by muscles. It's also needed to build certain amino acids and to turn others into hormones, among them one that synthesizes niacin (an important B vitamin) out of tryptophan (an essential amino acid). The body uses pyridoxine to build red blood cells and maintain nerve tissue. Pyridoxine also plays a role in the metabolism of polyunsaturated fats. **DEFICIENCY SYMPTOMS:** Mouth sores, nausea, nervousness, anemia, convulsions. The good news, however, is that B₆ deficiencies aren't common and usually occur only with an overall B-complex deficiency. **PRECAUTIONS:** Too much pyridoxine can be quite toxic, causing temporary or permanent nerve damage. But this happens only when high dosages are taken over prolonged periods to relieve the symptoms of premenstrual syndrome or mental illness. Still, heavy drinkers or those on the pill, diuretics or penicillamine may need to up their intake of B₆ (check with your doctor or registered dietitian). Processing destroys much of the B₆ present in food: As much as 70 percent may be lost in the making of cereal and 75 percent in the milling of refined flour (this vitamin is not replaced in enriched foods). Canned vegetables may have lost even more B₆—as much as 90 percent. Luncheon meats lose 50 to 70 percent in the processing, even frozen fruits 15 percent. Heat and ultraviolet light take a toll, too. **GOOD SOURCES:** Fish, meat, poultry, unprocessed whole grains, legumes, potatoes, sweet potatoes, nuts, avocados, bananas and brewer's yeast.

RDA FOR VITAMIN B₆ (PYRIDOXINE)

Babies:	
Birth to 6 months	0.3 mg per day
6 months to 1 year	0.6 mg per day
Children:	
1 to 3 years	1 mg per day
4 to 6 years	1.1 mg per day
7 to 10 years	1.4 mg per day
Men and Boys:	
11 to 14 years	1.7 mg per day
15 to 51+ years	2 mg per day
Women and Girls:	
11 to 14 years	1.4 mg per day
15 to 18 years	1.5 mg per day
19 to 51+ years	1.6 mg per day
Pregnant Women:	2.2 mg per day
Nursing Mothers:	2.1 mg per day

B₁₂, Vitamin; Cobalamin: Working in concert with folacin (a B vitamin also known as folic acid), B₁₂ is used in the production of red blood cells. It also helps build and maintain protective nerve sheaths. **DEFICIENCY SYMPTOMS:** Pernicious anemia, muscle and nerve paralysis. In order to absorb B₁₂ efficiently, the body relies on INTRINSIC FACTOR, a protein manufactured in the stomach. As one grows older, the production of intrinsic factor slows and may cease altogether. In such cases, the only way to get enough B₁₂ is via injection. And what about B₁₂ supplements as a quick fix for that dragged-out feeling? There's no proof that they work. **PRECAUTIONS:** Foods cooked at intense heat or in an alkaline solution (with baking soda, for example) will lose a certain amount of B₁₂. Pasteurized milk has lost about 10 percent of this precious vitamin. Because no plants contain B₁₂, vegetarians should include some animal protein (dairy products or eggs, for example) in their diets, use B₁₂-fortified soy milk or take a supplement. Two other factors reducing the absorption of B₁₂: Hypothyroidism, iron and/or pyridoxine deficiencies. **GOOD SOURCES:** Meats, fish, poultry, dairy products, eggs.

RDA FOR VITAMIN B₁₂ (COBALAMIN)

Babies:	
Birth to 6 months	0.3 mcg per day
6 months to 1 year	0.5 mcg per day
Children:	
1 to 3 years	0.7 mcg per day
4 to 6 years	1 mcg per day
7 to 10 years	1.4 mcg per day
Men and Boys:	
11 to 51+ years	2 mcg per day
Women and Girls:	
11 to 51+ years	2 mcg per day
Pregnant Women:	2.2 mcg per day
Nursing Mothers:	2.6 mcg per day

B₁₅, Vitamin: See DMG.

Baby Bottle Syndrome: See NURSING BOTTLE SYNDROME.

Baby Foods: See INFANT NUTRITION.

Bacalhau, Bacalao: Dried salt cod. The Portuguese, who began fishing for cod along Newfoundland's Grand Banks shortly after Columbus discovered America, are credited with learning to salt the fish at sea, then to sun dry them until stiff as boards. They are also credited—by Escoffier no less—with introducing dried salt cod to Europe. For years *bacalhau* was a staple among the poor of Portugal, who, it's said, devised 365 different ways to prepare it. One for each day of the year. Today, however, with supplies severely depleted, cod is no longer poor man's meat and much of that eaten today in Portugal is imported from Norway. Dried salt cod must be soaked well before it's cooked—not only to tenderize it and mute the fishy flavor but also to leach out most of the salt.

NUTRIENT CONTENT OF 3 OUNCES COOKED DRIED BACALHAU (SALT COD)	
(85 grams)	
91 calories	438 mg sodium
20 g protein	33 mg potassium
1 g fat, 0 saturated	0 g dietary fiber
56 mg cholesterol	13 RE vitamin A
0 g carbohydrate	0.02 mg thiamin
24 mg calcium	0.10 mg riboflavin
195 mg phosphorus	2.3 mg niacin
0.9 mg iron	0 mg vitamin C

Bacon: True bacon comes from pork bellies and it's leaner than it once was because geneticists have learned to breed slimmer hogs and packers are trimming the carcasses more closely. Most supermarkets today sell slab bacon as well as slices of varying thickness. Thin-sliced bacon averages 35 slices to the pound; medium sliced or regular, 16 to 20 slices per pound; thick sliced, 12 to 15 slices per pound. Some packers now cure bacon with minimal sodium nitrate (see NITRATES, NITRITES), the preservative that can combine with protein (amino acids) to form nitrosamines, which have caused cancer in laboratory animals. Reduced-sodium bacons are also widely available. Read labels carefully. There are many specialty bacons, among them: **double-smoked German bacon** (lean, deeply smoky but mellow), **Danish bacon** (mild and sweet), **Irish bacon** (intensely smoky) and **home-cured bacon** (heavily salted and smoked)—even **turkey bacon,** which is lower in fat and calories than regular bacon. Many specialty bacons, when bought by the slab, may show a thick encrust-

ation of salt and ash. Sometimes there may even be mold. No harm done. Simply rinse (or scrub) away the salt, mold and ash. **NOTE:** If you're using a heavily salty bacon in a recipe, reduce the amount of salt called for in the recipe. Or blanch the bacon briefly in boiling water to remove some of the salt. See also CANADIAN BACON; PANCETTA.

NUTRIENT CONTENT OF 2 SLICES COOKED BACON	
(about 1/2 ounce; 13 grams)	
73 calories	202 mg sodium
4 g protein	62 mg potassium
6 g fat, 2 saturated	0 g dietary fiber
11 mg cholesterol	0 RE vitamin A
0 g carbohydrate	0.09 mg thiamin
2 mg calcium	0.04 mg riboflavin
43 mg phosphorus	0.9 mg niacin
0.2 mg iron	4 mg vitamin C

NUTRIENT CONTENT OF 2 SLICES COOKED TURKEY BACON	
(about 2/3 ounce; 18 grams)	
68 calories	412 mg sodium
5 g protein	72 mg potassium
5 g fat, 1 saturated	0 g dietary fiber
18 mg cholesterol	NA RE vitamin A
1 g carbohydrate	NA mg thiamin
2 mg calcium	NA mg riboflavin
82 mg phosphorus	NA mg niacin
0.4 mg iron	NA mg vitamin C

Bacon Drippings: Frugal cooks like to recycle bacon drippings. They add rich meaty flavor, it's true. But they also add considerable sodium, saturated fat and cholesterol and, if heated to the smoke point, a noxious compound called ACROLEIN.

Bacteria: Restaurant and other institutional chefs, home cooks and anyone else involved in the preparation of food must be vigilant in their war on the bacteria that cause food poisoning. And all eaters must be aware of potential problems. Unfortunately, bacteria can contaminate food without making their presence known—until it's too late. Those most apt to cause grief:

Campylobacter jejuni: This bug causes a severe gastrointestinal upset that lasts a week or more. **BACTERIAL**

SOURCE: Raw poultry and meat, unpasteurized milk. **SYMPTOMS OF CAMPYLOBACTERIOSIS:** Abdominal cramps, diarrhea, fever and, in intense episodes, bloody stools. **HOW SOON SYMPTOMS OCCUR:** Within two to five days. **PREVENTIVES:** Use pasteurized milk only; cook poultry well done and red meat until it shows the *merest* tinge of pink in the center (160°F. on a meat thermometer). Hamburger and meat loaves should be brown clear through. Also, keep counters, cutting boards and implements scrupulously clean, and wash hands well after handling raw meat or poultry.

Clostridium botulinum: The bacterium itself doesn't kill, but the toxin it produces causes the deadly botulism. **BACTERIAL SOURCE:** Improperly canned low-acid foods (soups; vegetables such as peas, beans and corn; ripe olives; tuna; liver pâté), also hams, luncheon meats, shellfish, sausage, smoked and salted fish. The spores of *C. botulinum* multiply in low-acid foods in the absence of air, producing a poison so powerful minute amounts of it can kill. Sadly, the *C. botulinum* toxin often gives no clue of its presence; the food may look, smell and taste okay. Most outbreaks of botulism can be traced to faulty home-canned food, but commercial processors are sometimes fallible, too. **SYMPTOMS OF BOTULISM:** Double vision, difficulty in speaking or swallowing, progressive respiratory paralysis. If symptoms occur, get medical help at once. **HOW SOON SYMPTOMS OCCUR:** Within four to thirty-six hours. **PREVENTIVES:** Fortunately, heat deactivates botulism toxin—usually ten minutes of hard boiling will do the job. Still, if you doubt the safety of a particular food or can of food, get rid of it immediately—where neither people nor animals can get at it. *Don't taste* and *do* wash your hands thoroughly with soap and hot water after handling any suspicious food. The best policy always: When in doubt, throw it out.

Clostridium perfringens: Nicknamed the cafeteria bug, *C. perfringens* is responsible for about 10 percent of all cases of food poisoning. **BACTERIAL SOURCE:** Perishable foods, especially large batches of meat or poultry left at room temperature for longer than two hours. **SYMPTOMS OF C. PERFRINGENS FOOD POISONING:** Vomiting, diarrhea, abdominal cramps. In most cases, symptoms last about a day and, except in the elderly or infirm, are rarely serious enough to require medical attention. **HOW SOON SYMPTOMS OCCUR:** Within eight to twelve hours. **PREVENTIVES:** Keep cold foods cold and hot foods hot. When refrigerating large batches of hot food, divide among small containers so the food will chill fast.

Escherichia coli: Always considered a benign, indeed beneficial bug that lived quietly in the intestine synthesizing B vitamins, *E. coli* has suddenly turned vicious. Or rather, a killer strain (*E. coli* 0157:h7) has surfaced, the culprit behind a hemorrhagic form of food poisoning that began appearing in the early 1980s in Canada and the United States. Those felled by the disease shared one thing: They'd all eaten rare hamburgers at fast-food restaurants. Sad to say, several children died from eating the tainted burgers. Recently, there's been a shocking increase in *E. coli* food poisonings (even traced to unpasteurized apple cider pressed from unwashed windfalls possibly contaminated with deer feces). The young are particularly hard hit by hemorrhagic *E. coli,* as are the elderly and infirm. **BACTERIAL SOURCE:** Unpasteurized milk, undercooked meats (particularly hamburgers and all-beef hot dogs). **SYMPTOMS OF HEMORRHAGIC E. COLI FOOD POISONING:** Vomiting, bloody diarrhea, intense abdominal cramps and, in young children, sometimes kidney failure. Old people may suffer strokes or seizures (from blood clots on the brain). This acute food poisoning can last ten days or more, it can require hospitalization and it can kill. **HOW SOON SYMPTOMS OCCUR:** Within three to four days. **PREVENTIVES:** Drink pasteurized milk only. Handle raw meats carefully and cook them thoroughly (with hamburgers, this means until brown in the center). Never thaw frozen meat at room temperature (freezing does not kill *E. coli*) or let raw meat stand at room temperature for more than two hours. When putting groceries away, refrigerate perishables immediately. Use ground meat within three days of purchase and frozen patties within four months. Finally, keep kitchen counters, cutting boards and utensils spotless. And wash your hands well in hot, soapy water after handling raw meat.

Listeria monocytogenes: This form of food poisoning seems to target pregnant women and their fetuses, infants, the elderly and cancer and AIDS patients, as well as others with weakened immune systems. But *anyone* can get listeriosis. **BACTERIAL SOURCE:** Unpasteurized milk and milk products; fresh, soft cheeses (particularly Mexican types like *queso blanco* and *queso fresco*), also feta, Brie, Camembert, Roquefort and other blues; seafood;

frozen cooked shrimp, crab and *surimi;* even such deli items as coleslaw and cold cuts. Finally, sloppy food handling, which can cause cross-contamination of food. **SYMPTOMS OF LISTERIOSIS:** Nausea, vomiting, fever, headache and, occasionally, miscarriage, meningitis, septicemia, infant or fetal death. **HOW SOON SYMPTOMS OCCUR:** Usually within two to three days of eating the contaminated food although the illness may take a month to develop. **PREVENTIVES:** Avoid unpasteurized milk and milk products. Cook all meat thoroughly (to 160°F. although chefs and devotees of juicily red meat will probably throw up their hands in horror). Cook all fish to 160°F. (no more raw or rare fresh fish) and cook all poultry to 180°F. Keep hot foods good and hot (above 140°F.) and cold foods well chilled (below 40°F.).

Salmonella: With salmonella now rampaging through America's henhouses, many favorite recipes—eggnog, mayonnaises or ice creams made with raw eggs—must be abandoned. Meringue pie toppings are risky, too, if made with fresh eggs, and soft-cooked eggs are out. Salmonella is not a single bacterium but a cast of thousands that accounts for about half the cases of food poisoning. Regardless of which salmonella is the culprit, all cause the same intestinal flulike symptoms. **BACTERIAL SOURCE:** Raw or undercooked poultry and eggs; raw milk and dairy products; raw or undercooked meats and shrimp; and, finally, untidy cooking procedures. **SYMPTOMS OF SALMONELLA POISONING:** Nausea, vomiting, stomach cramps, fever, headache. **HOW SOON SYMPTOMS OCCUR:** Within six to forty-eight hours. **PREVENTIVES:** Rinse poultry, meat and shrimp well in cold water before you cook them (this sends some of the bugs down the drain). Never taste anything containing raw egg (no more bowl licking!); cook eggs until the yolks set and poultry until a meat thermometer, inserted in the fleshiest part of a thigh, not touching bone, registers 180°F. Cook meat to an internal temperature of 160°F. or more. Finally, keep counters, cutting boards, knives and other implements immaculate, washing them with hot soapy water or perhaps a diluted bleach solution as soon as you've finished working with raw eggs, meat or poultry. Lather your hands well, too.

Shigella: The medical name for the dysentery this pathogen causes is **shigellosis. BACTERIAL SOURCE:** Dairy products; poultry; potato, pasta and other bland salads. Contaminated by careless cooks or handlers, food, if not refrigerated, allows shigella to grow, and outbreaks of shigellosis will surely follow. **SYMPTOMS OF SHIGELLOSIS:** Diarrhea, abdominal cramps, vomiting, fever and sometimes blood, mucus and/or pus in stools. **HOW SOON SYMPTOMS OCCUR:** Within one to seven days. **PREVENTIVES:** Keeping the cook and kitchen squeaky clean; also refrigerating all perishables promptly and properly.

Staphylococcus aureus: The "*turista* bug" that so often plagues travelers. Actually, it's not the bug that makes you sick but the toxin it manufactures. *S. aureus* lives in the respiratory tract, so if a chef or waiter sneezes into food—particularly a protein-rich one—he contaminates it (he also contaminates it if he has infected sores on his hands). If the food is then not kept hot enough or cold enough, the bugs will thrive, producing their special brand of poison. Once staph toxins are present in food, no amount of cooking will destroy them. **BACTERIAL SOURCE:** Meats, poultry, egg products, cream-filled cakes and pastries, gelatins, cream sauces, creamed foods and bland salads (potato, macaroni, chicken, tuna, shrimp, etc.) that are allowed to stand too long at room temperature or, worse, as sometimes happens on cruise ships, are left to languish on a buffet under the downpouring sun. Such foods are warm and moist, the perfect breeding ground for bacteria. **SYMPTOMS OF STAPHYLOCOCCAL FOOD POISONING:** The "trots," stomach cramps, vomiting, fever. **HOW SOON SYMPTOMS OCCUR:** Anywhere from a half hour to eight hours after eating contaminated food. The good news is that these bouts rarely last more than a day or two and although they can make you wish you were dead, they're almost never fatal. **PREVENTIVES:** Keep hot foods hissing hot, cold foods icy cold. Also, thaw frozen food in the refrigerator, never at room temperature. Finally, refrigerate leftovers ASAP.

Vibrio vulnificus: This microbe lives in coastal waters and in warm weather can infect seafood and, ultimately, those who eat it. People at greatest risk are those with weakened immune systems, scanty stomach acid or liver problems. *Vibrio* infections strike abruptly with chills and fever. The best preventive? Avoid raw fish or shellfish taken in summer from shallow inshore waters.

Yersinia enterocolitica: Both food- and waterborne, *Y. enterocolitica* has occasionally infected livestock (beef, lamb and pork) and is passed along to humans through improperly cooked meat. It thrives at room temperature, even in the refrigerator but, fortunately, is destroyed by heat. **BACTERIAL SOURCE:** Raw meat, water, improperly handled nonfat dry milk reconstituted, tofu packed in contaminated water, chocolate syrup, raw vegetables, unpasteurized milk and milk products. **SYMPTOMS OF Y. ENTEROCOLITICA FOOD POISONING:** Fever, diarrhea and intense abdominal pain on the lower, right-hand side that mimics appendicitis (more than a few healthy appendixes have been removed because of wrong diagnoses). *Y. enterocolitica* infections, a major cause of enterocolitis in children, have also led to terminal ileitis, liver and spleen abscesses, septicemia and arthritis. **HOW SOON SYMPTOMS OCCUR:** Two to three days after eating or drinking contaminated food or water. **PREVENTIVES:** Keep kitchen and kitchen equipment immaculate, paying particular attention to implements and cutting boards used to prepare food that will be eaten raw. Avoid unpurified water, unpasteurized milk and milk products. Cook all meats thoroughly (to 160°F.).

The problem of harmful bacteria in the American food supply has become so acute that the USDA began posting safe-handling labels on all packages of fresh and frozen meat and poultry in 1994.

Of course, not all bacteria are bad. Many are beneficial—make that *indispensable*—to the food industry. For example, lactic acid bacteria are used in the manufacture of sour cream, buttermilk, yogurt, cheese, even sauerkraut. And acetobacter is used in the production of vinegar.

Bad Breath: What causes halitosis? Often it's nothing more than poor dental hygiene—bits of food stuck between the teeth. But something more serious may be responsible. Periodontal disease, for example, gastrointestinal and respiratory problems (especially inflamed or infected sinuses). Dry mouth, the culprit behind "morning breath," can cause bad breath, too (drinking more water may help, or chewing sugarless gum). Finally, smoking is a major cause of halitosis, as are drinking alcoholic beverages and eating garlic and onions. Apart from avoiding these, the best preventives are flossing, brushing and rinsing well with mouthwash every time you eat and, once a week, brushing with a thin paste of baking soda and hydrogen peroxide, which makes your mouth wonderfully sweet.

Bagels: Sometimes called "Jewish doughnuts," bagels are small, savory, yeast-raised, ring-shaped buns that are boiled, then baked. They were introduced to America by Jewish immigrants, probably early in the twentieth century.

Says John Mariani in *The Dictionary of American Food and Drink,* "The bagel was first mentioned in American print only in 1932." He believes its origins are "lost somewhere in the history of the Ashkenazi Jews, who brought Yiddish culture to America." Originally a staple in Jewish delica-

---

NUTRIENT CONTENT OF 1 EGG BAGEL
(about 2½ ounces; 68 grams)

189 calories	343 mg sodium
7 g protein	46 mg potassium
1 g fat, 0 saturated	2 g dietary fiber
16 mg cholesterol	22 RE vitamin A
36 g carbohydrate	0.36 mg thiamin
9 mg calcium	0.16 mg riboflavin
57 mg phosphorus	2.3 mg niacin
2.7 mg iron	0 mg vitamin C

NUTRIENT CONTENT OF 1 PLAIN BAGEL
(about 2½ ounces; 68 grams)

187 calories	363 mg sodium
7 g protein	69 mg potassium
1 g fat, 0 saturated	2 g dietary fiber
0 mg cholesterol	0 RE vitamin A
36 g carbohydrate	0.37 mg thiamin
50 mg calcium	0.21 mg riboflavin
65 mg phosphorus	3.1 mg niacin
2.4 mg iron	0 mg vitamin C

NUTRIENT CONTENT OF 1 WHOLE-WHEAT BAGEL
(about 2½ ounces; 68 grams)

143 calories	270 mg sodium
6 g protein	176 mg potassium
1 g fat, 0 saturated	5 g dietary fiber
0 mg cholesterol	0 RE vitamin A
30 g carbohydrate	0.20 mg thiamin
19 mg calcium	0.12 mg riboflavin
169 mg phosphorus	2.1 mg niacin
1.9 mg iron	0 mg vitamin C

tessens, where customers breakfasted on bagels, cream cheese and lox (smoked salmon), bagels are now available in nearly every American supermarket, freshly baked, packaged or frozen—and in dozens of permutations (whole wheat, honey and raisin, onion, garlic). To purists, however, the best bagels are plain.

Baked Beans: Some food historians believe that Native Americans invented baked beans. But novelist Kenneth Roberts wrote that baked beans were for centuries a traditional Sabbath dish among Sephardic Jews and that New England clipper-ship captains might have picked the recipe up on their travels. If so, that version would surely not have contained salt pork. Whatever the recipe's origin, Bostonians claim baked beans as their own. And they are plenty finicky about the recipe. Adding tomatoes, for example (which many Americans do), is a sacrilege. Classic Boston baked beans contain nothing more than dried beans, water, salt, dry mustard, molasses, brown sugar and salt pork. Even onion is optional. The secret? Baking the beans in a clay pot so long and slowly the starches begin to caramelize. The original recipe drips with fat (13 grams

Slimmed-Down Boston Baked Beans

Makes 8 Servings

1 pound dried navy or pea beans, washed and picked over

3 quarts cold water, approximately

2 ounces salt pork, in 1 piece

1½ teaspoons dry mustard

1½ teaspoons ground ginger

1¼ teaspoons salt

3 tablespoons molasses

2 tablespoons firmly packed dark brown sugar

1 large yellow onion, coarsely chopped

3 garlic cloves, slivered (not traditional but the garlic pumps up the flavor)

SOAK THE BEANS overnight in half the water. Drain well, measure soaking water, and add enough of the remaining water to total 1 quart. Bring beans and water to a boil in a large heavy kettle, adjust heat so mixture bubbles gently, cover, and cook, stirring now and then, 1 hour or until beans are almost tender.

TOWARD THE END of the cooking, preheat oven to 400°F. Drain beans, reserving 2 cups cooking water. Place one third of the salt pork in a 2-quart bean pot, then add beans. Combine reserved cooking water with all remaining ingredients except the remaining salt pork and mix into beans. Score rind of the remaining salt pork in crisscross fashion and push about 1 inch into the beans.

COVER AND BAKE 1 hour. Lower oven temperature to 250°F. and bake beans, still covered, for 4 hours, stirring up from the bottom every hour. Uncover and bake beans 1 hour more or until crusty-brown on top. Serve at once.

APPROXIMATE NUTRIENT COUNTS PER SERVING

242 calories	44 g carbohydrate	3.8 mg iron	0.28 mg thiamin
12 g protein	12 g dietary fiber	348 mg sodium	0.09 mg riboflavin
3 g fat, 1 saturated	118 mg calcium	639 mg potassium	0.9 mg niacin
2 mg cholesterol	221 mg phosphorus	0 RE vitamin A	2 mg vitamin C

per serving, 5 of them saturated), calories (nearly 400 per serving) and sodium (1,064 milligrams!). Here's a more healthful variation that remains true to the original.

NUTRIENT CONTENT OF 1 CUP CANNED PORK AND BEANS	
(9 ounces; 253 grams)	
311 calories	1,181 mg sodium
16 g protein	536 mg potassium
7 g fat, 3 saturated	18 g dietary fiber
10 mg cholesterol	30 RE vitamin A
49 g carbohydrate	0.20 mg thiamin
138 mg calcium	0.08 mg riboflavin
274 mg phosphorus	1.5 mg niacin
4.6 mg iron	5 mg vitamin C

Baker's Yeast: See YEAST.

Baking: Nothing mellows and intensifies the flavor of food like baking or cooking food uncovered in the dry heat of an oven. There's an added advantage, too. This dry method of cooking requires no liquid, which might leach out valuable vitamins and minerals. The downside? Baking is slow, thus heat-sensitive vitamin C and certain of the B-complex, especially thiamin (B_1), are more apt to be destroyed than when cooked quickly.

Baking Powder: Introduced in the mid-1800s, baking powders were one of America's first convenience foods. All are mixtures of starch, baking soda and acid salts. There are three basic types. First, single-acting **tartrate powders** (made with cream of tartar), which fizz the instant liquid is mixed into a batter but go flat just as fast. In the hands of a skillful cook, they produce exceptionally fine cakes. Second are the slower-acting **phosphate powders** (sometimes labeled "double-acting"), which react first with moisture, then again with heat. Finally, there is the **sodium-aluminum-sulfate** or **SAS-phosphate** variety. The most widely available today, this combination baking powder is truly double-acting and very nearly foolproof. All three types leaven by producing carbon dioxide gas. Indispensable as baking powders are, they do up one's intake of sodium (1 teaspoon baking powder equals 325 to 350 milligrams). Fortunately, low-sodium baking powders (averaging 200 milligrams per teaspoon) are now available.

Baking powders made with calcium salts boost the body's supply of calcium (1 teaspoon supplies 60 to 175 milligrams) and the SAS-phosphate type increases the level of aluminum.

Baking Soda: Nothing more than **bicarbonate of soda** (**sodium bicarbonate**), which in the presence of heat and water (or, better yet, a mild acid like buttermilk or sour milk) forms carbon dioxide gas, a splendid leavener of batters and doughs. The disadvantage of baking soda is that it's loaded with sodium (476 mg per ½ teaspoon). It's alkaline (as anyone knows who's taken it for acid indigestion) and has the power to turn certain green vegetables bright green. Years ago, cooks routinely added a pinch of soda to a pot of snap beans or garden peas. Unwise, because soda destroys vitamin C.

Bamboo Shoots: Only certain species of this largest of the grasses are edible; some contain prussic acid and are highly poisonous (even edible bamboo shoots must be parboiled five minutes—or until they no longer taste bitter—to rid them of hydrocyanic acid). What most Americans know are canned bamboo shoots, although the fresh are beginning to show up in high-end groceries as well as Asian markets. Delicate of flavor but nicely crunchy, fresh bamboo shoots are extremely low in calories, fat and sodium. They are also a stellar source of potassium. **SEASON:** Winter and spring.

NUTRIENT CONTENT OF 1 CUP SLICED BOILED (OR CANNED-IN-WATER) BAMBOO SHOOTS	
(about 4¼ ounces; 120 grams)	
14 calories	5 mg sodium
2 g protein	640 mg potassium
0 g fat, 0 saturated	1 g dietary fiber
0 mg cholesterol	0 RE vitamin A
2 g carbohydrate	0.02 mg thiamin
14 mg calcium	0.06 mg riboflavin
24 mg phosphorus	0.4 mg niacin
0.3 mg iron	0 mg vitamin C

Banana Peppers: See SWEET PEPPERS under PEPPERS, CAPSICUMS.

Bananas: Believed to be indigenous to Asia, bananas are also thought to be one of the first fruits cultivated by man. Alexander the Great saw them growing in the Indus Valley three hundred years before Christ. A thousand years later, Arabs introduced bananas to Egypt, whence they moved west across the continent. Portuguese explorers discovered them on Africa's Atlantic coast in the fifteenth century. Prince Henry the Navigator ordered specimens transplanted on the Portuguese island of Madeira where they flourish to this day. Bananas are nutritious and easily digested, which is why they so often show up in the diets of infants and invalids. Because of their high potassium content, physicians often prescribe bananas to patients on diuretics. **SEASON:** Year-round.

NUTRIENT CONTENT OF 1 MEDIUM-SIZE BANANA

(about 4 ounces; 114 grams)

104 calories	1 mg sodium
1 g protein	451 mg potassium
1 g fat, 0 saturated	2 g dietary fiber
0 mg cholesterol	9 RE vitamin A
27 g carbohydrate	0.05 mg thiamin
7 mg calcium	0.11 mg riboflavin
23 mg phosphorus	0.6 mg niacin
0.4 mg iron	10 mg vitamin C

Banana Squash: See SQUASH.

Barbecue, Barbecuing: Some say the word comes from the French *barb à queue,* meaning "from beard to tail," which is how Frenchmen saw New World natives cooking game. Others insist *barbecue* derives from *barbacoa,* the Spanish name for the rack on which Spanish explorers found West Indians grilling meat and fish. Both explanations seem plausible for cooking food over hot coals is one of the oldest-known methods of cooking. Today, barbecuing is a highly complex business—of marinating meat, poultry or fish in mysterious blends, burying them whole in fiery pits or grilling them over hot coals with liberal lashings of secret sauces. Recipes vary, techniques vary, even the foods being barbecued differ. In Texas it's beef or *cabrito* (kid). In North Carolina it's pork, although turkey is gaining ground. And on patios across America it's everything from burgers to chicken. Pit-barbecued meats literally ooze fat. The charcoal-grilled are leaner, but they may be suffused with the carcinogenic fumes that form as fats sputter into the fire.

Barbecue Sauces: These both tenderize and flavor meat. Southerners prefer an explosive oil and vinegar baste; Southwesterners thick red sauces that don't stint on chiles; and Californians sophisticated mixes spiked with soy sauce and fresh ginger. Middle America settles for bland and ketchupy bottled sauces. None is a nutritional powerhouse, as the following table proves.

NUTRIENT CONTENT OF 1 TABLESPOON BOTTLED BARBECUE SAUCE

(about ½ ounce; 16 grams)

12 calories	127 mg sodium
0 g protein	27 mg potassium
0 g fat, 0 saturated	0 g dietary fiber
0 mg cholesterol	14 RE vitamin A
2 g carbohydrate	0 mg thiamin
3 mg calcium	0 mg riboflavin
3 mg phosphorus	0.1 mg niacin
0.1 mg iron	1 mg vitamin C

Bariatrics: A branch of medicine devoted to the prevention, control and treatment of obesity.

Barley: Is this the world's oldest cultivated grain? Many food historians believe so, pointing to the fact that the ancients made barley breads long before they learned to grow and mill wheat. Probably these were leaden ash cakes because barley lacks the gluten (protein) necessary to build the framework of leavened breads. Most of the barley sold in supermarkets today is pearled, meaning that some of the nutrient-rich husk has been removed. It's available in **small-, medium-** and **large-pearl** (also sometimes labeled **fine, medium** and **coarse**) and is an economical extender of soups and stews. **Whole-grain barley** is also available, mostly through health-food stores. It can be boiled, like oatmeal, into a hearty hot cereal. Home consumption of barley pales, however, beside its use by brewers and distillers. Scotch whisky and beer couldn't be made without it. Indeed, **barley malt** is so key to the making of fine German beer that Duke Wilhelm IV of Bavaria instituted a *Rheinheitsgebot* (purity law) in 1516. Generally recognized as the world's first consumer protection law, it decreed that beer could be brewed only from barley malt, hops and water. It is still in force today.

NUTRIENT CONTENT OF 1 CUP COOKED PEARL BARLEY

(about 5¼ ounces; 157 grams)

193 calories	5 mg sodium
4 g protein	146 mg potassium
1 g fat, 0 saturated	9 g dietary fiber
0 mg cholesterol	1 RE vitamin A
44 g carbohydrate	0.13 mg thiamin
17 mg calcium	0.10 mg riboflavin
85 mg phosphorus	3.2 mg niacin
2.1 mg iron	0 mg vitamin C

NUTRIENT CONTENT OF 1 CUP COOKED WHOLE-GRAIN BARLEY

(about 7 ounces; 200 grams)

270 calories	1 mg sodium
7 g protein	230 mg potassium
2 g fat, 0 saturated	14 g dietary fiber
0 mg cholesterol	1 RE vitamin A
59 g carbohydrate	0.16 mg thiamin
26 mg calcium	0.10 mg riboflavin
230 mg phosphorus	2.8 mg niacin
2.1 mg iron	0 mg vitamin C

Basal Metabolism, Basal Metabolic Rate (BMR):

Basal metabolism is the amount of energy the body uses to perform such vital chores as breathing; circulation of the blood; digestion; liver, kidney and endocrine gland function as well as to maintain muscle tone and body temperature. It's measured under basal conditions; that is, at neutral temperatures (68°F. to 77°F.) with the body at total mental and physical rest (twelve to sixteen hours after eating). BMR tests are also conducted in quiet, peaceful atmospheres with the patient lying down. The reason for such tests is to determine metabolism efficiency, which may, among other things, shed light on why one can't lose—or gain—weight. The basal metabolic rate, or **resting metabolic rate** (**RMR**) as it's commonly phrased

today, means the amount of energy the body burns per hour under basal conditions. For healthy men, the norm is about 1 kcal (the amount of heat needed to raise the temperature of 1 kilogram [2.2 pounds] water 1 degree Celsius) per kilogram of body weight per hour; and for healthy women, 0.9 kcal per kilo of body weight per hour. But BMR rates vary widely. Age, health, nutritional state, pregnancy, growth rate, endocrine activity, body size, shape, weight, indeed even individual body composition all affect the BMR.

Base: See ALKALI.

Basic Four Food Groups: Now replaced by the FOOD GUIDE PYRAMID, these groupings of food by type were used throughout the 1970s and 1980s as a guide to good eating. The trouble with the Basic Four, nutritionists now believe, was that they gave equal emphasis to each group: (1) Milk; (2) Meat; (3) Fruits and Vegetables; (4) Breads and Cereals. Today, with the emphasis on eating less fat, cholesterol and protein, the pyramid casts meats and dairy foods in supporting roles and makes stars of vegetables, fruits and grains.

Basil: No Italian could cook without this pungent member of the mint family. Actually, there are several species of basil, but those best known to Americans are **sweet basil,** the tiny-leafed **bush basil** and rich maroon **opal basil.** Unlike other herbs, which are used sparingly, basil figures prominently in such classics as pesto and impacts on their nutritive value. This basil/garlic/Parmesan/*pignoli* (pine nut) paste has become as popular a pasta sauce in this country as marinara or Alfredo and, like them, is sold in plastic tubs in high-end supermarkets. Pesto has one enormous shortcoming, however: It *oozes* fat. Here's a considerably lighter processor version.

Basmati: See RICE.

Bass: See SEA BASS; STRIPED BASS.

BBS (Baby Bottle Syndrome): See NURSING BOTTLE SYNDROME.

Low-Fat Processor Pesto

Makes 4 Servings

2 cups firmly packed fresh basil leaves

1 large garlic clove, slivered

1 tablespoon fruity olive oil

1 tablespoon *pignoli* (pine nuts)

3 tablespoons freshly grated Parmesan cheese

¼ cup low-fat (1 percent) cottage cheese

½ cup reduced-sodium chicken broth

¼ teaspoon freshly ground black pepper

PLACE ALL INGREDIENTS in a food processor fitted with the metal chopping blade and churn 30 seconds. Scrape down the work bowl and churn 60 seconds longer, until uniformly smooth. Use as a sauce for trenette, fettuccine, or other long, slim pasta.

APPROXIMATE NUTRIENT COUNTS PER SERVING

91 calories	2 g carbohydrate	1.2 mg iron	0.04 mg thiamin
6 g protein	1 g dietary fiber	155 mg sodium	0.07 mg riboflavin
7 g fat, 2 saturated	110 mg calcium	167 mg potassium	0.8 mg niacin
4 mg cholesterol	99 mg phosphorus	92 RE vitamin A	4 mg vitamin C

B-complex: A family of vitamins, all water soluble, somewhat related in function and often occurring together in foods. They include **vitamin B$_1$** (thiamin), **vitamin B$_2$** (riboflavin), **vitamin B$_6$** (pyridoxine), **vitamin B$_{12}$** (cobalamin), **niacin** (nicotinic acid), **folacin** (folic acid, also called pteroylglutamic acid or PGA), **pantothenic acid** and **biotin.** All are covered in individual entries.

Bean Curd: See TOFU.

Beans, Dried: A glance at the nutrient content of any of the dried beans listed below explains why they're known as poor man's meat, why they've nourished the world since the beginning of time. All are legumes, second only to cereals as a source of food. Add to that the fact that beans are easily grown and, when dried, virtually imperishable. Small wonder Native Americans treated them with reverence and planted them with ceremony. Many beans are New World natives: **black** ("turtle") **beans, great northern beans, lima beans, kidney beans, navy** or **pea beans** and **pinto beans.** But there are Old World varieties, too. The big three of Asia are **adzuki** (small red beans that are not only dried but also ground into a sweet paste called *yokan*), **mung** and **soybeans** (fresh versions of the last two are discussed in separate entries). Europe can claim only two beans—one is the **fava** (also called **broad bean, horse bean, Scotch bean** or **Windsor**), the bean known to Western Europe before Columbus; it's thought to be indigenous to the Mediterranean rim. The other European bean is the **chickpea** or **garbanzo,** a favorite of ancient Egyptians, Greeks and Hebrews. Then there are **black-eyed peas** (cowpeas), which are also beans, thought to have originated somewhere in Central Africa. Nutritionally speaking, all dried beans are powerhouses of energy and abundant sources of such minerals as iron, phosphorus and potassium. They are respectable sources of protein (albeit incomplete protein) and, in the case of soybeans, a more than respectable source. Best of all, most are fat free and all, unless canned, extremely low in sodium. Read labels.

NUTRIENT CONTENT OF 1 CUP BOILED DRIED ADZUKI BEANS

(about 8 ounces; 230 grams)

294 calories	18 mg sodium
17 g protein	1,224 mg potassium
0 g fat, 0 saturated	12 g dietary fiber
0 mg cholesterol	2 RE vitamin A
57 g carbohydrate	0.26 mg thiamin
64 mg calcium	0.15 mg riboflavin
386 mg phosphorus	1.7 mg niacin
4.6 mg iron	0 mg vitamin C

NUTRIENT CONTENT OF 1 CUP BOILED DRIED CHICKPEAS (GARBANZO BEANS)

(about 5½ ounces; 164 grams)

267 calories	12 mg sodium
15 g protein	477 mg potassium
4 g fat, 0 saturated	10 g dietary fiber
0 mg cholesterol	5 RE vitamin A
45 g carbohydrate	0.19 mg thiamin
80 mg calcium	0.10 mg riboflavin
276 mg phosphorus	0.9 mg niacin
4.7 mg iron	2 mg vitamin C

NUTRIENT CONTENT OF 1 CUP BOILED DRIED BLACK BEANS

(about 6 ounces; 172 grams)

227 calories	2 mg sodium
15 g protein	611 mg potassium
1 g fat, 0 saturated	10 g dietary fiber
0 mg cholesterol	2 RE vitamin A
41 g carbohydrate	0.42 mg thiamin
46 mg calcium	0.10 mg riboflavin
241 mg phosphorus	0.87 mg niacin
3.6 mg iron	0 mg vitamin C

NUTRIENT CONTENT OF 1 CUP BOILED DRIED GREAT NORTHERN BEANS

(about 6¼ ounces; 177 grams)

209 calories	4 mg sodium
15 g protein	692 mg potassium
1 g fat, 0 saturated	11 g dietary fiber
0 mg cholesterol	0 RE vitamin A
37 g carbohydrate	0.28 mg thiamin
120 mg calcium	0.10 mg riboflavin
292 mg phosphorus	1.2 mg niacin
3.8 mg iron	2 mg vitamin C

NUTRIENT CONTENT OF 1 CUP BOILED DRIED BLACK-EYED PEAS (COWPEAS)

(about 6 ounces; 171 grams)

198 calories	7 mg sodium
13 g protein	475 mg potassium
1 g fat, 0 saturated	16 g dietary fiber
0 mg cholesterol	3 RE vitamin A
36 g carbohydrate	0.35 mg thiamin
41 mg calcium	0.09 mg riboflavin
267 mg phosphorus	0.8 mg niacin
4.3 mg iron	1 mg vitamin C

NUTRIENT CONTENT OF 1 CUP BOILED DRIED LARGE LIMA BEANS

(about 6½ ounces; 188 grams)

216 calories	4 mg sodium
15 g protein	955 mg potassium
1 g fat, 0 saturated	14 g dietary fiber
0 mg cholesterol	0 RE vitamin A
39 g carbohydrate	0.30 mg thiamin
32 mg calcium	0.10 mg riboflavin
209 mg phosphorus	0.8 mg niacin
4.5 mg iron	0 mg vitamin C

NUTRIENT CONTENT OF 1 CUP BOILED DRIED MUNG BEANS

(about 7 ounces; 202 grams)

212 calories	4 mg sodium
14 g protein	538 mg potassium
1 g fat, 0 saturated	5 g dietary fiber
0 mg cholesterol	4 RE vitamin A
39 g carbohydrate	0.33 mg thiamin
55 mg calcium	0.12 mg riboflavin
199 mg phosphorus	1.2 mg niacin
2.8 mg iron	2 mg vitamin C

NUTRIENT CONTENT OF 1 CUP BOILED DRIED RED KIDNEY BEANS

(about 6¼ ounces; 177 grams)

225 calories	4 mg sodium
15 g protein	713 mg potassium
1 g fat, 0 saturated	15 g dietary fiber
0 mg cholesterol	1 RE vitamin A
40 g carbohydrate	0.28 mg thiamin
50 mg calcium	0.10 mg riboflavin
251 mg phosphorus	1.0 mg niacin
5.2 mg iron	2 mg vitamin C

NUTRIENT CONTENT OF 1 CUP BOILED DRIED NAVY BEANS

(about 6½ ounces; 182 grams)

258 calories	2 mg sodium
16 g protein	670 mg potassium
1 g fat, 0 saturated	16 g dietary fiber
0 mg cholesterol	0 RE vitamin A
48 g carbohydrate	0.37 mg thiamin
127 mg calcium	0.11 mg riboflavin
286 mg phosphorus	1.0 mg niacin
4.5 mg iron	2 mg vitamin C

NUTRIENT CONTENT OF 1 CUP BOILED DRIED SMALL WHITE BEANS

(about 6¼ ounces; 179 grams)

254 calories	4 mg sodium
16 g protein	829 mg potassium
1 g fat, 0 saturated	14 g dietary fiber
0 mg cholesterol	0 RE vitamin A
46 g carbohydrate	0.42 mg thiamin
130 mg calcium	0.11 mg riboflavin
303 mg phosphorus	0.5 mg niacin
5.1 mg iron	0 mg vitamin C

NUTRIENT CONTENT OF 1 CUP BOILED DRIED PINTO BEANS

(about 6 ounces; 171 grams)

234 calories	3 mg sodium
14 g protein	800 mg potassium
1 g fat, 0 saturated	20 g dietary fiber
0 mg cholesterol	0 RE vitamin A
44 g carbohydrate	0.32 mg thiamin
82 mg calcium	0.16 mg riboflavin
274 mg phosphorus	0.7 mg niacin
4.5 mg iron	4 mg vitamin C

NUTRIENT CONTENT OF 1 CUP BOILED DRIED SOYBEANS

(about 6 ounces; 172 grams)

298 calories	2 mg sodium
29 g protein	886 mg potassium
15 g fat, 2 saturated	6 g dietary fiber
0 mg cholesterol	1.7 RE vitamin A
17 g carbohydrate	0.27 mg thiamin
175 mg calcium	0.49 mg riboflavin
421 mg phosphorus	0.7 mg niacin
8.8 mg iron	3 mg vitamin C

Beans, Fresh: This includes not only those beans that are eaten pods and all, like greens, but also those that are shelled, like favas and black-eyed peas.

Black-eyed Peas (Cowpeas): Believed to be native to Central Africa—and, like peanuts and sesame seeds, to have been brought to the Deep South by slaves—fresh black-eyed peas remain a staple there. Usually they bubble slowly on the back of the stove with a ham bone or lump of fatback and are served in bowls with fresh corn bread. Often, too, they're teamed with rice in that Low Country classic hoppin' John. See also BEANS, DRIED.

NUTRIENT CONTENT OF 1 CUP BOILED FRESH BLACK-EYED PEAS	
(about 6 ounces; 172 grams)	
160 calories	7 mg sodium
5 g protein	690 mg potassium
1 g fat, 0 saturated	12 g dietary fiber
0 mg cholesterol	130 RE vitamin A
34 g carbohydrate	0.17 mg thiamin
211 mg calcium	0.24 mg riboflavin
84 mg phosphorus	2.3 mg niacin
1.9 mg iron	4 mg vitamin C

Cranberry Beans: Also called **shellouts,** these are America's second most popular shell beans (limas are first). A particular favorite in New England (though most are grown in Michigan), cranberry beans look like giant wax beans that have been stained here and there with cranberry juice. Their pods are leathery but, if gathered young enough, the beans inside are creamily sweet and tender. They need only to be boiled gently, drained,

NUTRIENT CONTENT OF 1 CUP BOILED CRANBERRY BEANS	
(about 6¼ ounces; 176 grams)	
240 calories	2 mg sodium
16 g protein	680 mg potassium
1 g fat, 0 saturated	18 g dietary fiber
0 mg cholesterol	NA RE vitamin A
43 g carbohydrate	0.37 mg thiamin
88 mg calcium	0.12 mg riboflavin
236 mg phosphorus	0.9 mg niacin
3.7 mg iron	NA mg vitamin C

then tossed with a lump of unsalted butter, salt and freshly ground pepper. Anything more, New Englanders insist, is lily gilding. **SEASON:** Summer.

Fava Beans, Broad Beans, Horse Beans, Scotch Beans, Windsors: Shelled fresh favas have only recently begun to make their mark in this country. These are the broad beans of the ancients, a protean food that sustained Eastern Mediterranean peoples in Old Testament times. Although best known for his geometry theorems, Pythagoras also founded a religion—Pythagoreanism—that forbade, among other things, the eating of fava beans. Not as crazy as it sounds. Scientists now know that because of a genetic defect, many people of Mediterranean origin can die from eating favas. Put simply, their bodies lack an enzyme (G6PD), allowing a toxin in fava beans to destroy their red blood cells (the condition is known as FAVISM). Those without this altered gene can eat favas with no ill effects. **SEASON:** Early summer.

NUTRIENT CONTENT OF 1 CUP BOILED FRESH FAVA BEANS	
(about 6 ounces; 170 grams)	
99 calories	72 mg sodium
8 g protein	340 mg potassium
1 g fat, 0 saturated	3 g dietary fiber
0 mg cholesterol	48 RE vitamin A
18 g carbohydrate	0.23 mg thiamin
32 mg calcium	0.16 mg riboflavin
128 mg phosphorus	2.1 mg niacin
2.6 mg iron	35 mg vitamin C

Green Beans: Whether called green beans, **string beans, snap beans** or **pole beans,** these long, slim beans are eaten pods and all. There are dozens of varieties (seed catalogs devote pages to them). In the old days, the seams of bean pods were woody or stringy, hence the nickname string beans. But geneticists have managed to breed the strings out. And with the tiny, tender, elegant *haricot vert,* French botanists have bestowed perfection upon this lowly all-American food (the very word *haricot,* believe it or not, is thought to derive from the Aztec *ayacotl*). Italian green beans are chunky, about twice the heft of their U.S. cousins, but rarely come to supermarkets fresh; the bulk of the crop is frozen. All fresh green beans are low in calories, fat and sodium but high in fiber, vitamins A and C and potassium. When canned, green beans lose some of their vitamin C and gain considerable salt. However, health-conscious canners now offer low- or no-salt-added options. The nutritive value of frozen green beans is largely intact, but their texture is so mushy finicky cooks won't give them freezer room. **SEASON:** Year-round but best in summer.

NUTRIENT CONTENT OF 1 CUP BOILED GREEN (SNAP) BEANS

(about 4½ ounces; 125 grams)

44 calories	4 mg sodium
2 g protein	373 mg potassium
0 g fat, 0 saturated	4 g dietary fiber
0 mg cholesterol	84 RE vitamin A
10 g carbohydrate	0.09 mg thiamin
58 mg calcium	0.12 mg riboflavin
49 mg phosphorus	0.8 mg niacin
1.6 mg iron	12 mg vitamin C

Lima Beans: Sometimes called the aristocrats of the family because of their buttery richness (not for nothing do Southerners call them **butter beans**), limas belong to the same big family as mung beans and adzukis. Unlike them, limas are native to Brazil and Peru. Today, there are dozens of varieties of limas, but two basic types: the large, starchy **Fordhooks** (boiled too long, they break apart like potatoes) and the sweeter, nuttier **baby limas**—everyone's favorite. All limas are low-sodium, high-fiber, high-carbohydrate foods with plenty of vitamins and minerals. **SEASON:** Summer.

NUTRIENT CONTENT OF 1 CUP BOILED BABY LIMA BEANS

(about 6 ounces; 170 grams)

210 calories	29 mg sodium
12 g protein	970 mg potassium
1 g fat, 0 saturated	14 g dietary fiber
0 mg cholesterol	63 RE vitamin A
40 g carbohydrate	0.24 mg thiamin
54 mg calcium	0.16 mg riboflavin
222 mg phosphorus	1.8 mg niacin
4.2 mg iron	17 mg vitamin C

Wax Beans: You might call them albino beans, because they look like green beans that have lost their color. For that reason, they contain considerably less vitamin A than green beans. Waxy in texture and slightly bitter in flavor, wax beans can nonetheless be cooked exactly like green beans and substituted for them in recipes. **SEASON:** Summer.

NUTRIENT CONTENT OF 1 CUP BOILED WAX BEANS

(about 4¾ ounces; 135 grams)

35 calories	18 mg sodium
2 g protein	151 mg potassium
0 g fat, 0 saturated	4 g dietary fiber
0 mg cholesterol	15 RE vitamin A
8 g carbohydrate	0.07 mg thiamin
61 mg calcium	0.10 mg riboflavin
32 mg phosphorus	0.6 mg niacin
1.1 mg iron	11 mg vitamin C

Winged Beans, Wing Beans: "Wonder beans" might be a better name for these tropical exotics because they're reasonable sources of protein, vitamins and certain minerals, but extremely low in calories and sodium. Southeast Asians have been eating them for years; indeed, that was about the only place winged beans were known until 1975 when the National Academy of Sciences issued a glowing report on their nutritional merits. Since then they've spread across the world. Every part of the winged bean is edible (leaves, shoots, flowers), but the pod is choicest. It's intensely green, elongated like a green bean but chunkier and more or less square in cross section because four fins or wings run the length of the bean. As for flavor, winged

NUTRIENT CONTENT OF 1 CUP BOILED WINGED BEANS

(about 2¼ ounces; 62 grams)

23 calories	3 mg sodium
3 g protein	170 mg potassium
0 g fat, 0 saturated	1 g dietary fiber
0 mg cholesterol	5 RE vitamin A
2 g carbohydrate	0.05 mg thiamin
38 mg calcium	0.05 mg riboflavin
16 mg phosphorus	0.4 mg niacin
0.7 mg iron	6 mg vitamin C

beans are blander than green beans, but meatier, too—more like limas (like limas, too, they're best when boiled). **SEASON:** Because they grow in the tropics, winged beans know no season. They don't often come to American markets, except in metropolitan areas. Supplies are expected to improve, however, once geneticists perfect a strain hardy enough to tolerate our colder climate. At present, anything below 40°F. will kill them.

Yard-Long Beans, Asparagus Beans, Chinese Long Beans, Long Beans: Probably native to Africa, but a staple in China, these green beans are only *half* a yard long. They look like mutant green beans but botanically are closer to black-eyed peas, which may explain their blandness. Chinese markets and upscale greengrocers sell yard-long beans by the bunch. Because they have so little flavor and firm up in cooking, yard-long beans are best when cut into manageable lengths and stir-fried. **SEASON:** Year-round.

NUTRIENT CONTENT OF 1 CUP YARD-LONG BEANS STIR-FRIED IN 1 TABLESPOON OIL	
(about 6½ ounces; 185 grams)	
169 calories	4 mg sodium
3 g protein	302 mg potassium
14 g fat, 2 saturated	2 g dietary fiber
0 mg cholesterol	47 RE vitamin A
10 g carbohydrate	0.09 mg thiamin
46 mg calcium	0.10 mg riboflavin
59 mg phosphorus	0.7 mg niacin
1.0 mg iron	17 mg vitamin C

Bean Sprouts: A staple of the Chinese kitchen, now quite at home in the American supermarket, is the sprouts of the **mung bean**—crunchy, faintly bittersweet and the color of pearls. The Chinese use other sprouts, too: the nutty, feathery shoots of the red **adzuki bean** as well as coarse and pungent **soybean** sprouts. These are protein-rich, but they also contain a toxin that can be harmful. Soybean sprouts shouldn't be eaten regularly or in large quantities. They should also be cooked—5 minutes is all it takes to deactivate their toxin. **SEASON:** Year-round.

NUTRIENT CONTENT OF 1 CUP RAW MUNG BEAN SPROUTS	
(about 3½ ounces; 104 grams)	
31 calories	6 mg sodium
3 g protein	154 mg potassium
0 g fat, 0 saturated	3 g dietary fiber
0 mg cholesterol	2 RE vitamin A
6 g carbohydrate	0.09 mg thiamin
14 mg calcium	0.13 mg riboflavin
56 mg phosphorus	0.8 mg niacin
0.9 mg iron	14 mg vitamin C

NUTRIENT CONTENT OF 1 CUP CANNED, DRAINED MUNG BEAN SPROUTS	
(about 4½ ounces; 125 grams)	
15 calories	175 mg sodium
2 g protein	34 mg potassium
0 g fat, 0 saturated	2 g dietary fiber
0 mg cholesterol	3 RE vitamin A
3 g carbohydrate	0.04 mg thiamin
18 mg calcium	0.09 mg riboflavin
40 mg phosphorus	0.3 mg niacin
0.5 mg iron	0 mg vitamin C

NUTRIENT CONTENT OF 1 CUP FRESH SOYBEAN SPROUTS	
(about 3½ ounces; 94 grams)	
76 calories	9 mg sodium
8 g protein	334 mg potassium
4 g fat, 1 saturated	2 g dietary fiber
0 mg cholesterol	1 RE vitamin A
6 g carbohydrate	0.19 mg thiamin
56 mg calcium	0.05 mg riboflavin
127 mg phosphorus	1.0 mg niacin
1.2 mg iron	8 mg vitamin C

Bean Thread Noodles: See CELLOPHANE NOODLES.

Beef: America came to the cattle business late; in fact, its first cows were Texas longhorns introduced by Spanish conquistadores in the sixteenth century. These angular animals foraged far and wide, gaining sinew with every step. Small wonder pork and chicken outranked beef in popularity.

Then, a hundred years ago, four developments revolutionized the American beef industry. First came the cross-breeding of longhorns with superior British stock, then came the railroads, then refrigerated railroad cars, then finally, the penning and finishing of steers on rations of grain. Pampered animals meant meat of supreme tenderness and, at long last, beef became America's number-one meat.

That may now change. There's been a lot of beef bashing lately: It's too fat; it's loaded with cholesterol; it's full of pesticides (see HERBICIDES, PESTICIDES), ANTIBIOTICS and HORMONES; it's contaminated with *E. coli* (see BACTERIA) and no longer safe to eat rare; slaughterhouse conditions are deplorable. And so on and so on. Some of the criticisms, leveled mostly by investigative reporters and consumer advocates, are true. Indeed, the problem of bacteria in beef has become so acute the USDA requires safe-handling labels on all packages of fresh and frozen beef (IRRADIATION will kill the bacteria but remains hotly controversial). Consumption of beef is off nearly 30 percent (since the early eighties), but the beef industry has come out slugging, determined to restore its good name. Cattle are being crossbred for leaner meat, and meatpackers are trimming off almost all the fat; 40 percent of the beef now sold is so closely trimmed it has no outer covering of fat. Still, as in days past, the highest grades—**Prime** and **Choice**—are the fattest. The leanest is **Select** (formerly **Good**). NOTE: Since 1987, when the USDA began calling Good beef Select, sales of it have quintupled.

Nutritionally speaking, beef provides impressive amounts of vitamin B$_{12}$, iron and zinc, three nutrients hard to come by elsewhere—particularly if you are vegetarian. Beef also supplies fair amounts of niacin, even some thiamin and riboflavin, all important B vitamins. But don't expect to get any fiber from beef or vitamin A or C (except for kidney and liver). So, except for those two organ meats, we've simplified the nutrient counts for beef and concentrate on calories, fat and cholesterol (items of current concern), plus protein and minerals. NOTE: The nutrient counts that follow are for Choice beef, the grade most widely available today. Lower grades contain less fat.

NUTRIENT CONTENT OF 3 OUNCES (85 GRAMS) BROILED, TRIMMED TOP ROUND STEAK

153 calories	5 mg calcium
27 g protein	209 mg phosphorus
4 g fat, 1 saturated	2.5 mg iron
71 mg cholesterol	52 mg sodium
0 g carbohydrate	376 mg potassium

NUTRIENT CONTENT OF 3 OUNCES (85 GRAMS) ROASTED, TRIMMED BEEF RUMP ROAST

170 calories	5 mg calcium
24 g protein	200 mg phosphorus
8 g fat, 3 saturated	2.4 mg iron
69 mg cholesterol	54 mg sodium
0 g carbohydrate	319 mg potassium

NUTRIENT CONTENT OF 3 OUNCES (85 GRAMS) BROILED, TRIMMED SIRLOIN STEAK

171 calories	9 mg calcium
26 g protein	208 mg phosphorus
7 g fat, 3 saturated	2.9 mg iron
76 mg cholesterol	56 mg sodium
0 g carbohydrate	342 mg potassium

NUTRIENT CONTENT OF 3 OUNCES (85 GRAMS) BRAISED, TRIMMED BOTTOM ROUND POT ROAST

178 calories	4 mg calcium
27 g protein	231 mg phosphorus
7 g fat, 2 saturated	2.9 mg iron
82 mg cholesterol	43 mg sodium
0 g carbohydrate	261 mg potassium

NUTRIENT CONTENT OF 3 OUNCES (85 GRAMS) BRAISED, TRIMMED CHUCK ARM POT ROAST

184 calories	8 mg calcium
28 g protein	229 mg phosphorus
7 g fat, 3 saturated	3.0 mg iron
86 mg cholesterol	56 mg sodium
0 g carbohydrate	245 mg potassium

NUTRIENT CONTENT OF 3 OUNCES (85 GRAMS) BROILED, TRIMMED FILET MIGNON

179 calories	6 mg calcium
24 g protein	202 mg phosphorus
9 g fat, 3 saturated	3.0 mg iron
71 mg cholesterol	54 mg sodium
0 g carbohydrate	357 mg potassium

NUTRIENT CONTENT OF 3 OUNCES (85 GRAMS) BROILED, TRIMMED FLANK STEAK (LONDON BROIL)

175 calories	6 mg calcium
23 g protein	200 mg phosphorus
9 g fat, 4 saturated	2.2 mg iron
57 mg cholesterol	71 mg sodium
0 g carbohydrate	351 mg potassium

NUTRIENT CONTENT OF 3 OUNCES (85 GRAMS) BROILED, TRIMMED T-BONE STEAK

181 calories	6 mg calcium
24 g protein	176 mg phosphorus
9 g fat, 4 saturated	2.6 mg iron
68 mg cholesterol	56 mg sodium
0 g carbohydrate	345 mg potassium

NUTRIENT CONTENT OF 3 OUNCES (85 GRAMS) BROILED, TRIMMED PORTERHOUSE STEAK

186 calories	6 mg calcium
24 g protein	181 mg phosphorus
9 g fat, 4 saturated	2.6 mg iron
68 mg cholesterol	56 mg sodium
0 g carbohydrate	346 mg potassium

NUTRIENT CONTENT OF 3 OUNCES (85 GRAMS) ROASTED, TRIMMED STANDING RIB

207 calories	9 mg calcium
23 g protein	181 mg phosphorus
12 g fat, 5 saturated	2.4 mg iron
68 mg cholesterol	61 mg sodium
0 g carbohydrate	318 mg potassium

NUTRIENT CONTENT OF 3 OUNCES (85 GRAMS) WELL-DONE BROILED LEAN HAMBURGER

225 calories	8 mg calcium
24 g protein	161 mg phosphorus
14 g fat, 5 saturated	2.4 mg iron
84 mg cholesterol	70 mg sodium
0 g carbohydrate	314 mg potassium

NUTRIENT CONTENT OF 3 OUNCES (85 GRAMS) SIMMERED BEEF TONGUE

240 calories	6 mg calcium
19 g protein	120 mg phosphorus
18 g fat, 8 saturated	2.9 mg iron
91 mg cholesterol	51 mg sodium
0 g carbohydrate	153 mg potassium

NUTRIENT CONTENT OF 3 OUNCES (85 GRAMS) SIMMERED BEEF HEART

149 calories	54 mg sodium
25 g protein	198 mg potassium
5 g fat, 1 saturated	0 g dietary fiber
164 mg cholesterol	317 RE vitamin A
0 g carbohydrate	0.16 mg thiamin
5 mg calcium	3.45 mg riboflavin
212 mg phosphorus	5.1 mg niacin
6.4 mg iron	1 mg vitamin C

NUTRIENT CONTENT OF 3 OUNCES (85 GRAMS) SIMMERED BEEF KIDNEY

122 calories	113 mg sodium
22 g protein	152 mg potassium
3 g fat, 1 saturated	0 g dietary fiber
328 mg cholesterol	317 RE vitamin A
1 g carbohydrate	0.16 mg thiamin
15 mg calcium	3.45 mg riboflavin
260 mg phosphorus	5.1 mg niacin
6.2 mg iron	1 mg vitamin C

NUTRIENT CONTENT OF 3 OUNCES (85 GRAMS) SAUTÉED CALF'S LIVER

208 calories	112 mg sodium
25 g protein	372 mg potassium
10 g fat, 4 saturated	0 g dietary fiber
280 mg cholesterol	4,784 RE vitamin A
3 g carbohydrate	0.21 mg thiamin
10 mg calcium	2.86 mg riboflavin
373 mg phosphorus	14.4 mg niacin
4.5 mg iron	18 mg vitamin C

Beefalo: Beef is fat and juicy, buffalo lean and mean. And beefalo? A crossbreed that's buffalo-lean but as succulent as beef. Only drawback: Beefalo is still a "boutique meat," not widely available and thus expensive.

NUTRIENT CONTENT OF 3 OUNCES (85 GRAMS) ROASTED BEEFALO

161 calories	70 mg sodium
26 g protein	390 mg potassium
5 g fat, 2 saturated	0 g dietary fiber
49 mg cholesterol	0 RE vitamin A
0 g carbohydrate	0.03 mg thiamin
20 mg calcium	0.09 mg riboflavin
213 mg phosphorus	4.2 mg niacin
2.6 mg iron	8 mg vitamin C

Beef Tea: A concentrated, nourishing beef broth made by simmering very lean beef (usually top round) in water several hours. The mixture is strained through cheesecloth and all solids discarded so that only essence of beef remains. In olden days, beef tea was given to new mothers and convalescents to build them up.

Bee Pollen: Athletes swear it pumps them up, this mixture of bee saliva, plant nectar and pollen. Scientists, on the other hand, say it bestows no known benefits on athletes and may actually cause severe allergic reactions in those sensitive to bee stings or to certain pollens. Proceed with caution.

Beer: Historians suspect that the world's first brewer was a careless Mesopotamian housewife who left bowls of bread outdoors in a cloudburst. Had she been more fastidious, had she pitched out the drenched loaves, who knows when man would have discovered the glories of beer? As it happens, the soggy mess was left under the downpouring sun to bubble and froth. Some intrepid soul thrust a cup into the suds, tasted them and pronounced them superb. And that, historians tell us, was the beginning of beer, which for centuries has unwearied the bones, raised the spirits, turned dullards into conversationalists and restored the sickly to health. From the Norman Conquest until the sixteenth century, England brewed its "national beverage" with barley, malt and spring water that had tumbled over rocks. No "poisonous" hops allowed—until the Germans proved there was nothing lethal about them and that they improved beer.

Beer was Everyman's beverage during America's infancy and adolescence. For good reason: It was safer than water and cheaper than wine. Still, brewing remained a cottage industry here until the turn of the nineteenth century when Germans settled in the Midwest and began mass-producing fine **lagers,** lighter beers with an alcoholic content of about 6 percent. Many of these old breweries are still going strong. But to keep up with the times, they've begun producing **light beers** with fewer calories and lower alcohol contents.

NUTRIENT CONTENT OF 12 FLUID OUNCES (356 GRAMS) LAGER BEER

145 calories	18 mg sodium
1 g protein	89 mg potassium
0 g fat, 0 saturated	2 g dietary fiber
0 mg cholesterol	0 RE vitamin A
13 g carbohydrate	0.02 mg thiamin
18 mg calcium	0.09 mg riboflavin
43 mg phosphorus	1.6 mg niacin
0.1 mg iron	0 mg vitamin C

NUTRIENT CONTENT OF 12 FLUID OUNCES (356 GRAMS) LIGHT BEER

99 calories	11 mg sodium
1 g protein	64 mg potassium
0 g fat, 0 saturated	1 g dietary fiber
0 mg cholesterol	0 RE vitamin A
5 g carbohydrate	0.03 mg thiamin
18 mg calcium	0.11 mg riboflavin
43 mg phosphorus	1.4 mg niacin
0.1 mg iron	0 mg vitamin C

Beeswax (additive): Extracted by melting the honeycomb, then sterilized, beeswax is used in the manufacture of chewing gum and candy as a flavoring, plasticizer and finisher. Considered safe when used within amounts approved by the FDA.

Beet Greens: This most nutritious part of the beet is what most people discard. If crisp and fresh, beet greens can be steamed in their own rinse water like spinach (even mixed half and half with spinach), then dressed with fruity olive oil, vinegar, salt and freshly ground pepper. When

Almost Fat-Free Chocolate-Beet Bundt Cake

Makes 16 Servings

Believe it or not, pureed beets substitute for butter in this dense dark cake. Before you scoff, try the recipe. It's good.

½ cup plus 2 tablespoons unsweetened Dutch-process cocoa powder

1½ cups sifted cake flour

1 cup sifted all-purpose flour

2 cups confectioners' sugar plus 2 teaspoons (optional) for dusting

1 cup firmly packed light brown sugar

2 teaspoons baking powder

½ teaspoon baking soda

¼ teaspoon salt

1 cup pureed cooked or canned beets (or baby food if you like)

1½ cups evaporated skim milk

2 tablespoons instant espresso powder

1 tablespoon vanilla extract

1 cup frozen fat-free egg product, thawed

PREHEAT OVEN TO 350°F. Coat a 9-inch (12-cup) Bundt pan with nonstick spray and dust with the 2 tablespoons cocoa, tapping out excess; set pan aside. Mix flours, sugars, the remaining ½ cup cocoa, baking powder, baking soda, and salt in a food processor fitted with the metal chopping blade for 10 seconds, then pulse quickly 2 to 3 times. Transfer to large mixing bowl and make well in center. Pulse beets, milk, espresso powder, and vanilla in processor 3 to 5 times; add egg product and pulse 2 to 3 times. Pour beet mixture into the well in dry ingredients and fold in gently. Batter should be lumpy. No matter if a few dry flecks show; they will vanish during baking. *Don't overmix or cake will be tough.* Pour batter into prepared pan and smooth top. Bake 50 to 55 minutes or until cake tester inserted midway between pan rim and tube comes out clean. Cool cake 20 minutes in upright pan on wire rack. Carefully loosen cake and invert on rack. Cool to room temperature, then dust, if desired, with confectioners' sugar. Cut into wedges with a sharp serrated knife.

APPROXIMATE NUTRIENT COUNTS PER SERVING
(with confectioners' sugar dusting)

204 calories	43 g carbohydrate	2.1 mg iron	0.17 mg thiamin
5 g protein	2 g dietary fiber	173 mg sodium	0.21 mg riboflavin
1 g fat, 0 saturated	139 mg calcium	278 mg potassium	1.3 mg niacin
1 mg cholesterol	160 mg phosphorus	43 RE vitamin A	1 mg vitamin C

young and tender, they can be tossed into a green salad. **SEASON:** May through October.

NUTRIENT CONTENT OF 1 CUP BOILED BEET GREENS	
(about 5 ounces; 144 grams)	
39 calories	18 mg sodium
4 g protein	89 mg potassium
0 g fat, 0 saturated	3 g dietary fiber
0 mg cholesterol	734 RE vitamin A
8 g carbohydrate	0.17 mg thiamin
18 mg calcium	0.42 mg riboflavin
59 mg phosphorus	0.7 mg niacin
0.1 mg iron	36 mg vitamin C

Beets: Historians trace beets to Italy and a chardlike plant. In the beginning (and up through the Roman Empire), beet greens were prized and the roots tossed. By the time of Charlemagne, who ordered beets planted in his domains, both tops and bottoms were appreciated. These early beets were most likely white or orange. Not until the sixteenth or seventeenth century were red beets introduced, but it was years before Everyman considered them safe to eat. Now things have come full circle. The buzz among gardeners and chefs is designer beets—the white, and, yes, the orange. Unlike red beets, they do not bleed when boiled. Correctly cooked, however, red beets bleed very little. The trick is to leave the skin and root end on, also an inch of the tops. The pigment in red beets is a litmuslike indicator. In the presence of acid, it turns crimson (which is why Harvard beets contain vinegar). But with an alkali, it turns blue. Though a little higher in sodium than other vegetables, beets are a good source of iron, dietary fiber and potassium. **SEASON:** Spring through fall although certain beets, the keepers, winter over fairly well in cold storage.

NUTRIENT CONTENT OF 1 CUP DICED BOILED BEETS	
(about 6 ounces; 170 grams)	
75 calories	131 mg sodium
3 g protein	518 mg potassium
0 g fat, 0 saturated	4 g dietary fiber
0 mg cholesterol	7 RE vitamin A
17 g carbohydrate	0.05 mg thiamin
27 mg calcium	0.07 mg riboflavin
65 mg phosphorus	0.6 mg niacin
1.3 mg iron	6 mg vitamin C

Behavior Modification: Psychologists believe that by controlling the environment and thus the factors that trigger behavior, behavior itself can be changed or modified. The technique works, in tandem with exercise and carefully regulated meals, in helping dieters lose weight, then keep the pounds off.

Belgian Endive: **Witloof** the Belgians call this chunky, tightly sheathed stalked chicory. This particular species, *Cichorium intybus,* originated somewhere in Middle Europe but the Belgians have made it their own by growing the stalks in trenches mounded with fine soil so the sun never touches—and greens—them. When dug, the endive emerges as pale and pearly as white asparagus. Much of the Belgian endive imported into this country is shipped directly from Flanders fields. Its flavor is slightly bitter, its texture crisply succulent, a welcome contrast to blander, more buttery greens. It does lack the vitamins A (beta-carotene) and C of *greener* greens, however. Most of us prefer endives sliced raw into salads or used as a low-cal dipper for fancy cocktail spreads, but Europeans like the stalks halved and braised in broth. The bitter roots of this chicory are what Creoles roast and mix with their coffee. **SEASON:** Year-round, with supplies peaking between September and May.

NUTRIENT CONTENT OF 1 MEDIUM-SIZE RAW BELGIAN ENDIVE	
(about 1¾ ounces; 53 grams)	
8 calories	4 mg sodium
1 g protein	96 mg potassium
0 g fat, 0 saturated	1 g dietary fiber
0 mg cholesterol	0 RE vitamin A
2 g carbohydrate	0.04 mg thiamin
NA mg calcium	0.07 mg riboflavin
11 mg phosphorus	0.3 mg niacin
0.3 mg iron	5 mg vitamin C

Bell Peppers: See SWEET PEPPERS under PEPPERS, CAPSICUMS.

Bel Paese: This soft, quick-ripening, uncooked Italian cheese takes its name from *Il Bel Paese (The Beautiful Country),* a nineteenth-century Italian travelogue written by Father Antonio Stoppani. Made from whole cow's milk, Bel Paese often shows up on American hors d'oeuvre and dessert-cheese platters. There are American knockoffs, but they pale beside the Italian original made near Lake Como. **NOTE:** Specific nutrient counts unavailable.

Benzene: A highly toxic organic solvent used in the manufacture of chemicals, paints and plastics that has contaminated drinking water near some of the industrial plants where it's used. Benzene is carcinogenic and, because it's highly volatile, it endangers not only those who drink benzene-contaminated water but also those who shower with it. The EPA maintains a hot line (1-800-426-4791; in Alaska and the District of Columbia, 202-382-5533) manned by specialists who can answer questions about drinking water safety. It also publishes a free pamphlet, *Is Your Drinking Water Safe?*, which can be ordered through the hot line.

Benzocaine (additive): This local anesthetic, added to diet candies and chewing gums, is said to numb the palate. The idea is to kill the appetite and make food less appealing—i.e., the food you don't eat can't make you fat. The truth? There's no proof benzocaine works.

Benzoic Acid (additive): The harmless compound left in flour after it's bleached with benzoyl peroxide. GRAS. See also SODIUM BENZOATE.

Benzopyrene: One of the carcinogenic compounds that not only exist naturally in food but also are created by cooking or processing. See PAHS.

Benzoyl Peroxide (additive): A white powder used to bleach flour and whiten certain cheeses. It quickly breaks down into benzoic acid, which is harmless. GRAS.

Beriberi: Acute thiamin (vitamin B_1) deficiency causes this debilitating, often fatal nerve disease. See B_1, VITAMIN.

Beta-carotene (provitamin; additive): A pigment in rose-yellow fruits and vegetables and a precursor of vitamin A (see A, VITAMIN). Beta-carotene not only occurs widely in nature (it's the orange of carrots, yams, winter squash, papayas, mangoes, etc.) but is also used by food processors. Increasing beta-carotene in the diet is now believed to re-

duce the risk of certain types of cancer and, perhaps, heart disease as well by minimizing arterial damage. However, heavy drinkers should know that alcohol makes beta-carotene toxic to the liver. GRAS. See also CAROTENE, CAROTENOIDS.

BHA (Butylated Hydroxyanisole), BHT (Butylated Hydroxytoluene) (additives): Similar chemical compounds used not only to prolong shelf life of food containing fat or oil but also added to breakfast cereals (they contain small amounts of fat), enriched rice, chewing gum and many convenience foods. Though "Generally Recognized as Safe" by the FDA, both BHA and BHT are increasingly controversial and there is pressure from consumer watchdogs for further testing. And yet . . . and yet . . . Dr. Andrew Dannenberg of Cornell Medical College recently demonstrated that these two additives may actually reduce the risk of cancer in much the same way that cruciferous vegetables (broccoli, brussels sprouts, cauliflower, etc.) do. His studies with lab animals show that both BHA and BHT energize a gene that helps zap carcinogens before they can cause tumors. There's even early evidence that BHA and BHT act similarly in human beings. A promising development, to be sure, but studies continue. See also PHENOLIC COMPOUNDS.

Bibb Lettuce: See SALAD GREENS.

Biceps Skinfold Measurement: See SKINFOLD TESTS.

Bifidobacteria: Occurring naturally in breast milk, this "good" bug helps prevent diarrhea in infants. And now, according to tests conducted recently at Johns Hopkins Children's Center, adding it to infant formulas along with *Streptococcus thermophilus* (a popular yogurt culture) may reduce the risk of infant diarrhea as well—by nearly 80 percent. To promote intestinal health, the Japanese routinely add *Bifocbacteri bifidum* to yogurts. And it's beginning to be used in dairy products here, too.

Bile, Bile Salts: The liver manufactures bile and stores it in the gallbladder, the muscular sac that lies alongside it. Here bile is concentrated and readied for its job in digesting fat. When the stomach releases fat into the duodenum and pancreatic enzymes have reduced it to fatty acids and glycerol, the gallbladder sends its bitter green bile along to perform the next step. Bile salts attack the fatty acids and glycerol, unusable in their present form, and rework them until they're water soluble and easily absorbed by the small intestine. Once absorbed, they're relinked as triglycerides, then repackaged as water-soluble lipoproteins and sent into the blood. Usually this digestive process moves smoothly. But if the cholesterol present in bile should harden into stones, and if these should get wedged in the bile duct linking gallbladder and duodenum, the stones will have to be dissolved by drugs or ultrasound treatment or be removed by a surgeon.

Bioelectrical Impedance: A zip-quick way to estimate percentage of total body fat. It works like this: A low-energy electric current is sent through the body. The fatter the person, the greater the impedance, or resistance to the current, and the more slowly it travels. The rate of speed is recorded, then translated into percentage of body fat.

Bioflavonoids, Bioflavins: Though sometimes touted as vitamin P, these are not true vitamins. Indeed, there's no clinical evidence that humans need bioflavonoids although some researchers suspect they may promote the absorption of vitamin C. They are found mostly in citrus pulp. See also PHYTOCHEMICALS.

Biological Value of Protein: Nothing more than a way to rate the efficiency with which protein foods deliver essential AMINO ACIDS to the body in the proper proportions and amounts. The more efficiently a protein supplies body tissues with what they need for growth, repair and maintenance, the higher its biological value (BV). Egg white protein, with a BV of 100, is the standard against which all other proteins are gauged. Milk has a BV of 93, rice 86 and beef only 75. That's a surprise.

Biotechnology: Red ripe winter tomatoes that taste like summer's best . . . fat-free steaks . . . pesticide-, herbicide-free farming . . . cow's milk that approaches mother's milk in nutritive value. The wave of the future? *Near* future is more like it because biotechnicians are already on-line at top U.S. universities. What, exactly, is biotechnology? Genetic engineering, yes. Cloning, yes. But the best definition is broader: Biotechnology is the use of plants, animals, microbes—or any portions thereof—to create useful products. Despite boycotts by antibiotech activists who fear dangerous allergens, organisms and pesticides may be transferred to the engineered foods, biotechnology promises to revolutionize farming, food processing, medicine. To provide cleaner fuels, make agrochemicals obsolete and clean up the environment. See also BOVINE SOMATOTROPIN and discussion of the new Flavr Savr tomato under TOMATOES, FRESH.

Biotin (vitamin): This sulfurous, water-soluble member of the B-complex is not only widely distributed in food but also manufactured in the lower digestive tract by bacteria. Biotin plays a key role in the body's metabolism of fats, carbohydrates and proteins. **DEFICIENCY SYMPTOMS:** Depression, dermatitis, hair loss, inflamed tongue, gray pallor, loss of appetite, nausea, vomiting. Deficiencies are almost unknown in the United States. **GOOD SOURCES:** Egg yolks, meats, liver, milk, nuts, legumes, cauliflower, whole grains, brewer's yeast and—hooray!—peanut butter and chocolate. **PRECAUTIONS:** Raw egg white contains a protein—AVIDIN—that bonds with biotin, forming a compound the body cannot assimilate. Avidin is destroyed, however, when the egg white is cooked. Being water soluble, biotin is apt to dissolve in the cooking water. Although there are no known ill effects from biotin overdose, moderation is the best policy.

ESTIMATED SAFE AND ADEQUATE DAILY DIETARY INTAKE OF BIOTIN (ESADDI)*	
Babies	10 to 15 mcg per day
Children (1 to 10 years)	20 to 30 mcg per day
11 years up	30 to 100 mcg per day

*Because the RDA committee had insufficient information upon which to base a specific allowance for biotin, it suggested a range of intake.

Biscuits: "Hot'ns" Southerners called these quick breads because they should be served hissing hot, split immediately, then sandwiched back together with a nubbin of sweet butter. Hardly what the doctor ordered. Unfortunately, biscuits owe their flakiness to a high percentage of shortening, which zooms their fat and calorie content toward the danger zone.

NUTRIENT CONTENT OF 1 SMALL BISCUIT
(about 1 ounce; 28 grams)

101 calories	165 mg sodium
2 g protein	34 mg potassium
5 g fat, 1 saturated	0 g dietary fiber
1 mg cholesterol	7 RE vitamin A
13 g carbohydrate	0.10 mg thiamin
67 mg calcium	0.09 mg riboflavin
47 mg phosphorus	0.8 mg niacin
0.8 mg iron	0 mg vitamin C

Bisulfites (additives): See SULFITES.

Bitter Almonds: Because they contain an unstable glucoside (carbohydrate derivative) that breaks down into prussic acid, bitter almonds are poisonous and illegal in the United States. However, oil of bitter almond, which contains no prussic acid, is a popular flavoring throughout Mediterranean Europe.

Black Beans: See BEANS, DRIED.

Blackberries: Members of the rose family, blackberries (or **brambles**) may be indigenous to Asia. Today, however, no fruit is more American. Blackberries grow wild over much of the continent and are a particular treat down South where children happily dodge the thorns in their haste to fill their pails. And cooks stir these black beauties into pies, crisps, cobblers, cordials, jams and jellies.
SEASON: Summer. See also DEWBERRIES.

NUTRIENT CONTENT OF 1 CUP BLACKBERRIES
(about 5½ ounces; 165 grams)

75 calories	0 mg sodium
1 g protein	282 mg potassium
1 g fat, 0 saturated	7 g dietary fiber
0 mg cholesterol	23 RE vitamin A
18 g carbohydrate	0.04 mg thiamin
46 mg calcium	0.06 mg riboflavin
30 mg phosphorus	0.6 mg niacin
0.8 mg iron	30 mg vitamin C

Black-eyed Peas: See BEANS, DRIED; BEANS, FRESH.

Blackstrap Molasses: See MOLASSES.

Blanching: See PARBOILING, BLANCHING.

Bland Diet: The old way to treat ulcers was to put patients on pap (any soft, semiliquid food), bland, boring purees, milk, cream, cottage cheese, custard, rice, crackers and so forth, which set easy in the stomach and allowed lesions to heal. The latest dietary theory is to let ulcer patients eat anything that doesn't cause problems but urge them to avoid foods that do (coffee, both caffeinated and decaffeinated, and caffeinated soft drinks, for example), also to eat three well-balanced meals a day but no before-bed snacks. These start gastric juices churning and cause searing acid reflux, the backing up of partially digested food into the esophagus.

Bleaching Agents (additives): These chemicals are used almost exclusively to whiten flour. One of the safest and most widely used today is BENZOYL PEROXIDE. Since its introduction in 1917, benzoyl peroxide has been extensively tested on laboratory animals and found to be harmless. Its main drawback: It destroys vitamin E, but there's little of that in flour anyway. A second popular bleaching agent, ACETONE PEROXIDE, merits further testing.

Blintzes: Sweet or savory filled thin pancakes that have gone so mainstream they're available in supermarket frozen-food bins. Traditionally, blintzes are made with flour and stuffed with lightly sweetened cottage cheese. But the supermarket variety is likely to be fruit filled.

NUTRIENT CONTENT OF 1 FRUIT-FILLED BLINTZ
(about 2½ ounces; 70 grams)

124 calories	152 mg sodium
4 g protein	75 mg potassium
5 g fat, 2 saturated	0 g dietary fiber
50 mg cholesterol	79 RE vitamin A
17 g carbohydrate	0.04 mg thiamin
33 mg calcium	0.12 mg riboflavin
54 mg phosphorus	0.3 mg niacin
0.8 mg iron	7 mg vitamin C

Bloating: See EDEMA; FLATULENCE.

Blood: Quite literally the body's lifeline, the fluid that distributes nutrients and oxygen to tissues where they're needed, disposes of carbon dioxide and routes waste to excretory organs for elimination. For the body, blood is an important line of defense against disease and performs myriad other functions.

Blood Pressure: As blood circulates, it presses against the walls of blood vessels. Because the heart contracts, then rests, then pumps and rests again—ad infinitum—physicians take both the **pumping** (systolic) blood pressure and the **resting** (diastolic). A normal reading is 120 (systolic) over 80 (diastolic), usually written 120/80. But blood pressure varies widely from person to person. Age, weight, health, emotion, exercise and occupation all affect blood pressure. Fat people are prone to high blood pressure (hypertension) as are those with kidney or cardiovascular disease. To bring blood pressure down, diuretics may be prescribed and salt (sodium) intake may be restricted to 1,000 to 2,000 milligrams a day. Further, patients are told to cut down on alcohol and coffee and, if obese, ordered to lose weight.

Blood Sausage: These dark, rich, chunky links (called **blood pudding** by the British) are made of hog's blood and studded with cubes of pork fat—hardly diet food. Most are fully cooked and some of the German ones are smoked.

NUTRIENT CONTENT FOR 1 SLICE BLOOD SAUSAGE	
(about 1 ounce; 25 grams)	
95 calories	170 mg sodium
4 g protein	10 mg potassium
9 g fat, 3 saturated	0 g dietary fiber
30 mg cholesterol	0 RE vitamin A
0 g carbohydrate	0.02 mg thiamin
2 mg calcium	0.03 mg riboflavin
6 mg phosphorus	0.3 mg niacin
1.6 mg iron	0 mg vitamin C

Blood Sugar: Sugar (glucose) fuels the body, but too little or too much of it in the blood is dangerous. The normal blood sugar level: 70 to 100 milligrams per 100 milliliters of blood. Healthy bodies keep the level fairly constant. But certain conditions dramatically raise blood sugar levels, among them diabetes; overactive pituitary, thyroid or adrenal cortex; inadequate insulin production; head injury; and multiple trauma. Other conditions lower blood sugar levels: underactive pituitary, thyroid or adrenal cortex; excess insulin; prolonged malnutrition (including that caused by ANOREXIA NERVOSA); pancreatic tumors; and improper kidney function. High-fiber diets help moderate blood glucose levels. Indeed, persons with diabetes given high-fiber diets have been able to reduce their dosage of insulin and, in some cases of non-insulin-dependent DIABETES, to eliminate it altogether.

Blueberries: These all-American berries are related to both heather and the wild huckleberry. They grow particularly well in the Northeast and are big business in the state of Maine. Though the blueberry season is short, commercially frozen unsweetened blueberries (a dandy substitute for the fresh) stretches it to twelve months. Blueberries are one of the more versatile berries, taking to cakes, shortcakes, pies, crisps, cobblers, preserves and waffle syrups with equal grace. They are low in calories and sodium but supply respectable (if not awesome) amounts of potassium, dietary fiber and vitamin C. **SEASON:** May through September.

NUTRIENT CONTENT OF 1 CUP BLUEBERRIES	
(about 5 ounces; 145 grams)	
81 calories	9 mg sodium
1 g protein	129 mg potassium
1 g fat, 0 saturated	3 g dietary fiber
0 mg cholesterol	15 RE vitamin A
20 g carbohydrate	0.07 mg thiamin
9 mg calcium	0.07 mg riboflavin
15 mg phosphorus	0.5 mg niacin
0.2 mg iron	19 mg vitamin C

Blue Cheese: The best American blue is **Maytag,** produced in Iowa by the family of washing machine fame. Made from the milk of Holstein-Friesian cows, this richly veined cheese is creamy and pleasantly biting. Ironically, the sharper, saltier imported **Danish blue** is better known in this country. See also GORGONZOLA; ROQUEFORT; STILTON.

NUTRIENT CONTENT OF 1 OUNCE (28 GRAMS) BLUE CHEESE	
100 calories	395 mg sodium
6 g protein	73 mg potassium
8 g fat, 5 saturated	0 g dietary fiber
21 mg cholesterol	65 RE vitamin A
1 g carbohydrate	0.01 mg thiamin
149 mg calcium	0.11 mg riboflavin
110 mg phosphorus	0.3 mg niacin
0.1 mg iron	0 mg vitamin C

NUTRIENT CONTENT OF 1 BOILED BOCKWURST (about 2¼ ounces; 65 grams)	
200 calories	718 mg sodium
9 g protein	176 mg potassium
18 g fat, 7 saturated	0 g dietary fiber
38 mg cholesterol	4 RE vitamin A
0 g carbohydrate	0.27 mg thiamin
10 mg calcium	0.11 mg riboflavin
95 mg phosphorus	2.7 mg niacin
0.4 mg iron	0 mg vitamin C

Bluefish: When the call goes out that the blues are running, fishermen along the Atlantic from Cape Cod to Florida dash to the sea. The fun is not only in bringing in these scrappy fish but also in eating them. Averaging 5 to 20 pounds, darkish and buttery of flesh, fresh-caught bluefish are supremely sweet and tender. Their natural oils are evenly distributed in their flesh, not concentrated in the liver—the case with cod and other lean fish. For that reason, bluefish are best cooked simply—with a minimum of fat. Experienced cooks broil or bake them.

NUTRIENT CONTENT OF 3 OUNCES (85 GRAMS) BROILED BLUEFISH FILLET	
135 calories	66 mg sodium
22 g protein	406 mg potassium
5 g fat, 1 saturated	0 g dietary fiber
65 mg cholesterol	117 RE vitamin A
0 g carbohydrate	0.06 mg thiamin
8 mg calcium	0.08 mg riboflavin
247 mg phosphorus	6.2 mg niacin
0.5 mg iron	0 mg vitamin C

Bockwurst: Short and chunky, this delicately seasoned frankfurterlike German sausage was originally served only in spring at bock-beer time. Today American meat packers mass-produce bockwurst right around the calendar. Like most sausages, bockwursts aren't very nutritious. Just look at their fat, saturated fat and sodium content.

Body Mass Index (BMI): Also called **Quetelet Index**, this is the body's weight (in kilos) divided by the square of its height (in meters). Ideal body weight for men and women is a BMI of 20 to 25 (BMIs below 18.5 suggest PROTEIN-CALORIE MALNUTRITION; the lower the number, the worse the condition and the greater the need for medical help). Adults with a BMI of 30 or more are classified as obese and are at increased risk for hypertension, coronary artery disease, certain types of cancer and non-insulin-dependent diabetes. Physicians usually advise their obese patients to lose weight—slowly—and begin a regular program of exercise.

Boiling: The good news: Boiling is a moist, low-fat method of cooking. The bad news: Water-soluble minerals and vitamins (C and most of the B-complex) leach out in the cooking water and are lost unless the cooking water is somehow recycled. The best preventive: Using as little water as possible, boil vegetables whole, in their skins, only until crisp-tender. As for meats and poultry, boiling melts the fat, which rises to the top of the broth and can be neatly skimmed off.

Bok Choy: See CHINESE CABBAGE.

Bologna: A highly fatty, highly processed pork-and-beef cold cut inspired by a Bolognese sausage. The sodium content soars off the charts, too.

NUTRIENT CONTENT OF 2 SLICES BOLOGNA

(about 2 ounces; 57 grams)

179 calories	578 mg sodium
7 g protein	102 mg potassium
16 g fat, 6 saturated	0 g dietary fiber
31 mg cholesterol	0 RE vitamin A
2 g carbohydrate	0.10 mg thiamin
7 mg calcium	0.08 mg riboflavin
52 mg phosphorus	1.5 mg niacin
0.9 mg iron	12 mg vitamin C

Bone Meal (nutrient supplement): Powdered bone taken to boost the amount of calcium and other bone minerals in the body. Ten years ago, many bone meals were contaminated with enough lead to be hazardous to your health. Then the FDA cracked down, limiting amounts of lead for bone-meal calcium supplements to 5 parts per million. The *United States Pharmacopeia* (which sets guidelines for the pharmaceutical industry) adopted even stricter limits—3 parts per million. Recent government testing of bone-meal supplements has shown drastic lead-level drops—to about that of other calcium supplements.

Borage-Seed Oil: Although a six-month study conducted at the University of Pennsylvania suggests that oral doses of borage-seed oil can significantly ease the pain and swelling of rheumatoid arthritis with minimal side effects, researchers insist further studies are needed and caution against indiscriminate use of over-the-counter borage-seed-oil supplements.

Boron: A trace mineral identified as a growth factor only in 1982. Boron reduces calcium loss in postmenopausal women and may help prevent osteoporosis. Some researchers believe it essential enough to warrant RDAs. Peanuts, prunes, dates, raisins, honey and wine are good sources.

Boston Lettuce: See SALAD GREENS.

Botulism: See CLOSTRIDIUM BOTULINUM under BACTERIA.

Bouillon, Broth: Moderate-protein, low-fat, low-calorie beverages made from meat (usually beef), poultry and/or vegetables. Fortified with a dice of vegetables, dumplings, noodles, even slivered pancakes (a German favorite), these make light main courses. Served cold in their pristine form, they're nutritious soft-drink substitutes. Choose low-sodium varieties.

NUTRIENT CONTENT OF 1 CUP CANNED CONDENSED BEEF BOUILLON/BROTH (MIXED AS DIRECTED WITH WATER)

(8 fluid ounces; 240 grams)

17 calories	782 mg sodium
3 g protein	129 mg potassium
1 g fat, 0 saturated	0 g dietary fiber
0 mg cholesterol	0 RE vitamin A
0 g carbohydrate	0.01 mg thiamin
14 mg calcium	0.05 mg riboflavin
31 mg phosphorus	1.9 mg niacin
0.4 mg iron	0 mg vitamin C

NUTRIENT CONTENT OF 1 CUP CANNED CONDENSED CHICKEN BOUILLON/BROTH (MIXED AS DIRECTED WITH WATER)

(8 fluid ounces; 244 grams)

39 calories	776 mg sodium
5 g protein	209 mg potassium
1 g fat, 0 saturated	0 g dietary fiber
0 mg cholesterol	0 RE vitamin A
1 g carbohydrate	0.01 mg thiamin
10 mg calcium	0.07 mg riboflavin
73 mg phosphorus	3.3 mg niacin
0.5 mg iron	0 mg vitamin C

Bourbon: This American whiskey is distilled from a mash that's 51 percent corn. Sour mash is a bourbon made using starters from the previous batch. For calorie counts, see ALCOHOL, ALCOHOLIC BEVERAGES.

Boursin: An herbed and garlicked brand-name triple-crème French cheese as smooth and white as cream cheese, but with considerably more character. Little boxes of Boursin, staples at every American supermarket, are de rigueur on many an hors d'oeuvre tray. Go easy—this stuff is 43 percent butterfat. **NOTE:** Specific nutrient counts unavailable.

Bovine Somatotropin (BST), Bovine Growth Hormone (BGH): Whichever name you use, this new biotech hormone, which increases milk production in dairy herds, is hotly disputed even though the FDA now allows its use and doesn't require dairies to tell consumers whether or not their milk comes from BST-treated cows. Cows produce BST naturally, but scientists, who've learned to synthesize it in the lab, have discovered that when injected into cows, it boosts milk production by as much as 25 percent. Not surprisingly, many dairymen, excited by the prospects, rushed to take part in FDA BST-testing procedures. One worry, voiced by a dairy-state senator, was that increased milk production at the superdairies would drive milk prices so low small farmers would be hurt, perhaps irreparably. For similar reasons, the European Community has proposed a seven-year ban on BST use by its member countries.

Boysenberries: Blackberry-raspberry hybrids named for the man who developed them in 1923—Rudolph Boysen. Though a bit mellower than blackberries, boysenberries are low in calories and contain no sodium at all. A good choice for dieters. **SEASON:** Summer.

NUTRIENT CONTENT OF 1 CUP BOYSENBERRIES
(about 5 ounces; 144 grams)

75 calories	0 mg sodium
1 g protein	282 mg potassium
1 g fat, 0 saturated	7 g dietary fiber
0 mg cholesterol	23 RE vitamin A
18 g carbohydrate	0.04 mg thiamin
46 mg calcium	0.06 mg riboflavin
30 mg phosphorus	0.6 mg niacin
0.8 mg iron	30 mg vitamin C

Bracken Fern: See FIDDLEHEAD FERNS.

Brains: Except for liver and kidneys, Americans are squeamish about eating animal organs. Brains scrambled with eggs were once popular breakfast fare down South. And French chefs now working here often prepare brains in black butter. Still, brains are rarely eaten elsewhere.

Beef, pork, veal and lamb brains are all available, the last two being choicest. Unfortunately, brains are fairly high in fat and loaded with cholesterol.

NUTRIENT CONTENT OF 2 OUNCES (57 GRAMS) BRAISED LAMB BRAINS

82 calories	76 mg sodium
7 g protein	116 mg potassium
6 g fat, 1 saturated	0 g dietary fiber
1,158 mg cholesterol	0 RE vitamin A
0 g carbohydrate	0.06 mg thiamin
7 mg calcium	0.14 mg riboflavin
191 mg phosphorus	1.4 mg niacin
1.0 mg iron	7 mg vitamin C

Braising: To braise is to brown a sinewy cut of meat or a tough old bird in a small amount of fat, then to add liquid, cover and simmer slowly until tender. Braising's only drawback: The rich brown pan gravy is often full of fat. No problem; skim it off.

Bran: The fiber-rich husk of seeds and grains. For a while, oat bran was touted as a miracle food, a sort of Roto-Rooter that could cleanse veins of cholesterol. Predictably, food manufacturers rushed to pump their breads and cereals full of oat bran. In truth, oat bran is no more effective at lowering cholesterol than several other brans—or, for that matter, other high-fiber foods. And the results are not as miraculous as claimed. Fiber is, however, definitely beneficial because it keeps the gastrointestinal tract in good working order (it also contains no calories). Some researchers believe insoluble fiber (the kind in wheat bran and many vegetables) may reduce the risk of colon cancer. Certainly, eating high-fiber foods helps dieters, if for no other reason than that they *feel* full. On the downside, too much fiber can cause diarrhea and, for some, more serious digestive problems. Fiber also blocks the body's ability to absorb calcium, a fact those bulking up on fiber should note.

Brandy: An alcoholic liquor distilled from wine or fermented fruit juices. The finest brandies are **Cognac** and **Armagnac**. For calorie counts, see ALCOHOL, ALCOHOLIC BEVERAGES.

BRAT Diet: When preschool children suffer from diarrhea, they're sometimes put on a banana, rice, applesauce (unsweetened) and toast diet, acronym BRAT. Being nutritionally incomplete, it shouldn't be used for more than two or three days.

Bratwurst: This coarsely textured pork sausage, aromatic of caraway, marjoram and nutmeg, should be browned before it's served. That's the German way.

NUTRIENT CONTENT OF 1 COOKED BRATWURST	
(about 3 ounces; 85 grams)	
256 calories	473 mg sodium
12 g protein	180 mg potassium
22 g fat, 8 saturated	0 g dietary fiber
51 mg cholesterol	0 RE vitamin A
2 g carbohydrate	0.43 mg thiamin
37 mg calcium	0.16 mg riboflavin
127 mg phosphorus	2.7 mg niacin
1.1 mg iron	1 mg vitamin C

Braunschweiger: See LIVERWURST.

Brazil Nuts: The seeds of an immense South American jungle tree, these large, brown-skinned, ivory-hued nuts are about 65 percent oil and 20 percent protein by weight. In Brazil, Brazil-nut oil is used for cooking.

NUTRIENT CONTENT OF 1 OUNCE (28 GRAMS) UNSALTED BRAZIL NUTS	
186 calories	1 mg sodium
4 g protein	170 mg potassium
19 g fat, 5 saturated	3 g dietary fiber
0 mg cholesterol	0 RE vitamin A
4 g carbohydrate	0.28 mg thiamin
50 mg calcium	0.04 mg riboflavin
170 mg phosphorus	0.5 mg niacin
1.0 mg iron	0 mg vitamin C

Bread: Germans and Scandinavians prefer rye breads; the French, Italians and most other Europeans, crusty, jaw-busting white or whole-wheat loaves. Until recently, Americans doted on white bread. And the squishier the

better. But boutique bakers have arrived, filling local shops and greenmarkets with cracked-wheat loaves, oatmeal, rye, mixed grain, sourdough, you name it. Even big industrial bakers are turning out a variety of whole-grain loaves and using harder wheats in their white bread to approximate the chewiness of Europe's best. **NOTE:** One slice of bread yields ½ cup soft crumbs, so it's easy to calculate the nutrient content of bread crumbs using the tables below. See also PITA BREAD; PUMPERNICKEL; RYE BREAD.

NUTRIENT CONTENT OF 1 SLICE CRACKED-WHEAT BREAD	
(about ⅞ ounce; 25 grams)	
65 calories	135 mg sodium
2 g protein	44 mg potassium
1 g fat, 0 saturated	1 g dietary fiber
0 mg cholesterol	0 RE vitamin A
12 g carbohydrate	0.09 mg thiamin
11 mg calcium	0.06 mg riboflavin
38 mg phosphorus	0.9 mg niacin
0.7 mg iron	0 mg vitamin C

NUTRIENT CONTENT OF 1 SLICE WHOLE-WHEAT BREAD	
(about 1¼ ounces; 35 grams)	
86 calories	184 mg sodium
3 g protein	88 mg potassium
1 g fat, 0 saturated	2 g dietary fiber
0 mg cholesterol	0 RE vitamin A
16 g carbohydrate	0.12 mg thiamin
25 mg calcium	0.07 mg riboflavin
80 mg phosphorus	1.3 mg niacin
1.2 mg iron	0 mg vitamin C

NUTRIENT CONTENT OF 1 SLICE FIRM WHITE BREAD	
(about 1¼ ounces; 33 grams)	
91 calories	163 mg sodium
3 g protein	40 mg potassium
1 g fat, 0 saturated	1 g dietary fiber
1 mg cholesterol	4 RE vitamin A
17 g carbohydrate	0.13 mg thiamin
32 mg calcium	0.08 mg riboflavin
34 mg phosphorus	1.1 mg niacin
0.9 mg iron	0 mg vitamin C

NUTRIENT CONTENT OF 1 SLICE SOFT WHITE BREAD

(about 1 ounce; 28 grams)

76 calories	143 mg sodium
2 g protein	30 mg potassium
1 g fat, 0 saturated	1 g dietary fiber
1 mg cholesterol	0 RE vitamin A
14 g carbohydrate	0.11 mg thiamin
24 mg calcium	0.07 mg riboflavin
28 mg phosphorus	0.9 mg niacin
0.8 mg iron	0 mg vitamin C

NUTRIENT CONTENT OF 1 SLICE OATMEAL BREAD

(about 7/8 ounce; 25 grams)

67 calories	150 mg sodium
2 g protein	36 mg potassium
1 g fat, 0 saturated	1 g dietary fiber
0 mg cholesterol	1 RE vitamin A
12 g carbohydrate	0.10 mg thiamin
17 mg calcium	0.06 mg riboflavin
32 mg phosphorus	0.8 mg niacin
0.7 mg iron	0 mg vitamin C

NUTRIENT CONTENT OF 1 SLICE FRENCH BREAD

(about 1 1/4 ounces; 35 grams)

96 calories	213 mg sodium
3 g protein	40 mg potassium
1 g fat, 0 saturated	1 g dietary fiber
0 mg cholesterol	0 RE vitamin A
18 g carbohydrate	0.18 mg thiamin
26 mg calcium	0.12 mg riboflavin
37 mg phosphorus	1.7 mg niacin
0.9 mg iron	0 mg vitamin C

NUTRIENT CONTENT OF 1 SLICE RAISIN BREAD

(about 7/8 ounce; 25 grams)

69 calories	98 mg sodium
2 g protein	57 mg potassium
1 g fat, 0 saturated	1 g dietary fiber
0 mg cholesterol	0 RE vitamin A
13 g carbohydrate	0.09 mg thiamin
17 mg calcium	0.10 mg riboflavin
27 mg phosphorus	0.9 mg niacin
0.7 mg iron	0 mg vitamin C

NUTRIENT CONTENT OF 1 SLICE ITALIAN BREAD

(about 1 ounce; 30 grams)

81 calories	175 mg sodium
3 g protein	33 mg potassium
1 g fat, 0 saturated	1 g dietary fiber
0 mg cholesterol	0 RE vitamin A
15 g carbohydrate	0.14 mg thiamin
23 mg calcium	0.09 mg riboflavin
31 mg phosphorus	1.3 mg niacin
0.9 mg iron	0 mg vitamin C

NUTRIENT CONTENT OF 1 SALTED BREADSTICK

(about 1 1/4 ounces; 35 grams)

135 calories	586 mg sodium
4 g protein	32 mg potassium
1 g fat, 0 saturated	1 g dietary fiber
1 mg cholesterol	0 RE vitamin A
26 g carbohydrate	0.23 mg thiamin
10 mg calcium	0.18 mg riboflavin
35 mg phosphorus	2.3 mg niacin
1.5 mg iron	0 mg vitamin C

NUTRIENT CONTENT OF 1 SLICE SOURDOUGH BREAD

(about 7/8 ounce; 25 grams)

69 calories	152 mg sodium
2 g protein	28 mg potassium
1 g fat, 0 saturated	1 g dietary fiber
0 mg cholesterol	0 RE vitamin A
13 g carbohydrate	0.13 mg thiamin
19 mg calcium	0.08 mg riboflavin
26 mg phosphorus	1.2 mg niacin
0.6 mg iron	0 mg vitamin C

NUTRIENT CONTENT OF 1 UNSALTED BREADSTICK

(about 1/3 ounce; 10 grams)

38 calories	70 mg sodium
1 g protein	9 mg potassium
0 g fat, 0 saturated	0 g dietary fiber
0 mg cholesterol	0 RE vitamin A
8 g carbohydrate	0.07 mg thiamin
3 mg calcium	0.05 mg riboflavin
10 mg phosphorus	0.6 mg niacin
0.4 mg iron	0 mg vitamin C

Breakfast: The most important meal of the day because it literally breaks the overnight fast. What exactly is a good breakfast? The menu might include fruit or fruit juice; protein (cereal with milk, egg, a low-fat meat, peanut butter or cottage cheese); a complex carbohydrate (cereal, bread or toast) and; for children, teens, pregnant women and breast-feeding moms, additional milk or other dairy food such as cheese or yogurt. This good-breakfast pattern applies to people of all ages.

Breast Feeding: Nursing not only bonds mother and baby, but it also bolsters the baby's immune system and, according to results of a recent study, reduces the risk of ear infection in newborns. Breast milk is highly nutritious and best meets babies' nutritional needs.

NUTRIENT CONTENT OF 1 CUP BREAST MILK
(8 fluid ounces; 246 grams)

171 calories	42 mg sodium
3 g protein	125 mg potassium
11 g fat, 5 saturated	0 g dietary fiber
34 mg cholesterol	157 RE vitamin A
17 g carbohydrate	0.03 mg thiamin
79 mg calcium	0.09 mg riboflavin
34 mg phosphorus	0.4 mg niacin
0.1 mg iron	12 mg vitamin C

Brewer's Yeast: As a dietary supplement, brewer's yeast (*Saccharomyces cerevisiae*) supplies the body with high-quality protein, thiamin, riboflavin, iron and phosphorus. In beer making, it's used to ferment sugars to alcohol.

NUTRIENT CONTENT OF 1 OUNCE (28 GRAMS) BREWER'S YEAST

80 calories	34 mg sodium
11 g protein	535 mg potassium
0 g fat, 0 saturated	9 g dietary fiber
0 mg cholesterol	0 RE vitamin A
11 g carbohydrate	4.43 mg thiamin
60 mg calcium	1.21 mg riboflavin
496 mg phosphorus	10.7 mg niacin
4.5 mg iron	0 mg vitamin C

Brick Cheese: See CHEDDAR.

Brie: The quintessential French cheese, some say, a cheese saluted by kings, counts and poets. The best Brie, fermented from clotted, unskimmed cow's milk, comes from Meaux in the department of Seine-et-Marne. Unripe, it can be dry and chalky; improperly ripened, creamy outside but dry at heart. But a perfect ripe Brie is liquid ivory, pungent, as smooth as butter on the tongue (its fat content must not drop below 44 percent). Like oysters, Brie is best in the *R* months, with September being the best month of all.

NUTRIENT CONTENT OF 1 OUNCE (28 GRAMS) BRIE

95 calories	178 mg sodium
6 g protein	43 mg potassium
8 g fat, 5 saturated	0 g dietary fiber
28 mg cholesterol	52 RE vitamin A
0 g carbohydrate	0.02 mg thiamin
52 mg calcium	0.15 mg riboflavin
53 mg phosphorus	0.1 mg niacin
0.1 mg iron	0 mg vitamin C

Brioche: The feathery yeast buns the French—and now the Americans—love to eat with their morning coffee. Unfortunately, they're loaded with calories, cholesterol, fat (a third of it saturated) and sodium.

NUTRIENT CONTENT OF 1 MEDIUM-SIZE BRIOCHE
(about 3 ounces; 88 grams)

307 calories	382 mg sodium
7 g protein	100 mg potassium
15 g fat, 5 saturated	2 g dietary fiber
79 mg cholesterol	30 RE vitamin A
35 g carbohydrate	0.37 mg thiamin
25 mg calcium	0.37 mg riboflavin
97 mg phosphorus	2.9 mg niacin
2.4 mg iron	0 mg vitamin C

Broad Beans: See FAVA BEANS under BEANS, FRESH.

Broccoflower: The newest "cabbage," a yellow-green "cauliflower" that's actually a broccoli-cauliflower hybrid. It shows up occasionally in big-city greenmarkets and high-end groceries. Though broccoflower's nutrient content has yet to be assessed, it is certainly a good source of vitamins A and C. **SEASON:** Year-round but more plentiful in summer.

Broccoli: This ancient member of the cabbage family, believed to be native to Italy (or at least the Mediterranean), is one of the cruciferous vegetables thought to re-duce the risk of cancer. Its intense green color signals that broccoli is a powerful source of vitamins A and C. It's low in calories and sodium, a protean source of minerals, easier to digest than cabbage and thus one of the most healthful vegetables known to man. Yet broccoli wasn't widely grown in this country until the 1920s, when Italians began emigrating to California. **SEASON:** Year-round.

Broccoli Rabe: A looser, leafier, more pungent form of broccoli that's equally nutritious. **SEASON:** Year-round.

Broiling, Grilling: The benefit of broiling and grilling (cooking under direct heat or over a gas or charcoal fire) is that they require no additional fat; indeed, they melt,

NUTRIENT CONTENT OF 1 CUP STEAMED BROCCOLI

(about 5¼ ounces; 156 grams)

44 calories	42 mg sodium
5 g protein	505 mg potassium
1 g fat, 0 saturated	4 g dietary fiber
0 mg cholesterol	228 RE vitamin A
8 g carbohydrate	0.09 mg thiamin
75 mg calcium	0.18 mg riboflavin
103 mg phosphorus	0.9 mg niacin
1.4 mg iron	123 mg vitamin C

Dry-Sautéed Broccoli Sesame

Makes 4 Servings

1 tablespoon roasted Asian sesame oil

1 tablespoon peanut oil

1 medium garlic clove, minced

One 1-inch cube fresh ginger, peeled and minced

⅛ to ¼ teaspoon crushed red pepper flakes

1 large bunch broccoli, washed, trimmed, and divided into small florets

1 teaspoon sugar

3 tablespoons water blended with ½ teaspoon cornstarch

1 tablespoon dry sherry or port

2 tablespoons soy sauce

COAT A LARGE heavy skillet or wok with nonstick spray, add sesame and peanut oils, and heat 1 minute. Add garlic, ginger, and red pepper and stir-fry 3 minutes, until garlic and ginger are golden but not brown. Add broccoli and sugar and stir-fry 1 to 2 minutes, just until broccoli turns bright green. Stir in the cornstarch paste, sherry, and soy sauce; cover and steam 3 to 4 minutes, until broccoli is crisp-tender. Toss well and serve.

APPROXIMATE NUTRIENT COUNTS PER SERVING

125 calories	12 g carbohydrate	1.8 mg iron	0.11 mg thiamin
6 g protein	5 g dietary fiber	563 mg sodium	0.22 mg riboflavin
7 g fat, 1 saturated	86 mg calcium	588 mg potassium	1.4 mg niacin
0 mg cholesterol	126 mg phosphorus	303 RE vitamin A	135 mg vitamin C

Sweet and Spicy Broccoli Rabe

Makes 4 Servings

Wonderful with broiled chicken, salmon, swordfish, or tuna.

¼ cup dried tomatoes (not packed in oil)

¼ cup seedless golden raisins

1 cup hot water

1 bunch (12 ounces) broccoli rabe, tough ends removed

2 teaspoons fruity olive oil

2 garlic cloves, slivered

¼ teaspoon salt, or to taste

¼ teaspoon crushed red pepper flakes

SOFTEN THE TOMATOES and raisins by soaking in hot water 20 minutes. Drain, reserving ½ cup soaking liquid. Coarsely chop the tomatoes and mix with raisins; set aside. Cook the broccoli rabe in a large kettle of boiling water until not quite tender, about 4 minutes; then drain well. Heat oil in a large heavy skillet 1 minute over low heat. Add the garlic and cook, stirring occasionally, until fragrant, about 3 minutes. Add the broccoli rabe, sprinkle with salt and red pepper, and stir to coat. Add the raisin-tomato mixture and reserved soaking liquid, and continue cooking until broccoli rabe is tender and juices are slightly reduced, about 4 minutes. Serve at once.

APPROXIMATE NUTRIENT COUNTS PER SERVING

87 calories	15 g carbohydrate	1.3 mg iron	0.07 mg thiamin
3 g protein	3 g dietary fiber	229 mg sodium	0.14 mg riboflavin
3 g fat, 0 saturated	50 mg calcium	441 mg potassium	1.0 mg niacin
0 mg cholesterol	75 mg phosphorus	169 RE vitamin A	62 mg vitamin C

then drain away some of the fat in meat, poultry or fish. The shortcomings? Meats may toughen and dry and if the heat is too intense—or the food too close to the flame—fat may reach the smoke point, producing hazardous fumes (see ACROLEIN; PAH). The high temps of broiling, grilling, even frying and roasting may also create heterocyclic aromatic amines (see HAAS). Like PAHs, these are suspected of being carcinogenic. See also CHARCOAL GRILLING.

Bromelin (additive): A natural enzyme found in pineapple that's used to tenderize beef, soften commercial bread doughs and clarify beer. Anyone who's tried to make a gelatin dessert with fresh pineapple knows that it won't set. Here's why: The bromelin breaks down (actually digests) the gelatin (a protein). Usually canned pineapple *will* gel because the heat used in canning inactivates most of the bromelin. Still, you may need to use 1½ times the amount of gelatin called for. Safe.

Brominated Vegetable Oil (BVO) (additive): Highly controversial, this lighter-than-water blend of bromine and corn, cottonseed, olive or sesame oil is used to stabilize fruit-flavored soft drinks and create an illusion of body. Rated GRAS when use is limited to 15 parts per million, brominated vegetable oil is nonetheless taking considerable heat from watchdog groups because bromine accumulates in body tissues. In one Canadian study, lab rats fed BVO-enriched rations for eighty days suffered heart, kidney, liver and thyroid damage. Consumer advocates want further testing and reevaluation of BVO.

Brownies: Almost the first thing children learn to bake because they're quick and practically foolproof, brownies have little to recommend them other than that deep-down, oh-so-satisfying chocolate flavor.

NUTRIENT CONTENT OF 1 MEDIUM-SIZE BROWNIE

(about 1¼ ounces; 36 grams)

157 calories	90 mg sodium
2 g protein	62 mg potassium
9 g fat, 3 saturated	1 g dietary fiber
27 mg cholesterol	13 RE vitamin A
18 g carbohydrate	0.06 mg thiamin
24 mg calcium	0.07 mg riboflavin
62 mg phosphorus	0.4 mg niacin
0.7 mg iron	0 mg vitamin C

Brown Rice: See RICE.

Brown Sugar: See SUGARS.

Brussels Sprouts: These delicate baby cabbages were first grown in the Belgian countryside near Brussels (hence their name). Soon they were the rage of royal courts. The French liked those no bigger than peas, and Belgians, even today, prefer those about the size of grapes. Like other cabbages, brussels sprouts contain cancer-fighting indoles as well as impressive amounts of vitamins A and C. **SEASON:** Year-round, with supplies peaking in fall.

NUTRIENT CONTENT OF 1 CUP BOILED BRUSSELS SPROUTS

(about 5¼ ounces; 156 grams)

61 calories	33 mg sodium
4 g protein	495 mg potassium
1 g fat, 0 saturated	7 g dietary fiber
0 mg cholesterol	112 RE vitamin A
14 g carbohydrate	0.17 mg thiamin
56 mg calcium	0.13 mg riboflavin
87 mg phosphorus	0.9 mg niacin
1.9 mg iron	97 mg vitamin C

Bûcheron: A rich and creamy French *chèvre* (goat cheese) shaped into little logs. Although now popular in the United States, nutrient counts aren't available for *Bûcheron*. You can be sure, however, that these snowy little links are neither low fat nor low calorie. Also that cholesterol levels soar.

Buckwheat, Kasha; Buckwheat Flour: Native to Central Asia, buckwheat arrived in Europe during the Middle Ages. It remains a staple across the Continent but is nowhere more popular than in Russia. There, whole buckwheat grains (groats) are toasted, then cooked with beaten egg, onion and sometimes mushrooms or walnuts in a kind of pilaf called *kasha* (indeed, the groats are often sold as kasha in American supermarkets). In Western Europe and America, buckwheat flour is more popular than groats, except among transplanted Eastern European Jews who continue to prepare kasha and *kasha varnishkas* (kasha mixed with bow-tie pasta) the way their forebears did. The

---

NUTRIENT CONTENT OF 1 CUP COOKED KASHA (ROASTED BUCKWHEAT)

(about 7 ounces; 198 grams)

182 calories	8 mg sodium
7 g protein	174 mg potassium
1 g fat, 0 saturated	5 g dietary fiber
0 mg cholesterol	0 RE vitamin A
39 g carbohydrate	0.08 mg thiamin
14 mg calcium	0.08 mg riboflavin
138 mg phosphorus	1.9 mg niacin
1.6 mg iron	0 mg vitamin C

NUTRIENT CONTENT OF 1 CUP BUCKWHEAT FLOUR

(about 3½ ounces; 98 grams)

328 calories	11 mg sodium
12 g protein	565 mg potassium
3 g fat, 1 saturated	8 g dietary fiber
0 mg cholesterol	0 RE vitamin A
69 g carbohydrate	0.41 mg thiamin
40 mg calcium	0.19 mg riboflavin
330 mg phosphorus	6.0 mg niacin
4.0 mg iron	0 mg vitamin C

Italians knead buckwheat flour into noodles (*pizzoccheri*), as do the Japanese (*soba*). But what Americans know and like best are buckwheat pancakes, almost as popular now as they were during their nineteenth-century heyday when painter James McNeill Whistler, of all people, served them to London society.

Bulgur: Bran- and germ-rich cracked wheat that's been parboiled. Used throughout the Middle East as a potato substitute, bulgur is also the key ingredient in *tabbouleh,* a garlicky cold salad that's dressed with olive oil.

NUTRIENT CONTENT OF 1 CUP COOKED BULGUR WHEAT
(about 6½ ounces; 182 grams)

151 calories	9 mg sodium
6 g protein	123 mg potassium
0 g fat, 0 saturated	8 g dietary fiber
0 mg cholesterol	0 RE vitamin A
34 g carbohydrate	0.10 mg thiamin
18 mg calcium	0.05 mg riboflavin
73 mg phosphorus	1.8 mg niacin
1.8 mg iron	0 mg vitamin C

Bulimia: A serious binge-purge eating disorder that afflicts those of insatiable appetite who are terrified of gaining weight. Bulimia often strikes young women who equate success with being bone thin. So they stuff themselves, then vomit and/or take laxatives. Repeated induced vomiting decays the teeth, inflames the esophagus, dehydrates the body and causes alkalosis and other metabolic imbalances. Laxative abuse may lead to rectal bleeding and calcium deficiency. In severe cases of bulimia, hospitalization is required and, for total recovery, a team effort by internists, psychiatrists and nutritionists. See also ANOREXIA NERVOSA.

Bulk: The old-fashioned word for fiber.

Bulking Agent (additive): A nonfood (cellulose, for example) that's used to increase the volume of food without adding any calories.

Burritos: A favorite new fast food that's crossed the border from Mexico. Burritos are nothing more than tortillas filled with cooked dried beans (usually pintos or kidneys),

cheese or meat. Many are high in fat, cholesterol, calories and sodium. But they also contribute significant amounts of iron, riboflavin and niacin. Not exactly junk food.

NUTRIENT CONTENT OF 1 BEAN BURRITO
(about 3¾ ounces; 109 grams)

224 calories	493 mg sodium
7 g protein	327 mg potassium
7 g fat, 3 saturated	4 g dietary fiber
2 mg cholesterol	16 RE vitamin A
36 g carbohydrate	0.32 mg thiamin
57 mg calcium	0.30 mg riboflavin
49 mg phosphorus	2.0 mg niacin
2.3 mg iron	1 mg vitamin C

NUTRIENT CONTENT OF 1 BEEF BURRITO
(about 3¾ ounces; 110 grams)

262 calories	746 mg sodium
13 g protein	370 mg potassium
10 g fat, 5 saturated	1 g dietary fiber
32 mg cholesterol	14 RE vitamin A
29 g carbohydrate	0.12 mg thiamin
42 mg calcium	0.46 mg riboflavin
87 mg phosphorus	3.2 mg niacin
3 mg iron	1 mg vitamin C

Butter: Man learned long ago that if he churned the milk of animals into fat, it would last longer. So butter's original use was as a way of preserving milk. Today, butter is the shortening of choice throughout America and northern

NUTRIENT CONTENT OF 1 TABLESPOON UNSALTED BUTTER
(½ ounce; 14 grams)

102 calories	2 mg sodium
0 g protein	4 mg potassium
12 g fat, 7 saturated	0 g dietary fiber
31 mg cholesterol	107 RE vitamin A
0 g carbohydrate	0 mg thiamin
3 mg calcium	0.01 mg riboflavin
3 mg phosphorus	0 mg niacin
0 mg iron	0 mg vitamin C

Note: If butter is salted, the sodium count zooms to 117 milligrams per tablespoon; all other nutrient counts remain the same.

Europe, but it is 80 percent fat, more than half of it saturated, and therein lies one problem (another is its cholesterol content). With doctors and nutritionists urging us all to cut down on fat—especially saturated fats—many health-conscious cooks are switching to soft margarines or cooking oils. But these lack the shortening power of butter and the sunny golden flavor. In the old days, the flavor of butter varied according to where the cows had grazed. Today it owes its flavor more to the lactic acid bacteria used to sour the cream from which it's made. Gourmets prefer unsalted or sweet butter, but it goes rancid faster than the salted. The USDA grades butter according to color, flavor and texture. Tops is AA, followed by A, B and C.

Butter Cakes: Not a good choice for those with an eye on their fat, calorie and cholesterol intake because butter cakes contain plenty of butter (and/or vegetable shortening) plus whole eggs, sometimes in abundance. ANGEL FOOD CAKES are the dieter's best friend.

Buttercup Squash: See SQUASH.

Butterfish: These small, dark- and buttery-fleshed East Coast fish are particular favorites in New York and Boston, where they are available both fresh and smoked. Connoisseurs say the only way to cook a butterfish is to broil it or bake it with the skin intact.

NUTRIENT CONTENT OF 3 OUNCES (85 GRAMS) BROILED OR BAKED BUTTERFISH	
159 calories	97 mg sodium
19 g protein	408 mg potassium
9 g fat, NA saturated	0 g dietary fiber
71 mg cholesterol	28 RE vitamin A
0 g carbohydrate	0.13 mg thiamin
24 mg calcium	0.16 mg riboflavin
262 mg phosphorus	4.9 mg niacin
0.5 mg iron	0 mg vitamin C

Butterhead Lettuce: See SALAD GREENS.

Buttermilk: Originally nothing more than the tart liquid left after butter was churned, buttermilk is now low-fat or skim milk that's clotted and soured with bacteria cultures (usually lactobacillus), then homogenized with carrageenan (Irish moss or seaweed), guar and carob gum until it's as thick and smooth as cream. In cold soups, buttermilk makes a dandy substitute for cream, it can double for whole milk in many quick breads and cakes (as long as ½ teaspoon of the baking powder is replaced by soda) and it can be buzzed into a superlative low-fat salad dressing. But, make a note, it is higher in sodium than sweet milk.

NUTRIENT CONTENT OF 1 CUP CULTURED BUTTERMILK	
(8 fluid ounces; 245 grams)	
99 calories	257 mg sodium
8 g protein	370 mg potassium
2 g fat, 1 saturated	0 g dietary fiber
9 mg cholesterol	20 RE vitamin A
12 g carbohydrate	0.08 mg thiamin
284 mg calcium	0.38 mg riboflavin
218 mg phosphorus	0.1 mg niacin
0.1 mg iron	2 mg vitamin C

Butternut Squash: See SQUASH.

Butter Substitutes: These shake-on powders liquefy on contact with moist, hot foods and look very much like melted butter. They ape the flavor of butter, too, some brands more convincingly than others. Most butter substitutes are alphabet soups of chemicals that horrify food purists. In truth, these are harmless mixtures of starches, oils and pigments that occur naturally in plants and animals: lecithin, a waxy substance found in egg yolks (among other places) that thickens and emulsifies; maldodextrin, starch obtained from corn; partially hydrogenated soybean and/or cottonseed oil; butter flavor plus spray-dried butter; salt; and, for color, turmeric and annatto, two spices sold by the jar in nearly every supermarket. Most butter substitutes average 3 to 4 calories per ½ teaspoon (about what's needed to season a single portion), less than 1 gram of fat and 0 cholesterol. Purists may scoff, but for those on low-fat, low-cholesterol and/or low-calorie diets, butter substitutes make butterless food far more appealing. **NOTE:** Some butter substitutes are higher in sodium than others, so scrutinize labels.

Butter Yellow: A toxic pigment once used to color butter and margarine that is now banned by the FDA.

Tangy Low-Fat Buttermilk Dressing

Makes About 3½ Cups

2½ cups buttermilk

¼ cup freshly grated Parmesan cheese

2 tablespoons olive oil

1 tablespoon ketchup

1 tablespoon Dijon mustard

1 tablespoon sweet paprika

1 small garlic clove, crushed

1½ teaspoons dried basil

1 teaspoon dried marjoram

1 teaspoon sugar

½ teaspoon freshly ground black pepper

1 tablespoon snipped fresh chives (optional)

1 tablespoon minced fresh parsley (optional)

CHURN ALL INGREDIENTS in a food processor fitted with metal chopping blade 30 seconds; scrape down work bowl and churn 30 to 45 seconds longer or until uniformly creamy. Store in tightly covered 1–quart preserving jar in refrigerator; dressing keeps well for about 5 days.

APPROXIMATE NUTRIENT COUNTS PER TABLESPOON

12 calories	1 g carbohydrate	0.1 mg iron	0.01 mg thiamin
1 g protein	0 g dietary fiber	27 mg sodium	0.02 mg riboflavin
1 g fat, 0 saturated	21 mg calcium	24 mg potassium	0 mg niacin
1 mg cholesterol	15 mg phosphorus	10 RE vitamin A	0 mg vitamin C

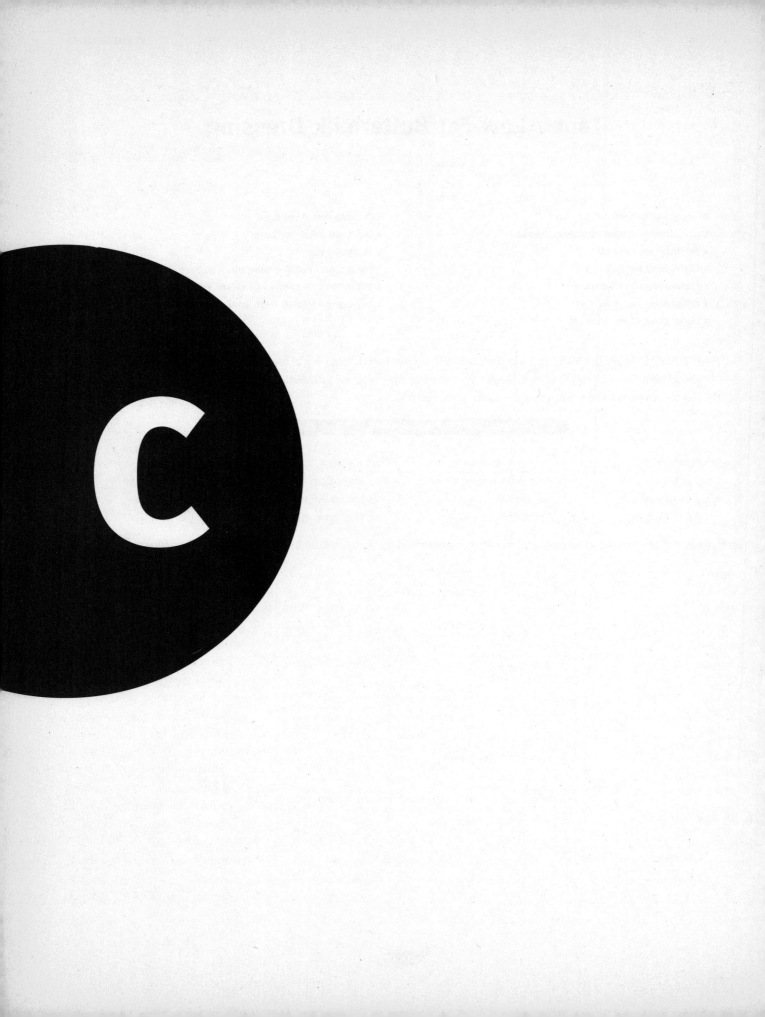

C, Vitamin; Ascorbic Acid: "It wrought so well that if all the physicians of Montpelier and Louaine had been there, with all the drugs of Alexandria, they would not have done as much in one yere as that tree did in six days." Thus spoke French explorer Jacques Cartier in 1535 on his second voyage to Newfoundland after seeing Native Americans cure his men of scurvy with a strong sassafras tea. In 1747, a British Navy surgeon experimenting with sailors' rations showed that those given oranges and lemons each day were cured of scurvy. Throughout the following years, British naval surgeons' medicine chests included concentrated syrup of lemon juice (or *lime,* as the Brits called it, which is why British sailors are known as limeys). Another 173 years would pass before researchers extracted this antiscorbutic substance from orange juice and named it vitamin C. We now know that ascorbic acid is a particularly versatile vitamin. It's integral to the building and maintenance of collagen, a protein or "glue" that holds the body's cells in place. It's indispensable to bones and teeth (for much the same reason), to blood vessels, to the healing of wounds. Further, vitamin C helps metabolize several amino acids and hormones. It's a powerful antioxidant, too, helping the body rid itself of carcinogenic by-products of metabolism called free radicals. There's even strong evidence that vitamin C may raise blood levels of HDL, or "good" cholesterol, which helps flush fatty deposits from the arteries, thereby reducing the risk of cardiovascular disease. Or so studies at the National Institute on Aging and the USDA indicate. But researchers are quick to point out that beyond 345 milligrams of vitamin C per day for men and 215 milligrams for women, the HDL boosting stops. **DEFICIENCY SYMPTOMS:** Inflamed gums; frequent, unexplained bruising; slow healing of cuts and burns; paleness and lassitude; intense fatigue; brittle bones; and ultimately, in severe, prolonged deficiencies, scurvy. **GOOD SOURCES:** Fresh fruits, especially citrus fruits, melons, kiwis, strawberries, and such vegetables as broccoli, sweet green and red peppers, tomatoes, brussels sprouts, cabbage and dark leafy greens like chard, kale, collards, spinach, mustard, turnip and beet tops. As a general rule, the darker or brighter the green pigment, the greater the vitamin C. **PRECAUTIONS:** Unfortunately, vitamin C is extremely unstable. Heat and air (oxygen) destroy it. Moreover, it's water soluble, meaning it can leach into cooking water and be lost if that water is dumped. The best idea is to cook vitamin C-rich foods in a small amount of water in a covered pan just until crisp-tender. Heavy smokers need extra vitamin C because nicotine doubles the rate of vitamin C depletion in the body.

RDA FOR VITAMIN C		
Babies:		
Birth to 6 months	30 mg per day	
6 months to 1 year	35 mg per day	
Children:		
1 to 3 years	40 mg per day	
4 to 6 years	45 mg per day	
7 to 10 years	45 mg per day	
Men and Boys:		
11 to 14 years	50 mg per day	
15 to 51+ years	60 mg per day	
Women and Girls:		
11 to 14 years	50 mg per day	
15 to 51+ years	60 mg per day	
Pregnant Women:	70 mg per day	
Nursing Mothers:		
First 6 months	95 mg per day	
Second 6 months	90 mg per day	

Note: Because nicotine lowers blood levels of vitamin C, smokers should get at least 100 milligrams of ascorbic acid each day.

Cabbage, Chinese: See CHINESE CABBAGE.

Cabbage, Green: Man has been eating cabbage for more than four-thousand years and cultivating it for about half that. According to Greek myth, the first cabbages sprang from the tears of Lycurgus, prince of Thrace, whom Dionysus caught trampling grapes. As punishment, he lashed Lycurgus to a grapevine. A curious outgrowth of this legend was the belief that eating cabbage would keep you from getting drunk. Aristotle was said "to dine well upon cabbage" before setting out for a night on the town, as indeed did Europeans right up through the Middle Ages. Despite all the lore that has accumulated about cabbages, man has always prized them for what they are: versatile, satisfying, highly nutritious and, yes, cheap vegetables. Diogenes, the ancient Greek philosopher, once advised a young courtier, "If you lived on cabbage, you would not be obliged to flatter the powerful." To which the courtier replied, "If you flattered the powerful, you would not be obliged to live upon cabbage." An Old World food, cabbage didn't reach the New until the mid-sixteenth century when French explorer Jacques Cartier planted it in Canada. English colonists later brought their own supply, and cabbages apparently then moved westward with the wagon trains. As one of the cruciferous vegetables believed by food researchers to reduce the risk of cancer, cabbage is enjoying new celebrity. **SEASON:** Year-round.

NUTRIENT CONTENT OF 1 CUP SHREDDED RAW GREEN CABBAGE

(about 2¼ ounces; 70 grams)

16 calories	12 mg sodium
1 g protein	112 mg potassium
0 g fat, 0 unsaturated	2 g dietary fiber
0 mg cholesterol	8 RE vitamin A
4 g carbohydrate	0.04 mg thiamin
32 mg calcium	0.02 mg riboflavin
16 mg phosphorus	0.2 mg niacin
0.4 mg iron	33 mg vitamin C

NUTRIENT CONTENT OF 1 CUP COOKED UNSEASONED GREEN CABBAGE

(about 5¼ ounces; 150 grams)

32 calories	28 mg sodium
1 g protein	308 mg potassium
0 g fat, 0 unsaturated	5 g dietary fiber
0 mg cholesterol	12 RE vitamin A
7 g carbohydrate	0.09 mg thiamin
50 mg calcium	0.08 mg riboflavin
36 mg phosphorus	0.3 mg niacin
0.6 mg iron	36 mg vitamin C

Cabbage, Red: Despite its rich ruby color, red cabbage contains about the same nutritive value as green cabbage. To heighten the redness, add a dash of vinegar or cranberry juice to the cooking water. Or do as Germans do and cook red cabbage in a mixture of vinegar and dry red wine. **SEASON:** Year-round.

Quick Curried Cabbage

Makes 6 Servings

2 tablespoons peanut oil
1 tablespoon mustard seeds
1 medium yellow onion, chopped
1 medium carrot, peeled and shredded
2 tablespoons finely minced red or green bell pepper
2 teaspoons finely minced fresh ginger
2 teaspoons curry powder

⅛ teaspoon ground cinnamon
⅛ teaspoon grated nutmeg
2 quarts thinly sliced, cored cabbage (a 2-pound head)
1 tablespoon tomato paste
½ teaspoon salt
⅛ teaspoon freshly ground black pepper

COAT A LARGE heavy skillet with nonstick spray, add the oil and mustard seeds, and heat about 2 minutes over moderately high heat until the seeds begin to sputter. Reduce heat to moderate; then add the onion, carrot, bell pepper, and ginger; and stir-fry 3 minutes, until limp. Stir in the curry powder, cinnamon, and nutmeg, and cook 1 minute. Add the cabbage, stir-fry 5 minutes until nicely glazed, reduce the heat to low, then add the tomato paste and cook, uncovered, stirring often, 5 to 10 minutes or until the cabbage is as tender as you like. Season with the salt and pepper, toss well, then serve.

APPROXIMATE NUTRIENT COUNTS PER SERVING

101 calories	12 g carbohydrate	1.5 mg iron	0.10 mg thiamin
3 g protein	4 g dietary fiber	229 mg sodium	0.08 mg riboflavin
6 g fat, 1 saturated	89 mg calcium	470 mg potassium	0.8 mg niacin
0 mg cholesterol	64 mg phosphorus	244 RE vitamin A	45 mg vitamin C

Confettied Health Slaw

Makes 6 Servings

3 tablespoons plain nonfat yogurt

2 tablespoons reduced-fat mayonnaise

1 tablespoon cider vinegar

2 teaspoons rinsed and drained small capers

2 teaspoons prepared horseradish

1 teaspoon sugar

1 teaspoon dried dill

¼ teaspoon salt

3 cups shredded red and/or green cabbage

1⅓ cups shredded carrots

IN A LARGE mixing bowl, combine all ingredients except the cabbage and carrots. Add the cabbage and carrots, and fold in thoroughly. Cover with plastic food wrap and refrigerate at least 1 hour. Stir well before serving.

APPROXIMATE NUTRIENT COUNTS PER SERVING

43 calories	7 g carbohydrate	0.6 mg iron	0.05 mg thiamin
2 g protein	2 g dietary fiber	136 mg sodium	0.06 mg riboflavin
1 g fat, 0 saturated	44 mg calcium	186 mg potassium	0.4 mg niacin
5 mg cholesterol	42 mg phosphorus	688 RE vitamin A	22 mg vitamin C

NUTRIENT CONTENT OF 1 CUP SHREDDED RAW RED CABBAGE

(about 2¼ ounces; 70 grams)

20 calories	8 mg sodium
1 g protein	144 mg potassium
0 g fat, 0 unsaturated	3 g dietary fiber
0 mg cholesterol	2 RE vitamin A
4 g carbohydrate	0.04 mg thiamin
36 mg calcium	0.02 mg riboflavin
30 mg phosphorus	0.2 mg niacin
0.3 mg iron	40 mg vitamin C

Cabbage, Savoy: As far as most Europeans are concerned, this loose, crinkly head is the only green cabbage fit to cook. Its flavor is milder and its texture more buttery than the smooth, pale, tight heads familiar to Americans. Savoy cabbage is usually steamed or boiled though it does make dandy slaw. Germans like to shred it, toss it with crisp bacon crumbles and bake it in a sort of quiche called kuchen. Like other cabbages, savoy is a good source of vitamin C and dietary fiber as well as being one of the cruciferous vegetables now thought to reduce one's risk of cancer. **SEASON:** Summer and fall.

NUTRIENT CONTENT OF 1 CUP COOKED UNSEASONED RED CABBAGE

(about 5¼ ounces; 150 grams)

32 calories	12 mg sodium
2 g protein	210 mg potassium
0 g fat, 0 unsaturated	5 g dietary fiber
0 mg cholesterol	2 RE vitamin A
7 g carbohydrate	0.06 mg thiamin
56 mg calcium	0.03 mg riboflavin
42 mg phosphorus	0.3 mg niacin
0.6 mg iron	52 mg vitamin C

NUTRIENT CONTENT OF 1 CUP COOKED UNSEASONED SAVOY CABBAGE

(about 5¼ ounces; 146 grams)

36 calories	34 mg sodium
3 g protein	268 mg potassium
0 g fat, 0 unsaturated	5 g dietary fiber
0 mg cholesterol	130 RE vitamin A
8 g carbohydrate	0.04 mg thiamin
44 mg calcium	0.02 mg riboflavin
48 mg phosphorus	0 mg niacin
0.6 mg iron	24 mg vitamin C

Cactus Pads, Nopales:

Hardly mainstream, except in Mexico, these fleshy cactus chunks (from the same species that supplies prickly pears) are appearing more and more frequently in high-end groceries. *Nopales* are a modest source of vitamin C and several minerals. Though okay raw, cactus pads are best when steamed or blanched, then tossed into salads or scrambled eggs. If overcooked, they're as slimy as okra. **SEASON:** Year-round.

NUTRIENT CONTENT OF 1 MEDIUM-SIZE RAW CACTUS PAD
(about 1¼ ounces; 35 grams)

14 calories	2 mg sodium
0 g protein	77 mg potassium
0 g fat, 0 unsaturated	1 g dietary fiber
0 mg cholesterol	2 RE vitamin A
3 g carbohydrate	0.01 mg thiamin
20 mg calcium	0.02 mg riboflavin
8 mg phosphorus	0.2 mg niacin
0.1 mg iron	5 mg vitamin C

NUTRIENT CONTENT OF 1 CUP COOKED CACTUS PADS
(about 5¼ ounces; 149 grams)

61 calories	352* mg sodium
1 g protein	293 mg potassium
1 g fat, 0 unsaturated	5 g dietary fiber
0 mg cholesterol	6 RE vitamin A
14 g carbohydrate	0.02 mg thiamin
79 mg calcium	0.08 mg riboflavin
36 mg phosphorus	0.6 mg niacin
0.5 mg iron	15 mg vitamin C

*This figure is for salted *nopales*. To lower the figure, reduce the salt: ½ teaspoon salt = 1,000 milligrams sodium.

Cadmium:

A fairly heavy metal, often absorbed from water run through galvanized pipes, that deactivates certain body enzymes. Like mercury and lead, cadmium remains in the tissues and too much of it can be toxic.

Caffeine:

People joke about "coffee nerves" but they're no laughing matter. Caffeine, an alkaloid that exists naturally in tea, kola nuts and chocolate as well as in coffee, is clearly toxic in high doses. It can cause heart palpitations, high blood pressure, vomiting, convulsions. It also saps the body's supply of calcium. Used in moderation, caffeine is a mild stimulant. And, according to a recent study conducted at Montreal University and its affiliate, Sainte-Justine Hospital, pregnant women who drink 1½ cups of coffee a day (or 5 cups of tea or 4 colas) may double their risk of miscarriage, and those downing 3 to 4 cups of coffee a day may triple it (even women drinking 3 to 4 cups of coffee a day the month *before* they conceive are twice as likely to lose their babies). Although further study is needed, the American College of Obstetricians and Gynecologists agrees that pregnant or about-to-be-pregnant women should cut back on coffee.

Average Caffeine Content of Some Popular Beverages

1 cup (5 fl oz) standard-brewed coffee = 80 mg (perk), 130 (drip)

1 cup (5 fl oz) instant coffee = 60 mg

1 cup (5 fl oz) decaf = 3 mg

1 cup (5 fl oz) tea (brewed 1 minute) = 28 mg

1 cup (5 fl oz) tea (brewed 5 minutes) = 46 mg

1 glass (12 fl oz) iced tea = 70 mg

1 cup (5 fl oz) instant tea = 30 mg

1 cup (5 fl oz) hot cocoa = 5 mg

1 glass (8 fl oz) chocolate milk = 5 mg

1 can (12 fl oz) cola = 38 mg

Calciferol: See D, VITAMIN.

Calcitonin:

A thyroid hormone that works in concert with vitamin D and a parathyroid hormone to maintain the body's delicate balance of calcium. Calcitonin's main job is to take calcium from the blood and deposit it in the bones.

Calcium:

This mineral, we've been taught since grammar school, builds strong bones and teeth. In fact, 99 percent of the body's supply of calcium goes into the formation and maintenance of bones and teeth. *Maintenance* is the key word here for calcium is constantly being shuttled from bones to meet other bodily needs (the transmission of nerve impulses, for example, the clotting of blood, the regulation of heart muscle rhythm and the absorption of vitamin B_{12}). Then, if there's an excess, it's redeposited. Hormones and vitamin D control the body's use of calcium; indeed, the body can't even absorb calcium without vitamin D. Recent studies suggest that calcium plays a far bigger role in the body than originally thought. It may be important in both preventing and treating high blood pressure (hypertension). It's been found to ease the symptoms of PMS, to reduce the risk of heart disease, strokes, colon cancer, even kidney stones. **DEFICIENCY SYMPTOMS:** Retarded growth and deformed or brittle bones in children, dental caries, osteoporosis in adults. **GOOD SOURCES:** All dairy products except butter; dried peas and beans; most dark leafy greens (beet and turnip tops, kale

RDA FOR CALCIUM*

Babies:

Birth to 6 months	400 mg per day
6 months to 1 year	600 mg per day

Children:

1 to 10 years	800 mg per day

Men and Boys:

11 to 24 years	1,200 mg per day
25 to 51+ years	800 mg per day

Women and Girls:

11 to 24 years	1,200 mg per day
25 to 51+ years	800 mg per day

Pregnant Women: 1,200 mg per day

Nursing Mothers: 1,200 mg per day

*New daily recommendations for calcium came out of the June 1994 NIH Consensus Conference, where it was agreed that the current RDAs for calcium (above) were too low (except for infants and children through five years of age). Here are the new higher figures:

NEW DAILY CALCIUM INTAKE (AS RECOMMENDED FOR OPTIMAL HEALTH AT THE 1994 NIH CONSENSUS CONFERENCE)

Children:

6 to 10 years	800 to 1,200 mg per day

Adolescents and Young Adults:

11 to 24 years	1,200 to 1,500 mg per day

Men:

25 to 65 years	1,000 mg per day
65+ years	1,500 mg per day

Women:

25 to 50 years	800 to 1,200 mg per day
50 to 60 years (on estrogen therapy)	1,000 mg per day
50 to 65 years (not on estrogen therapy)	1,500 mg per day
65+ years	1,500 mg per day

Pregnant Women: 1,200 to 1,500 mg per day

Nursing Mothers: 1,200 to 1,500 mg per day

and collards but not spinach or Swiss chard); the soft bones of canned fish. **PRECAUTIONS:** A high-protein diet can accelerate calcium loss, as can too much sodium or caffeine, postmenopausal hormone changes, lack of exercise and certain steroids. Fiber interferes with the absorption of calcium (particularly bean, nut, wheat bran or seed fiber). And oxalic acid, present in spinach, Swiss chard, rhubarb, almonds and chocolate, combines with calcium to form calcium oxalate, a chemical salt the body can't use. On the other hand, too much calcium blocks the absorption of iron and zinc.

Calcium Alginate: See ALGINATES.

Calcium Benzoate (additive): These water-soluble white crystals are used as a preservative in margarine. Their use is limited to 0.1 percent of the weight of the finished product or, if used in tandem with sorbic acid, to 0.2 percent. Though generally considered safe, calcium benzoate is combustible and, when overheated, sends forth acrid, noxious fumes.

Calcium Bromate (additive): This crystalline white powder is used to bleach flour and condition dough. GRAS.

Calcium Carbonate (additive; dietary supplement): The active ingredient in certain antacids, calcium carbonate occurs widely in rocks and minerals, limestone being an important source. For the body, it is the most usable form of calcium available. As a dietary supplement, calcium carbonate tablets are more effective if spaced throughout the day than if swallowed in a single massive dose.

Calcium Disodium EDTA (additive): An antioxidant used to clarify beverages and retard staling of sandwich spreads, mayonnaises, margarines and salad dressings. It's also used to prevent canned clams, crab and other shellfish from discoloring. Although the body absorbs only about 5 percent of the calcium disodium EDTA swallowed, many believe that this additive is overdue for testing to resolve any questions about its safety. When heated, it gives off toxic nitrous oxide fumes.

Calcium Enriched: Milk is what's usually had calcium added (or yogurt). And though there's no official standard regulating just *how* enriched it is, cartons of "calcium-enriched milk" in supermarket coolers are fortified with 50 percent of the Daily Value (DV) or Reference Daily Intake (RDI) for calcium, which works out to 500 milligrams per cup (8 fluid ounces). But the calcium content of other foods is being boosted, too: flour, breads, cereals. There are even calcium-enriched orange juices on the market and a calcium-enriched cola on the way.

Calcium Lactate (additive): This calcium salt of lactic acid is used to keep canned fruits and vegetables firm, also to pump up the volume of whipped toppings, meringues and angel food cakes. GRAS.

Calcium Propionate (additive): A preservative used in yeast breads to retard molding. It also supplements the body's supply of calcium. GRAS.

Calcium Salts (additives): Calcium carbonate, calcium caseinate, calcium chloride, calcium citrate, calcium phosphates and calcium sulfates are calcium salts. Most are gelling or firming agents and acid neutralizers; the phosphates are leaveners. Most are GRAS.

Calcium Silicate (additive): Its purpose is to keep baking powders and table salts from caking. GRAS, but, make a note, further studies are due because inhaling calcium silicate may trigger respiratory problems.

Calcium Sorbate (additive): A mold inhibitor used primarily in processed cheeses, mayonnaises, cakes, syrups and jellies. GRAS.

Calcium Stearoyl Lactylate (additive): Although it is considered safe, no in-depth studies have been conducted on this chemical. Its purpose is twofold: To condition bread doughs and, as a whipping agent, to increase the volume of squirt-can, nondairy "whipped cream" and of dehydrated and frozen egg whites. What is known is that body enzymes reduce calcium stearoyl lactylate to lactic acid and stearic alcohol—both harmless. See also DOUGH CONDITIONERS.

Calorie: People talk about calories; they damn them, but few know what a calorie is: a unit used to measure energy, specifically the amount of heat necessary to raise the temperature of 1 gram of water 1 degree Celsius. What concerns dieters, however, is food energy, correctly measured with the **Calorie** (with a capital *C*) or **kilocalorie** (kcal), meaning 1,000 calories. However, most dietitians, nutritionists and other food professionals simply use *calorie* (small *c*) when they mean *kilocalorie*. Are all calories created equal? Yes, even though the body seems to pack on fat calories faster than others. As someone said when wolfing down a bowl of superpremium ice cream, "I might as well just glue it on my hips." There's good reason for this. Gram for gram, fat contains more calories (food energy) than either protein or carbohydrate.

1 g fat = 9 calories

1 g protein = 4 calories

1 g carbohydrate = 4 calories

1 g alcohol = 7 calories

How many calories should you consume each day? It depends on your age, height, weight, whether you're active or sedentary, whether you're trying to gain weight, lose weight or maintain weight. And certainly, your basal metabolic rate (see BASAL METABOLISM) is a factor. You gain weight when you consume more calories than your body needs, and lose when you consume fewer. Although there are no hard-and-fast rules, we offer these ballpark figures as a guideline.

MEDIAN RECOMMENDED DAILY CALORIE INTAKES*

Infants:	
Up to 6 months	650
6 months to 1 year	850
Boys and Girls:	
1 to 3 years	1,300
4 to 6 years	1,800
7 to 10 years	2,000
Men:	
11 to 14 years	2,500
15 to 18 years	3,000
19 to 24 years	2,900
25 to 50 years	2,900
51+ years	2,300
Women:	
11 to 50 years	2,200
51+ years	1,900
Pregnant Women:	
First trimester	2,200
Second and third trimesters	2,500
Nursing Mothers:	2,500

*These are average figures only and recommended for moderately active people. Adapted from *Recommended Dietary Allowances,* Tenth Edition (Washington, D.C.: National Academy Press, 1989).

Camembert: Created two hundred years ago by a Norman farmer's wife, this buttery but pungent mold-ripened round is today the most widely exported French cheese. Napoleon, an early fan, kissed the waitress who first served it to him, then named the cheese after the village where this auspicious occasion took place. Although there are plenty of imitations made elsewhere, only Norman Camembert fermented from unpasteurized whole milk is queen. It averages 21 percent butterfat.

NUTRIENT CONTENT OF 1 OUNCE (28 GRAMS) CAMEMBERT

85 calories	239 mg sodium
6 g protein	53 mg potassium
7 g fat, 4 saturated	0 g dietary fiber
20 mg cholesterol	71 RE vitamin A
0 g carbohydrate	0.01 mg thiamin
110 mg calcium	0.14 mg riboflavin
98 mg phosphorus	0.1 mg niacin
0.1 mg iron	0 mg vitamin C

Campylobacter jejuni, Campylobacteriosis: See BACTERIA.

Canadian Bacon: Pork tenderloin that has been cured and smoked like ham. As bacons go, it is ultralean. Because of its lack of fat, Canadian bacon should be sautéed in a nonstick skillet or, better yet, steamed in the skillet with about ¼ cup water.

NUTRIENT CONTENT OF 2 SLICES GRILLED CANADIAN BACON
(about 1½ ounces; 47 grams)

87 calories	726 mg sodium
11 g protein	183 mg potassium
4 g fat, 1 saturated	0 g dietary fiber
27 mg cholesterol	0 RE vitamin A
1 g carbohydrate	0.39 mg thiamin
5 mg calcium	0.09 mg riboflavin
139 mg phosphorus	3.3 mg niacin
0.4 mg iron	10 mg vitamin C

Cancer (diet and): Cancer, first of all, is not a single disease but a large family of them, often characterized by tumors or tumorlike growths. Is there a link between diet and cancer? There have been studies galore—of the Japanese diet, the Japanese American diet, the Finnish diet, the Seventh Day Adventists' lacto-ovo-vegetarian diet—in attempts to link particular eating patterns with cancer or the lack of it. **THE CONCLUSIONS, SO FAR:** Low-fat, high-fiber diets lower the risk of breast, ovary and colon cancer; diets loaded with vitamin A/beta-carotene-rich fruits and vegetables (carrots, mangoes, yams, dark leafy greens) bolster the immune system and, specifically, lower the risk of lung cancer (even of smokers). Vitamin C not only seems to be an all-around cancer fighter but also prevents the conversion of the nitrites present in many vegetables, as well as in cured hams and bacons, to carcinogenic nitrosamines. Too much iron, on the other hand, may increase the risk of colon and rectal cancers, and serious overloads of iron may cause liver cancer. For those who want to lower their risk of cancer, the Food and Nutrition Board of the National Academy of Sciences presently suggests (without officially recommending) a diet that's:

- Low in *all* fat (and that includes polysaturates, which may be more guilty of promoting cancer than saturated fats).

- High in citrus fruits and both the beta-carotene-rich (orange/yellow/dark green) vegetables and the cruciferous (the cabbage) family. These, of course, are high-fiber, too.

- Low in smoked and cured meats and fish.

- Low in possible carcinogens—nitrite-cured meats, for example, because cooking produces NITROSAMINES; moldy peanuts, which may contain a carcinogenic mycotoxin called AFLATOXIN. There's been much *Sturm und Drang* about additives, but in truth these may be only bit players. Cyclamates (artificial sweeteners suspected of being carcinogenic) have been off the market for years. Today, saccharin is the only additive still approved for use that's a possible carcinogen.

- Low in mutagens (possibly carcinogenic chemicals that cause cellular mutations in the body). Among these are: PAHs (polycyclic aromatic hydrocarbons produced when meat is cooked at high heat) and tannins (strong tea contains large doses of tannin).

- Moderate in alcohol (although few people realize it, alcohol can be as carcinogenic as nitrosamines and mycotoxins like aflatoxin). For women, this means no more than 12 ounces of beer a day *or* 5 ounces of wine *or* 1½ ounces of whiskey. For men, moderate drinking means about twice that—2 bottles of beer a day *or* 2 glasses of wine *or* 2 (1½-ounce) shots of whiskey.

It's important, too, to monitor drinking water (sometimes the source of powerful carcinogens), to vary the diet as much as possible, not to pig out and to keep weight under control (obesity may raise the risk of some cancers). And never underestimate the benefits of exercise. It may reduce the risk of breast cancer, according to a new Los Angeles study conducted by the University of Southern California School of Medicine. And the younger you are, the better. For example, the study found that teenage girls who exercise three to four hours a week can cut their chances of getting breast cancer by half. Older women who work out regularly improve their odds, too, but not so dramatically.

Candy: The trouble with candy is that kids love it; indeed, some never outgrow their sweet tooth. If indulgent parents keep candy jars well stocked, children are likely to snack on candy (few candies offer little more than empty calories), then turn up their noses come dinnertime when nutritious food is put on the table. Sticky candies—caramels, gumdrops, toffees, taffies—are particularly bad because they stick to the teeth and accelerate decay. Chocolates actually inhibit the formation of plaque and cavities somewhat, but they're full of fat, much of it saturated. Candies are poor choices for hypoglycemics (those with low blood sugar) because they send blood sugar levels soaring, then plummeting.

Canning: When Napoleon sounded the call for ways to provision French troops with rations that would prevent scurvy (see C, VITAMIN), Nicolas Appert sealed food in jars, then subjected them to intense heat for many minutes. An effective way to conserve food, it turned out, although the high temperatures destroyed not only some of the vitamin C but much of the thiamin (B₁), too. Canning still destroys some vitamin C and thiamin although methods have improved significantly and modern canned foods (whether put up in metal cans, plastic or paperboard cartons, flexible pouches or glass jars) offer a nutritious alternative to fresh and frozen food. If glass jars are used instead of opaque containers, the food loses some of its riboflavin (B₂), a vitamin that succumbs to light. A further problem with canned foods is that many of them are excessively salty. Choose low- or reduced-sodium brands or rinse canned tuna, salmon, sardines, anchovies and whole or diced vegetables in cool running water to sluice away some of the salt. Occasionally there are faulty batches of canned food

and desperate recalls by the manufacturer because of possible bacterial contamination (see BACTERIA). Reject any cans that are severely dented or bulging. Do not taste any canned food that you suspect may be spoiled. Dispose of it at once where neither people nor animals can get at it.

Canola Oil: When canola oil first appeared on grocery shelves a few years back, everyone wondered what a canola was. Not a nut or a seed, it turns out, but the acronym of the Canadian company that developed it—*can* for Canada, *ol* for oil, and *a* just to give the word a flourish. Canola is rapeseed oil, a liquid fat pressed from the seeds of a member of the mustard family that's long been known in Europe. Early on, canola got good press in the United States because it's extremely low in saturated fatty acids (4 percent), relatively high in monounsaturates (55 percent) and polyunsaturates (35 percent). It's a thin, pale oil, and though it's okay for sautéing, it hasn't got much oomph. Today, with the nutritional benefits of polyunsaturated fatty acids in question (they don't protect and maintain blood levels of "good" cholesterol, or HDL, the way monounsaturated fatty acids do and there's even some worry that they may be carcinogenic), some nutritionists now suggest replacing canola with olive oil. Canola's lower than olive oil in polyunsaturates but higher in the monounsaturates that boost blood levels of "good" cholesterol, thereby lowering total cholesterol. In many quarters, it's already become the cooking oil of choice—even for sweets. See also OLIVE OIL.

Cantaloupe: See MELONS.

Capers: The pickled or brined buds of a wild, sprawling Mediterranean bush that have been used for centuries as a condiment. Although this book is not a dictionary of food, we include capers because their tart, resiny/lemony flavor is so intense it punches up the flavor of low-fat sauces and salad dressings. The choicest of all are the tiny *non pareilles* and for most seasoning jobs, a tablespoon of them is all that's needed. **NOTE:** As for nutritive value, capers offer very little other than sodium—up to 150 to 170 milligrams per tablespoon depending upon how they were processed. If you've been told to cut down on salt, better skip the capers. Or drain and rinse them very well.

Capon: A cock castrated while young so that it becomes fleshier, fatter. Capons average 4 to 7 pounds and roast to supreme succulence. Now with everyone trying to cut down on fat, will capons become extinct? Not likely, though there may be less demand for them. See also CHICKEN.

NUTRIENT CONTENT OF 3 OUNCES (85 GRAMS) ROASTED CAPON (WITH SKIN)

194 calories	41 mg sodium
24 g protein	216 mg potassium
10 g fat, 3 saturated	0 g dietary fiber
72 mg cholesterol	17 RE vitamin A
0 g carbohydrate	0.06 mg thiamin
12 mg calcium	0.14 mg riboflavin
208 mg phosphorus	7.1 mg niacin
1.2 mg iron	0 mg vitamin C

Cappuccino: This cinnamon-dusted Italian hot coffee/milk drink is becoming as popular in America as pizza.

NUTRIENT CONTENT OF 1 CUP CAPPUCCINO (DRY MIX + WATER)

(8 fluid ounces; 242 grams)

82 calories	137 mg sodium
1 g protein	159 mg potassium
3 g fat, 2 saturated	0 g dietary fiber
0 mg cholesterol	0 RE vitamin A
14 g carbohydrate	0.02 mg thiamin
10 mg calcium	0.01 mg riboflavin
36 mg phosphorus	0.4 mg niacin
0.2 mg iron	0 mg vitamin C

Caprenin: A new fat substitute that apes the flavor and "mouth feel" of chocolate. Synthesized from fats the body only partly absorbs, it contains 40 percent fewer calories that cocoa butter but, alas, no less saturated fat.

Capsaicin, Capsaicinoids: The fiery ingredients in chiles and other hot red and green peppers. Extracted, purified and added to rub-on creams, capsaicin has been used with some success to ease the pain of arthritis, osteoarthritis, cluster headaches, neuralgia, diabetic neuropathy and mastectomies. Unlike conventional rubefacients, which merely "warm" and relax muscles, capsaicin depletes the nerve endings' supply of substance P, a messenger of pain that shoots impulses to the central nervous system. The newest development is that researchers are experimenting with capsaicin as a treatment for the pressure and congestion of sinusitis and rhinitis—so far with impressive results. There is even some talk—but no proof, alas—that capsaicin may ratchet up the metabolism.

Carambolas: Now being grown in Florida, these pleated, waxy-skinned yellow Asian fruits now appear with some regularity in upscale groceries. Star-shaped when sliced (they're also called **star fruit**), carambolas can be crisply sweet or turn-your-mouth-inside-out sour. A good sniff should tell you which you're buying—the sweet are pleasantly flowery. How to describe a carambola's flavor? It's part apple, part grape. **SEASON:** September till mid-February.

NUTRIENT CONTENT OF 1 MEDIUM-SIZE CARAMBOLA

(about 4½ ounces; 130 grams)

42 calories	2 mg sodium
1 g protein	207 mg potassium
0 g fat, 0 saturated	2 g dietary fiber
0 mg cholesterol	63 RE vitamin A
10 g carbohydrate	0.04 mg thiamin
6 mg calcium	0.03 mg riboflavin
20 mg phosphorus	0.5 mg niacin
0.3 mg iron	27 mg vitamin C

Caramels: See CANDY.

Carbohydrate Loading: See ENERGY BOOSTERS.

Carbohydrates: Put simply, these are sugars and starches. Body fuel. When runners bulk up on carbohydrates before a marathon, they know what they're doing. Our bodies run on carbs much the way cars run on gas. Complex carbohydrates (those in pasta, the runner's favorite, potatoes, rice, dried peas and beans, grains) are nothing more than fancy configurations of hundreds, often thousands of glucose (simple sugar) molecules. Our bodies don't break these down into usable form very fast, especially if fiber is also present. Nutritionally speaking, all carbohydrates fall into one of three basic groups:

Monosaccharides (simple sugars): These include FRUCTOSE (fruit sugar) and GLUCOSE, often called blood sugar because it's what all carbohydrates are broken down into in the body. Only glucose circulates in the blood, providing energy to organs, glands, muscles, indeed to every cell. Finally, there is GALACTOSE, which rarely stands alone but does combine with other simple sugars, notably with glucose to form LACTOSE (milk sugar).

Disaccharides (double sugars): Nothing more than bonded pairs of simple sugars. There is sucrose (table sugar), GLUCOSE plus FRUCTOSE; LACTOSE (milk sugar), glucose plus GALACTOSE; and MALTOSE (malt sugar), two linked glucose molecules.

Polysaccharides (complex carbohydrates): Elaborate chains of GLUCOSE molecules, which from a nutritional standpoint are far and away the most important because they digest more slowly than simple or double sugars. Found in peas, beans, grains, potatoes and other starchy plants, they come freighted with dietary fiber, vitamins and minerals.

As far as calories are concerned, however, all carbohydrates are created equal. The monosaccharides, disaccharides and polysaccharides all weigh in at 4 calories per gram. Still, for all their pluses, too many carbs, like too much fat or protein, will put on the pounds. What nutritionists now recommend: Make 55 to 60 percent of your daily calories "carbohydrate calories."

Carbon: A nonmetallic element present in all organic compounds and that includes food. Carbohydrates, for example, are composed of carbon, hydrogen and oxygen.

Carbonated Beverages: The bubbles in seltzer, colas and other soft drinks are merely carbon dioxide, pumped in under pressure. Carbonated beverages are slightly acid, many are intensely sweet, thus regular use may, over time, etch the teeth and encourage cavity formation. Because soft drinks are extremely high in phosphates, nutritionists once believed they impaired the body's ability to absorb calcium and that women were in particular jeopardy. But after a number of new tests, nutritionists have done a one-eighty. Soft-drink phosphates, they now agree, pose no problem.

What does is caffeine. Extracted from kola nuts, it's integral to colas. And though the government strictly regulates its use (the total caffeine content must not exceed 0.02 percent, by weight, of the finished product), anyone downing half a dozen or more colas a day risks elevated blood pressure, increased anxiety, sweating and inability to concentrate. Some research (albeit controversial) points to a correlation between caffeine abuse and fibrocystic breast disease, cardiovascular disease and heart attack. Four (12-ounce) colas a day are considered moderate caffeine use—not risky.

The single biggest soft-drink problem is that many people—children and teenagers especially—use them to the exclusion of all other beverages. That means they're missing out on milk and the nutrients it supplies. Soft drinks offer little more than phosphorus, sugar or suspect artificial sweeteners. And what about the old theory that fizzy drinks are good for upset stomachs and acid indigestion? A little sparkling water or ginger ale, slowly sipped, may ease the symptoms. Certainly, it will do no harm. Indeed, two British surgeons recently found that carbonated drinks help break up pieces of unchewed food that sometimes get trapped in a narrow esophagus.

Carboxymethyl Cellulose (CMC) (additive): This water-soluble gum is used to thicken, bind and stabilize salad dressings, sauces, puddings, ice creams and baked goods. Because the body can't absorb it, it's considered safe when used in moderate amounts (0.05 to 0.5 percent, by weight, of the finished product).

Carcinogen: Any substance that can cause cancer. Carcinogens exist in the food we eat, the tobacco smoke we inhale, the water we drink, the air we breathe.

Cardiovascular Disease: See CORONARY HEART DISEASE.

Cardoons: These primitive artichokes, much appreciated in Italy and once popular among American colonists, had plummeted from favor. Now they're on the comeback trail and show up not only at specialty greengrocers but also,

NUTRIENT CONTENT OF 1 CUP STEAMED CARDOONS	
(about 7 ounces; 200 grams)	
44 calories	352 mg sodium
2 g protein	784 mg potassium
0 g fat, 0 saturated	NA g dietary fiber
0 mg cholesterol	24 RE vitamin A
10 g carbohydrate	0.04 mg thiamin
144 mg calcium	0.06 mg riboflavin
46 mg phosphorus	0.6 mg niacin
1.4 mg iron	4 mg vitamin C

sometimes, in big-city supermarkets. Though prickly, cardoons look more like celery than artichokes. Their flavor, however, is definitely artichoke. But bitterer. If young, tender and not overly astringent, cardoons can be sliced into salads or served, like celery, with a cocktail dip. Otherwise, they should be steamed and sauced. **SEASON:** Winter and early spring.

Cariogenic: Anything that promotes tooth decay. When it comes to food, candies—especially caramels, taffies, toffees, gumdrops that stick to the teeth—might be called hypercariogenic. Those who snack on candies are at particular risk if they don't brush their teeth after each piece of candy.

Carnitine: A nitrogen-based nutrient needed by the body to oxidize (metabolize) complex fatty acids. The liver and kidneys manufacture carnitine out of two amino acids (glutamine and methionine); meat and dairy foods provide more of it. Those most apt to lack carnitine are formula-fed babies. For that reason, infant formulas are fortified with carnitine. Contrary to popular opinion, athletes aren't likely to improve their performances by bulking up on carnitine. Some supplements—those containing D-carnitine—may actually weaken the muscles because D-carnitine decreases the body's own supply of it. L-carnitine supplements are believed to be safe. Just don't expect them to turn you into Superman or Wonder Woman.

Carob: For years health faddists have been substituting carob powder for cocoa. Like cocoa, it comes from the pod of a tropical tree. Unlike cocoa, carob is low in fat (1 percent versus 23 percent) but high in sugar (48 percent versus 5 percent). To some, carob tastes unpleasantly perfumy. Certainly it lacks the finesse, the deeply satisfying flavor of cocoa.

NUTRIENT CONTENT OF 1 TABLESPOON CAROB POWDER
(about 1/5 ounce; 6 grams)

25 calories	239 mg sodium
0 g protein	53 mg potassium
0 g fat, 0 saturated	1 g dietary fiber
0 mg cholesterol	0 RE vitamin A
6 g carbohydrate	0 mg thiamin
22 mg calcium	0.03 mg riboflavin
6 mg phosphorus	0.1 mg niacin
0.2 mg iron	0 mg vitamin C

Carob-Seed Gum, Locust Bean Gum (additive): Once used by Egyptians to make mummy bindings stick, carob-seed gum is today a popular thickener and texturizer for commercial ice creams, salad dressings, sauces and pie fillings. It's also used to improve the plasticity of doughs. Though considered safe by the FDA, carob-seed gum is a mild laxative and thus, consumer watchdogs believe, merits further testing. GRAS.

Carotene, Carotenoids: Vivid yellow and orange pigments that give sweet potatoes, winter squash, carrots, apricots, papayas and other fruits and vegetables their intense color (they are also abundant in broccoli and such dark leafy greens as kale, collards and spinach). In addition, these pigments are widely used by food processors to color butter, margarine, shortening, nondairy creamers, whipped toppings and cake mixes. Of the 600-odd carotenoids so far identified, BETA-CAROTENE, which the body converts to vitamin A, is far and away the best known, yet it accounts for only 25 percent of the edible carotenoids. Not all carotenoids end up in the body as vitamin A; still, many are such powerful antioxidants that their anticarcinogenic properties may actually exceed that of beta-carotene. Some of them also help protect against cardiovascular disease and such eye conditions as macular degeneration. Medical researchers now believe that the different carotenoids working in concert, not isolated forms of beta-carotene are what do the job. Mother always told us to eat our fruits and vegetables, and it turns out Mother knew best. Among the less well-known (but no less powerful) carotenoids present in food are **alpha-carotene** (found in carrots), a vitamin A precursor that may boost the immune system and lower the risk of lung cancer; **beta-cryptoxanthin** (mangoes, oranges, papayas, tangerines), also a precursor of vitamin A; **canthaxanthin** (a natural food color), which strengthens the immune system and reduces the risk of skin cancer in lab rats; **lutein** (broccoli, dark leafy greens), which decreases the risk of lung cancer; and **lycopene** (the red pigment in tomatoes), which also reduces the risk of cancer, specifically bladder and colon cancers.

Carp: Asians have relished these fat freshwater fish almost since the beginning of time. In Europe, their popularity dates to the Middle Ages, when monks built immense carp ponds to provide them with "meat" in an age when fast days outnumbered feast days. Carp remains a particular favorite in Germany, where it's cooked in beer for Christmas

Eve and in red wine for New Year's Eve. Not many Americans appreciate carp because its flavor is often musky. It deserves to be used for something other than gefilte fish.

NUTRIENT CONTENT OF 3 OUNCES (85 GRAMS) BAKED CARP (WITHOUT SKIN)

138 calories	54 mg sodium
19 g protein	363 mg potassium
6 g fat, 1 saturated	0 g dietary fiber
72 mg cholesterol	8 RE vitamin A
0 g carbohydrate	0.12 mg thiamin
44 mg calcium	0.06 mg riboflavin
452 mg phosphorus	1.8 mg niacin
1.4 mg iron	1 mg vitamin C

Carrageenan (additive): Obtained from Irish moss (a seaweed), carrageenan is a stabilizer/emulsifier used to add creaminess to sherbets, ice creams, assorted chocolate products, salad dressings and aerosol whipped creams. GRAS.

Carrot Juice: The vegetarian's favorite tipple and a nutritional powerhouse it is. Too much of it, however, can turn the skin yellow.

Carrots: Carrots may be one of the earliest foods eaten by man. Native to Asia, they were being cultivated throughout the Mediterranean long before Christ was born. Greeks wrote of them, though not with particular

Braised Carrots and Onion with Bulgur

Makes 4 Servings

- 2 tablespoons fruity olive oil
- 1 medium yellow onion, coarsely chopped
- 2 medium carrots, peeled and coarsely shredded
- 1 teaspoon curry powder
- ¼ teaspoon freshly ground coriander seeds (preferably green Indian coriander)
- 1 cup bulgur
- ¼ cup dried currants (optional)
- 1¾ cups chicken broth
- ½ teaspoon salt, or to taste
- ¼ teaspoon freshly ground black pepper, or to taste

COAT A MEDIUM heavy saucepan with nonstick spray, add the oil, and heat 1 minute. Add the onion and carrots and stir-fry 8 to 10 minutes over moderate heat, until golden. Add the curry powder, coriander, and bulgur and stir-fry 2 to 3 minutes, just until the bulgur glistens and looks translucent. Add the currants, if you like, and the broth and bring to a simmer. Adjust the heat so the mixture bubbles gently, then simmer uncovered for about 20 minutes or until all liquid is absorbed and the bulgur is firm-tender. Season with salt and pepper and serve with pork or lamb in place of potatoes.

APPROXIMATE NUTRIENT COUNTS PER SERVING

250 calories	40 g carbohydrate	1.9 mg iron	0.12 mg thiamin
8 g protein	8 g dietary fiber	636 mg sodium	0.11 mg riboflavin
8 g fat, 1 saturated	44 mg calcium	441 mg potassium	3.6 mg niacin
0 mg cholesterol	169 mg phosphorus	814 RE vitamin A	2 mg vitamin C

fondness (the Romans preferred turnips). Carrots were one of the vegetables Charlemagne ordered to be planted throughout his dominions and one of the Old World vegetables the English introduced to the New. Today, of course, they're as common as peas or beans. Carrots owe their brilliant color to beta-carotene, a vitamin A precursor that's known to be anticarcinogenic (see CAROTENE), and are second only to beets in natural sugars. **SEASON:** Year-round.

NUTRIENT CONTENT OF 1 CUP BOTTLED CARROT JUICE
(8 fluid ounces; 246 grams)

98 calories	71 mg sodium
2 g protein	718 mg potassium
0 g fat, 0 saturated	3 g dietary fiber
0 mg cholesterol	6,332 RE vitamin A
23 g carbohydrate	0.23 mg thiamin
59 mg calcium	0.14 mg riboflavin
103 mg phosphorus	1.0 mg niacin
1.1 mg iron	21 mg vitamin C

NUTRIENT CONTENT OF 1 MEDIUM-SIZE RAW CARROT
(about 2½ ounces; 72 grams)

31 calories	25 mg sodium
1 g protein	233 mg potassium
0 g fat, 0 saturated	2 g dietary fiber
0 mg cholesterol	2,025 RE vitamin A
7 g carbohydrate	0.07 mg thiamin
19 mg calcium	0.04 mg riboflavin
32 mg phosphorus	0.7 mg niacin
0.4 mg iron	7 mg vitamin C

Shredded Carrots Scrambled with Red Onion, Lemon, and Lime

Makes 6 Servings

A beta-carotene-rich stir-fry from the South of France.

2 tablespoons fruity olive oil
1½ pounds carrots, peeled and coarsely shredded
1 large red onion, coarsely chopped
1 medium garlic clove, minced
½ teaspoon dried marjoram

¼ teaspoon dried thyme
2 tablespoons fresh lemon juice
2 tablespoons fresh lime juice
¼ teaspoon salt, or to taste
⅛ teaspoon freshly ground black pepper, or to taste

COAT A LARGE heavy skillet with nonstick cooking spray, add the oil, and heat 1 minute over moderately high heat. Add the carrots and onion, and stir-fry 3 minutes. Add the garlic, marjoram, and thyme and stir-fry 3 to 5 minutes, until vegetables are crisp-tender. Sprinkle with the lemon and lime juices, salt, and pepper, and serve hot or cold.

APPROXIMATE NUTRIENT COUNTS PER SERVING

98 calories	14 g carbohydrate	0.8 mg iron	0.05 mg thiamin
1 g protein	3 g dietary fiber	159 mg sodium	0.07 mg riboflavin
5 g fat, 1 saturated	40 mg calcium	281 mg potassium	0.6 mg niacin
0 mg cholesterol	39 mg phosphorus	2,561 RE vitamin A	8 mg vitamin C

NUTRIENT CONTENT OF 1 CUP COOKED UNSEASONED SLICED CARROTS

(about 5¼ ounces; 156 grams)

70 calories	104 mg sodium
2 g protein	354 mg potassium
0 g fat, 0 saturated	4 g dietary fiber
0 mg cholesterol	3,830 RE vitamin A
16 g carbohydrate	0.06 mg thiamin
48 mg calcium	0.08 mg riboflavin
48 mg phosphorus	0.8 mg niacin
1.0 mg iron	4 mg vitamin C

Casaba: See MELONS.

Casein: The major protein in milk. It's now used to fortify processed cheeses, breads and cereals.

Cashews: In 1500, Portuguese explorer Pedro Alvarez Cabral discovered these tropical nuts in Brazil and carried them to India, where they are now grown on a wide scale. Like all nuts, cashews are extremely rich in fat. They're 47 percent fat, 22 percent carbohydrate, 21 percent protein and packed with potassium and phosphorus. Small wonder they've sustained people for ages.

NUTRIENT CONTENT OF ½ CUP UNSALTED OIL-ROASTED CASHEWS

(about 2¼ ounces; 65 grams)

374 calories	11* mg sodium
11 g protein	345 mg potassium
31 g fat, 2 saturated	4 g dietary fiber
0 mg cholesterol	0 RE vitamin A
19 g carbohydrate	0.28 mg thiamin
27 mg calcium	0.11 mg riboflavin
277 mg phosphorus	1.2 mg niacin
2.7 mg iron	0 mg vitamin C

*If nuts are salted, add 407 milligrams sodium per ½ cup.

Cassava: Next to the sweet potato, the cassava, also called **manioc,** is the most important food crop grown in the tropics and subtropics. There are more than 150 varieties but just two basic types: **Bitter cassavas,** which contain high levels of deadly cyanide, and **sweet cassavas** (with little or no cyanide, these only need to be cooked). Bitter cassavas must be soaked (usually after being pounded to pulp) or fermented to rid them of poison. Cassavas are endlessly versatile. They can be boiled like potatoes or ground and baked in thin cakes. They can even be made into TAPIOCA.

NUTRIENT CONTENT OF 1 CUP COOKED UNSEASONED CASSAVA

(about 5 ounces; 137 grams)

267 calories	450 mg sodium
4 g protein	837 mg potassium
14 g fat, 3 saturated	1 g dietary fiber
0 mg cholesterol	185 RE vitamin A
33 g carbohydrate	0.22 mg thiamin
110 mg calcium	0.12 mg riboflavin
80 mg phosphorus	1.5 mg niacin
4.1 mg iron	38 mg vitamin C

Catalyst: A substance that accelerates a chemical reaction without itself being permanently changed. Catalysts are effective in tiny doses and are recycled rather than depleted. For example, to speed the breakdown of protein into amino acids, the stomach secretes hydrochloric acid, which acts as a catalyst. The amino acids then move into the small intestine, where they are absorbed and used to maintain body tissue.

Cataracts (diet and): This clouding of the lens of the eye usually—but not always—occurs in older people. It impairs vision and can, unless treated, lead to blindness. The latest protocol is to remove the clouded lens and replace it with a plastic implant. Scientists have observed possible links between cataracts and excessive dietary protein, fat, sugar (particularly lactose or milk sugar) and calories. They further suspect that deficiencies of vitamins B_2 (riboflavin) and E, also of the minerals selenium and zinc, may play a role. More promising are the results of a recent Harvard study of more than fifty thousand women: Those whose diets were fortified by beta-carotene were 40 percent less apt to require cataract surgery than those who consumed little of this important antioxidant. Subsequent studies in Finland suggest that two additional antioxidants—vitamins C and E—may also lower the risk of cataracts. **CAUTION, SMOKERS:** You are more apt to develop cataracts than nonsmokers because smoke is thought to destroy antioxidants circulating in the body.

Catfish: How Southerners dote on "cats," fresh caught, breaded, fried and sent forth with a big basket of hush puppies. Now that cats are being farm raised in the Deep South, fish lovers all over the country can sink their teeth into these sweet-meated fish. They are surprisingly lean and delicate, unlike those pulled from brown rivers, which taste mostly like mud.

NUTRIENT CONTENT OF 3 OUNCES (85 GRAMS) FRIED, BREADED, SKINNED CATFISH	
228 calories	458 mg sodium
18 g protein	325 mg potassium
12 g fat, 3 saturated	1 g dietary fiber
78 mg cholesterol	27 RE vitamin A
10 g carbohydrate	0.07 mg thiamin
57 mg calcium	0.16 mg riboflavin
212 mg phosphorus	2.4 mg niacin
1.5 mg iron	0 mg vitamin C

Cauliflower: What Mark Twain called "a cabbage with a college education" probably comes from Asia. It was known in Roman times but apparently never crossed the Alps into northern Europe until the Renaissance. Not much later, the English brought cauliflower to the American colonies. Because of its buttery texture, filling nature and mild, almost meaty flavor, this elegant member of the cabbage family has managed to satisfy people in meatless times. Indeed, in northern Europe it was once popular Lenten food. Among cauliflower's blessings: It is extremely low in calories and sodium but high in vitamin C and potassium. **SEASON:** Year-round.

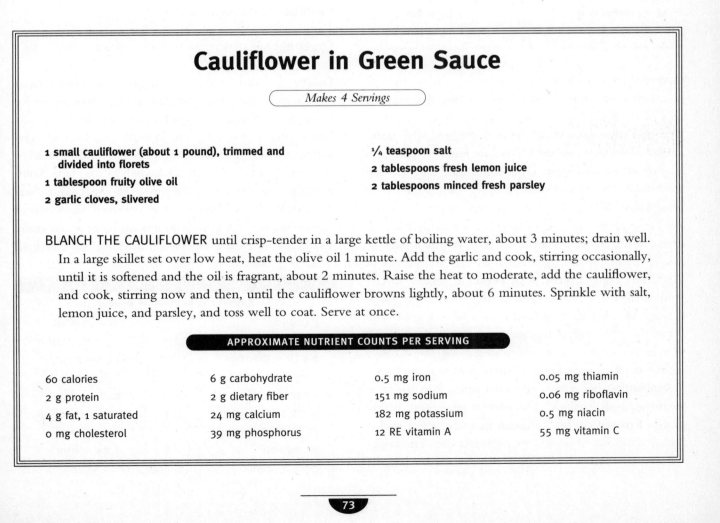

Cauliflower in Green Sauce

Makes 4 Servings

1 small cauliflower (about 1 pound), trimmed and divided into florets

1 tablespoon fruity olive oil

2 garlic cloves, slivered

¼ teaspoon salt

2 tablespoons fresh lemon juice

2 tablespoons minced fresh parsley

BLANCH THE CAULIFLOWER until crisp-tender in a large kettle of boiling water, about 3 minutes; drain well. In a large skillet set over low heat, heat the olive oil 1 minute. Add the garlic and cook, stirring occasionally, until it is softened and the oil is fragrant, about 2 minutes. Raise the heat to moderate, add the cauliflower, and cook, stirring now and then, until the cauliflower browns lightly, about 6 minutes. Sprinkle with salt, lemon juice, and parsley, and toss well to coat. Serve at once.

APPROXIMATE NUTRIENT COUNTS PER SERVING			
60 calories	6 g carbohydrate	0.5 mg iron	0.05 mg thiamin
2 g protein	2 g dietary fiber	151 mg sodium	0.06 mg riboflavin
4 g fat, 1 saturated	24 mg calcium	182 mg potassium	0.5 mg niacin
0 mg cholesterol	39 mg phosphorus	12 RE vitamin A	55 mg vitamin C

NUTRIENT CONTENT OF 1 CUP RAW CAULIFLOWER FLORETS
(about 3½ ounces; 100 grams)

24 calories	14 mg sodium
2 g protein	356 mg potassium
0 g fat, 0 saturated	2 g dietary fiber
0 mg cholesterol	2 RE vitamin A
5 g carbohydrate	0.08 mg thiamin
28 mg calcium	0.06 mg riboflavin
46 mg phosphorus	0.6 mg niacin
0.6 mg iron	46 mg vitamin C

NUTRIENT CONTENT OF 1 CUP COOKED UNSEASONED CAULIFLOWER FLORETS
(about 4¼ ounces; 124 grams)

30 calories	8 mg sodium
2 g protein	400 mg potassium
1 g fat, 0 saturated	3 g dietary fiber
0 mg cholesterol	2 RE vitamin A
6 g carbohydrate	0.08 mg thiamin
34 mg calcium	0.06 mg riboflavin
44 mg phosphorus	0.7 mg niacin
0.5 mg iron	55 mg vitamin C

Caviar: Although the roe of many fish have for years been passed off as caviar, the FDA decreed in 1966 that only the eggs of sturgeon could be sold as caviar in this country. This near-prehistoric family of fish, armored with plates instead of scales, sometimes lives one hundred years and may weigh a ton or more. Once so plentiful they jammed the Hudson River at spawning time, sturgeon are now being killed off by polluted waters. Not only in the Western Hemisphere but also in the Caspian and Black seas, source of the choice beluga caviar. The **beluga** is the biggest of the different sturgeons and its eggs are the size of BBs. Next come **osetra,** then **sevruga,** smaller species with smaller roe. Colors vary, too—from near black through silvery gray to golden brown to true gold. The last of these was called the czar's caviar because nearly all of this rare **sterlet roe** was reserved for the Russian court—or, if taken in Persian waters, for the shah of Iran.

Malosol is not a type of caviar but a Russian term meaning "lightly salted" (the best caviar *is* only lightly salted). **Pressed caviar** is inferior in every way, a sticky, fishy paste made of broken or imperfect roe. The bright red-orange "berries" of salmon roe cannot, by law, be called caviar but they are much appreciated. Other "caviars" include the gritty black lumpfish eggs popular throughout Scandinavia and the small orange-gold herring roe. As for nutritive value, all caviar is oily and extremely high in sodium because it must be salted if it's to last more than a day. It's loaded with cholesterol, too. The good news? Caviar contains plenty of iron and vitamin A. See also FISH ROE.

NUTRIENT CONTENT OF 1 OUNCE (28 GRAMS) BLACK CAVIAR

71 calories	425 mg sodium
7 g protein	51 mg potassium
5 g fat, 1 saturated	0 g dietary fiber
167 mg cholesterol	159 RE vitamin A
1 g carbohydrate	0.05 mg thiamin
78 mg calcium	0.18 mg riboflavin
101 mg phosphorus	0 mg niacin
3.4 mg iron	0 mg vitamin C

Cavities: See DENTAL HEALTH.

Cayenne: See HOT PEPPERS under PEPPERS, CAPSICUMS.

Celery: The first celery was a wild stalky plant that thrived in bogs along the eastern Mediterranean. Once prized for its decorative leaves, celery wasn't much eaten by the ancients. And didn't come into its own until modern agricultural methods produced crisp, sweet, succulent stalks or ribs as individual branches are known in the trade. Until recently, most of the celery grown in this country was mounded with dirt so the sun-deprived stalks stayed creamy white. Today, with Americans more nutritionally aware, green **Pascal celery** is outselling the bleached.

NUTRIENT CONTENT OF 1 MEDIUM-SIZE RIB CELERY
(about 1½ ounces; 40 grams)

6 calories	35 mg sodium
0 g protein	115 mg potassium
0 g fat, 0 saturated	1 g dietary fiber
0 mg cholesterol	5 RE vitamin A
1 g carbohydrate	0.02 mg thiamin
16 mg calcium	0.02 mg riboflavin
10 mg phosphorus	0.1 mg niacin
0.2 mg iron	3 mg vitamin C

Chlorophyll (the green pigment), most people now understand, generally means more vitamins A and C. **Season:** Year-round.

NUTRIENT CONTENT OF 1 CUP COOKED UNSEASONED SLICED CELERY

(about 5¼ ounces; 150 grams)

26 calories	136 mg sodium
1 g protein	426 mg potassium
0 g fat, 0 saturated	2 g dietary fiber
0 mg cholesterol	20 RE vitamin A
6 g carbohydrate	0.06 mg thiamin
63 mg calcium	0.07 mg riboflavin
38 mg phosphorus	0.5 mg niacin
0.6 mg iron	9 mg vitamin C

Celery Cabbage: See CHINESE CABBAGE.

Celery Root, Celeriac: This big, bulbous species with fibrous brown skin has always been more popular in Europe than here. It is the celery of celery remoulade, and

NUTRIENT CONTENT OF 1 CUP RAW SHREDDED CELERY ROOT

(about 5½ ounces; 160 grams)

62 calories	156 mg sodium
2 g protein	468 mg potassium
1 g fat, 0 saturated	7 g dietary fiber
0 mg cholesterol	0 RE vitamin A
14 g carbohydrate	0.08 mg thiamin
67 mg calcium	0.09 mg riboflavin
179 mg phosphorus	1.1 mg niacin
1.1 mg iron	13 mg vitamin C

NUTRIENT CONTENT OF ½ CUP BOILED UNSEASONED CELERY ROOT

(about 3½ ounces; 100 grams)

25 calories	61 mg sodium
1 g protein	173 mg potassium
0 g fat, 0 saturated	4 g dietary fiber
0 mg cholesterol	0 RE vitamin A
6 g carbohydrate	0.03 mg thiamin
26 mg calcium	0.04 mg riboflavin
66 mg phosphorus	0.4 mg niacin
0.4 mg iron	4 mg vitamin C

when pureed and mixed half and half with mashed potatoes, it is superb. Because of its meaty, mellow flavor, Germans slice celery root, blanch it quickly in acidulated water (for it darkens when cut), bread it and fry it like schnitzel. **Season:** Autumn through early spring.

Celiac Disease, Celiac Sprue: See GLUTEN INTOLERANCE.

Cellophane Noodles, Bean Thread Noodles: These fine, translucent noodles made from mung-bean starch are so fragile they need only a quick soaking in hot water or frizzle in hot oil before they're used. To the Chinese, long noodles symbolize long life, so they are not cut but slurped.

NUTRIENT CONTENT OF 1 CUP COOKED CELLOPHANE NOODLES

(about 6¾ ounces; 190 grams)

160 calories	9 mg sodium
0 g protein	5 mg potassium
0 g fat, 0 saturated	0 g dietary fiber
0 mg cholesterol	0 RE vitamin A
39 g carbohydrate	0.07 mg thiamin
14 mg calcium	0 mg riboflavin
15 mg phosphorus	0.1 mg niacin
1 mg iron	0 mg vitamin C

Cellulose: A fibrous, complex carbohydrate that humans cannot digest. It occurs naturally in many grains, fruits and vegetables and contains no calories or other nutrients but is an important source of dietary fiber. Powdered cellulose is often added to low-calorie liquid meals to give them bulk.

Cèpes: See MUSHROOMS.

Cereals: One of the most important food groups and one of the largest, too, as a cruise down any supermarket aisle quickly proves. There are brans, flakes, puffs, granules, shreds, mini biscuits, whole grains plus assorted high-calorie granolas and mueslis (grain/fruit/nut combos). There are wheat cereals, rice, corn, oat and any number of blends—to say nothing of shelves of the sugar-coated, frosted or honeyed varieties beloved by children. There are ready-to-eat cereals and those that must be cooked, not to mention scores of instants that need only be mixed with hot liquid and heated briefly. Most nutritionists favor simple whole-grain cereals, and the less adulterated (the less sugary, the less salty) the better. Fans of processed cereals should read labels carefully to make sure that their favorites provide adequate amounts of iron and B vitamins and that they're low in fat, sugar and sodium. See also entries for individual grains: CORN; OATS; RICE; WHEAT; etc.

Chamomile Tea: The dried yellow flowers of chamomile, a Eurasian medicinal plant of ancient lineage, are steeped in hot water to obtain an infusion that's pleasantly but pungently grassy. Caffeine free, chamomile tea is not only a digestive but also a mild tranquilizer and soporific. But make a note, chamomile belongs to the ragweed family, so anyone sensitive to ragweed—also to such other family members as asters and chrysanthemums—may be allergic to chamomile.

Chanterelles: See MUSHROOMS.

Chaparral: This toxic herb was marketed as a "fountain of youth," as a blood cleanser, even as an acne cure—*after* the FDA ordered all chaparral products pulled off the market. The teas and tablets compounded of chaparral, a shrub native to the American Southwest, are known to cause acute toxic hepatitis, a life-threatening liver disease. Anyone taking chaparral in any form should stop. *At once.*

Charcoal: Used in the food and wine industries to clarify grape juice, sherries and other wines; also to decolorize, deodorize and purify fats, especially such refined animal fats as lard.

Charcoal Grilling: It's the great American summer pastime, firing up the backyard grill and charcoal broiling everything from T-bones to burgers to fish to skewered vegetables. What few people realize is that charcoal grilling may be hazardous to their health if done too often. Many forms of cooking—but grilling in particular—cause known carcinogens, polycyclic aromatic hydrocarbons (see PAHS), to form. There are, however, ways to lower the risk:

1. Trim as much fat from food as possible before grilling. Better yet, choose low-fat foods. Fat melts as food grills, drippings sputter down upon the coals raising clouds of smoke, which deposit carcinogenic PAHs on the food.

2. Douse flare-ups the instant they occur.

3. Minimize cooking times by partially cooking food before it goes on the grill.

4. Grill over less intense heat and at a greater distance from the coals.

5. Don't char or overbrown food.

6. Don't use oily bastes.

7. Grill food in foil or pans whenever possible.

8. Never use wads of paper or kindling to fuel grills or even as starters.

9. If tossing aromatic wood chips onto the coals, use only hard wood, not soft woods and especially not resinous ones like cedar, pine or MESQUITE.

Chard, Swiss Chard: Two vegetables for the price of one: Fleshy ivory stalks that can be cooked like asparagus and dark beta-carotene-rich green leaves that are best steamed or stir-fried like spinach. Once cooked, the two are often tossed together, then seasoned. Italians, who adore chard, have devised more ways to cook it than anyone else. Into frittatas it goes, and savory custards, soups, stuffings and steaming bowls of pasta. Scarcely surprising given the fact that this ancient vegetable probably originated in Italy—or at least in the Mediterranean area. **SEASON:** Spring through fall.

NUTRIENT CONTENT OF 1 CUP STEAMED UNSEASONED CHARD (LEAVES AND STEMS)	
(about 6¼ ounces; 175 grams)	
35 calories	313 mg sodium
3 g protein	961 mg potassium
0 g fat, 0 saturated	4 g dietary fiber
0 mg cholesterol	549 RE vitamin A
7 g carbohydrate	0.06 mg thiamin
102 mg calcium	0.15 mg riboflavin
58 mg phosphorus	0.6 mg niacin
4.0 mg iron	32 mg vitamin C

Chayote, Christophene, Cho-Cho, Mirliton, Vegetable Pear: For all its exotic names, this tropical/subtropical fruit belongs to the squash family. Being savory rather than sweet, chayotes are cooked like vegetables and served as a side dish. Called mirlitons or vegetable pears in the Deep South where they're grown, chayotes look like waxy, deeply furrowed apple-green pears. Raw, their flesh is crisp; cooked it is squash soft. In texture and flavor chayotes resemble pattypan squash more than they do yellow crooknecks or zucchini. They do contain some vitamin C and they are exceptionally low in calories and contain almost no sodium. **SEASON:** Year-round, with supplies at their peak in winter.

NUTRIENT CONTENT OF 1 CUP BOILED OR STEAMED UNSEASONED CHAYOTE

(about 5½ ounces; 160 grams)

38 calories	1 mg sodium
1 g protein	276 mg potassium
1 g fat, 0 saturated	1 g dietary fiber
0 mg cholesterol	8 RE vitamin A
8 g carbohydrate	0.04 mg thiamin
21 mg calcium	0.06 mg riboflavin
46 mg phosphorus	0.7 mg niacin
0.4 mg iron	13 mg vitamin C

Cheddar: Not a single cheese but an extended family of them. To connoisseurs, "the one and only" is an English farmhouse Cheddar made of whole, unpasteurized, sweet milk from cows that have drunk nothing more than pure water and grazed on grasses free of dandelions, daisies or other bitter flora that would alter the flavor. True Cheddars come from Somerset; they're made of summer milk (meaning between May and October) and they're never rushed but allowed to age slowly for about two years. They are buttery, moist, dense and biting but never bitter. Nearly every country where Englishmen have settled makes one sort of Cheddar or another, and in America each region has developed its own. New England Cheddars are white; down South they're red-orange; in the

NUTRIENT CONTENT OF 1 OUNCE (28 GRAMS) CHEDDAR

114 calories	176 mg sodium
7 g protein	28 mg potassium
9 g fat, 6 saturated	0 g dietary fiber
30 mg cholesterol	86 RE vitamin A
0 g carbohydrate	0.01 mg thiamin
204 mg calcium	0.11 mg riboflavin
145 mg phosphorus	0 mg niacin
0.2 mg iron	0 mg vitamin C

Midwest pale orange; and on the West Coast as pale as ivory. Monterey Jack is a Cheddar, as are Colby, "rat cheese," "brick cheese," cracker-barrel cheese and, of course, the pungent white Vermont Cheddar (even processed AMERICAN CHEESE is a Cheddar type). Made of whole milk, Cheddars run to fat, cholesterol and calories. But they're protein rich, too, and contain plenty of vitamin A, calcium and phosphorus. As for the low-fat, fat-free fakes, cheese lovers find them about as appealing as erasers, although these synthetics are improving.

Cheese: See entries for individual types—BRIE; CAMEMBERT; CHEDDAR; ROQUEFORT; etc.

Cheesecake: Although innovative American chefs are constantly dreaming up variations on the theme (pumpkin cheesecake, for example, or hazelnut and bourbon), there are two classics only: the **Lindy's** (Jewish) type made with cream cheese and the less caloric **Italian cheesecake** made of ricotta or cottage cheese. Neither is what the doctor ordered because saturated fats, cholesterol and calories all soar. Here's a slimmed-down version good enough for company.

Cheese Food: A highly processed blend of pasteurized cheese whey, whole and skim milk and cream. By law, its cheese content must be at least 51 percent pure cheese. **Cheese spread,** lower in fat but higher in moisture (from 47 to 60 percent by weight) and vegetable gums (allowable up to 0.8 percent), is soft enough at room temperature to spread. See also AMERICAN CHEESE.

Chelation Therapy: A chelate is a chemical compound that acts somewhat like a mop. In medical conditions where there's too much iron in the body, a chelate is used to soak up the excess and flush it from the body. Chelation therapy, on the other hand, is a quack remedy for atherosclerosis and assorted other diseases, including cancer. It consists of large, repeated, intravenous doses of EDTA, a lab-synthesized amino acid.

Chemotherapy (diet and): Chemotherapy is one of the treatments now being used to control or cure a variety of cancers. It consists of a series of "chemical cocktails" administered intravenously or by mouth that are toxic

Skinnier Cheesecake

Makes 24 Servings

CRUST:

2½ cups graham cracker crumbs (20 double crackers, each 4½ × 2¼ inches)

3 tablespoons light brown sugar

½ teaspoon ground cinnamon

½ teaspoon freshly grated nutmeg

4 tablespoons extralight olive oil

3 tablespoons evaporated skim milk

1 teaspoon butter extract

TOPPING:

½ cup light sour cream

½ cup low-fat plain yogurt

⅓ cup granulated sugar

1 teaspoon vanilla extract

FILLING:

2 packages (8 ounces each) low-fat cream cheese (Neufchâtel)

1 cup low-fat cottage cheese

1 cup nonfat ricotta

½ cup light sour cream

½ cup evaporated skim milk

¾ cup sugar

⅔ cup fat-free frozen egg product, thawed

1 tablespoon vanilla extract

FOR CRUST: PULSE crumbs, brown sugar, cinnamon, and nutmeg in a food processor fitted with the metal chopping blade. Drizzle oil, evaporated milk, and butter extract evenly over crumbs and churn 10 seconds. Using the back of a tablespoon, pat mixture firmly over bottom and halfway up sides of a 10-inch springform pan; set aside.

FOR FILLING: PREHEAT oven to 325°F. Churn all ingredients in food processor 1½ minutes until smooth. Pour into crust, set on baking sheet, and bake 35 minutes. Remove from oven and cool 10 minutes. Raise oven temperature to 400°F.

FOR TOPPING: WHILE cake bakes, whisk topping ingredients together. When pie has cooled 10 minutes, carefully smooth topping over filling with a rubber spatula so it touches crust all around. Bake pie 10 minutes longer, cool on rack 1 hour, and chill overnight. Carefully remove pan sides and cut pie into slim wedges.

APPROXIMATE NUTRIENT COUNTS PER SERVING

204 calories	24 g carbohydrate	1 mg iron	0.05 mg thiamin
7 g protein	0 g dietary fiber	235 mg sodium	0.20 mg riboflavin
9 g fat, 4 saturated	81 mg calcium	129 mg potassium	0.6 mg niacin
16 mg cholesterol	100 mg phosphorus	73 RE vitamin A	0 mg vitamin C

enough to kill malignant cells. Some cancer patients sail through chemotherapy with no side effects. Others suffer nausea, vomiting, diarrhea, mouth sores, esophagitis, weight loss. The "chemical recipe," the treatment's du-ration and the general health of the patient all determine the side effects. Because these side effects duplicate those of radiation treatment, the diet plan is also similar. See also RADIATION THERAPY.

Cherimoya, Custard Apple, Annona: This ancient Inca fruit looks like a leathery, many-faceted green apple. But its flavor, trapped in custardy flesh, is part pineapple, part mango, part banana. Now being grown in California, cherimoyas are more widely available than ever. Occasionally they even show up in high-dollar supermarkets. **SEASON:** Winter and early spring.

NUTRIENT CONTENT OF 1 LARGE CHERIMOYA
(about 1¼ pounds; 547 grams)

514 calories	NA mg sodium
7 g protein	NA mg potassium
2 g fat, NA saturated	14 g dietary fiber
0 mg cholesterol	6 RE vitamin A
131 g carbohydrate	0.55 mg thiamin
125 mg calcium	0.60 mg riboflavin
218 mg phosphorus	7.1 mg niacin
2.7 mg iron	49 mg vitamin C

Cherries: Native to Eurasia, cultivated since long before Christ, cherries came to the American colonies with the English. Though more than a thousand varieties of this fruit are grown today, there are only two types: **sweet** and

NUTRIENT CONTENT OF 1 CUP PITTED SWEET CHERRIES
(about 5 ounces; 145 grams)

104 calories	1 mg sodium
2 g protein	325 mg potassium
1 g fat, 0 saturated	2 g dietary fiber
0 mg cholesterol	31 RE vitamin A
24 g carbohydrate	0.07 mg thiamin
21 mg calcium	0.09 mg riboflavin
28 mg phosphorus	0.6 mg niacin
0.6 mg iron	10 mg vitamin C

NUTRIENT CONTENT OF 1 CUP PITTED SOUR CHERRIES
(about 5¼ ounces; 155 grams)

77 calories	5 mg sodium
2 g protein	268 mg potassium
1 g fat, 0 saturated	2 g dietary fiber
0 mg cholesterol	199 RE vitamin A
19 g carbohydrate	0.05 mg thiamin
24 mg calcium	0.06 mg riboflavin
23 mg phosphorus	0.6 mg niacin
0.5 mg iron	16 mg vitamin C

sour. Sweet cherries (the maroon **Bings** and pink-blushed yellow **Royal Anns,** to name two top sellers) are usually shipped to market fresh from the Great Lakes states and Pacific Northwest, where they're grown, although some of the Royal Anns wind up as maraschinos. The bulk of the sour-cherry crop is canned either whole or as pie filling. **SEASON:** Summer.

Chestnuts: In the first half of this century, blight decimated the American chestnut. It was a tall, stately tree valued more for its timber than its fruit (nut), which was always inferior to the *marron* of the European chestnut. Known to the ancients, the *marron* has sustained rich and poor down the centuries. It is eaten raw, roasted, boiled and mashed like potatoes, even steamed with bitter greens (a Roman favorite). It is dried, ground to flour and baked into bread; candied; sweetened, pureed; and mixed with whipped cream in an awesome dessert known as *mont blanc* (white mountain). Though called nuts, chestnuts are anything but oily. In fact, the bulk of their calories come from carbohydrates.

NUTRIENT CONTENT OF 5 OUNCES (142 GRAMS) ROASTED SHELLED CHESTNUTS

350 calories	3 mg sodium
5 g protein	846 mg potassium
3 g fat, 1 saturated	7 g dietary fiber
0 mg cholesterol	3 RE vitamin A
76 g carbohydrate	0.30 mg thiamin
42 mg calcium	0.30 mg riboflavin
153 mg phosphorus	1.9 mg niacin
1.3 mg iron	37 mg vitamin C

Chewing Gum Base, Chicle: Nothing more than the latex of the sapodilla tree, which is boiled down until thick.

Chicken: The first chicken was a wild red fowl that fluttered and squawked about the jungles of India four thousand years ago. The natives, impressed by the bird's color, courage and dash, lured it down from the trees and tamed it. Before long the chicken showed up in China. And by the time of King Tutankhamen (1358 B.C.), it had arrived in Egypt, where, according to inscriptions in the boy pharaoh's tomb, it was a bird of royal plumage. The first farmers to fatten chickens for the table were ancient Greeks on the Aegean island of Cos (which also gave us romaine lettuce, the cult of Aesculapius, Hippocrates and modern medicine). The Romans, who adopted most things Greek, plumped chickens on rations of barley and milk and, as in today's poultry industry, immobilized the birds in elevated cages so they'd be meltingly tender. By the Middle Ages, chickens were common throughout Europe. The French Abbey of St. Riquier listed, as part of its annual income, 10,000 capons, 10,000 chickens and 75,000 eggs. Hardly chicken feed. Today, with people obsessing about saturated fats, chicken is more popular than ever.

And there's a chicken for every pot: tender, young **broiler-fryers** (7 to 9 weeks; 2 to 3½ pounds), **roasters** (about 16 weeks; 3½ to 6 pounds), **capons** (see CAPON; 16 weeks, 4 to 7 pounds), **hens,** sometimes called heavy hens (tough old birds; 4½ to 6 pounds). There are whole chickens, halves, quarters, pieces, and even, these days, chicken scaloppine.

Unfortunately, salmonella (see BACTERIA) has swept through America's henhouses, infecting both the chicken and the egg, and growers haven't been able to stop its forward march. In addition, *Campylobacter jejuni* outbreaks are on the rise. Indeed, the problem of bacteria in poultry has become so acute the USDA now requires safe-handling labels on all packages of fresh and frozen chicken. Luckily,

NUTRIENT CONTENT OF ½ FRIED, FLOURED CHICKEN BREAST (WITH SKIN AND BONE)
(about 4¼ ounces; 118 grams)

218 calories	75 mg sodium
31 g protein	253 mg potassium
9 g fat, 3 saturated	0 g dietary fiber
88 mg cholesterol	15 RE vitamin A
2 g carbohydrate	0.08 mg thiamin
16 mg calcium	0.13 mg riboflavin
228 mg phosphorus	13.5 mg niacin
1.2 mg iron	0 mg vitamin C

NUTRIENT CONTENT OF ½ POACHED OR STEAMED CHICKEN BREAST (WITH SKIN AND BONE)
(about 4 ounces; 110 grams)

202 calories	68 mg sodium
30 g protein	195 mg potassium
8 g fat, 1 saturated	0 g dietary fiber
83 mg cholesterol	26 RE vitamin A
0 g carbohydrate	0.05 mg thiamin
14 mg calcium	0.13 mg riboflavin
172 mg phosphorus	8.6 mg niacin
1.0 mg iron	0 mg vitamin C

NUTRIENT CONTENT OF 1 POACHED OR STEAMED CHICKEN THIGH (WITH SKIN AND BONE)
(about 3¼ ounces; 90 grams)

198 calories	61 mg sodium
20 g protein	144 mg potassium
13 g fat, 4 saturated	0 g dietary fiber
71 mg cholesterol	38 RE vitamin A
0 g carbohydrate	0.05 mg thiamin
10 mg calcium	0.16 mg riboflavin
118 mg phosphorus	4.1 mg niacin
1.1 mg iron	0 mg vitamin C

NUTRIENT CONTENT OF ½ POACHED OR STEAMED CHICKEN BREAST (SKINNED AND BONED)
(about 3 ounces; 85 grams)

128 calories	54 mg sodium
24 g protein	158 mg potassium
3 g fat, 1 saturated	0 g dietary fiber
65 mg cholesterol	5 RE vitamin A
0 g carbohydrate	0.04 mg thiamin
11 mg calcium	0.10 mg riboflavin
140 mg phosphorus	7.1 mg niacin
0.8 mg iron	0 mg vitamin C

NUTRIENT CONTENT OF 1 POACHED OR STEAMED CHICKEN THIGH (SKINNED AND BONED)
(about 3 ounces; 85 grams)

165 calories	64 mg sodium
21 g protein	155 mg potassium
8 g fat, 2 saturated	0 g dietary fiber
76 mg cholesterol	16 RE vitamin A
0 g carbohydrate	0.06 mg thiamin
9 mg calcium	0.19 mg riboflavin
126 mg phosphorus	4.4 mg niacin
1.2 mg iron	0 mg vitamin C

thorough cooking kills the bugs and makes chicken safe to eat (USDA poultry specialists recommend cooking the dark meat to an internal temperature of 180°F. and white meat to 170°F.). White meat, as the following charts show, is leaner than dark, especially if the skin is removed. As far as fat content is concerned, it doesn't matter whether you skin the chicken before you cook it or after. Skin fat melts and drains away as the bird cooks; it doesn't penetrate the meat. What cooking with the skin on does do is seal in the juices, thus chicken broiled or roasted with the skin intact will be more succulent than a bird cooked "nude."

NUTRIENT CONTENT OF 1 FRIED, FLOURED CHICKEN THIGH (WITH SKIN AND BONE)

(about 4 ounces; 115 grams)

324 calories	110 mg sodium
34 g protein	294 mg potassium
18 g fat, 6 saturated	0 g dietary fiber
120 mg cholesterol	36 RE vitamin A
4 g carbohydrate	0.12 mg thiamin
16 mg calcium	0.32 mg riboflavin
232 mg phosphorus	8.6 mg niacin
1.8 mg iron	0 mg vitamin C

Chicken Scallops in Dijon Sauce

Makes 4 Servings

4 boneless and skinless chicken breasts (3 to 4 ounces each), pounded thin as for scaloppine

¼ teaspoon salt

¼ teaspoon dried thyme

¼ teaspoon freshly ground black pepper

¼ cup all-purpose flour

1 tablespoon olive oil

¼ cup dry vermouth

1 tablespoon plus 1 teaspoon Dijon mustard

½ cup evaporated skim milk

¼ teaspoon cornstarch, blended with 1 teaspoon cold water

2 tablespoons light sour cream

2 tablespoons snipped fresh chives or finely minced scallion tops

SPRINKLE CHICKEN PIECES lightly on both sides with salt, thyme, and pepper, then dredge lightly in flour. Spray a large heavy skillet well with nonstick cooking spray, add the olive oil, and heat 1 minute over moderate heat. Brown chicken 2 to 3 minutes per side, then remove to a heated platter to keep warm. Pour vermouth into skillet and heat, stirring about 1 minute and scraping up browned bits. Stir in mustard, then evaporated milk, and boil 1 to 2 minutes until lightly thickened. Blend in cornstarch mixture and boil 1 minute. Remove from heat and stir in sour cream and chives. Spoon over chicken and serve.

APPROXIMATE NUTRIENT COUNTS PER SERVING

202 calories	7 g carbohydrate	1.2 mg iron	0.08 mg thiamin
23 g protein	0 g dietary fiber	350 mg sodium	0.20 mg riboflavin
7 g fat, 2 saturated	122 mg calcium	302 mg potassium	8.9 mg niacin
61 mg cholesterol	231 mg phosphorus	62 RE vitamin A	1 mg vitamin C

Chicken Livers: Like all liver, these are chockablock with iron, vitamin A and, alas, cholesterol. The good news is that they are low in sodium and, if well trimmed, low in fat and saturated fat, too.

NUTRIENT CONTENT OF 2 OUNCES (57 GRAMS) SIMMERED CHICKEN LIVERS

88 calories	29 mg sodium
14 g protein	80 mg potassium
3 g fat, 1 saturated	0 g dietary fiber
358 mg cholesterol	2,785 RE vitamin A
1 g carbohydrate	0.09 mg thiamin
8 mg calcium	1.0 mg riboflavin
176 mg phosphorus	2.5 mg niacin
4.8 mg iron	9 mg vitamin C

Chickpeas: See BEANS, DRIED.

Chicory: See SALAD GREENS.

Chiffon Cakes: Invented by a professional baker in the 1920s, these feathery, high-rising cakes went mass America in the late 1940s and early 1950s, thanks to the boost given them by processors of vegetable oil. Chiffon cakes were tailor-made, the dream marketing tool because they substituted vegetable oil for butter. Quite a bit of oil—sometimes as much as a cup. They owe their volume to the fact that the eggs are separated and the stiffly beaten whites folded in at the end. Because of all the oil, egg yolks, sugar and flour they contain, chiffon cakes are loaded with fat, cholesterol and calories.

Chiles: See HOT PEPPERS under PEPPERS, CAPSICUMS.

Chinese Cabbage, Bok Choy, Pak Choi: There are two Chinese cabbages: **bok choy (pak choi)**—or **Chinese white cabbage,** to give its correct name—and **Chinese** or **celery cabbage.** Although both belong to the cabbage family, both are long, more like Swiss chard than our round cabbages. They're blander than red or green cabbage, but they're not without bite. Both can be eaten raw, but brief cooking enhances their flavor without destroying their texture. Of the two, bok choy is more nutritious because its leaves are darker green. It is, in fact, a stellar source of beta-carotene. **SEASON:** Year-round.

NUTRIENT CONTENT OF 1 CUP RAW SHREDDED BOK CHOY
(about 2½ ounces; 70 grams)

9 calories	46 mg sodium
1 g protein	176 mg potassium
0 g fat, 0 saturated	1 g dietary fiber
0 mg cholesterol	210 RE vitamin A
2 g carbohydrate	0.03 mg thiamin
74 mg calcium	0.05 mg riboflavin
26 mg phosphorus	0.4 mg niacin
0.6 mg iron	32 mg vitamin C

NUTRIENT CONTENT OF 1 CUP COOKED SHREDDED BOK CHOY
(about 6 ounces; 170 grams)

20 calories	58 mg sodium
3 g protein	631 mg potassium
0 g fat, 0 saturated	3 g dietary fiber
0 mg cholesterol	437 RE vitamin A
3 g carbohydrate	0.05 mg thiamin
158 mg calcium	0.11 mg riboflavin
49 mg phosphorus	0.7 mg niacin
1.8 mg iron	44 mg vitamin C

Chinese Long Beans: See YARD-LONG BEANS under BEANS, FRESH.

Chinese Restaurant Syndrome: Palpitations, tingling, headache, flushes, numbness, weakness. All are symptoms of what has come to be called Chinese restaurant syndrome. The culprit is MONOSODIUM GLUTAMATE (MSG), the flavor enhancer Chinese chefs use with abandon. Not everyone is MSG sensitive (in late 1995, scientific advisers to the FDA concluded that MSG was safe for nearly everyone). And those who are can minimize—or eliminate—the unpleasantness of Chinese restaurant syndrome by eating MSG-free food before they sit down to a big Asian feast.

Chipotle: See HOT PEPPERS under PEPPERS, CAPSICUMS.

Chitterlings, Chitlins: The intestines of young pigs, the very soul of soul food. Chitterlings are a cheap source of protein and iron but unfortunately aren't particularly nutritious except for their iron content. They're low in sodium but high in fat, saturated fat and cholesterol.

**NUTRIENT CONTENT OF 3 OUNCES (85 GRAMS)
BOILED CHITTERLINGS**

258 calories	33 mg sodium
9 g protein	7 mg potassium
25 g fat, 9 saturated	0 g dietary fiber
122 mg cholesterol	0 RE vitamin A
0 g carbohydrate	0 mg thiamin
23 mg calcium	0.07 mg riboflavin
40 mg phosphorus	0.1 mg niacin
3.2 mg iron	0 mg vitamin C

Chlorella: Microscopic blue-green ALGAE sold by health-food stores as a vitamin- and mineral-packed "natural" nutritional supplement. It is available as both granules and tablets. Like SPIRULINA, chlorella possesses none of the magical powers attributed to it.

Chloride, Chlorine Dioxide, Chlorine: Not only are chlorines popular water purifiers and flour bleachers, but chlorine is also an essential nutrient supplied by chloride ions (a part of table salt, or sodium chloride). Chlorides are integral to the production of hydrochloric acid, an important component of gastric juice, the digestive fluid in the stomach. They're also necessary for the assimilation of vitamin B_{12}.

Chlorogenic Acid: A chemical present in tomatoes that appears to detox cancer-causing nitrosamines in the body. See PHYTOCHEMICALS.

Chlorophyll: The green pigment in plants sometimes used as a food coloring, which plays a pivotal role in photosynthesis, the process by which plants, using the sun's energy, convert carbon dioxide to carbohydrates and oxygen. Blanching or quick, intense heat heightens the green in vegetables, as does a pinch of baking soda. But soda also destroys some of the thiamin and vitamin C; too much of it, moreover, will turn vegetables slimy. Chlorophyll can be used as an indicator of the beta-carotene and vitamin C content of many foods. Generally speaking, the greener the fruit or vegetable, the richer it is in both beta-carotene and vitamin C.

Chlorosucrose, Sucralose: A new artificial sweetener said to be 600 times sweeter than sugar. Unlike aspartame, it can be used in baked goods. Chlorosucrose is still awaiting FDA approval.

Chocolate: Like tomatoes and potatoes, chocolate made it north from Latin America the roundabout way. Columbus, we're told, found a canoe of cocoa beans near Yucatán on his fourth voyage but found them bitter. Only when Cortés pushed deep into Mexico and joined Moctezuma in a cup of cocoa did the conquistadores take notice. Cortés sent cocoa beans home to Spain together with instructions for processing them and a recipe for Moctezuma's drink—*chocolatl*. Still, chocolate didn't find universal favor until Louis XIII's Spanish-born queen made it stylish at the French court.

Only with the invention of the steam engine could chocolate be mass-produced and priced within reach of Everyman. Today, the average American eats more than 12 pounds of chocolate a year and drinks heaven knows how many gallons of cocoa. The myriad chocolates now available include **unsweetened, semisweet** (with sugar and additional cocoa butter), **bittersweet** (a smoother, more refined semisweet), **milk chocolate** (a chocolate/powdered milk/sugar blend) and **white chocolate** (sweetened cocoa butter). All solid chocolate is high in fat, much of it saturated; it also contains small amounts of caffeine.

**NUTRIENT CONTENT OF 1 OUNCE (28 GRAMS)
UNSWEETENED CHOCOLATE**

145 calories	1 mg sodium
3 g protein	235 mg potassium
16 g fat, 9 saturated	4 g dietary fiber
0 mg cholesterol	1 RE vitamin A
8 g carbohydrate	0.01 mg thiamin
22 mg calcium	0.07 mg riboflavin
109 mg phosphorus	0.4 mg niacin
1.9 mg iron	0 mg vitamin C

**NUTRIENT CONTENT OF 1 OUNCE (28 GRAMS)
SEMISWEET CHOCOLATE**

144 calories	1 mg sodium
1 g protein	92 mg potassium
10 g fat, 5 saturated	2 g dietary fiber
0 mg cholesterol	1 RE vitamin A
16 g carbohydrate	0 mg thiamin
9 mg calcium	0.02 mg riboflavin
43 mg phosphorus	0.1 mg niacin
0.7 mg iron	0 mg vitamin C

Dark and Delicious Pots de Crème

Makes 6 Servings

Not all chocolate desserts are saturated with fat, calories, and cholesterol. These quick and creamy chocolate puddings prove the point.

1½ cups firmly packed part-skim or nonfat ricotta

6 tablespoons sugar or 4 packets (1 g each) sugar substitute

¼ cup unsweetened Dutch-process cocoa powder

2 tablespoons coffee liqueur, or 1 tablespoon each coffee liqueur and brandy

1 tablespoon instant espresso powder

2 teaspoons vanilla extract

2 to 3 tablespoons evaporated skim milk

PLACE ALL INGREDIENTS except evaporated milk in a food processor fitted with the metal chopping blade and churn 5 seconds; scrape down work bowl and churn 5 seconds more. With motor running, add evaporated milk down the feed tube, 1 tablespoon at a time, just until mixture is consistency of chocolate pudding. Continue churning 8 to 10 seconds, until absolutely smooth. Divide among six 4- to 5-ounce ramekins and serve at once or chill until ready to serve.

APPROXIMATE NUTRIENT COUNTS PER SERVING
(if made with sugar and part-skim ricotta)

169 calories	21 g carbohydrate	0.9 mg iron	0.02 mg thiamin
8 g protein	1 g dietary fiber	81 mg sodium	0.14 mg riboflavin
5 g fat, 3 saturated	180 mg calcium	199 mg potassium	0.3 mg niacin
19 mg cholesterol	146 mg phosphorus	73 RE vitamin A	0 mg vitamin C

APPROXIMATE NUTRIENT COUNTS PER SERVING
(if made with sugar substitute and part-skim ricotta)

123 calories	9 g carbohydrate	0.9 mg iron	0.02 mg thiamin
9 g protein	1 g dietary fiber	81 mg sodium	0.14 mg riboflavin
5 g fat, 3 saturated	180 mg calcium	199 mg potassium	0.3 mg niacin
19 mg cholesterol	146 mg phosphorus	73 RE vitamin A	0 mg vitamin C

APPROXIMATE NUTRIENT COUNTS PER SERVING
(if made with sugar substitute and nonfat ricotta)

83 calories	8 g carbohydrate	0.6 mg iron	0.01 mg thiamin
10 g protein	1 g dietary fiber	34 mg sodium	0.10 mg riboflavin
1 g fat, 0 saturated	134 mg calcium	199 mg potassium	0.3 mg niacin
0 mg cholesterol	94 mg phosphorus	124 RE vitamin A	0 mg vitamin C

NUTRIENT CONTENT OF 1 OUNCE (28 GRAMS) MILK CHOCOLATE

147 calories	27 mg sodium
2 g protein	109 mg potassium
9 g fat, 5 saturated	1 g dietary fiber
0 mg cholesterol	8 RE vitamin A
16 g carbohydrate	0.02 mg thiamin
65 mg calcium	0.10 mg riboflavin
65 mg phosphorus	0.1 mg niacin
0.3 mg iron	0 mg vitamin C

Chocolate Milk: Low-fat chocolate milk is the big seller in many schools, sometimes accounting for 80 percent of all milk sold at lunch. There used to be some worry that the oxalic acid of the chocolate would bind with the calcium of the milk, making it useless to the body. Recent tests refute that. In fact, chocolate milk is an excellent source of calcium. It is also, however, about 5 percent sugar.

NUTRIENT CONTENT OF 1 CUP LOW-FAT (1 PERCENT) CHOCOLATE MILK

(8 fluid ounces; 242 grams)

157 calories	151 mg sodium
8 g protein	425 mg potassium
3 g fat, 2 saturated	4 g dietary fiber
7 mg cholesterol	148 RE vitamin A
26 g carbohydrate	0.10 mg thiamin
285 mg calcium	0.42 mg riboflavin
255 mg phosphorus	0.3 mg niacin
0.6 mg iron	2 mg vitamin C

NUTRIENT CONTENT OF 1 CUP LOW-FAT (2 PERCENT) CHOCOLATE MILK

(8 fluid ounces; 242 grams)

178 calories	150 mg sodium
8 g protein	423 mg potassium
5 g fat, 3 saturated	4 g dietary fiber
17 mg cholesterol	143 RE vitamin A
26 g carbohydrate	0.09 mg thiamin
285 mg calcium	0.41 mg riboflavin
255 mg phosphorus	0.3 mg niacin
0.6 mg iron	2 mg vitamin C

Chocolate Syrup: Apart from flavor, everybody's favorite ice cream topping hasn't got much going for it.

NUTRIENT CONTENT OF 1 TABLESPOON THIN CHOCOLATE SYRUP

(about ¾ ounce; 19 grams)

41 calories	18 mg sodium
0 g protein	42 mg potassium
0 g fat, 0 saturated	0 g dietary fiber
0 mg cholesterol	1 RE vitamin A
11 g carbohydrate	0 mg thiamin
3 mg calcium	0.01 mg riboflavin
24 mg phosphorus	0.1 mg niacin
0.4 mg iron	0 mg vitamin C

Cholecalciferol: See D, VITAMIN.

Cholecystitis: Inflammation of the gallbladder, which can be chronic or acute. Sometimes an infection is to blame, sometimes gallstones, sometimes adhesions or a tumor. Whatever the cause, cholecystitis is not pleasant. In acute cases, there's intense pain under the right rib, spreading as far as the lower abdomen and shoulder. There may also be nausea and/or vomiting, chills and fever and jaundice. As a part of the treatment, doctors usually recommend a twenty-four-hour fast, then two to three days of clear liquids, then soft foods and thereafter a diet moderately low in fat, spicy seasonings and any other food that causes discomfort.

Cholelithiasis: A ten-dollar word for the formation or presence of gallstones (see GALLBLADDER, GALLSTONES).

Cholesterol: Our bodies cannot function without cholesterol. This waxy lipid (fat) is used to manufacture estrogen and testosterone, vitamin D, bile, skin oils, nerve- and brain-cell sheaths (indeed, the body's richest concentration of cholesterol is in the brain). Our livers make all the cholesterol we need—some 1,000 milligrams a day. And our diets add another 400 to 500 milligrams. Under optimum conditions, cholesterol constantly shuttles back and forth between the liver and body cells, where it's needed aboard lipoproteins (these, too, are synthesized in the liver). The reason for the recent cholesterol bashing is that it can build up as plaque in the arteries, clog them and, ultimately, cause heart attacks and strokes.

So what's this about "good" cholesterol and "bad"? Actually it's less the cholesterol itself that's good or bad than the lipoproteins on which it hitches rides through the bloodstream. **High-density lipoprotein (HDL)**, the "good," removes cholesterol from the cells and zooms it back to the liver, where it's either reprocessed or excreted. **Low-density lipoprotein (LDL)**, the "bad," is sloppier, more sluggish. On its round-trips from liver to cells, it drops cholesterol along the way, which sticks to artery walls, hardens and, over time, accumulates to the point of blockage.

Scientists now know that foods high in saturated fats do more to raise the levels of "bad" cholesterol in the blood than such cholesterol-laden foods as eggs, liver and steak. They know, too, that obesity, cigarette smoking, steroid use and sedentary lifestyles also elevate "bad" cholesterol levels.

Avoiding saturated animal fats (butter, cheese, meat) and a trio of tropical oils (coconut, palm and palm kernel), increasing exercise and dietary fiber, upping your vitamin C intake (to about 5 times the RDA if you're a man, and to 3½ times if you're a woman; see C, VITAMIN), losing weight and swearing off cigarettes all will increase blood levels of "good" cholesterol, or HDL, and, at the same time, lower the "bad." So will avoiding hard margarines; the trans fatty acids formed when vegetable oils are hydrogenated to give margarines the consistency of butter dramatically raise levels of "bad" cholesterol in the blood (soft and squeeze margarines less so). And it seems the trimmer you are, the faster your blood cholesterol will drop once you begin eating healthy (or so scientists participating in a U.S./Dutch study report).

The best fats to use for cooking are oils high in monounsaturated fatty acids, because these raise "good" cholesterol levels, which in turn flush out the "bad." Highest marks go to olive oil, with canola and peanut oil not far behind. Until recently, highly polyunsaturated oils were just what the doctor ordered. Now that they're suspected of being carcinogenic, the monounsaturates—and olive oil especially—are the oils of choice. See MONOUNSATURATED FATTY ACID.

Many physicians and dietitians still caution patients to limit their cholesterol intake to 300 milligrams a day, the amount generally recommended for good heart health. And here's a mental crutch to help you keep tabs on dietary cholesterol: *No food of plant origin contains cholesterol. Ever.*

What about too little blood cholesterol? Is that dangerous? Researchers now believe that people with cholesterol levels below 160 are at greater risk of liver cancer, nonmalignant lung disease, brain hemorrhage, even alcoholism and suicide although they can't say why. Nor can they explain why some people have basement blood cholesterol levels although they suspect it has more to do with heredity than diet.

The latest salvo in the cholesterol controversy comes from a new Yale University College of Medicine study, which suggests that men and women over the age of seventy needn't fret about their cholesterol levels (unless they already have cardiovascular disease). This five-year study of 997 men and women with an average age of seventy-nine showed that those with high blood cholesterol levels suffered no more heart attacks than those with normal—or even low—levels. Further, the death rate among the high-cholesterol group—from heart trouble or any other disease—was no greater than for those with "healthier" cholesterol levels. Earlier cholesterol studies had focused upon middle-agers, mostly men. *And here blood cholesterol levels do still count.*

The consensus among the Yale researchers is that golden-agers with high cholesterol counts may somehow be immune to cholesterol damage. That the bullet's missed them. They also suggest that the side effects of powerful cholesterol-lowering drugs may be more damaging to the seventy-and-up group than high blood cholesterol itself.

This new Yale study, needless to add, is getting plenty of flak, and many medical researchers believe that further tests are necessary before its results can be taken as gospel.

BLOOD SERUM CHOLESTEROL LEVELS (IN MILLIGRAMS PER DECILITER) AND HOW THEY RATE*

	Total Cholesterol	HDL	LDL
Desirable	Below 200 mg	45 to 65 mg	Below 130 mg
Borderline	200 to 239 mg	35 to 45 mg	130 to 159 mg
At risk	240 mg or more	Below 35 mg	160 mg or more

*Table adapted from "Recommendations for All Adults" by the National Cholesterol Education Program.

Choline: A B vitamin cousin widely distributed in food that aids metabolism. Though choline isn't considered an essential nutrient, health hucksters attribute magical memory-boosting powers to it. The truth: Although physicians have found large doses of choline (given in tandem with lecithin) helpful to patients with loss of memory or muscular coordination, the average person needs no supplementary choline. Indeed, megadoses of it can cause gastrointestinal upset, anorexia, sweating and, over time, nerve and cardiovascular distress.

Chromium: A mineral that makes the body more sensitive to insulin, regulates cholesterol and fatty acid production in the liver, and aids in the digestion of protein. If chromium is lacking, blood levels of cholesterol and fatty acids rise, glucose is poorly metabolized, and, in severe deficiencies, there may be nerve damage. **GOOD SOURCES:** Brewer's yeast, liver, meat, mushrooms, nuts, oysters, peanut butter, potatoes, unpeeled apples, whole grains, beer and wine.

Chromium Picolinate: "Lose the fat," the ads promise. "Keep the muscle. . . . Maintain a normal, healthy metabolism." Is it any wonder that this chromium compound is flying off the shelves of pharmacies and health-food stores? For several years the supplement of choice of the hard-body set (because it's safer than anabolic steroids), chromium picolinate has recently gone mainstream as a weight-loss aid. But does it really build muscle and melt fat? Are these little white pills the answer to a prayer for those who diet in vain, losing a few pounds only to pile them all back on? **HERE ARE THE FACTS:** Chromium picolinate is not a diet aid; it's a nutrient, a more easily digested form of CHROMIUM. Although chromium is essential to the metabolism of fats, proteins and carbohydrates and also helps insulin provide blood sugar (glucose) to body cells more efficiently, there is no proof that it builds muscles, boosts energy, accelerates fat loss, curbs the appetite or cures a sweet tooth. Nutritionists agree that chromium picolinate is safe but stress that it's unnecessary for anyone who gets the 50 to 200 micrograms of chromium per day that the National Academy of Sciences recommends for adults.

Cider: See APPLE CIDER.

Cider Vinegar: See VINEGAR.

Cigarette Smoking: We all know that cigarette smoking can be hazardous to our health, but the surgeon general's warning, printed on all cigarette packages, is only part of the story. Smoking raises cholesterol levels in the blood and elevates blood pressure, too. It increases the risk of cancer and cataracts and doubles the depletion of vitamin C in the body. Heavy smokers should get an extra 100 milligrams of ascorbic acid each day to counter the effects of nicotine.

Ciguatera Poisoning: An insidious form of food poisoning carried by several tropical or subtropical saltwater fish: amberjack (other jacks, too), barracuda, grouper, hogfish, king mackerel, moray eel, red snapper, sea bass and triggerfish, with the first three—plus eel and snapper—posing the worst threat (Dade County, Florida, which includes Miami, now bans the sale of barracuda). What happens is this: A protozoan attaches itself to coral algae and produces a poison called ciguatoxin. Small fish eat the algae, poison and all; bigger fish eat the small fish, which are in turn gobbled up by still bigger fish. And so it goes up the food chain, the oil-soluble ciguatoxin becoming more concentrated each step of the way. Although ciguatera poisoning isn't new, outbreaks are becoming more common. Travelers roam the globe zeroing in on sun spots in Florida, the Caribbean, Hawaii and the South Pacific; tropical fish are air shipped to trendy restaurants in New York, San Francisco and elsewhere; and sportfishermen are reeling in—and sometimes eating—deep-sea giants.

The trouble with ciguatoxin is that there's no way to detect its presence in fish. And no way to destroy it. Cooking doesn't help, nor do soaking, smoking, pickling, canning, freezing, drying. Symptoms of ciguatera poisoning usually occur within six hours of eating contaminated fish: first diarrhea, abdominal cramps, nausea and vomiting; then tingling on the bottoms of the feet, the palms, in the mouth; then aches, shooting pains and sometimes a bizarre sensation reversal—cold feels hot, hot feels cold.

Misdiagnoses are common—flu, chronic fatigue syndrome, even MS. And unless a doctor "nails" the disease early, there's nothing to do but let it run its course, which can take months. Florida physicians specializing in ciguatera poisoning have had some luck reversing the symptoms, early on, with hefty intravenous doses of mannitol, a sugar alcohol. They believe, too, that Prozac and other antidepressants at least ease the symptoms.

Clearly, the best medicine is prevention. Avoid eating any of the fish known to carry ciguatoxin—and this means at home as well as abroad. If you must eat these problem fish, make sure they're small enough to fit on your plate—head and all. Never settle for fillets, which may have been cut from a 150-pounder loaded with ciguatoxin.

Cirrhosis (diet and): Often brought on by prolonged alcohol abuse (but sometimes by malaria, syphilis, blocked bile ducts or malnutrition), cirrhosis is a progressive liver disease in which liver cells die and are replaced by fibrous connective tissue. In the early stages of cirrhosis, the first step is to ban alcohol, then to regenerate liver tissue by bulking up on carbohydrates and protein (50 percent over the RDA is the usual diet). If there's edema, sodium intake must be slashed to about 500 milligrams a day. In advanced cirrhosis when the liver can't perform its role in protein metabolism, protein must be restricted, sometimes to as little as 40 grams a day. If there are esophageal varices (varicose veins), coarse or fibrous foods are off-limits, too.

Citric Acid (additive): Obtained from citrus fruits, this is one of the safest, most widely used food additives in the United States. It's cheap, it's an effective antioxidant, it imparts tartness. Tons of citric acid are mixed into prepared foods each year—everything from soft drinks to cheese.

Citrus Red 2 (artificial coloring): It's not called Citrus Red because it's extracted from citrus fruits but because growers long used it to mask green spots on oranges. A carcinogenic coal-tar dye, it can now be used only to color Florida orange rinds and in limited amounts (less than 2 parts per million by weight of whole fruit). To overcome consumer fears, some Florida growers are no longer using Citrus Red 2. And to counter skepticism about their mottled green oranges, they've mounted a TV ad blitz to prove they're sweetly ripe inside.

Clam Juice: Cooks who don't want the fuss of making fish or shellfish stock from scratch find that a 50-50 blend of bottled clam juice and water makes a dandy substitute in soups and stews. And those eager to take the sizzle out of summer enjoy cooling off with a half and half mix of bottled clam juice and canned beef broth on the rocks. Available in 8-ounce bottles almost everywhere, "canned" clam juice is heavily salted and flavor-enhanced with HYDROLYZED VEGETABLE PROTEIN, an additive the FDA considers safe.

NUTRIENT CONTENT OF 1 CUP BOTTLED CLAM BROTH
(8 fluid ounces; 242 grams)

5 calories	516 mg sodium
1 g protein	358 mg potassium
0 g fat, 0 saturated	0 g dietary fiber
7 mg cholesterol	22 RE vitamin A
0 g carbohydrate	0.02 mg thiamin
31 mg calcium	0.05 mg riboflavin
274 mg phosphorus	0.4 mg niacin
0.7 mg iron	2 mg vitamin C

Clams: Of the dozen-and-some different clams found in offshore American waters, the two most popular are East Coast **softshell clams** (steamers) and **quahogs** or **hardshell clams** (littlenecks and cherrystones are the smallest quahogs). If the middens of clamshells found up and down the Atlantic seaboard are any indication, Native Americans were clam eaters without peer. It was they who buried quahogs (the word is derived from the Narraganset) in earthen pits alongside ears of corn and came up with the

NUTRIENT CONTENT OF 6 MEDIUM-SIZE SHUCKED RAW CLAMS
(about 3 ounces; 85 grams)

58 calories	94 mg sodium
6 g protein	192 mg potassium
2 g fat, 0 saturated	0 g dietary fiber
46 mg cholesterol	77 RE vitamin A
3 g carbohydrate	0.09 mg thiamin
38 mg calcium	0.14 mg riboflavin
117 mg phosphorus	1.1 mg niacin
5.6 mg iron	9 mg vitamin C

NUTRIENT CONTENT OF 9 SMALL STEAMED, SHUCKED CLAMS
(about 3 ounces; 85 grams)

58 calories	94 mg sodium
6 g protein	192 mg potassium
2 g fat, 0 saturated	0 g dietary fiber
46 mg cholesterol	185 RE vitamin A
3 g carbohydrate	0.13 mg thiamin
38 mg calcium	0.14 mg riboflavin
117 mg phosphorus	1.0 mg niacin
5.6 mg iron	19 mg vitamin C

clambake. Today our clam supply is threatened by polluted waters, also by the RED TIDE, a warm-weather plague of microscopic planktons that makes most mollusks toxic. At such times, many states ban fishing. As for polluted waters, they are an ongoing problem. The lesson here: Unless you know local clamming grounds to be clean, cook clams before eating. Serving them on the half shell is flirting with hepatitis.

NUTRIENT CONTENT OF 3 OUNCES (85 GRAMS) BREADED, FRIED CLAMS

167 calories	355 mg sodium
8 g protein	208 mg potassium
11 g fat, 2 saturated	0 g dietary fiber
69 mg cholesterol	77 RE vitamin A
10 g carbohydrate	0.09 mg thiamin
53 mg calcium	0.21 mg riboflavin
135 mg phosphorus	1.8 mg niacin
5.9 mg iron	9 mg vitamin C

Clay, Eating of: See PICA.

Clostridium botulinum: See BACTERIA.

Clostridium perfringens: See BACTERIA.

Club Soda, Seltzer: See CARBONATED BEVERAGES.

CMC: See CARBOXYMETHYL CELLULOSE.

Coal-Tar Dyes: See COLORINGS.

Cobalamin: See B_{12}, VITAMIN.

Cobalt: This mineral, an important part of cobalamin or vitamin B_{12}, is integral to the development of red blood cells, also to enzymes involved with cell metabolism in general. The best sources of cobalt are meats, particularly organ meats like liver and kidneys. Few people, other than strict vegetarians (vegans), are apt to be deficient in it.

Cocaine (diet and): Users of cocaine and crack (addictive, energizing drugs extracted from the leaves of the coca plant) suffer appetite and weight loss, stomach cramps, diarrhea and malnutrition. Once detoxed, they are put on calorie-dense, high-complex-carbohydrate diets to build them up.

Cocarcinogen: Something, either a chemical or an environmental factor, that reinforces or encourages the action of a carcinogen and results in a malignancy.

Cochineal (additive): A natural red pigment obtained from insects used to color food. GRAS.

Cocoa: In the mid-nineteenth century a Dutch scientist named Conrad J. van Houten discovered a way to defat cocoa beans and press them into dry cakes that could be pulverized. He called his chocolate powder cocoa. Today, there are two principal types of cocoa: **all-purpose** and **Dutch process** (darker and richer because it's been treated with lye). Both are significantly lower in fat than CHOCOLATE and thus good bets for dieters.

NUTRIENT CONTENT OF 1 TABLESPOON UNSWEETENED ALL-PURPOSE COCOA POWDER

(about 1/5 ounce; 5 grams)

12 calories	1 mg sodium
1 g protein	82 mg potassium
1 g fat, 0 saturated	2 g dietary fiber
0 mg cholesterol	0 RE vitamin A
3 g carbohydrate	0 mg thiamin
7 mg calcium	0.01 mg riboflavin
39 mg phosphorus	0.1 mg niacin
0.8 mg iron	0 mg vitamin C

NUTRIENT CONTENT OF 1 TABLESPOON DUTCH PROCESS COCOA POWDER

(about 1/5 ounce; 5 grams)

12 calories	1 mg sodium
1 g protein	135 mg potassium
1 g fat, 0 saturated	2 g dietary fiber
0 mg cholesterol	0 RE vitamin A
3 g carbohydrate	0.01 mg thiamin
6 mg calcium	0.03 mg riboflavin
39 mg phosphorus	0.1 mg niacin
0.8 mg iron	0 mg vitamin C

Cocoa Butter: The fat of chocolate. It's highly saturated, and when extracted from the chocolate and blended with sugar, milk solids and flavorings, it becomes WHITE CHOCOLATE.

Coconut Oil: Pressed from the nut kernels of the coconut palm, this oil changes from liquid to butter-hard in the space of a few degrees Celsius. Coconut oil is used in commercial breads, cookies, cakes and candies. But because the public is wising up to the fact that coconut oil is highly saturated, manufacturers are beginning to use less of it.

Coconuts: To us, the coconut may seem frivolous, but to a third of the world it is meat and drink. Because coconuts drift thousands of miles across open ocean taking root wherever they fetch up, no one knows where they originated although the South Pacific is a good guess. Columbus found no coconuts in the New World. Marco Polo tasted them in India and was impressed. Still, these tropical exotics made no culinary impact on Western Europe until the turn of the eighteenth century. And then only because a British explorer brought Australian coconuts home to England and began extolling their virtues. That, to be sure, was before our nutritional consciousness had been raised, before we began counting calories and grams of fat. Co-

conuts have plenty of both. Their fat, moreover, is highly saturated. So is the fat in coconut milk, a creamy liquid squeezed from freshly shredded coconut. Coconut cream is something else again, a sweet, thick blend sold by the can that's popular for mixed drinks. As for the liquid inside every ripe coconut, that's coconut juice. Fresh coconuts seldom show up in supermarkets nowadays, so what most of us know best is shredded and flaked coconut—presweetened, bagged and ready to fold into cakes, cookies and candies.

NUTRIENT CONTENT OF ½ CUP COMMERCIALLY FLAKED OR SWEETENED COCONUT
(about 1½ ounces; 39 grams)

171 calories	8 mg sodium
1 g protein	125 mg potassium
12 g fat, 11 saturated	7 g dietary fiber
0 mg cholesterol	0 RE vitamin A
16 g carbohydrate	0.01 mg thiamin
6 mg calcium	0.01 mg riboflavin
40 mg phosphorus	0.1 mg niacin
0.7 mg iron	0 mg vitamin C

NUTRIENT CONTENT OF 1 (2 × 2 × ½-INCH) PIECE FRESH SHELLED, PEELED COCONUT
(about 1¾ ounces; 45 grams)

159 calories	9 mg sodium
2 g protein	160 mg potassium
15 g fat, 13 saturated	4 g dietary fiber
0 mg cholesterol	0 RE vitamin A
7 g carbohydrate	0.03 mg thiamin
6 mg calcium	0.01 mg riboflavin
51 mg phosphorus	0.2 mg niacin
1.1 mg iron	2 mg vitamin C

NUTRIENT CONTENT OF ½ CUP CANNED COCONUT MILK
(4 fluid ounces; 113 grams)

223 calories	15 mg sodium
2 g protein	249 mg potassium
24 g fat, 21 saturated	1 g dietary fiber
0 mg cholesterol	0 RE vitamin A
3 g carbohydrate	0.03 mg thiamin
20 mg calcium	0 mg riboflavin
109 mg phosphorus	0.7 mg niacin
3.7 mg iron	1 mg vitamin C

Cod: The world's most important saltwater fish, lean and white of flesh, delicate of flavor and now, sad to say, overfished. Shortly after Columbus discovered America, the Portuguese were scooping up tons of cod on Newfoundland's Grand Banks, salting them, then carrying them home to sun dry on the beaches of Portugal until as stiff as boards (see BACALHAU). In early Massachusetts, cod was so important (as both food and income) it found its way onto corporate signs and seals, family crests, even stationery. It was the foundation of the New England fishing industry (not for nothing is Boston called the land of the bean and the cod) and remains an important catch to this day. Cod comes in all sizes—from **scrod** averaging 1½ to 2½ pounds to giants of 25 pounds or more. Scrod are usually broiled or sautéed in a nubbin of butter; larger cod are more likely to be cut into steaks and steamed or to be slipped into chowder. For approximate nutrient counts, see FISH, LEAN WHITE.

Cod-Liver Oil: Like all lean fish, cod has its oils concentrated in the liver. Cod-liver oil, the most important of all the fish-liver oils, is a potent source of vitamins A and D.

Before vitamin pills were commonplace, mothers often force-fed their children a teaspoon or two of cod-liver oil every morning—mint-flavored, if the kids were lucky. Today, it is fed to livestock.

Coenzyme Q, Coenzyme Q-10, Ubiquinone: A fatty substance, chemically similar to vitamins E and K, that's found in almost all living cells and also easily synthesized by the body. Its role is to help break nutrients down, releasing energy to fuel respiration. **DIETARY SOURCES:** Meats, fish and fowl; vegetable oils and soybeans. Health-food stores hype coenzyme Q-10 heavily as a fountain of youth and preventive of heart disease, among other things. Though preliminary studies suggest that it may work like an antioxidant, it should never be used indiscriminately, only as a doctor advises.

Coenzymes: Small molecules that enable enzymes to do their job, by either bonding with the enzyme or becoming part of it. Many of the B vitamins are coenzymes, among them **thiamin, riboflavin, niacin** and **pyridoxine.**

Coffee: It causes cancer . . . heart attacks . . . infertility . . . ulcers . . . birth defects. These are just a few of the bashes aimed at coffee in recent years. A study will surface indicting coffee on one count or another only to be shot down by a second study. So far no one has proved that two or three cups of coffee a day are harmful, although everyone agrees that coffee is a mild stimulant (see CAFFEINE) and that habitual coffee drinkers often become cranky, headachy, even nauseated if deprived of their cuppas. Decaf (brewed from beans that are 97 percent caffeine free), is becoming the coffee of choice (four times as many people drink it today as twenty-five years ago). But it's taken some heat, too. A recent Stanford study puts forth pretty convincing evidence that drinking decaffeinated coffee significantly raises the amount of "bad" cholesterol (LDL) in the blood. What *next*? Clearly, moderation is the best policy when it comes to drinking coffee—decaf or otherwise. Most people consider coffee a nutritional cipher. Actually, it does contain traces of calcium, iron and phosphorus as well as some of the B-complex. As for calories, there are about 5 in each cup of *black* coffee.

Colas: See CARBONATED BEVERAGES.

Colds: Viral infections of the respiratory tract characterized by a sore throat, coughing, sniffles, a stuffy nose and sometimes a fever as well. How does the old saying go? "Starve a fever, feed a cold"? And what about megadoses of vitamin C? Do they keep you cold-free? Does sucking zinc tablets stop a cold in its tracks? The truth is not so dramatic. Vitamin C may reduce the severity of the symptoms of a cold, but nutritionists say it will not prevent colds. Nor will gobbling zinc tablets, although mild zinc deficiencies do seem to weaken the immune system. Grandmother was right. "Feeding a cold" is the way to go. Chicken soup opens the head, as do garlic, horseradish and hot chile peppers.

Colic: There is no known cause or cure for these bouts of inconsolable crying that afflict so many babies (most often those less than four months old). The good news is that the colic won't last forever and doesn't seem to impair infants in any way.

Collagen: The main protein in connective tissue, bones and hooves. The reason tough cuts of meat become tender when cooked with liquid is that the collagen is converted to gelatin. Indeed, all that's needed to extract gelatin from bones and hooves is to crack them and boil them in water.

Collards: This nonheading Old World cabbage with intense green leaves is more nutritious than its paler cousins. Food historians believe collards were brought to the Deep South by slaves. This vegetable is still a Southern staple, particularly among African Americans who have beatified it as soul food. Usually collards are cooked to death with

NUTRIENT CONTENT OF 1 CUP BOILED/STEAMED COARSELY CHOPPED COLLARDS	
(about 4½ ounces; 128 grams)	
34 calories	21 mg sodium
2 g protein	168 mg potassium
0 g fat, 0 saturated	4 g dietary fiber
0 mg cholesterol	349 RE vitamin A
8 g carbohydrate	0.03 mg thiamin
30 mg calcium	0.07 mg riboflavin
10 mg phosphorus	0.4 mg niacin
0.2 mg iron	15 mg vitamin C

lots of water and a chunk of ham or fatback—a sure way to destroy much of the vitamin C. Steaming collards quickly like spinach will preserve most of the vitamins, as will shredding them and tossing, Portuguese-style, into potato soup at the very last minute. *Caldo verde* ("green soup") the Portuguese call this oniony, garlicky emerald soup. It's the national dish and they eat it almost every day. **SEASON:** Year-round, with supplies peaking between December and April.

Colorings (additives): The FDA has approved thirty-three different pigments for coloring food, twenty-six of them natural pigments. These, however, are more expensive and less stable than the intense palette of artificial colors synthesized from coal tar, so food processors use the synthetics almost exclusively. The trouble is, some artificial colorings are carcinogenic and those still in use are under intense scrutiny—Red No. 3 (used to dye maraschino cherries and pistachios) and Yellow No. 5, to name two. Artificial colorings may make soft drinks, instants and mixes, cold cuts, hot dogs and so on cosmetically pretty, but they may also be hazardous to your health. **THOSE NOW DEFINITELY BANNED:** Red Nos. 1, 2, 4 and 32; Orange Nos. 1 and 2; Yellow Nos. 1, 2, 3 and 4; Butter Yellow; Green Nos. 1 and 2; Violet No. 1; and Sudan 1.

Colostrum: The "premilk" new mothers produce two or three days after delivery before true lactation begins. Colostrum is higher in protein than fully developed breast milk, also in antibodies that boost the newborn's immunity and such nutrients as chloride, iodine, potassium, sodium, sulfur and zinc. It's lower, however, in lactose (milk sugar) and fat. These two increase, along with water-soluble vitamins (C and the B group) as breast feeding progresses while the amount of proteins and fat-soluble vitamins (A, D, E and K) decrease. The body, so to speak, tailors mother's milk to fit the baby's changing nutritional needs.

Comfrey, Comfrey Tea: A medicinal herb used for a variety of ailments since medieval days. The leaves, dried and infused into tea, were sipped to relieve respiratory congestion and indigestion. Comfrey poultices were applied to speed the healing of wounds and broken bones, which explains why this herb was also called **boneset** and **knitbone. CAUTION:** Although comfrey teas and potions still have their champions, botanists point out that comfrey, taken internally, is highly toxic, and that frequent use may, over time, damage—perhaps even destroy—the liver. Canada now bans the sale of many comfrey products.

Complementary Proteins: See PROTEIN.

Complete Proteins: See PROTEIN.

Complex Carbohydrates: See CARBOHYDRATES.

Conch: Pronounced *konk*. This mollusk proliferates throughout the Caribbean and Gulf of Mexico and is an important food there. Like abalone and octopus, conch is tough and must be pounded until tender. Or ground—often the case—and cooked in chowders or fritters. Conch tastes quite like clams although it's a bit milder and sweeter. Although no nutrient counts are available for conch, it is surely a high-protein, low-fat food with plenty of minerals—iron, potassium and the like.

Condensed Milk: See MILK.

Congeners: By-products of wine and liquor making that give the different wines and spirits their individuality. Congeners are responsible for aromas, flavors and yes, hangovers, too. According to one study, brandy causes the worst hangovers, then red wine, then rum, then Scotch, bourbon or other whiskey, then white wine, then gin.

Constipation (diet and): A sluggish or inactive bowel, usually temporary. Although diet can't cure constipation, it can certainly ease the symptoms. For **atonic constipation** (caused by lack of intestinal muscle tone), plenty of water and dietary fiber (with the emphasis on whole grains, legumes, fresh fruits and vegetables) is the way to spell r-e-l-i-e-f. With **spastic constipation,** the best diet minimizes fiber, which can irritate and distend the intestines.

Convenience Foods: They're great time-savers and they simplify cleanup, but they're expensive. More important, they often aren't as nutritious as food cooked from scratch. Too many convenience foods—the instants, mixes, canned goods, TV dinners, indeed all but the simplest frozen foods—may be loaded with fat, sugar and/or salt, so scrutinize labels. Handling is a problem with frozen foods, too, because some are allowed to thaw in transit or storage. (Reject any frozen food that feels soft or misshapen; it's probably thawed, then refrozen, and may be contaminated with bacteria as well as be of poor quality.) Many convenience foods, moreover, brim with a scary pharmacopoeia of additives. The FDA, to be sure, regulates the use of additives to keep our food supply safe (*not* carefully enough, consumer advocates howl).

Copper: This mineral plays many vital roles in the body. It's used in the manufacture of red blood cells, bones and COLLAGEN; the healing of wounds; the absorption and transport of iron; the metabolism of fatty acids; even the creation of ribonucleic acid (RNA). Copper deficiencies are rare in human beings, but animal tests show that lack of copper can cause, among other things, anemia, nervous disorders, infertility and skeletal defects. Although there are no RDAs for copper, the amount judged safe and adequate for adults is 1.5 to 3 milligrams per day. **GOOD SOURCES:** Wheat (although some copper is lost in the milling), peanuts (again, losses when peanuts are churned into peanut butter), shellfish, liver, cereals, nuts and legumes. And here's a chemical curiosity: If you use a copper pot to cook red cabbage, beets or other food rich in red pigments called ANTHOCYANINS, it will turn a revolting shade of slate blue.

Corn: The miracle of corn is that it survived the centuries to become a world staple. It's the most helpless of plants, incapable of propagating itself, so from earliest times on, man has had to do that job himself. The Jemez Indians of New Mexico will show you a spindly grass at Bandelier National Monument and tell you, "From this we got corn." Botanists, however, have long known that the teosintes, wild annual grasses that grow over much of Mexico and Guatemala, are corn's closest relatives. What clinched the kinship was the recent discovery that a particular teosinte, the balsas or *guerrero,* not only had the same biochemical and genetic makeup as corn but could be interbred with it. The first European to encounter corn was probably Leif Eriksson, who landed just south of Cape Cod in the year 1000 and commented upon the cornfields. In the New World, Columbus found both corn and cornmeal, which he described as "a very well-tasted flour made of a kind of grain called maize." His high regard for maize, however, was not shared by his fellow Europeans, who considered corn fit only for animals. Many Europeans still

do. Americans, on the other hand, can't get enough of it, especially sweet corn on the cob, rushed from stalk to kettle and served neath a thick buttery rub. Corn is a high-fiber, high-carbohydrate food, a fair source of vitamin A (if the corn is yellow). Low-sodium and low-fat, it contains traces of iron, vitamin C and some of the Bs. **SEASON:** Mid- to late summer.

NUTRIENT CONTENT OF 1 MEDIUM-SIZE BOILED/STEAMED EAR OF YELLOW CORN

(about 2¾ ounces; 77 grams)

83 calories	13 mg sodium
3 g protein	192 mg potassium
1 g fat, 0 saturated	3 g dietary fiber
0 mg cholesterol	17 RE vitamin A
19 g carbohydrate	0.17 mg thiamin
2 mg calcium	0.06 mg riboflavin
79 mg phosphorus	1.2 mg niacin
0.5 mg iron	5 mg vitamin C

NUTRIENT CONTENT OF 1 CUP BOILED/STEAMED WHOLE-KERNEL YELLOW CORN

(about 5¾ ounces; 164 grams)

178 calories	28 mg sodium
5 g protein	408 mg potassium
2 g fat, 0 saturated	8 g dietary fiber
0 mg cholesterol	18 RE vitamin A
42 g carbohydrate	0.36 mg thiamin
4 mg calcium	0.12 mg riboflavin
168 mg phosphorus	2.6 mg niacin
1.0 mg iron	10 mg vitamin C

NUTRIENT CONTENT OF 1 CUP CANNED CREAM-STYLE YELLOW CORN

(about 9 ounces; 256 grams)

186 calories	730 mg sodium
4 g protein	344 mg potassium
1 g fat, 0 saturated	3 g dietary fiber
0 mg cholesterol	24 RE vitamin A
46 g carbohydrate	0.06 mg thiamin
8 mg calcium	0.14 mg riboflavin
130 mg phosphorus	2.5 mg niacin
1.0 mg iron	12 mg vitamin C

Corn Dog: A hot dog dipped in corn batter and deep-fat-fried—a uniquely American form of junk food. Corn dogs drip with calories, fat, cholesterol and sodium. And though they do contain some minerals, vitamins A and B-complex, their nutritional minuses outweigh the pluses.

NUTRIENT CONTENT OF 1 CORN DOG
(about 6 ounces; 175 grams)

460 calories	973 mg sodium
17 g protein	263 mg potassium
19 g fat, 5 saturated	NA g dietary fiber
79 mg cholesterol	37 RE vitamin A
56 g carbohydrate	0.28 mg thiamin
102 mg calcium	0.70 mg riboflavin
166 mg phosphorus	4.2 mg niacin
6 mg iron	0 mg vitamin C

Corned Beef: Before refrigeration, before freezing, before canning even, people preserved meat by soaking it in brine, often a solution of saltpeter, sugar and spices. When beef—usually brisket—is cured this way, it's called corned beef. Aside from the nitrates (and potential carcinogens) it contains, corned beef is loaded with sodium, fat (mostly saturated) and cholesterol. Brisket isn't the only cut of beef that's corned. Tongue often is, and in a way, beef hot dogs, too. All are poor choices for anyone with heart disease, high blood pressure or kidney problems.

NUTRIENT CONTENT OF 3 OUNCES (85 GRAMS) TRIMMED, COOKED CORNED-BEEF BRISKET

213 calories	962 mg sodium
15 g protein	123 mg potassium
16 g fat, 6 saturated	0 g dietary fiber
83 mg cholesterol	0 RE vitamin A
0 g carbohydrate	0.02 mg thiamin
7 mg calcium	0.15 mg riboflavin
106 mg phosphorus	2.6 mg niacin
1.6 mg iron	14 mg vitamin C

Cornell Bread: Some years ago, New York State mental hospitals sounded the call for a supernutritious bread because patients were eating bread to the exclusion of everything else. Cornell nutritionist Clive McCay set to work and developed a firm, chewy loaf, bulking up the protein, vitamins and minerals with wheat germ, nonfat dry milk and soy flour. See page 95 for the recipe.

Cornish Game Hens: See ROCK CORNISH HENS.

Cornmeal: Southerners insist on stone-ground meal—preferably white. The rest of the country settles for the granular yellow stuff—or worse, corn bread mixes, most of which are full of sugar and salt. To produce cornmeal, white or yellow kernels are dried, their hull (outer husk) and germ are removed, then the rest of the kernel (flint) is ground. Unfortunately, many vitamins and minerals are sacrificed in the hulling and degerming. So to approximate the nutrient level of whole kernels, most cornmeal is now enriched with iron, calcium, thiamin, riboflavin and niacin in amounts set by the government. Whole-corn meals are also available at many health-food stores but should be refrigerated to prolong their short shelf life (the oily germ quickly goes rancid). See also GRITS.

NUTRIENT CONTENT OF 1 CUP ENRICHED SELF-RISING YELLOW CORNMEAL
(about 4¼ ounces; 122 grams)

489 calories	1,858 mg sodium
12 g protein	235 mg potassium
2 g fat, 0 saturated	7 g dietary fiber
0 mg cholesterol	57 RE vitamin A
103 g carbohydrate	0.94 mg thiamin
483 mg calcium	0.53 mg riboflavin
858 mg phosphorus	6.3 mg niacin
6.5 mg iron	0 mg vitamin C

NUTRIENT CONTENT OF 1 CUP WHOLE-GRAIN YELLOW CORNMEAL
(about 4¼ ounces; 122 grams)

440 calories	43 mg sodium
10 g protein	350 mg potassium
4 g fat, 1 saturated	13 g dietary fiber
0 mg cholesterol	57 RE vitamin A
94 g carbohydrate	0.47 mg thiamin
7 mg calcium	0.25 mg riboflavin
294 mg phosphorus	4.4 mg niacin
4.2 mg iron	0 mg vitamin C

Note: The nutrients for 1 cup whole-grain white cornmeal are identical except that it contains zero vitamin A.

Corn Oil: This sun-gold oil is pressed from the germ of corn kernels. Food processors use it for mayonnaises, margarines and baked goods. And though it doesn't make a

Cornell Bread

Makes two 9 × 5 × 3-inch Loaves, 16 Slices per Loaf

1½ cups warm water (105° to 115°F.)

1 envelope (1 scant tablespoon) active dry yeast

½ cup milk, scalded

3 tablespoons sugar

3 tablespoons unsalted butter or margarine

2 teaspoons salt

6 tablespoons soy flour

6 tablespoons nonfat dry milk

2 tablespoons wheat germ

5 cups unbleached all-purpose flour, approximately

PLACE WATER IN a large warm bowl, sprinkle in yeast, and stir to dissolve; set aside. Combine milk, sugar, butter, and salt in a bowl. Cool to lukewarm and stir into yeast mixture. Mix in soy flour, dry milk, wheat germ, and 3 cups flour, beating hard. Beat in remaining flour, 1 cup at a time, to form a soft but manageable dough. Turn out onto a floured cloth and knead 8 to 10 minutes, until smooth and springy, adding only enough flour to keep dough from sticking. Shape dough into ball, place in a buttered large bowl, then turn in bowl so surface is buttered, too. Cover with a cloth and let rise in a warm, dry spot, away from drafts for 1 hour or until doubled in bulk.

PUNCH DOUGH DOWN, let rest 5 minutes, then knead lightly 2 minutes on floured cloth. Shape into 2 loaves, place in greased 9 × 5 × 3-inch loaf pans, cover, and let rise 50 to 60 minutes, or until almost doubled in bulk. Toward the end of rising, preheat oven to 400°F. Bake loaves 35 to 40 minutes or until nicely browned and hollow sounding when tapped. Remove bread from pans and cool upright on wire racks before cutting.

APPROXIMATE NUTRIENT COUNTS PER SLICE

97 calories	17 g carbohydrate	1.1 mg iron	0.15 mg thiamin
3 g protein	1 g dietary fiber	140 mg sodium	0.14 mg riboflavin
2 g fat, 0 g saturated	20 mg calcium	74 mg potassium	1.2 mg niacin
1 mg cholesterol	45 mg phosphorus	21 RE vitamin A	0 mg vitamin C

very tasty salad, it is a good all-round cooking oil. The fatty-acid breakdown in corn oil looks like this: 13 percent saturated, 62 percent polyunsaturated and 25 percent monounsaturated. As for nutrient content: 1 tablespoon of corn oil contains 14 grams of fat, 120 calories and 0 cholesterol.

Cornstarch: A fine snow-white powder made from the endosperm of corn kernels. When heated with liquid, cornstarch has about twice the thickening power of flour although—make a note—if the liquid is acid (citrus juice, apple or cherry juice, for example) its thickening power is diminished by about half. The advantage of using corn-starch as a thickener is that it forms a sparkling, near-clear sauce—not true of flour-based sauces, which are always milky. Cornstarch has other important uses, too. It's what gives Scottish shortbread its dissolve-on-the-tongue texture and accounts for the wispy coatings on such deep-fried foods as tempura. As for nutritive value: 1 tablespoon cornstarch = 29 calories and 7 grams of carbohydrate. There are also traces of protein, fat, sodium and potassium but they're too tiny to matter.

Corn Syrup: Made by partially hydrolyzing cornstarch, this viscous sweetener contains maltose (malt sugar), dextrose (another name for glucose) plus several complex carbohydrates. **Light corn syrup** is a blend of light corn syrup, high-fructose corn syrup, salt and vanilla; **dark corn syrup** is a mix of dark corn syrup, refiner's syrup, caramel flavoring, salt, sodium benzoate (a preservative) and caramel color. As for nutrients, corn syrup offers little other than calories, carbohydrate and sodium. For example, 1 tablespoon light corn syrup contains 60 calories, 15 grams carbohydrate and 30 milligrams sodium. The counts for dark corn syrup are identical except that its sodium count is slightly higher—40 milligrams instead of 30.

Coronary Heart Disease (CHD)   (diet and):

Silent and sneaky, coronary heart disease is this nation's number-one killer. Its most likely targets? Cigarette smokers, those with a family history of CHD or with diabetes, high blood pressure and/or too many extra pounds. The last three are diet related. The lengthy FRAMINGHAM HEART STUDY, begun in 1949, proved that men with blood CHOLESTEROL averaging 260 or more were three times as likely to suffer heart attacks as those with cholesterol levels down around 195. In 1988, the U.S. surgeon general concluded not only that high blood cholesterol was a major factor in CHD but, more important, that it could be modified by eating less fat, especially saturated fats. These increase blood cholesterol levels, which in turn accelerate the formation of artery-clogging plaques. The surgeon general's report further recommended that only 30 percent of the day's calories come from fat, with the emphasis on lowering saturated fat (some cardiologists would like to see the limit lowered to 20 percent, even 10).

What this means is drinking skim milk instead of whole, substituting soft margarines (or butter substitutes) for butter, using cooking oils high in monosaturated fatty acids that elevate blood levels of HDL, or "good," cholesterol, which flush fatty deposits from the veins, and lower those of the "bad," or LDL, which increase arterial plaque build-up. It also means eating ices instead of ice creams, low-fat mayonnaises instead of the oil-rich, lean fish and skinned chicken breasts instead of steak and hamburger.

In addition to telling patients to cut down on fat, some physicians advise reducing salt (to help lower blood pressure) and eating fewer cholesterol-laden foods (egg yolks, liver, kidneys, etc.) although the food cholesterol is now considered less a culprit than saturated fat.

The latest devlopment—actually new support for an old theory—is that a buildup in the blood of the amino acid homocysteine may injure blood vessels. This in turn can cause hardening of the arteries and possibly heart attacks and strokes. Lowering homocysteine levels is apparently as easy as consuming more folic acid, a B vitamin that is present in orange juice, many fresh fruits and dark green leafy vegetables. Some scientists believe that getting adequate vitamin B_6 may also play a role in lowering homocysteine levels. See also FOLIC ACID and HOMOCYSTEINE.

Cortisol, Cortisone: Steroid hormones synthesized in the adrenal glands that are vital to the metabolism of carbohydrate, protein and fat. Too much cortisol or cortisone whets the appetite, depletes the body's supply of calcium and elevates blood sugar levels. Cortisone, sometimes prescribed as a medication to relieve the pain of rheumatoid arthritis, can be addicting.

Cottage Cheese: "Mary, Mary, quite contrary, eating her cottage cheese." It doesn't sing like "curds and whey," but what nursery rhyme Mary was eating *was* cottage cheese. Or perhaps a simple precursor of it. Today, there's **pot cheese** (sour and dry), **farmer's cheese** (cottage cheese still made on the farm), **cream-style** (with cream mixed in), **sweet-curd** (with much of the sour lactic acid rinsed out), **California style** (small curd), **low-fat, reduced-sodium** and **no-salt,** not to mention cottage cheeses of assorted flavors. All begin with fresh cow's milk, which is heated, clabbered (either with rennet or by bacterial action), drained and cut. These are soft, fresh cheeses—highly perishable. Despite all the confusing label names and descriptions, all cottage cheeses are categorized according to their milk-fat content and fall into one of three groups: **creamed** (with 4 percent milk fat or more),

NUTRIENT CONTENT OF ½ CUP CREAMED COTTAGE CHEESE	
(about 3¾ ounces; 105 grams)	
109 calories	425 mg sodium
13 g protein	89 mg potassium
5 g fat, 3 saturated	0 g dietary fiber
16 mg cholesterol	51 RE vitamin A
3 g carbohydrate	0.02 mg thiamin
62 mg calcium	0.17 mg riboflavin
139 mg phosphorus	0.1 mg niacin
0.2 mg iron	0 mg vitamin C

low fat (½ to 2 percent milk fat) or **dry-curd** (less than ½ percent milk fat). All are high-protein foods rich in riboflavin, phosphorus and, alas, sodium, too. Unfortunately, much of the calcium is drained off with the whey.

NUTRIENT CONTENT OF ½ CUP LOW-FAT COTTAGE CHEESE

(about 3¾ ounces; 105 grams)

82 calories	469 mg sodium
14 g protein	97 mg potassium
1 g fat, 1 saturated	0 g dietary fiber
5 mg cholesterol	13 RE vitamin A
3 g carbohydrate	0.02 mg thiamin
69 mg calcium	0.19 mg riboflavin
151 mg phosphorus	0.1 mg niacin
0.2 mg iron	0 mg vitamin C

NUTRIENT CONTENT OF ½ CUP DRY-CURD COTTAGE CHEESE

(about 2⅔ ounces; 73 grams)

62 calories	10 mg sodium
13 g protein	24 mg potassium
0 g fat, 0 saturated	0 g dietary fiber
5 mg cholesterol	12 RE vitamin A
1 g carbohydrate	0.02 mg thiamin
23 mg calcium	0.10 mg riboflavin
76 mg phosphorus	0.1 mg niacin
0.2 mg iron	0 mg vitamin C

Cottonseed Oil: Extracted from cotton seeds, this oil is slow to turn rancid, one reason processors like it for shortenings, cooking oil blends and margarines. As for composition, 27 percent of the fatty acids in cottonseed oil are saturated, 54 percent polyunsaturated and 19 percent monounsaturated—not as healthful a mix as in olive or canola oil. Its fat, calorie and cholesterol counts, however, are identical to other oils. Thus 1 tablespoon of cottonseed oil equals 14 grams of fat, 120 calories and 0 cholesterol.

Coumarin: A perfumy artificial vanilla flavoring extracted from the tonka bean that's more powerful than vanilla itself. Among its derivatives are a series of blood thinners or anticoagulants frequently prescribed to heart patients and warfarin, a rat poison. Once a food additive (a vanilla fla-

voring cheaper than the real thing), it has been banned by the FDA since 1954. But it is still widely sold in Mexico as "genuine vanilla extract."

Couscous: Sometimes called **Moroccan pasta,** couscous is nothing of the sort. It is the hard golden heart of semolina wheat dried and reduced to granules (*couscous* is the Arabic word for semolina). Across North Africa, couscous is the starch of choice, the perfect sop for a huge repertoire of lamb and chicken stews. In the United States, many cooks like to use couscous as a substitute for rice, potatoes and, yes, even pasta. It's available in most supermarkets—often in instant form, which needs nothing more than to be covered with boiling broth or water and left to stand for five minutes.

NUTRIENT CONTENT OF 1 CUP BOILED COUSCOUS

(about 6⅓ ounces; 179 grams)

201 calories	9 mg sodium
7 g protein	104 mg potassium
0 g fat, 0 saturated	5 g dietary fiber
0 mg cholesterol	0 RE vitamin A
42 g carbohydrate	0.11 mg thiamin
15 mg calcium	0.05 mg riboflavin
39 mg phosphorus	1.8 mg niacin
0.7 mg iron	0 mg vitamin C

Cowpeas: See BEANS, DRIED; BEANS, FRESH.

Crab Apples: Too acid to eat raw, most of these tiny apples are boiled into jelly or preserved whole and sent forth as edible garnishes. They are fairly low in calories but do contain a little calcium and phosphorus and some po-

NUTRIENT CONTENT OF 1 CUP CRAB APPLE SLICES

(about 3¾ ounces; 110 grams)

84 calories	1 mg sodium
0 g protein	213 mg potassium
0 g fat, 0 saturated	1 g dietary fiber
0 mg cholesterol	4 RE vitamin A
22 g carbohydrate	0.03 mg thiamin
20 mg calcium	0.02 mg riboflavin
17 mg phosphorus	0.1 mg niacin
0.4 mg iron	9 mg vitamin C

tassium and vitamin C. The canned variety also contains considerable sugar and artificial food color. Read labels carefully.

Crabs: To East Coasters, nothing beats a **blue crab,** "the beautiful swimmer" of Chesapeake Bay—especially the just molted softshells of spring and summer. But West Coasters insist that their **Dungeness** is bigger and better in every way. For years professional chefs competed in a blue crab/Dungeness cook-off to determine, once and for all, which crab was better. One year a San Francisco chef would win; the next year a New York or Baltimore chef. And so it went—and goes—for the argument isn't likely to end anytime soon. **Alaska king crabs** and **snow crabs** aren't really in the running (nor are Florida's all-claw **stone crabs**); they come to us frozen. Still, they have their champions in mid-America, where blue crabs and Dungeness are a rarity.

Crackers: By the end of the eighteenth century, **soda crackers**—so called because they made a cracking sound when chewed—were well known in America. So were **common** or **pilot crackers,** a blander version New Englanders liked to crumble into their chowders. Today supermarket shelves overflow with crackers of every size, shape and flavor. They're the favorite scooper-upper for cocktail dips, the preferred "canvas" for spreads, the accompaniment of choice for soups, the quintessential snack

NUTRIENT CONTENT OF 3 OUNCES (85 GRAMS) STEAMED/BOILED BLUE CRAB

87 calories	237 mg sodium
17 g protein	275 mg potassium
2 g fat, 0 saturated	0 g dietary fiber
85 mg cholesterol	2 RE vitamin A
0 g carbohydrate	0.09 mg thiamin
88 mg calcium	0.04 mg riboflavin
175 mg phosphorus	2.8 mg niacin
0.8 mg iron	3 mg vitamin C

NUTRIENT CONTENT OF 3 OUNCES (85 GRAMS) STEAMED/BOILED DUNGENESS CRAB

94 calories	321 mg sodium
19 g protein	347 mg potassium
1 g fat, 0 saturated	0 g dietary fiber
65 mg cholesterol	26 RE vitamin A
1 g carbohydrate	0.05 mg thiamin
50 mg calcium	0.17 mg riboflavin
149 mg phosphorus	3.1 mg niacin
0.4 mg iron	3 mg vitamin C

NUTRIENT CONTENT OF 1 OUNCE (28 GRAMS) SODA CRACKERS (SALTINES)

123 calories	369 mg sodium
3 g protein	36 mg potassium
3 g fat, 1 saturated	1 g dietary fiber
0 mg cholesterol	0 RE vitamin A
20 g carbohydrate	0.16 mg thiamin
34 mg calcium	0.13 mg riboflavin
30 mg phosphorus	1.5 mg niacin
1.5 mg iron	0 mg vitamin C

NUTRIENT CONTENT OF 3 OUNCES (85 GRAMS) STEAMED/BOILED ALASKA KING CRAB

82 calories	911 mg sodium
17 g protein	222 mg potassium
1 g fat, 0 saturated	0 g dietary fiber
45 mg cholesterol	7 RE vitamin A
0 g carbohydrate	0.05 mg thiamin
50 mg calcium	0.05 mg riboflavin
238 mg phosphorus	1.1 mg niacin
0.6 mg iron	6 mg vitamin C

NUTRIENT CONTENT OF 1 OUNCE (28 GRAMS) RICH ROUND CRACKERS (RITZ)

143 calories	240 mg sodium
2 g protein	38 mg potassium
7 g fat, 1 saturated	1 g dietary fiber
0 mg cholesterol	0 RE vitamin A
17 g carbohydrate	0.12 mg thiamin
34 mg calcium	0.10 mg riboflavin
65 mg phosphorus	1.2 mg niacin
1.0 mg iron	0 mg vitamin C

that needs only a quick daub of peanut butter or cheese. Soda crackers aren't particularly nutritious (many are frighteningly high in sodium). The rich round crackers everyone adores, moreover, are high in fat. The latest development is that manufacturers, aware of the public's obsession with all things healthful, are offering low-sodium versions of their best-sellers. Will low-fat be next? See also GRAHAM CRACKERS.

NUTRIENT CONTENT OF 1 OUNCE (28 GRAMS) THIN WHEAT CRACKERS

135 calories	247 mg sodium
2 g protein	56 mg potassium
6 g fat, 2 saturated	2 g dietary fiber
6 mg cholesterol	1 RE vitamin A
18 g carbohydrate	0.14 mg thiamin
9 mg calcium	0.10 mg riboflavin
51 mg phosphorus	1.2 mg niacin
1.0 mg iron	0 mg vitamin C

NUTRIENT CONTENT OF 1 OUNCE (28 GRAMS) 100 PERCENT STONED-WHEAT CRACKERS

114 calories	155 mg sodium
2 g protein	34 mg potassium
4 g fat, 1 saturated	3 g dietary fiber
0 mg cholesterol	0 RE vitamin A
19 g carbohydrate	0.15 mg thiamin
7 mg calcium	0.09 mg riboflavin
54 mg phosphorus	1.3 mg niacin
0.9 mg iron	0 mg vitamin C

NUTRIENT CONTENT OF 1 OUNCE (28 GRAMS) PLAIN MATZO CRACKERS

112 calories	1 mg sodium
3 g protein	32 mg potassium
0 g fat, 0 saturated	1 g dietary fiber
0 mg cholesterol	0 RE vitamin A
24 g carbohydrate	0.11 mg thiamin
4 mg calcium	0.08 mg riboflavin
25 mg phosphorus	1.1 mg niacin
0.9 mg iron	0 mg vitamin C

NUTRIENT CONTENT OF 1 OUNCE (28 GRAMS) ANIMAL CRACKERS

126 calories	111 mg sodium
2 g protein	28 mg potassium
4 g fat, 1 saturated	NA g dietary fiber
0 mg cholesterol	0 RE vitamin A
21 g carbohydrate	0.10 mg thiamin
12 mg calcium	0.09 mg riboflavin
32 mg phosphorus	1.0 mg niacin
0.8 mg iron	0 mg vitamin C

Cranberries: Originally called "crane berries" because the graceful birds inhabiting New England bogs doted on these tart scarlet berries (or perhaps because the pistil of the plant's flower is as slim as a crane's beak), cranberries are native to North America. Native Americans called them *i-bimi,* meaning "bitter berry," pounded them into paste and mixed them into pemmican. Cranberries have been an important commercial crop for more than 150 years, with Massachusetts, New Jersey and Wisconsin being the biggest producers. No one knows for sure whether the Pilgrims ate cranberries that first Thanksgiving although it's likely the local Native Americans contributed them to the spread. Certainly cranberries are now as traditional to Thanksgiving as turkey and pumpkin pie. Too tart to eat raw, cranberries are cooked into sauce or squeezed, sweetened and sold as a beverage, either plain or blended with apple or other fruit juice (and yes, the old folk remedy—drinking cranberry juice to cure or prevent cystitis—does appear to work; see URINARY TRACT INFECTIONS). The

NUTRIENT CONTENT OF ¼ CUP WHOLE OR JELLIED CRANBERRY SAUCE
(about 2½ ounces; 68 grams)

105 calories	20 mg sodium
0 g protein	18 mg potassium
0 g fat, 0 saturated	2 g dietary fiber
0 mg cholesterol	1 RE vitamin A
27 g carbohydrate	0.01 mg thiamin
3 mg calcium	0.02 mg riboflavin
4 mg phosphorus	0.1 mg niacin
0.2 mg iron	1 mg vitamin C

latest form of cranberry is the "craisin," sun-dried and sweet enough to eat out of hand. **SEASON:** Late fall and early winter (but you can pop plastic bags of fresh cranberries into a 0°F. freezer and use them year-round).

NUTRIENT CONTENT OF 1 CUP CRANBERRY JUICE COCKTAIL (WITH SUGAR AND VITAMIN C)

(8 fluid ounces; 240 grams)

147 calories	10 mg sodium
0 g protein	61 mg potassium
0 g fat, 0 saturated	1 g dietary fiber
0 mg cholesterol	1 RE vitamin A
38 g carbohydrate	0.01 mg thiamin
8 mg calcium	0.04 mg riboflavin
3 mg phosphorus	0.1 mg niacin
0.4 mg iron	108 mg vitamin C

NUTRIENT CONTENT OF 1 CUP LOW-CALORIE CRAN-APPLE JUICE (WITH EXTRA VITAMIN C)

(8 fluid ounces; 240 grams)

46 calories	5 mg sodium
0 g protein	65 mg potassium
0 g fat, 0 saturated	0 g dietary fiber
0 mg cholesterol	0 RE vitamin A
11 g carbohydrate	0 mg thiamin
17 mg calcium	0.05 mg riboflavin
7 mg phosphorus	0.1 mg niacin
0.1 mg iron	77 mg vitamin C

Cranberry Beans: See BEANS, FRESH.

Crayfish, Crawfish: The Cajuns have a lovely legend about crawfish. When the French living in Nova Scotia (then Acadia) were deported for refusing to swear alle-

NUTRIENT CONTENT OF 3 OUNCES (85 GRAMS) STEAMED/BOILED CRAYFISH

97 calories	58 mg sodium
20 g protein	298 mg potassium
1 g fat, 0 saturated	0 g dietary fiber
151 mg cholesterol	13 RE vitamin A
0 g carbohydrate	0.04 mg thiamin
26 mg calcium	0.07 mg riboflavin
280 mg phosphorus	2.5 mg niacin
2.7 mg iron	3 mg vitamin C

giance to the British Crown, they say lobsters followed the ships south to Louisiana, and by the time the crustaceans arrived they were so puny they'd turned into crawfish. Today many Cajuns maintain their own crawfish ponds lest they run short. Fortunately for the rest of the United States, crayfish are being commercially farmed and shipped cross-country.

Cream: In the good old days, cooks used to skim off the top milk, which of course was cream. Today there are many different creams, each categorized as to fat content. **Heavy (whipping) cream** must contain at least 36 per-

NUTRIENT CONTENT OF 1 TABLESPOON HEAVY CREAM

(about ½ ounce; 14 grams)

52 calories	6 mg sodium
0 g protein	11 mg potassium
6 g fat, 3 saturated	0 g dietary fiber
21 mg cholesterol	63 RE vitamin A
0 g carbohydrate	0 mg thiamin
10 mg calcium	0.02 mg riboflavin
9 mg phosphorus	0 mg niacin
0 mg iron	0 mg vitamin C

NUTRIENT CONTENT OF 1 TABLESPOON LIGHT CREAM

(about ½ ounce; 14 grams)

29 calories	6 mg sodium
0 g protein	18 mg potassium
3 g fat, 2 saturated	0 g dietary fiber
10 mg cholesterol	27 RE vitamin A
1 g carbohydrate	0.01 mg thiamin
14 mg calcium	0.02 mg riboflavin
12 mg phosphorus	0 mg niacin
0 mg iron	0 mg vitamin C

NUTRIENT CONTENT OF 1 TABLESPOON HALF-AND-HALF

(about ½ ounce; 14 grams)

20 calories	6 mg sodium
1 g protein	19 mg potassium
2 g fat, 1 saturated	0 g dietary fiber
6 mg cholesterol	16 RE vitamin A
1 g carbohydrate	0.01 mg thiamin
16 mg calcium	0.02 mg riboflavin
14 mg phosphorus	0 mg niacin
0 mg iron	0 mg vitamin C

cent milk fat; **light whipping cream,** 30 to 36 percent; **light (coffee) cream,** 18 to 30 percent; and **half-and-half,** a milk-and-cream blend, 10½ to 18 percent. As for squirt-can whipped creams, these may contain no cream or milk at all. Often they are synthesized out of such highly saturated tropical oils as coconut (scrutinize labels); still, they contain no cholesterol. See also CRÈME FRAÎCHE; NONDAIRY CREAMERS; SOUR CREAM.

Cream Cheese: This may be America's oldest packaged food; Philadelphia brand cream cheese, in its protective wrapper, went on sale in 1885. Before that cream cheeses were so perishable they could be bought only near the dairies where they were made. Today's cream cheese, a blend of cow's milk and cream, has a fat content of about 33 percent. It is creamy smooth (often thanks to the addition of vegetable gum), bland and only faintly tart. Whipped cream cheese is just that—cream cheese that's had a lot of air beaten in to make it softer and easier to spread. Because of its greater volume, whipped cream cheese is, measure for measure, somewhat less fatty and caloric than compact blocks of cream cheese. NEUFCHÂTEL is genuinely lighter because it contains one-third less milk fat. So, too, is the brand-new fat-free cream cheese.

NUTRIENT CONTENT OF 1 OUNCE (28 GRAMS) CREAM CHEESE	
99 calories	84 mg sodium
2 g protein	34 mg potassium
10 g fat, 6 saturated	0 g dietary fiber
31 mg cholesterol	124 RE vitamin A
1 g carbohydrate	0.01 mg thiamin
23 mg calcium	0.06 mg riboflavin
30 mg phosphorus	0 mg niacin
0.3 mg iron	0 mg vitamin C

NUTRIENT CONTENT OF 1 OUNCE (28 GRAMS) LIGHT CREAM CHEESE (NEUFCHÂTEL)	
70 calories	115 mg sodium
3 g protein	47 mg potassium
6 g fat, 4 saturated	0 g dietary fiber
20 mg cholesterol	63 RE vitamin A
1 g carbohydrate	0.01 mg thiamin
32 mg calcium	0.08 mg riboflavin
41 mg phosphorus	0 mg niacin
0.5 mg iron	0 mg vitamin C

NUTRIENT CONTENT OF 1 OUNCE (28 GRAMS) NONFAT CREAM CHEESE (PHILADELPHIA FREE)	
25 calories	170 mg sodium
4 g protein	NA mg potassium
0 g fat, 0 saturated	0 g dietary fiber
5 mg cholesterol	80 RE vitamin A
1 g carbohydrate	NA mg thiamin
0 mg calcium	0.06 mg riboflavin
NA mg phosphorus	NA mg niacin
NA mg iron	0 mg vitamin C

Creamers, Nondairy: See NONDAIRY CREAMERS.

Cream of Tartar: A white, acid powder extracted from grapes that's used as a leavening. Cream of tartar also helps to stabilize egg whites beaten to soft or stiff peaks. A pinch is all that's needed.

Crème Fraîche: A rich, nutty sour cream popular in France. It's nothing more than sweet double cream that's naturally fermented by lactic acid bacteria. It's less tart, less acidic than U.S. sour cream, richer, too (with about 35 percent milk fat, it's only slightly less rich than heavy cream). Some U.S. dairies now produce crème fraîche and upscale groceries stock it. You can also approximate the flavor and consistency of crème fraîche by warming ½ cup sour cream with 1 cup heavy cream to about 80°F., then letting the mixture stand overnight at room temperature with the lid on askew. Mix well and store tightly covered in the refrigerator. **NOTE:** Nutrient counts for crème fraîche are unavailable, but it's reasonable to say they would approximate those of heavy cream (see CREAM).

Cremini: See MUSHROOMS.

Crenshaw: See MELONS.

Cretinism: Stunted growth and mental retardation in children caused by the mother's not getting enough iodine during pregnancy. These children suffer from hypothyroidism (a sluggish or inactive thyroid) and, in addition to being dwarfed and retarded, often have protruding bellies and pale, pasty skin. See also IODINE.

Crohn's Disease (diet and): A chronic, long-term inflammation of the intestines, usually the lower reaches of the small intestine, that can develop, over time, into cancer. At the outset—and many people develop Crohn's while in their twenties—there's sharp burning in the lower right abdomen, diarrhea and sometimes weight loss. The inflamed spots may heal, never to return. Or they may recur and spread. In the more advanced stages of Crohn's, there may be intestinal bleeding, even perforation of the intestinal wall, which can lead to peritonitis. Crohn's is not believed to be infectious and a predisposition to it may be hereditary. **BEST DIET:** Calories and protein should be increased by 50 percent and a multivitamin/mineral supplement taken. In some cases, dietary fat is restricted; also colas, grapefruit juice and tea.

Croissants: Crescent-shaped French breakfast rolls that are supremely short and flaky thanks to the chips of butter rolled into the yeast dough. Croissants have taken America by such storm that they're staples at many fast-food restaurants and doughnut shops, where—horrors—they're offered in assorted flavors; including chocolate. Unfortunately, croissants are loaded with saturated fat, calories, cholesterol and sodium. And as if this weren't sinful

enough, many fast-food joints now offer an artery-clogging breakfast special: croissants filled with a fried egg and a slice of bacon.

Cruciferous Vegetables: Cabbages and such cousins as broccoli, brussels sprouts, cauliflower, rutabagas and turnips. All contain cancer-fighting INDOLES. These vegetables all have cross-shaped flowers, which is why they're called cruciferous.

Cucumbers: Native to northern India, cucumbers have been cultivated for thousands of years. Columbus introduced them to the New World, where the natives loved them and sped their growing zone from Mexico into North America. Today there are two basic types of cucumbers: **eating cucumbers** (the heavily waxed supermarket staple plus the cellophane-sealed English or hothouse cucumber) and the smaller, firmer, wartier **pickling cucumbers** (or **kirbies**). Pickling cucumbers make splendid eating, but standard cucumbers don't pickle well. They're too mushy. Cucumbers are largely water although they do contain some vitamins—mostly in the skin, which, if waxed, should be removed. Their biggest plus is that they're unusually low in calories and sodium, fat free, filling and perfect for dieters. **SEASON:** Year-round for eating cucumbers, summer for pickling cucumbers.

NUTRIENT CONTENT OF 1 MEDIUM-SIZE PLAIN CROISSANT

(about 2 ounces; 57 grams)

231 calories	424 mg sodium
5 g protein	67 mg potassium
12 g fat, 7 saturated	2 g dietary fiber
43 mg cholesterol	78 RE vitamin A
26 g carbohydrate	0.22 mg thiamin
21 mg calcium	0.14 mg riboflavin
60 mg phosphorus	1.3 mg niacin
1.2 mg iron	0 mg vitamin C

NUTRIENT CONTENT OF 1 MEDIUM-SIZE CHOCOLATE CROISSANT

(about 2 ounces; 57 grams)

233 g calories	257 mg sodium
5 g protein	109 mg potassium
14 g fat, 8 saturated	2 g dietary fiber
56 mg cholesterol	104 RE vitamin A
24 g carbohydrate	0.15 mg thiamin
30 mg calcium	0.19 mg riboflavin
81 mg phosphorus	1.4 mg niacin
1.6 mg iron	0 mg vitamin C

NUTRIENT CONTENT OF 1 MEDIUM-SIZE (8-INCH) UNPEELED CUCUMBER

(about 10¾ ounces; 301 grams)

39 calories	6 mg sodium
2 g protein	433 mg potassium
0 g fat, 0 saturated	3 g dietary fiber
0 mg cholesterol	63 RE vitamin A
8 g carbohydrate	0.07 mg thiamin
42 mg calcium	0.07 mg riboflavin
60 mg phosphorus	0.7 mg niacin
0.8 mg iron	16 mg vitamin C

Cuprous Iodide (additive): One of the chemicals used to "iodize" salt, a practice developed early this century to reduce the incidence of GOITER (the two most often used compounds are sodium iodide and potassium iodide). Cuprous iodide adds copper as well as iodine. GRAS for use in table salt when limited to 0.01 percent by weight.

Curcamin: An anticarcinogen occurring naturally in food.

Cured Meats and Fish: Curing, one of the earliest methods of food preservation, remains popular today for beef (see CORNED BEEF), pork and oily fish like eel, herring, salmon and sardines. The food may be salted or salted *and* smoked. What goes into the cure—both the ingredients and the technique—are often deep, dark secrets, the case with Smithfield hams. The reason there's been such a flurry of excitement recently about cured meats is that they contain nitrites. These prevent the growth of *Clostridium botulinum* (see BACTERIA), the "bug" responsible for botulism, a fatal form of food poisoning. So far, so good. The downside is that when heated, nitrites combine with amino acids (the building blocks of protein) to form cancer-causing NITROSAMINES. With that in mind, many food processors are using fewer nitrites for curing and further reducing nitrite levels by adding two powerful antioxidants—vitamins C and E. These grab some of the nitrite so there's less of it to be turned into nitrosamine. If the meat or fish is smoked, more carcinogens are added. The lesson here: Keep your consumption of smoked and cured meats within reason or moderation.

Currants, Dried: A misnomer, for dried currants are actually small raisins. No matter. They are high-energy foods, delicious eaten out of hand or stirred into batters for breads, cakes and cookies.

NUTRIENT CONTENT OF ½ CUP DRIED CURRANTS

(about 2½ ounces; 72 grams)

204 calories	6 mg sodium
3 g protein	642 mg potassium
0 g fat, 0 saturated	5 g dietary fiber
0 mg cholesterol	5 RE vitamin A
53 g carbohydrate	0.12 mg thiamin
62 mg calcium	0.10 mg riboflavin
90 mg phosphorus	1.2 mg niacin
2.3 mg iron	3 mg vitamin C

Currants, Fresh: There are **red currants, black currants** and **white currants.** All are exceptionally tart and thus perfect for preserves and puddings. Red and white currants are native to northern Europe; black currants to North America. Fresh currants rarely come to market but do make brief appearances at big-city greengrocers of the gourmet ilk. They're extremely fragile and so expensive they ought to be sold by the karat. **SEASON:** June to September.

NUTRIENT CONTENT OF ½ CUP FRESH RED CURRANTS

(about 2 ounces; 56 grams)

31 calories	1 mg sodium
1 g protein	154 mg potassium
0 g fat, 0 saturated	2 g dietary fiber
0 mg cholesterol	7 RE vitamin A
8 g carbohydrate	0.02 mg thiamin
18 mg calcium	0.03 mg riboflavin
24 mg phosphorus	0.1 mg niacin
0.6 mg iron	23 mg vitamin C

Custard Apple: See CHERIMOYA.

Cyclamate: An artificial sweetener banned in 1969 because it was found to cause bladder tumors in lab rats.

Cysteine, Cystine: Once considered a nonessential amino acid, cysteine has been upgraded to semiessential because if there's enough of it in the diet, the body can use it in place of methionine (an essential amino acid) to make protein. Also, two molecules of cysteine can bond, forming cystine, another amino acid, albeit a nonessential one. Good sources of cysteine are meat, fish, fowl, soybeans, oats and wheat. Food manufacturers use cysteine as an antioxidant to safeguard the vitamin C content of processed foods. And bakers mix it into doughs to speed kneading. Cystine, on the other hand, is used as a dough strengthener as well as a dietary supplement. See also AMINO ACIDS.

Cytotoxic Testing: An allergy test that consists of taking a person's white blood cells, mixing a few of them with a dried food extract, then another batch with another food extract and so on, then monitoring each reaction under a microscope. It's an unreliable method of determining food allergies and a complete waste of money.

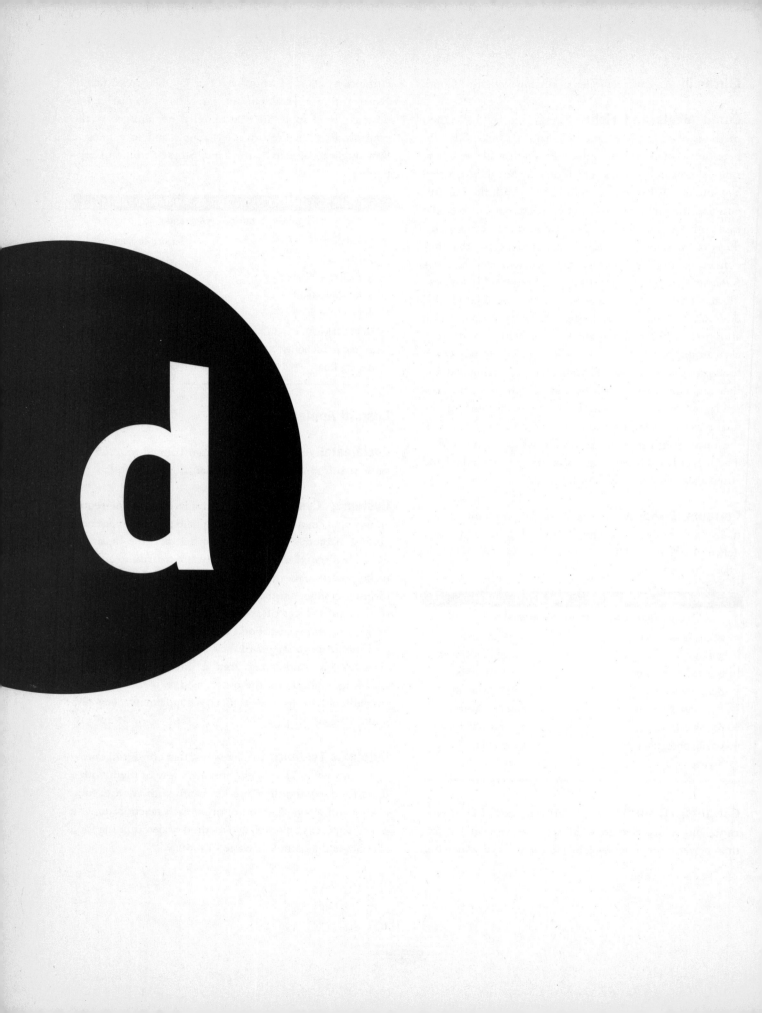

D, Vitamin: When parents send their children out in the sun to play, they're not just trying to get them out of the house. They know that sunlight forms vitamin D in the skin (actually, it's ultraviolet radiation that does it). Indeed, most people can manufacture enough vitamin D in summer to last them through the winter and there's little danger of ODing on sunlight vitamin D because the body limits the amount formed. Why is vitamin D important? It facilitates the absorption of calcium in the body, regulates calcium and phosphorus metabolism in the body and thus helps build strong bones and teeth. In the old days, children in cold climates with limited sunshine often suffered from rickets, an acute vitamin D deficiency most often manifested as bowlegs and deformed ribs. Now that milk's fortified with vitamin D, rickets is almost unheard of. The standard measurement for the vitamin D content of foods, also for determining the RDAs, is micrograms of cholecalciferol (another name for vitamin D). **DEFICIENCY SYMPTOMS:** Calcium loss, soft bones and teeth and, in severe cases, rickets. Blacks synthesize vitamin D from sunlight much more slowly than fair-skinned people, which explains why rickets was so prevalent among black children in New York and other northern cities until the 1920s. About that time scientists began administering daily doses of vitamin D-rich cod-liver oil and effecting "magical cures." **GOOD SOURCES:** Sunshine, cod-liver oil, fortified milk and dairy products, butter, margarine, eggs, liver and such oily fish as salmon. **NOTE:** Because few foods contain vitamin D and because the dairy fortification program has almost eradicated deficiencies, we don't include food-by-food vitamin D contents in this book as we do for other important vitamins. **PRECAUTIONS:** Being fat soluble, vitamin D is stored in the body and too much of it is highly toxic, causing stunted growth, weight loss and calcification of soft tissues. Beware of supplements. Also note that most yogurts and cheeses are made from unfortified milk. Finally, be aware that certain medications—barbiturates, cholesterol-lowering drugs, cortisone, certain anticonvulsants—block the metabolism of vitamin D.

Daikon: See RADISHES.

Daily Reference Values: See DRVS.

Daily Values: See DVS.

Daminozide (pesticide): The chemical name for the now-banned pesticide ALAR.

Dandelion Greens: The blight of lawns is not only edible but also highly nutritious. Dandelion leaves, named *dents de lion* by the French, who thought their jagged edges looked like sharp lion's teeth, have a biting flavor akin to arugula and, as their rich green color (chlorophyll) suggests, plenty of beta-carotene. Dandelion greens can be tossed raw into salads or cooked along with spinach, collards, turnip greens and/or beet tops. **SEASON:** Spring and summer although the tenderest greens will be those that have just sprouted.

RDA FOR VITAMIN D

Babies:

Birth to 6 months	7.5 mcg cholecalciferol per day

Children:

6 months to 10 years	10 mcg cholecalciferol per day

Men and Boys:

11 to 24 years	10 mcg cholecalciferol per day
25 to 51+ years	5 mcg cholecalciferol per day

Women and Girls:

11 to 24 years	10 mcg cholecalciferol per day
25 to 51+ years	5 mcg cholecalciferol per day

Pregnant Women:

	10 mcg cholecalciferol per day

Nursing Mothers:

	10 mcg cholecalciferol per day

NUTRIENT CONTENT OF 1 CUP CHOPPED RAW DANDELION GREENS

(about 2 ounces; 56 grams)

25 calories	42 mg sodium
2 g protein	218 mg potassium
0 g fat, 0 saturated	1 g dietary fiber
0 mg cholesterol	770 RE vitamin A
5 g carbohydrate	0.10 mg thiamin
103 mg calcium	0.14 mg riboflavin
36 mg phosphorus	0.4 mg niacin
1.7 mg iron	19 mg vitamin C

NUTRIENT CONTENT OF 1 CUP BOILED OR STEAMED DANDELION GREENS

(about 3¾ ounces; 104 grams)

35 calories	46 mg sodium
2 g protein	244 mg potassium
1 g fat, 0 saturated	1 g dietary fiber
0 mg cholesterol	1,228 RE vitamin A
7 g carbohydrate	0.14 mg thiamin
147 mg calcium	0.18 mg riboflavin
44 mg phosphorus	0.5 mg niacin
1.9 mg iron	19 mg vitamin C

Dasheens, Taro: Although not well known here, these big, fibrous brown-skinned tubers with ivory to lilac flesh are more precious than potatoes in much of the tropical world. Toxic when raw (even their juice can irritate the skin), dasheens must always be cooked. As starchy as potatoes, dasheens are not as versatile. Dry when baked, they require plenty of gravy. Boiled, they go gluey (the Polynesians and Hawaiians make them into a paste called *poi*). It's best to cook dasheens, mash or puree them, then fold into soufflés or mix with beaten egg and shape into cakes that can be fried. No matter how you prepare them, dasheens will turn from ivory to mauve when cooked. In the tropics, dasheens are dried and milled into flour, then mixed into a variety of flat breads much as stone-ground cornmeal is down South. **SEASON:** Year-round.

NUTRIENT CONTENT OF ½ CUP COOKED SLICED DASHEENS OR TARO

(about 2¼ ounces; 61 grams)

94 calories	10 mg sodium
1 g protein	319 mg potassium
0 g fat, 0 saturated	3 g dietary fiber
0 mg cholesterol	0 RE vitamin A
23 g carbohydrate	0.07 mg thiamin
12 mg calcium	0.02 mg riboflavin
50 mg phosphorus	0.3 mg niacin
0.5 mg iron	3 mg vitamin C

Dates: Although desert nomads and camel caravans have been known to subsist on dates for days, they are mostly instant energy. Their greatest advantage to these peoples, however, is that they are eminently portable and practically imperishable. We like their candylike sweetness and if not eating them out of hand, stir them into batters for breads, cakes and cookies.

NUTRIENT CONTENT OF 3 LARGE PITTED DATES

(about 1 ounce; 25 grams)

86 calories	1 mg sodium
1 g protein	162 mg potassium
0 g fat, 0 saturated	1 g dietary fiber
0 mg cholesterol	1 RE vitamin A
18 g carbohydrate	0.02 mg thiamin
8 mg calcium	0.03 mg riboflavin
10 mg phosphorus	0 mg niacin
0.3 mg iron	0 mg vitamin C

DDT (dichlorodiphenyltrichloroethane): Though this pesticide was banned for agricultural use in the United States in 1972, its residues remain in the soil, the water, even the flesh of humans and animals. Long known to be carcinogenic, DDT has recently been implicated as a cause of breast cancer by a study conducted at Mount Sinai Medical Center in New York City. The results, published in April 1993, show that women with high blood levels of DDT residues were four times as apt to get breast cancer as those with low levels. Though many scientists remain skeptical, citing a complex mix of cancer-causing factors, both environmental and hereditary, the Mount Sinai study adds another piece to the puzzle.

Decaffeinated Coffee: Three different chemicals are used to decaffeinate COFFEE: methylene chloride, ethyl acetate (a somewhat toxic compound found naturally in fruits and vegetables that's also used to decaffeinate tea) and a combination of water and either carbon dioxide or coffee oils. Methylene chloride, for years the preferred method, has now been shown to cause cancer when inhaled by lab animals. And although the FDA has yet to ban it (the amount of methylene chloride left in coffee is negligible; besides, coffee is drunk, not inhaled), most major coffee makers are switching to the safer chemicals. Just how much caffeine is removed in the process? Ninety-seven percent.

Deep-Fat Frying: How we Americans love doughnuts, french fries, crunchy Southern fried chicken. Anything, in fact, that comes brown and crisp from the deep-fat fryer. If the temperature of the oil is just right, we delude ourselves into thinking we really aren't getting much fat. Wrong! Even if a portion of fries adds only 1 tablespoon of fat (most contain more), that's 13 additional grams of fat if lard is the frying medium and 14 grams if it's vegetable oil. Fat we don't need, not to mention 115 to 120 calories. If the frying medium is vegetable shortening, much of that fat is saturated, and if it's lard, it's not only highly saturated but also contains 12 milligrams of cholesterol per tablespoon.

Dehydrated Foods: Before freezing, before canning, there was drying, an ancient method of food preservation discovered, probably by accident: Food left in the sun to dry didn't spoil. **Sun drying** is still used to turn grapes into raisins and plums into prunes. Most foods, however, are now dried indoors under controlled conditions. It's faster, more efficient and there's less risk of contamination. The only real disadvantage of dehydration is that much of the vitamin C is destroyed (and unless sulfur compounds are added, apricots, peaches and other quick-to-darken fruits discolor). Not so with **freeze-drying.** In this newest, supereffective method of food preservation, 99 percent of the vitamin C remains intact. So far, however, this intricate four-step process is too expensive to use on a grand scale and is limited mostly to astronaut rations, coffee and orange juice.

Delaney Clause: Incorporated into the 1958 Food Additive Amendment to the Food, Drug, and Cosmetic Act adopted in 1938, this clause bans the addition to food— even in minute amounts—of any substance known to cause cancer in animals or humans. At this same time, the Food and Drug Administration drew up a list of additives "Generally Recognized as Safe" (see GRAS). Many food industry professionals now feel the Delaney Clause is unrealistic and are lobbying for an update or repeal of it.

Delicata: See WINTER SQUASH under SQUASH.

Dendê: A bright orange palm oil, beloved by Brazilians, that's so high in saturated fat it's semisolid at room temperature. *Dendê* very quickly turns rancid—or at least that bottled in Brazil does.

Dental Health (diet and): Despite the great strides that have been made during the past few decades in improving the dental health of American children, the battle isn't

won. Schoolchildren surveyed during one year averaged more than three missing, decayed or filled permanent teeth, and among seventeen-year-olds the average was more than eight. In many cases, diet is to blame. To simplify: Candy is bad but cheese is good. Fruit yogurts are bad; plain yogurt is good. Unsweetened grains are good, granola—and especially granola bars—are bad. As bad as sticky candies, dentists say. The culprits in tooth decay are sugars and starches, which mouth bacteria turn into tooth-eroding acids. For good dental health, limit your sweets to 10 percent of your day's calories and eat more high-fiber foods. Don't snack, especially on caramels or other sticky candies; instead, make sweets part of the meal. Don't sip soft drinks all day long (the sugar-sweetened variety is especially hard on the teeth) and don't suck lemon drops, which are a sort of double whammy—acidic as well as sweet. The foods most dentists consider good for the teeth are milk, cheese, plain yogurt, fresh or water-packed canned fruits, unsweetened frozen fruits and fruit juices, most vegetables and grains. The bad guys? Dried fruits; jams and jellies; sugar-sweetened dairy products and fruit juices; soft drinks and candies.

Dermatitis (diet and): Acute vitamin A, C or niacin deficiencies can cause severe dermatitis (skin rashes and sores), as can too much vitamin A, E or niacin. Food allergies or sensitivities often induce hives, the most common culprits being beans, chocolate, citrus fruits, condiments, corn, eggs, nuts, peanuts (which are actually legumes), pork, seafood, strawberries and tomatoes. Yellow Dye No. 5 can bring on bouts of hives, too, as can sodium benzoate, a preservative; aspirin, and such salicylate-rich foods as apples, peaches and potatoes. Hyperallergenic people may even react to blueberries, bananas, green peas and licorice. Indeed for some, merely touching dasheens (or taro), mangoes, oil of orange or cinnamon produces poison ivylike rashes. In one study, eczema, always considered more hereditary than dietary, has been improved by subtracting certain foods from the diet. And in another by adding a dietary supplement, evening-primrose oil. But further research is needed.

DES (diethylstilbesterol): This synthetic female hormone/growth promoter mixed into animal feed was banned in 1972 after it was discovered that the daughters of women given DES in the 1950s and 1960s to prevent miscarriages were developing vaginal cancer. Cries of alarm rang across the country, forcing the FDA to ban DES. Seeing their profits plummet, cattle raisers and sheep ranchers raised such a howl the FDA took a second look at DES and a compromise was reached. DES could be used (either in animal feed or as ear implants) as long as it was withdrawn two weeks before the animals were slaughtered. Through radioactive tracers the FDA is able to measure even minute amounts of residual DES in animals, all of which, it turns out, is concentrated in the liver. Amounts average 5 to 10 parts per billion, so little, the FDA says, you'd have to eat 220 pounds of beef liver a day to get a single milligram of DES. Compared to the 65 milligrams per day once prescribed to miscarriage-prone women, the amount of DES actually present in meat seems inconsequential. Still, the hue and cry continues, especially now that the European Community has banned the import of meat from DES-treated animals.

Designer Foods: Lean beef and pork? Soups with pumped-up beta-carotene? These are just a few of the designer foods already available. Others are on the way as researchers identify anticarcinogens and other protective compounds that occur naturally in food, learn how to isolate them, then add them to a variety of other foods. It's the hottest new food trend. Newer still is the umbrella term approved by the Food and Nutrition Board of the Institute of Medicine and sanctioned by the American Dietetic Association—FUNCTIONAL FOODS, which are defined as "foods with ingredients thought to prevent disease." These include not only designer foods but also PHYTOCHEMICALS and NUTRACEUTICALS. The term *functional foods* sounds so "official," so flat-footed. Certainly it lacks the ring of *designer foods, phytochemicals* or *nutraceuticals.* So these more colorful, original terms will no doubt continue to be used in some quarters.

Dewberries: Trailing BLACKBERRIES cultivated in the New World since the time of Columbus. Dewberries are larger than wild blackberries and their seeds smaller, which makes them a better choice for jams and jellies, pies and cobblers. In flavor and nutritive value, however, dewberries and wild blackberries are identical. **SEASON:** Late summer.

Dexfenfluramine: A powerful appetite suppressant widely prescribed in Europe as a weight-loss aid. A variation of fenfluramine, it discourages snacking, particularly on carbohydrates. But dexfenfluramine remains highly controversial. Tests by the National Institute of Mental Health/National Institute on Drug Abuse showed that lab monkeys given high doses of dexfenfluramine for just four days exhibited brain and nerve damage that was clearly evident a year and a half later. A newer study conducted by the Environmental Protection Agency (EPA) refutes those findings. According to EPA tests, dexfenfluramine does cause a shortfall of serotonin, a vital brain neurotransmitter. But, the EPA researchers add, the drop is only temporary and causes no permanent damage. More tests will surely follow before the Food and Drug Administration approves dexfenfluramine for use by Americans struggling to peel off the pounds.

Dextrins (additives): Flavor carriers extracted from starch used primarily in dry drink mixes, soups and gravies. Unlike many additives, dextrins actually have some nutritive value—about the same as cornstarch. GRAS.

Dextrose: Another name for glucose. See CARBOHYDRATES.

DHA (docosahexaeonic acid): One of the omega-3 fatty acids found in fish that are extremely effective in reducing blood cholesterol levels and the risk of arterial plaque formation by making blood platelets less apt to clump.

DHEA (dehydroepiandrosterone): Preliminary studies suggest that this hormone generated by the adrenal glands may bolster the immune system and help strengthen the bones and muscles of the elderly. Like MELATONIN, the body's production of DHEA peaks during puberty, then ebbs with age. Not so long ago, health-food stores sold DHEA supplements. The FDA banned its sale over the counter once high dosages of it were shown to cause liver damage. Today DHEA is available only with a doctor's prescription.

Diabetes (diet and): Diabetes mellitus occurs when the pancreas fails to manufacture the insulin needed to convert glucose (sugar) into energy or when the body can't utilize the insulin that is produced. Either way, blood sugar levels can rise dangerously (the norm is 70 to 150 milligrams per 100 milliliters of blood) and, if left untreated, can overload the kidneys, causing kidney failure, blindness, heart disease or death. In the United States, diabetes is the third major killer (after heart disease and cancer) and the second leading cause of blindness. There are two main types of diabetes: first, **insulin-dependent diabetes** (IDDM) or Type I, sometimes also called **juvenile-onset diabetes,** a serious disease that afflicts some 10 percent of the nation's diabetes sufferers; and second, **non-insulin-dependent diabetes** (NIDDM), Type II or **adult-onset diabetes.** Less serious than Type I, the latter diabetes usually strikes overweight men and women with family histories of diabetes and can often be controlled by diet and exercise. All people with diabetes must watch what they eat. Yet there's good news. In 1994, the American Diabetes Association established new dietary guidelines that should make life "sweeter" for people with diabetes.

Told for years to avoid simple sugars and concentrate on the more slowly digested complex carbohydrates (potatoes, pasta, rice, etc.), researchers now believe that the body digests the two with equal efficiency. So they've devised a list of carbohydrate choices that allow people with diabetes options they've never had, even to enjoy the occasional cookie or dish of ice cream. What counts now is *total carbohydrates.* It's important for a person with diabetes to remember that a sweet should not simply be added to the diet; it should be substituted for another carbohydrate food. The new guidelines focus on the whole patient, with lifestyle, beliefs and background all a part of the picture. Diets are now being tailor-made for the individual patient. This means much greater flexibility for people with diabetes, an abandoning of the old, rigid meal patterns. Ask your doctor or registered dietitian about the new dietary guidelines and recommendations for exercise or contact your local branch of the American Diabetes Association. As a general rule, the new guidelines suggest that protein account for 10 to 20 percent of the calories consumed each day, fat for no more than 30 percent; carbohydrate should supply the rest. All people with diabetes should monitor their blood sugar levels frequently and carefully. And do as their doctors advise.

Diacetyl Tartaric Acid Ester of Monoglycerides and Diglycerides (additive): Bakers use this emulsifier to improve the volume of breads and rolls, to soften the crumb and slow staling. Confectioners use it to thicken chocolate and make it stick as a covering, and food processors use it to whiten nondairy coffee creamers. In use since 1950, this synthetic compound is due careful testing to prove its safety—or lack of it. GRAS.

Diallyl Disulfide: One of the chemicals that give garlic, leeks and other members of the onion family their pungent flavor and odor. Now believed to be anticarcinogenic, diallyl disulfide is being intensively researched.

Diarrhea (diet and): The cause of the diarrhea (frequent loose or watery stools) determines the diet. If it's food poisoning or a viral infection, the first job is to restore water and electrolyte loss, so bland liquids, salty soups, boiled rice or potatoes, bananas, dry toast and salty crackers are in order. A recent report on traveler's diarrhea in the *British Medical Journal* suggests that not drinking the water while abroad and eating only cooked foods may not keep you *turista*-free because the bacteria that make you sick also exist in swimming pools, rivers, surf, even hot foods. Taking antibiotics as preventives isn't recommended for anyone except high-risk patients or those on intense business schedules who must keep going.

If, on the other hand, the cause of the diarrhea is diverticulitis (inflammation of pouches in the large intestine), a high-fiber diet may help prevent future bouts. And if the cause is sprue, a condition that literally greases the intestines by blocking the absorption of fats, the first order of business is to determine the cause of the sprue (often an intolerance for wheat), then build a new diet, omitting problem foods.

Dietary Fiber: See FIBER, DIETARY.

Dietary Guidelines: The U.S. departments of Agriculture and Health and Human Services set forth these seven guidelines to good eating:

1. Eat as broad a variety of foods as possible. For good health, you need forty different nutrients each day—vitamins and minerals, proteins, carbohydrates and, yes, fats, too. See FOOD GUIDE PYRAMID.

2. Maintain a healthful weight.

3. Eat fewer fats (no more than 30 percent of the day's calories should come from fat), fewer saturated fats (limit them to 10 percent of the total fat intake) and watch out for cholesterol (don't exceed 300 milligrams per day).

4. Bulk up on grains, fresh fruits and vegetables.

5. Cut down on sweets, especially between-meals sweets. And hold the sugar, too.

6. Use a lighter hand with the salt shaker and eat fewer sodium-rich foods (frozen dinners and canned foods are notoriously high in salt). The American Heart Association

recommends no more than 3,000 milligrams of sodium a day and *Diet and Health* (a National Academy of Sciences report), 2,400 milligrams.

7. Drink alcohol in moderation. For women, that means no more than 12 ounces of beer per day *or* 5 ounces of wine *or* 1½ ounces whiskey; for men, about twice that.

Needless to say, diet alone won't make you healthy. Too many other factors play a role: heredity, active or passive lifestyle, stress, use of medications, whether or not you smoke, drink, do drugs. But a daily diet planned around these seven steps will surely help to keep you fit.

Dietary Risk Evaluation System (DRES): A computerized system developed by the EPA to measure, by area and population subgroup, chemical pollutants, potential exposures and risks.

Dietetic Technician: A food and nutrition-trained associate who works in health care or food service under a dietitian's supervision. He must have completed a prescribed course of study in an accredited school as well as a supervised practice. He may elect to take a special registration exam.

Diethylpropion: See DIET PILLS.

Dieting, Yo-yo or Seesaw (dangers of): Despite the fact that a new study conducted by a government task force questions whether a life of losing/gaining/losing/gaining may throw your metabolism so out of kilter you can no longer shed pounds without going on a near-starvation diet, many nutritionists and physicians continue to believe that it does. And they caution that such dire measures pose a risk of malnutrition as well as high blood pressure. Further, some nutritionists now believe that each of us is born with a predetermined number of fat cells and that these constantly cry out for food. When you lose weight, your fat cells shrink, but their appetite for food never does, which is why so many of us regain all the weight we've lost—*plus* some. Most of us, some nutritionists theorize, are genetically programmed to be a certain weight at a certain age. SET-POINT for body fatness, they call it. They further admit it's extremely difficult for most people to diet below this set-point unless exercise becomes a major part of the daily routine—the case with TV talk-show diva Oprah Winfrey. See also LEPTIN.

Dietitian, Registered (R.D.): A nutritionist whose particular area of expertise is the human diet. Many dietitians work in hospitals, in the community, in schools, colleges and universities both as teachers and as hands-on practitioners. To obtain an R.D., a student must graduate from a college or university after completing a program of dietetics that has been accredited by the American Dietetic Association, complete a 900-hour supervised practice or internship, then pass the association's registration examination. To remain an R.D. in good standing, he must maintain competency through continuing education. CAVEAT: The fields of dietetics, food and nutrition are overrun by poseurs waving credentials bought from diploma mills, many of them in California, where food-fad-driven quackery is rampant. Before seeking advice or plunking down hard-earned money, always do a reality check on the nutritionist or dietitian.

Diet Pills: People forever waging the battle of the bulge dream of a pill that will magically melt the pounds away. Many tablets claim to do just that, but the truth isn't so rosy. In 1990, the FDA released an updated list of ineffective or unsafe over-the-counter diet aids. There were 111 in all and they included everything from soy lecithin and sea kelp to grapefruit extract and guar gum. This last, FDA sleuths believe, was the ingredient in the now-banned Cal-Ban 3000, which sent eight to the hospital to have blobs of guar gum surgically removed from their esophagi and gastrointestinal tracts. One of the eight died. The FDA admits that it's almost impossible to police the diet industry as closely as it should and urges consumers to educate themselves. Here are the facts about the major types of diet pills now on the market, both those that require a prescription and those sold over the counter (see also LEPTIN):

Amphetamines: Often called **uppers** or **speed,** amphetamines stimulate the central nervous system. They also kill the appetite and jump-start the metabolism. So for a couple of weeks you *will* lose weight. But as your body adjusts to the speed, you will regain the lost weight— and then some—unless the dosage is increased. And therein lies the danger. Amphetamines are not only addictive but also fraught with serious side effects: extreme nervousness, heart palpitations, diarrhea (or constipation), high blood pressure, sweating, nausea, vomiting. Recognizing the harm amphetamines can do, few doctors prescribe them nowadays, preferring to put patients on gentler amphetaminelike appetite suppressants, among them **diethylpropion, mazindol, phentermine** and **fenfluramine.** DEXFENFLURAMINE, widely prescribed in Europe, has yet to receive FDA approval. As for over-the-counter diet pills, they're largely **phenylpropanolamine (PPA)**, a speed-related chemical that can cause dizziness, hypertension and nervousness. If you read the fine print, you'll note that anyone with heart, kidney or thyroid disease, with diabetes or high blood pressure is cautioned not to use PPA. In fact, there's a move to make PPA available by prescription only.

Fiber Pills: These supposedly "blow up" in the stomach and make you feel full so you eat less. But they don't really work. Most contain **methylcellulose,** which the body can't metabolize, or **glucomannon,** extracted from konjac root, which the Japanese have long used for weight control.

Orlistat, Tetrahydrolipstatin: This "fat" pill is considered a magic bullet by the you-can-never-be-too-rich-or-too-thin set. Orlistat isn't for the already slim who yearn to shed 5 or 10 pounds in a hurry for bikini season. Or for those who want to have their cake and eat it, too. It's for the clinically obese who are at least 20 percent over their ideal weight. Orlistat does not make calorie cutting obsolete. Exercise either. Weight-control specialists believe that if orlistat is to be effective, it must be used in tandem with a sound weight-loss/exercise regimen. By blocking the action of three enzymes (lipases) that break dietary fat into fatty acids and glycerol, which can be assimilated by the body, three orlistat pills a day prevent the body from metabolizing about a third of the fat eaten. Translated into calories, this equals 225 to 270 fat calories per day. What isn't yet known is how orlistat affects nutrition in general. It does lower fat levels in the blood (but not abnormally so). It also lowers blood levels of at least one fat-soluble vitamin: E (again, not abnormally). How it affects the absorption of the other essential fat-soluble vitamins—A and D—has not been determined. Studies continue at the Duke University School of Medicine and elsewhere and it may be years before orlistat is available—and then by prescription only.

Starch Blockers: Banned by the FDA in 1982, these pills containing a protein extracted from kidney beans were supposed to keep the body from metabolizing carbohydrates. They didn't.

Thyroid Hormone: This does send metabolism into overdrive, but what the body burns is precious muscle tissue, not fat. Too much thyroid, moreover, can throw the neurological system out of whack.

Water Pills: Nothing more than diuretics, which make you lose fluid (and thus weight). But the loss is only temporary. Frequent or prolonged use of diuretics can damage the heart. See also CHROMIUM PICOLINATE and EPHEDRINE.

Diets: Mention the word *diet* and thoughts turn immediately to reducing diets, especially those that promise to melt the excess pounds overnight. But there are many other types of diets, too, most of them planned to alleviate specific medical conditions. **NOTE:** Because most of these diets are part of the treatment for specific medical conditions, they should always be supervised by a physician and/or registered dietitian—never undertaken independently.

Diabetic Diets: See DIABETES.

Eat More, Weigh Less Diet: Although this low-fat diet became a nineties fad, it is not a fad diet. Developed by Dean Ornish, M.D., of the Preventive Medicine Research Institute of Sausalito, California, it was originally designed to reverse coronary heart disease. Those participating in Ornish's Life Choice Program also lost significant amounts of weight. As a result, Ornish wrote *Eat More, Weigh Less*, which soared to the top of the best-seller lists and quickly popularized his mostly vegetarian regimen as the Eat More, Weigh Less diet. For details, see ORNISH DIET

Elimination Diet: To pinpoint specific allergies, doctors will subtract "suspicious" foods from the diet, one at a time. If they don't discover the culprit, they may then administer a diet elimination test. That is, they will totally rework the diet, beginning with foods that rarely cause allergic reactions. If, after a couple of weeks, the patient remains symptom free, they'll introduce new foods at four-day intervals, with such known troublemakers as eggs, milk and wheat coming last. This way the allergenic foods can usually be identified.

Fad Diets: Let's see, we've had the Westchester Diet, the Beverly Hills Diet, the Drinking Man's Diet, the Rice Diet, the Liquid Diet, the Grapefruit and Coffee Diet. And on and on. If any of these diets worked—took the weight off safely and kept it off—there wouldn't be another diet of the month. You will lose weight on most of the fad diets, it's true. But the minute you tumble off the diet, you'll regain those pounds in a hurry—and then some. The reason fad diets don't work over time is that they're gimmicky, unbalanced, boring. More important, they fail to address the real problem: bad eating habits. Too much fat. Too much sugar. The sad truth is there's no magic, fast or easy way to lose weight. You didn't pack on the pounds in a week or a month, so don't expect to shed them that fast. The only way to lose weight permanently is to readjust eating habits—forever. It's a lifestyle change that's needed, not a "diet." And that change should include a regular program of exercise as well as a well-balanced daily diet rich in whole grains, fruits and vegetables. See FOOD GUIDE PYRAMID.

Gluten-Free Diet: See GLUTEN INTOLERANCE.

High-Calorie Diets: Yes, there *are* people who need to gain weight. The diet prescribed for them is usually high in complex carbohydrates and protein. But unsaturated fats may be increased, too, to make sure calories consumed are greater than calories burned. During World War II, youths too skinny to pass military physicals often bulked up on milk shakes. But that was before anyone worried about cholesterol and saturated fats. Knew much about them, either. Today, dietitians prefer to tailor the diet to the individual patient, increasing the calories as needed—even doubling the daily quota, if necessary, to produce safe but steady weight gain.

High-Fiber Diets: A normal diet that includes an extra portion of high-fiber carbohydrate—whole grains, for example, dried peas or beans. Although all of us are now being urged to increase our fiber intake, high-fiber diets are aimed in particular at those with chronic DIVERTIC-ULOSIS as well as at people with constipation, diabetes or simply too many pounds.

Lactose-Restricted Diet: See LACTOSE INTOLERANCE.

Low-Calorie Diets: The goal here is to burn more calories than you eat so pounds begin to drop away. Most doctors and dietitians discourage patients from losing more than a pound or two a week. They also discourage fad diets, some of which are dangerous. A sound reducing diet always includes a wide variety of foods, even some fat. Just less of everything. If you trim calories by 500 a day, you'll lose about a pound a week. A reducing diet of less than 1,200 calories a day may be nutritionally unbalanced and isn't recommended *except* under strict medical supervision.

Low-Carbohydrate Diets: Because of a genetic defect in their metabolism, some people can't handle certain CAR-BOHYDRATES (sugars)—for example, galactose (a simple sugar). Others, because they lack the intestinal enzyme lactase, can't digest lactose (milk sugar). So these sugars must be restricted in the diet or eliminated altogether. Hypoglycemics, moreover, are told to avoid concentrated sweets and stick to complex carbohydrates, fiber and protein, which slowly release glucose into the bloodstream and thus help keep blood sugar levels steady. Finally, young epileptic children are sometimes, as a last resort, prescribed ketogenic (high-fat, low-carbohydrate) diets, which seem to lessen the intensity and frequency of seizures that medicines can't control.

Low-Cholesterol Diets: People with high blood cholesterol are often put on low-cholesterol diets (300 milligrams per day or less) although many nutritionists now believe that dietary cholesterol does less than saturated fats to raise blood cholesterol levels. Certainly anyone with a cholesterol problem should cut down on saturated fats by eating smaller portions of meat, fish and poultry (two 2- to 3-ounce servings a day are the usual recommendation). Also by substituting lean white fish or poached, skinned chicken breast for red meat, skim milk for whole, low-fat cheeses for the regular, olive oil or soft margarine for butter and, by eating fewer eggs. Fortunately, there are many products available today to make the job easier.

Low-Fat Diets: Like low-cholesterol diets, these are often recommended for those with high blood cholesterol. Also for those with high blood pressure, gallstones, pancreatitis, cystic fibrosis or just too much excess baggage. Dietitians zero in on saturated fats because reducing them automatically reduces blood cholesterol levels. Some nutritionists believe fat calories should account for no more than 10 percent of the day's total calorie intake; others think less than 30 percent more realistic. They further recommend that the fat calories break down thus: no more than 10 percent each from saturated and polyunsaturated fats, 10 to 15 percent from monounsaturated fats. See also ORNISH DIET.

Low-Fiber Diets: These are more correctly called **minimum-** or **low-residue diets.** Post-bowel-op patients as well as those suffering from acute diverticulitis or bouts of bowel obstruction are often put on low-fiber diets to give the bowel a rest. The strictest low-fiber diets are nutritionally balanced, low-residue liquid formulas. Other low-fiber diets, depending upon the gravity of the medical problem, range from avoiding whole grains, dried peas and beans, cereals, nuts and seeds, unpeeled fruits and vegetables to forgoing all of the above *plus* tough cuts of meat, shellfish full of sinewy connective tissue (octopus, squid and certain crustaceans), prune juice, coconut, potatoes, indeed any fruits and vegetables that haven't been reduced to juice. It may even mean cutting down on milk and dairy products—any food, in fact, that exacerbates a particular condition. Your dietitian and doctor know best.

Low-Protein Diets: Those with acute kidney or liver disease are often told to avoid milk, meat and other high-protein foods and eat more fruits and low-protein vegetables (green beans, the cabbage family, celery, cucumber, summer squash, tomatoes, etc.), breads and cereals, even such high-energy foods as jams, jellies and hard candies.

Low-Sodium Diets: Salt and high-sodium foods (cured meats and fish, smoked meats and fish); sausages; canned soups, meats, fish and vegetables; cheese; pickles and bottled sauces are severely restricted or even off-limits for people with high blood pressure, congestive heart failure, chronic edema, cirrhosis and kidney disease. Moreover, little or no salt can be used in cooking or to season foods. Baking powder and soda may be taboo, too, as may breads and cakes made with them. For such people, total sodium intake is limited to 2,000 to 3,000 milligrams a day (not much when you learn that ½ teaspoon salt equals 1,000 milligrams). People with less serious medical conditions may be put on a **no–extra–salt diet** (also called the **no–salt–added** or **NAS** diet), which allows 3,000 to 4,000 milligrams sodium a day. But even this means no salt shakers at table and using low-sodium mustards, steak sauces and other condiments.

Very Low-Calorie Diets: Sometimes, for medical reasons, seriously obese patients must lose weight fast. So they're put on a high-protein, low-carbohydrate, vitamin- and mineral-fortified daily diet containing less than 800 calories. There's rapid, dramatic weight loss: Most women drop 2 to 4 pounds a week, men 3 to 5. Some nutritionists question the safety of these diets, even when they're supervised by a physician. Moreover, those who lose weight this way rarely keep it off. See also LEPTIN.

Digestive Blockers, Starch Blockers: See DIET PILLS.

Diglyceride (additive): This emulsifier, derived from two fatty acids and glycerol, is what makes commercial ice creams, puddings, margarines, shortenings and peanut butters supremely creamy. Diglyceride is also used to plasticize doughs and stabilize nondairy coffee creamers. GRAS.

Dill: Herbs aren't our primary concern here, but the clean lemony/salty tang of this feathery herb makes it a dandy substitute for salt. Both fresh dill and dillweed are compatible with fish and shellfish, poultry, lamb, eggs, beets, carrots, green beans, the whole cabbage family (even coleslaw), cucumbers and summer squash. Popular throughout Scandinavia, Germany, Russia and the rest of Eastern Europe, dill is probably native to Asia. It's an ancient herb and, in olden days, mothers used a mild dill tea to soothe colicky babies.

Dioctyl Sodium Sulfosuccinate (DSS) (additive):
Called a wetting agent in the food industry, this chemical is added to powdered gelatins, drink mixes and cocoas to make them dissolve more quickly and completely in liquids. It's also used as a stabilizer in chewing gums and canned milks. DSS is moderately toxic. It can irritate the skin and eyes, and when heated it gives off noxious fumes. The FDA limits the amount of DSS that can be used, varying the amount from food to food, but still rates it GRAS.

Dioxins: With progress come problems. In the old days, milk was delivered in glass bottles, coffeemakers used washable felt filters (if any at all), nuke-and-eat dinners didn't exist and most of us ate off china plates. Enter paper products and, with them, dioxins—powerful carcinogens formed when paper is bleached with chlorine. Dioxins can migrate—albeit in minute quantities—into food. The FDA has decreed that milk drunk from bleached paper cartons isn't hazardous to your health. Still, some people continue to buy milk in glass bottles or transfer cartoned milk to glass jars the minute they get home from the grocery to minimize the risk of dioxins' migrating into their milk. They use unbleached coffee filters and paper plates (if at all) and they avoid TV dinners whenever possible—or at least don't cook them in their original containers. The good news is that responsible paper manufacturers are beginning to use less chlorine. At present, the greatest source of dietary dioxin comes from bottom-feeding fish that swim the Great Lakes, an area of intense industrial activity.

Disaccharides: Double sugars, which, when hydrolyzed (split by absorbing molecules of water), yield two simple sugars. See CARBOHYDRATES.

Disodium 5'-Guanylate (DSG) (additive): An MSG-like flavor booster that's twice as effective as MSG and often used in conjunction with it. Processed foods most likely to contain it are canned soups, meats and vegetables; spreads; sauces; and a wide variety of snacks. GRAS.

Disodium 5'-Inosinate (additive): Another flavor enhancer, a close chemical relative of DSG that's used in much the same way. But it's only half as potent. GRAS.

Disodium Phosphate (additive): This multipurpose additive, a mildly alkaline salt of phosphoric acid, is used to shortcut pasta cooking times, to stabilize evaporated milk, whipped toppings and nondairy coffee creamers, also to accelerate setting or thickening times of instant puddings and sauces. Disodium phosphate also masquerades under assorted aliases: **sodium phosphate, dibasic; disodium monohydrogen orthophosphate;** and **disodium monophosphate.** GRAS.

Diuretic: Anything that increases urine production. Some foods and beverages are said to be naturally diuretic—asparagus and coffee, to name two. Physicians prescribe diuretic pills (often furosemide and Hydrodiuril) to patients with edema, heart, liver or kidney disease. And foolhardy dieters pop them to lose weight fast. The pounds do drop away. But it's water that's being lost. And potassium. *Not* fat. Anyone using diuretics should eat plenty of potassium-rich foods like bananas and oranges.

Diverticulitis: Infected or inflamed diverticuli, which are small pouches on the walls of the colon (most older Americans have them to some degree). Diverticulitis can be excruciating and cause vomiting, fever, rectal bleeding. Once the infection is tamed by antibiotics, the patient is put on a high-fiber prevention diet.

Diverticulosis: Pouching or the formation of diverticuli on the walls of the bowel. Sixty-six percent of Americans beyond the age of sixty have diverticulosis and so does a third of the population over forty-five, although few suffer enough to even know it. Others, however, experience alternate bouts of diarrhea and constipation, gas and discomfort low on the left side of the abdomen. Nutritionists believe that a meat-heavy diet exacerbates diverticulosis and a high-fiber one alleviates it.

DMG (dimethylglycine): Also sometimes marketed as **pangenic acid** or **vitamin B$_{15}$** (both meaningless), this so-called energy booster is popular among U.S. athletes, particularly football players, who sometimes gobble as much as 300 milligrams of this nonessential amino acid at game time. DMG's champions swear it jump-starts the body's metabolism of oxygen and hones mental alertness. However, a recent University of Alabama study of sixteen marathon runners dosed with DMG showed that they performed no better than the DMG-less racers. CONCLUSION: DMG may do no harm, but it's no miracle ergonomic aid, either. Save your money.

Dolomite Pills (nutrient supplement): Dolomite (**calcium magnesium carbonate,** to give its chemical name) is extracted from limestone and marble. It's powdered, pressed into pills and sold by many health-food stores as a calcium/magnesium supplement. Some dolomite pills are contaminated with such toxic metals as arsenic, mercury and lead. Even if the pills are uncontaminated, the form of calcium and magnesium they contain isn't easily assimilated by the body and actually blocks the absorption of other minerals.

Dough Conditioners (additives): Bakers like to toughen the gluten (wheat protein) in their breads so they're sturdier and easier to work, and one way to do it is to use a dough conditioner. Most are mineral mixes—usually calcium salts, phosphates and sulfates—and some are sodium-rich. Among the widely used dough conditioners are **calcium** and **sodium stearoyl lactylates** and **sodium stearoyl fumarate.** GRAS.

Doughnut: One of America's most beloved junk foods. As far as nutritive value is concerned, *olykoeks* (oil cakes) is an apter name for these deep-fried Dutch fritters because most of them ooze fat. The original recipe, brought to New England by Pilgrims after a stay in Holland, had no holes. In *The Dictionary of American Food and Drink,* John Mariani says, "The Pennsylvania Dutch were probably the first to make doughnuts with holes in their centers, a perfect shape for 'dunking' in coffee." That might not have been the only reason for punching holes in the blobs of dough. Solid doughnuts were always doughy in the middle because the centers never cooked as fast as the edges. Rings, some long-ago cook discovered, simply cooked more evenly. Although early doughnuts were plain, the list of varieties available today is long and getting longer. Doughnuts still come plain, but better sellers are the gussied up—sugar dusted, frosted, jelly filled, honey dipped, glazed or coated with candy sprinkles. Further, they may be yeast raised or leavened with baking powder like cake. Given the number of franchised doughnut shops strewn across this country, Americans can't get their fill of these greasy little nuts of dough. Here's a sobering look at their nutrient content.

NUTRIENT CONTENT OF 1 MEDIUM-SIZE PLAIN CAKELIKE DOUGHNUT

(about 1³/₄ ounces; 51 grams)

211 calories	273 mg sodium
3 g protein	64 mg potassium
12 g fat, 2 saturated	1 g dietary fiber
19 mg cholesterol	9 RE vitamin A
25 g carbohydrate	0.11 mg thiamin
22 mg calcium	0.12 mg riboflavin
135 mg phosphorus	0.9 mg niacin
1.0 mg iron	0 mg vitamin C

NUTRIENT CONTENT OF 1 MEDIUM-SIZE GLAZED YEAST-RAISED DOUGHNUT

(about 2 ounces; 60 grams)

242 calories	205 mg sodium
4 g protein	65 mg potassium
14 g fat, 4 saturated	1 g dietary fiber
4 mg cholesterol	11 RE vitamin A
27 g carbohydrate	0.22 mg thiamin
26 mg calcium	0.13 mg riboflavin
56 mg phosphorus	1.7 mg niacin
1.2 mg iron	0 mg vitamin C

NUTRIENT CONTENT OF 1 MEDIUM-SIZE JELLY-FILLED YEAST-RAISED DOUGHNUT

(about 2¹/₄ ounces; 65 grams)

221 calories	190 mg sodium
4 g protein	51 mg potassium
12 g fat, 3 saturated	1 g dietary fiber
17 mg cholesterol	12 RE vitamin A
25 g carbohydrate	0.20 mg thiamin
16 mg calcium	0.09 mg riboflavin
55 mg phosphorus	1.4 mg niacin
1.2 mg iron	1 mg vitamin C

Drug-Nutrient Interaction: Many medications affect metabolism in one way or another, blocking perhaps the absorption of certain vitamins or minerals. Diuretics flush potassium from the body. Too many antacids deplete the supply of phosphate; oral contraceptives can cause low blood levels of some B-complex vitamins. Drug-nutrient interaction is a complex subject and it's best to ask your doctor *and* pharmacist if the medications you're taking can interfere with the way your body metabolizes food and, if so, what you should do about it.

DRVs (Daily Reference Values): To guide consumers and simplify the new food labels (in force since May 1994), the FDA developed a table of DRVs. Based on a 2,000-calories-a-day diet, the DRVs suggest amounts of fat, saturated fat, cholesterol, carbohydrate, fiber and sodium generally considered to be healthful for anyone over the age of four (assuming, of course, they are in good health). These figures, it should be stressed, are not RDAs officially established by the National Research Council, National

Academy of Sciences, Washington, D.C. They are merely guidelines or reference points. For example, if a food manufacturer claims that his product is "high-fiber," it must contain at least 20 percent of the DRV for fiber. Here's the table of DRVs the FDA has developed:

DAILY REFERENCE VALUES (DRVs)	
(based on a 2,000-calories-a-day diet)	
Total fat	65 g
Saturated fat	20 g
Cholesterol	300 mg
Total carbohydrate	300 g
Fiber	25 g
Sodium	2,400 mg

Although this table will appear on food labels, the values will be referred to as Daily Values (see DVs), not as DRVs.

Drying (as means of food preservation): See DE-HYDRATED FOODS.

Dry Milk Powder: See MILK.

Duck, Duckling: All ducks and ducklings raised in America for the table today are descended from a single small flock of white Pekins introduced to Long Island, New York, about one hundred years ago. Although now grown in several other states, most ducks are still sold as Long Island ducklings. And ducklings are just what they are:

NUTRIENT CONTENT OF 3 OUNCES (85 GRAMS) ROASTED DUCK MEAT (WITH SKIN)	
292 calories	52 mg sodium
17 g protein	177 mg potassium
25 g fat, 8 saturated	0 g dietary fiber
73 mg cholesterol	55 RE vitamin A
0 g carbohydrate	0.15 mg thiamin
10 mg calcium	0.23 mg riboflavin
135 mg phosphorus	4.2 mg niacin
2.3 mg iron	0 mg vitamin C

young birds of seven to eight weeks, weighing 4 to 5 pounds. Ducks are older (ten weeks or more), bigger (over 5 pounds), fatter and tougher. All ducks and ducklings con-

tain a lot of fat and bone, so you should allow about 1¼ pounds of dressed bird per person (the amount of meat they get won't be much more than 3 or 4 ounces). The biggest problem in cooking ducks is ridding them of all the fat, most of which is underneath the skin. The standard technique is to prick the ducks with a sharp-pronged fork as they roast so the fat melts and runs down into the bottom of the pan. TIP: Always cook duck on a rack so it doesn't fry in its drippings.

NUTRIENT CONTENT OF 3 OUNCES (85 GRAMS) ROASTED DUCK MEAT (WITHOUT SKIN)	
171 calories	55 mg sodium
20 g protein	214 mg potassium
10 g fat, 4 saturated	0 g dietary fiber
76 mg cholesterol	20 RE vitamin A
0 g carbohydrate	0.22 mg thiamin
10 mg calcium	0.40 mg riboflavin
173 mg phosphorus	4.4 mg niacin
2.3 mg iron	0 mg vitamin C

Duodenal Ulcers: See PEPTIC ULCERS.

Durum Wheat: A strain of hard wheat with a high gluten content that's used for making pasta. Doughs made of durum wheat are tough, elastic and easily shaped. Moreover, they don't disintegrate when boiled.

DVs (Daily Values): The FDA, in its infinite wisdom, has decided that DRVs and RDIs are terms too confusing to appear on food labels. So it's hit upon the shorter, more inclusive DV, or Daily Value, which will encompass both standards. Get used to it. RDIs (Reference Daily Intakes) are suggested daily amounts of vitamins and minerals that the FDA developed based on the old U.S. Recommended Daily Allowances (USRDAs).

Dysphagia: The inability to swallow easily—or at all. A diet of purees and thick liquids is usually recommended; however, those less seriously afflicted can usually handle finely chopped or bite-size meats and vegetables if accompanied by thin liquids.

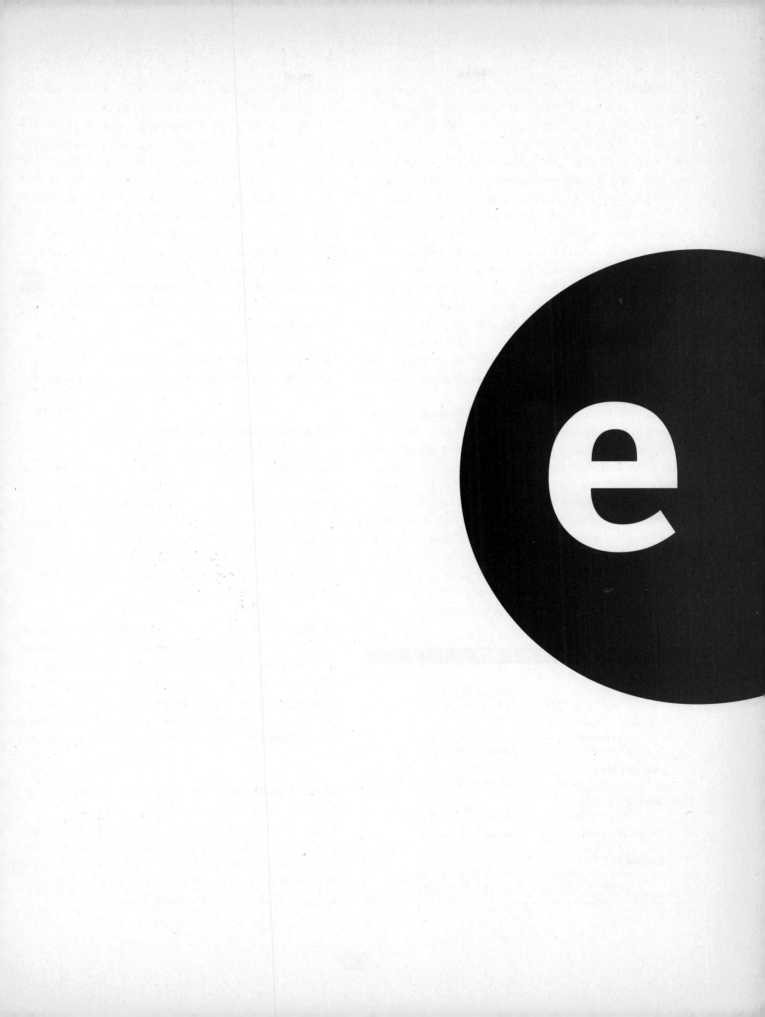

E, Vitamin: This powerful antioxidant, circulating in the blood and detoxing free radicals (destructive by-products of metabolism), prevents damage to cell membranes, thereby reducing the risk of heart disease and cancer. Further, vitamin E keeps "bad" cholesterol (LDL) from turning into even worse cholesterol—*oxidized LDL*—which initiates buildup of arterial plaque (atherogenesis) and can lead, ultimately, to serious heart disesae. Finally, it also speeds healing in burn and post-op patients and, recent studies suggest, seems to ease the pain and swelling of osteoarthritis and rheumatoid arthritis, to reduce the risk of cataracts, to bolster the immune system, even to slow the progress of Parkinson's disease. Is E, then, the "everything vitamin," the elixir of health and fountain of youth man has been seeking for centuries? No nutritionist or medical researcher will climb out on *that* limb; still a number of them do admit to taking vitamin E supplements—just in case.

A fat-soluble vitamin (like A, D and K), vitamin E exists in the form of **tocopherols** and **tocotrienols.** Four different tocopherols have been identified, and although the most active is **alpha-tocopherol,** researchers now believe there's a symbiotic relationship among the different tocopherols, that all work in concert to promote good health. The unit of measurement for vitamin E is the D-alpha-tocopherol equivalent, abbreviated α-TE and computed in milligrams. **DEFICIENCY SYMPTOMS:** Anemia. **GOOD SOURCES:** Vegetable oils (particularly those pressed from wheat germ, barley, corn and soybeans), peanut butter, liver, leafy greens, wheat germ, whole grains and nuts.

RDA FOR VITAMIN E	
Babies:	
Birth to 6 months	3 mg α-TE per day
6 months to 1 year	4 mg α-TE per day
Children:	
1 to 3 years	6 mg α-TE per day
4 to 10 years	7 mg α-TE per day
Men and Boys:	
11 to 51+ years	10 mg α-TE per day
Women and Girls:	
11 to 51+ years	8 mg α-TE per day
Pregnant Women:	10 mg α-TE per day
Nursing Mothers:	
First 6 months	12 mg α-TE per day
Second 6 months	11 mg α-TE per day

PRECAUTIONS: Milling removes almost all of the vitamin E in grains, and the refining of vegetable oils robs them of at least a fourth of their vitamin E content. Foods lose vitamin E during prolonged storage, also when frozen or cooked at intense heat (frying and deep-fat frying are singularly destructive). If you smoke, you'll need extra vitamin E to counteract the stress put on your lungs. Finally, air pollution may increase your need for vitamin E. *Is there a danger in taking too much vitamin E?* Yes, if you're on blood-thinning or anticlotting drugs. Megadoses of vitamin E will depower them and may also cause gastrointestinal upsets. Compared to two other fat-soluble vitamins—A and D—however, vitamin E seems to be relatively nontoxic.

Eating Disorder: A portmanteau term that includes a variety of eating problems. See ANOREXIA NERVOSA; BULIMIA.

Eat More, Weigh Less Diet: See ORNISH DIET.

Echinacea: An old herbal remedy and patent medicine ingredient extracted from the purple coneflower. Once prescribed for everything from snakebite to tired blood, echinacea is again news, this time as a therapy for colds, flu and chronic fatigue syndrome. Though German scientists think it may have antiinfective/inflammatory powers, no U.S. studies are planned. Echinacea extracts are of questionable value and composition.

Eclampsia: A serious, potentially fatal form of pregnancy-induced hypertension. No one knows what causes it. **SYMPTOMS:** Edema, protein in the urine, convulsions, even coma and death. In the old days, doctors would put eclampsia patients on low-sodium diets and diuretics. Today, knowing that sodium is necessary and that diuretics may be harmful, doctors prescribe good nutrition and bed rest.

Eczema (diet and): The itching and skin rashes of eczema may be caused by food allergies, according to a recent Duke University study. Children seem allergic in particular to eggs and milk, with peanuts, peas, rye and wheat also occasionally causing problems. Children often outgrow their allergies. Not so adults, whose bouts of eczema are apt to be triggered by these same foods.

Edam: One of the "cannonball" cheeses of Holland (the other is GOUDA), encased in a coating of crimson. It's a Cheddar-rich cheese made from the milk of Friesian cows. Aged about two years and pale yellow in color, Edam is mild to sharp, full bodied and moderately hard. The Dutch have been breakfasting on Edam, black bread and coffee for years.

NUTRIENT CONTENT OF 1 OUNCE (28 GRAMS) EDAM CHEESE	
101 calories	273 mg sodium
7 g protein	53 mg potassium
8 g fat, 5 saturated	0 mg dietary fiber
25 mg cholesterol	72 RE vitamin A
0 g carbohydrate	0.01 mg thiamin
207 mg calcium	0.11 mg riboflavin
152 mg phosphorus	0 mg niacin
0.1 mg iron	0 mg vitamin C

Edema: Often called **water retention,** this buildup of bodily fluid, most noticeable in swollen ankles and feet, can be caused by something as simple as PMS (premenstrual syndrome) or eating too many salty foods. But something more serious may be responsible: kidney disease, cirrhosis of the liver, congestive heart failure or malnutrition (particularly protein malnutrition and/or beriberi, the disease brought on by acute thiamin deficiency; see B_1, VITAMIN). To correct edema, physicians, depending on the cause of the water retention and often working with registered dietitians, restructure the diet, balancing the intake of protein, fluid and/or sodium and potassium.

Eel: Americans have never been keen on this oily, snake-like fish caught in both fresh and salt water. Europeans, however, dote upon eel, particularly Scandinavians and Germans, who prefer it smoked; the French, who bubble it into heady stews; and the Portuguese, who construct effigies of their beloved *lampreia* (lamprey) out of *doces d'ovos* (egg sweets). Polluted waters are not only diminishing the supplies of eel but also jeopardizing their safety because of alarming buildups of lead, mercury and other toxic metals in their flesh.

NUTRIENT CONTENT OF 3 OUNCES (85 GRAMS) SMOKED EEL	
280 calories	89 mg sodium
16 g protein	359 mg potassium
24 g fat, 6 saturated	0 g dietary fiber
55 mg cholesterol	411 RE vitamin A
0 g carbohydrate	0.19 mg thiamin
15 mg calcium	0.31 mg riboflavin
171 mg phosphorus	1.2 mg niacin
0.6 mg iron	0 mg vitamin C

Efamol: Another name for EVENING-PRIMROSE OIL, which is said to provide relief from premenstrual syndrome (see PMS).

Egg Noodles: By weight, these flat strands of pasta must be at least 5½ percent egg. Usually they're made with flour milled from durum wheat (the hardest of the hard), water and whole eggs, either fresh or dehydrated. However, to lower the fat and cholesterol counts a bit, some manufacturers make an imitation noodle using the whites only (scrutinize labels). Available in wide, medium and narrow widths, egg noodles are an economical way to plump up stews and boost soups and casseroles into the main-dish category. They're a superb potato substitute, too, particularly if the meat has gobs of gravy. And in a pinch, noodles can double for fettuccine, taking with equal grace to pesto, meat and marinara sauces.

NUTRIENT CONTENT OF 1 CUP BOILED EGG NOODLES (about 5¾ ounces; 160 grams)	
213 calories	11 mg sodium
8 g protein	45 mg potassium
2 g fat, 0 saturated	4 g dietary fiber
53 mg cholesterol	10 RE vitamin A
40 g carbohydrate	0.30 mg thiamin
19 mg calcium	0.13 mg riboflavin
110 mg phosphorus	2.4 mg niacin
2.5 mg iron	0 mg vitamin C

Eggplant: Thomas Jefferson, that great gardener and gatherer of exotic seeds, introduced eggplant to America. Not, however, with much success. Only in recent years have Americans begun to cook eggplant in earnest—but still mostly as eggplant Parmesan or *baba ganouj* (poor man's caviar). Few people prize eggplant more than those living on the Mediterranean's eastern rim, but then it was the Arabs who discovered this unusual vegetable in India, where it's said to have originated four thousand years ago. The eggplants we know best are the plump, deep purple, pear-shaped ones, but there are others. White ones the size of goose eggs, slim lavender ones no bigger than bananas, striated melons, even finger-size babies. But these are boutique items, seen only in pricey big-city greengroceries. All eggplants are highly perishable, so buy them just before you cook them. **SEASON:** Year-round.

NUTRIENT CONTENT OF 1 CUP BOILED EGGPLANT CUBES
(about 3½ ounces; 96 grams)

27 calories	3 mg sodium
1 g protein	238 mg potassium
0 g fat, 0 saturated	3 g dietary fiber
0 mg cholesterol	6 RE vitamin A
6 g carbohydrate	0.07 mg thiamin
5 mg calcium	0.02 mg riboflavin
22 mg phosphorus	0.6 mg niacin
0.3 mg iron	1 mg vitamin C

NUTRIENT CONTENT OF 1 CUP STIR-FRIED EGGPLANT CUBES
(about 3½ ounces; 100 grams)

107 calories	4 mg sodium
1 g protein	209 mg potassium
8 g fat, 1 saturated	2 g dietary fiber
0 mg cholesterol	6 RE vitamin A
6 g carbohydrate	0.08 mg thiamin
35 mg calcium	0.02 mg riboflavin
32 mg phosphorus	0.6 mg niacin
0.6 mg iron	1 mg vitamin C

Eggs: Once called "nature's perfect food," eggs have gotten a bum rap recently—on two counts. First, doctors damned eggs for their cholesterol content (one very nearly supplies the day's suggested quota) and limited their heart patients to one or two eggs a week (nutritionists now believe the saturated fats in food are more harmful than the cholesterol). Second, eggs became contaminated with salmonella (see BACTERIA), which made many people mighty sick. With salmonella still rampaging through America's

henhouses, the surest ways to avoid food poisoning are to wash all implements, work surfaces and, yes, hands, well after handling raw eggs; to avoid tasting anything containing raw eggs (no more bowl licking for the kids!); and to cook all eggs thoroughly, be they for meringues, hollandaise or breakfast. Salmonella food poisoning has become so prevalent in the Northeast that New Jersey recently banned the serving of sunny-side-up eggs in its restaurants. Still, the egg remains a nutritional powerhouse, delivering impressive amounts of protein, vitamin A and riboflavin. Though few people know it, eggs are low in calories, even in saturated fat and sodium.

NUTRIENT CONTENT OF 1 LARGE EGG
(about 1¾ ounces; 50 grams)

75 calories	63 mg sodium
6 g protein	61 mg potassium
5 g fat, 2 saturated	0 g dietary fiber
212 mg cholesterol	96 RE vitamin A
1 g carbohydrate	0.03 mg thiamin
25 mg calcium	0.25 mg riboflavin
89 mg phosphorus	0 mg niacin
0.7 mg iron	0 mg vitamin C

NUTRIENT CONTENT OF 1 LARGE EGG YOLK
(about ⅔ ounce; 17 grams)

59 calories	7 mg sodium
3 g protein	16 mg potassium
5 g fat, 2 saturated	0 g dietary fiber
212 mg cholesterol	96 RE vitamin A
0 g carbohydrate	0.03 mg thiamin
23 mg calcium	0.11 mg riboflavin
81 mg phosphorus	0 mg niacin
0.6 mg iron	0 mg vitamin C

NUTRIENT CONTENT OF 1 LARGE EGG WHITE
(about 1¼ ounces; 33 grams)

16 calories	55 mg sodium
3 g protein	45 mg potassium
0 g fat, 0 saturated	0 g dietary fiber
0 mg cholesterol	0 RE vitamin A
0 g carbohydrate	0 mg thiamin
2 mg calcium	0.15 mg riboflavin
4 mg phosphorus	0 mg niacin
0 mg iron	0 mg vitamin C

Egg Substitutes: Formulas vary from manufacturer to manufacturer, but most of these viscous liquids, frozen in ½- to 1-cup cardboard cartons, are largely egg white with natural colors added to mimic the sunny yellow of beaten eggs and gums or other stabilizers blended in to approximate their texture. Some egg substitutes contain fat, others none at all, so read labels carefully. With ¼ cup thawed egg substitute equaling one whole egg, they're a snap to use. Egg substitutes work splendidly in sauces, cakes, cookies, puddings and ice creams. Best of all they're pasteurized, so salmonella isn't a worry.

NUTRIENT CONTENT OF ¼ CUP NONFAT LIQUID EGG SUBSTITUTE (EQUIVALENT OF 1 EGG)
(2 fluid ounces; 57 grams)

25 calories	80 mg sodium
5 g protein	NA mg potassium
0 g fat, 0 saturated	0 g dietary fiber
0 mg cholesterol	60 RE vitamin A
1 g carbohydrate	0.04 mg thiamin
24 mg calcium	0.78 mg riboflavin
NA mg phosphorus	0 mg niacin
0.9 mg iron	0 mg vitamin C

Eicosapentaenoic Acid: See EPA.

Elastin: The yellow connective tissue in meat that no amount or method of cooking will tenderize. The cuts of meat most apt to contain elastin come from well-exercised parts of the animal—neck, legs (shanks) and tail.

Elbow Breadth: A simple test used to determine frame size, which in turn is used to determine ideal body weight. Here's how it works. With fingers splayed, crook your elbow at a right angle, then swivel your wrist away from your body. With calipers or the thumb and index finger of the other hand, measure the distance between the two bones on either side of the crooked elbow. Here are the norms (adapted from a Metropolitan Life Insurance Company table):

WOMEN

Height (in 1-inch heels)	Elbow Breadth (in inches)
5 feet to 5 feet 3 inches	2¼ to 2½
5 feet 4 inches to 5 feet 11 inches	2⅜ to 2⅝
6 feet or more	2½ to 2¾

MEN

Height (in 1-inch heels)	Elbow Breadth (in inches)
5 feet 4 inches to 5 feet 7 inches	2⅝ to 2⅞
5 feet 8 inches to 5 feet 11 inches	2¾ to 3
6 feet to 6 feet 3 inches	2¾ to 3⅛
6 feet 4 inches or more	2⅞ to 3¼

Measurements lower than those given in the table indicate a small frame; measurements higher, a large frame.

Elderberries: It's too bad these wild deep purple berries aren't more popular because they're powerful sources of vitamin C, potassium and dietary fiber. Too tart to eat raw, elderberries are superb stirred into quick breads, cobblers, pies and jams. Elder bushes grow across much of the United States, often tree-tall. In the old days, the creamy flowers (in bloom in June and July) were plucked and fermented into wine. Elderberries come a bit later and are yours for the picking. Since the Middle Ages, superstitions have surrounded the elder. In medieval England, legend had it that Judas hanged himself from an elder, and crowns of elder came to symbolize shame. **SEASON:** August.

NUTRIENT CONTENT OF 1 CUP ELDERBERRIES
(about 5¼ ounces; 145 grams)

105 calories	NA mg sodium
1 g protein	406 mg potassium
1 g fat, 0 saturated	10 g dietary fiber
0 mg cholesterol	87 RE vitamin A
27 g carbohydrate	0.10 mg thiamin
55 mg calcium	0.09 mg riboflavin
57 mg phosphorus	0.7 mg niacin
2.3 mg iron	52 mg vitamin C

Elderly Persons (diet and): Senior citizens, who should make an extra effort to eat a varied, balanced meal three times a day, often lapse into habits that are hazardous to their health—snacking on junk food, settling for TV dinners or fast food, catching meals wherever, whenever they can. Perhaps they've lost a spouse, lost their appetite or sense of taste. Perhaps they can't get to the store to shop. Perhaps they are scraping by to make ends meet. Perhaps they've been put on strict diets. Or maybe food no longer interests them. Whatever the reason, too many elderly people are poorly nourished and their health suffers. For good health, seniors should eat or drink *each day:*

- *At least five servings of fruits and vegetables,* aiming for as much variety as possible and making sure to include beta-carotene-rich bright yellow or orange yams, carrots, winter squash, apricots, mangoes and papayas along with plenty of citrus fruits, berries, melons and green vegetables for vitamin C. Fruits and vegetables are preferable to juices because they contain fiber. They are also the foods to snack on instead of candies, chips and nuts.

- *At least six servings of grains, whole-grain cereals and breads.* These complex carbohydrates contain not only most of the B-complex but also plenty of fiber, essential to good digestion. As the fiber intake increases, so, too, should the consumption of liquids.

- *At least two servings of milk and dairy products* with the emphasis on low-fat milks, yogurts and cheeses and, if there's a lactose intolerance, low-lactose versions as well.

- *Two servings of lean meats and/or meat alternatives a day.* These include poultry, fish, eggs, tofu, dried peas and beans, and other protein-, vitamin- and mineral-rich foods. To maximize the absorption of iron from these foods by the body, it's wise to accompany them with fruits and vegetables high in vitamin C.

For good health, seniors should drink plenty of liquids throughout the day (especially in hot weather or when eating high-fiber foods). They should also cut down on fats, refined sugars and alcohol. These extras are loaded with calories and the body's demand for them ebbs with age. Elders should keep active, adopt a regular program of exercise even if it's nothing more than taking a stroll every day. Moderate amounts of exercise increase fitness—and appetite. Finally, seniors who live alone should seek company at mealtime, invite a friend in for lunch or dinner or go to a restaurant or fellowship center. Those who break bread with family or friends are usually better nourished than those who eat alone. Those unable to get out should contact their local MEALS-ON-WHEELS office.

Seniors who enjoy cooking might prepare double or triple some of their favorite recipes, then package them in single or double portions, date and store in the freezer. NOTE: For safe storage, the freezer must maintain a steady 0°F. and the refrigerator, 40°F.

Electrolytes, Electrolyte Balance: The body utilizes minerals as salts; these dissolve in bodily fluids, forming positively and negatively charged ions—or electrolytes—

that are integral to the transmission of nerve impulses and proper muscular function. Electrolytes also maintain the body's delicate acid/alkaline ratio, known as electrolyte balance. Although all dietary minerals are converted by the body to electrolytes, the heavy hitters are **sodium** (plus its balancer, **chloride**) and **potassium** (together with its regulator, **phosphate**). These electrolytes, working in tandem with the kidneys, not only regulate the amount of water in body fluids and cells but also balance the number of positively and negatively charged ions. If the balance tips too far one way or the other, if bodily fluids become too acid or too alkaline, you die.

Elimination Diet: A test used by physicians to try to pinpoint food allergies. The patient begins with a core diet of carefully selected foods unlikely to cause trouble. If after two weeks no signs of allergy appear, additional foods are added, one every four days, ending with that notoriously allergenic trio—milk, eggs and wheat. If the patient remains asymptomatic, or if the core diet doesn't relieve symptoms at the outset, the allergist assumes that food isn't the culprit.

Ellagic Acid: A phytochemical (beneficial compound that's neither vitamin nor mineral) found in nuts, vegetables, apples and other fruits that's believed to help prevent cancer. Specifically, it depowers two carcinogens present in our food supply—AFLATOXIN and BENZENE.

Emmentaler: This ivory-hued giant cheese has been a staple in the Emmental Valley of Switzerland ever since the sixteenth century. Made of cow's milk, it's shot through with holes, exported in wheels of 145 pounds or more and is prized for its slightly sweet, slightly salty, nut-

NUTRIENT CONTENT OF 1 OUNCE (28 GRAMS) EMMENTALER CHEESE	
106 calories	74 mg sodium
8 g protein	32 mg potassium
8 g fat, 5 saturated	0 g dietary fiber
26 mg cholesterol	72 RE vitamin A
1 g carbohydrate	0.01 mg thiamin
271 mg calcium	0.10 mg riboflavin
171 mg phosphorus	0 mg niacin
0 mg iron	0 mg vitamin C

like flavor. Germany makes a superb Emmentaler, too; indeed, the one from Allgau is Germany's most famous hard cheese. The Swiss and German Emmentalers are high-protein cheeses averaging 25 to 30 percent butterfat. They slice and shred neatly and, if well aged, melt velvet smooth, which explains why they're not only eaten out of hand but also slipped into a variety of soups, salads and savory kuchen.

Emulsifier: A category of additives widely used in processed foods. Basically, the function of an emulsifier is to keep oil and water or other nonfat liquid from separating, to keep them in emulsion (smoothly blended). But the food industry uses emulsifiers not only to keep oils from separating out of peanut butters, processed meats and salad dressings but also to retard the staling of bread, to make nondairy creamers dissolve on contact with hot coffee, to stabilize whipped toppings so they mount to stratospheric heights, to prevent starches from crystallizing and to ensure the creaminess of ice creams.

Endive, Belgian: See BELGIAN ENDIVE.

Endive, Curly; Curly Chicory; Frisée: See SALAD GREENS.

Endorphins: Sometimes called the body's natural pain-killers, these morphinelike hormones produced by the brain play a larger role. They are thought to trigger hunger pangs and also to heighten our pleasure in eating.

Endosperm: The meaty, protein- and starch-rich inner kernel of whole grains. In wheat, the endosperm comprises 83 percent of the kernel, contains three fourths of the protein, about a third of the riboflavin and a tenth of the niacin. The bran or husk encloses the endosperm and at its heart lies the germ. When wheat is milled, the endosperm is separated from the germ and bran, which contain most of the nutrients, then it is pulverized into flour.

Energy: Without energy, the body cannot function—at work, at play, at rest. But that's not all. Energy—to be specific, chemical energy—fuels such bodily processes as metabolism of food and helps maintain body temperature. Once food is eaten, the body, through a complex series of chemical reactions, breaks proteins, fats, carbohydrates and

alcohol down into glucose, which drives the body. Reduced to a simple equation: Glucose + oxygen = carbon dioxide (which we exhale), water (some of which we excrete) and energy. See also BASAL METABOLISM.

Energy Balance, Caloric Balance: Usually the ideal, which occurs when energy intake (or calories taken as food) equals energy (calorie) expenditure. People in energy balance will maintain their weight at a constant level. On the other hand, when the energy intake exceeds the outgo, the pounds begin to pile on. And when the number of calories burned is greater than those consumed, weight is lost. To give some notion of the body's energy demands, here are a few figures. A 125-pound woman burns 1 calorie a minute just sleeping or sitting and watching TV, 3 calories per minute making beds and 14 calories per minute walking upstairs. A 175-pound man burns about 1½ times that; a 250-pounder, approximately double.

Energy Boosters: To improve their performance, athletes often bulk up on pasta and potatoes before important games or competitions. The technical name for it is **carbohydrate loading,** and it's effective most of the time for athletes who compete in events lasting 1½ to 2 hours or more. Here's how it works: Six days before the event, the athlete follows a specific workout regimen, perhaps an hour a day for the first two days, forty minutes for each of the next two days and twenty minutes each for the last two days. At the same time, he eats more carbohydrates. For the first three days, about half his day's calories will come from carbohydrates and for the last three, some 75 percent. This carbohydrate loading doubles or triples the amount of muscle glycogen (stored energy). There are disadvantages, however. Glycogen can hold up to four times its weight in water and that means extra pounds, particularly for those who tend to retain water on high-carbohydrate diets.

Phosphate loading, or taking high doses of phosphate pills, won't work miracles either, although some athletes swear they've greater endurance. And what about **vitamin B_{12}** pills as energy boosters? No one's proved they pump you up.

Then there are all the pills and potions lining the shelves of health-food stores. Do these energy boosters work? Are they safe? Here's the story on the most popular of them: GINSENG (benefits unproved); MA HUANG (it's EPHED-

RINE, a stimulant and dangerous for anyone with heart or thyroid disease, high blood pressure, diabetes); CAFFEINE (it's the "magic" ingredient, usually extracted from kola nuts, in several energy boosters); CHROMIUM (integral to insulin production, it may create a fleeting "lift," but there's no evidence of its being a true energizer); SPIRU-LINA (it contains some vitamin B₁₂, generally believed to be a pumper-upper but it isn't); and BEE POLLEN (all it's known to do is trigger allergic reactions).

Energy Requirement: Here's an easy way to determine your ideal body weight, then compute your daily energy (calorie) requirement. First, jot down your height; then, if you're a woman, allow 100 pounds for the first 5 feet; if you're a man, 106 pounds. Next add 5 pounds for each additional inch (6 pounds per inch if you're a man). The total will be your ideal weight. Now for your energy requirements: If you're sedentary, multiply your ideal body weight by 13; if moderately active, by 15; and if very active, by 17. The figure you get is the number of calories you should consume each day to maintain your ideal weight. To lose a pound a week, eat 500 fewer calories a day; to gain a pound a week, eat 500 more calories per day.

English Muffins: According to John Mariani in *The Dictionary of American Food and Drink,* these flat, chewy, yeast-raised rounds made of refined wheat flour, malted barley, farina and vinegar were first made in America, not England. Commercially, at least, although the baker *was* English, a recent transplant named Samuel Bath Thomas, who turned his mother's tea-cake recipe into the English muffins we all know and adore. That was more than one hundred years ago.

NUTRIENT CONTENT OF 1 PLAIN ENGLISH MUFFIN	
(about 2 ounces; 57 grams)	
134 calories	264 mg sodium
4 g protein	75 mg potassium
1 g fat, 0 saturated	2 g dietary fiber
0 mg cholesterol	0 RE vitamin A
26 g carbohydrate	0.25 mg thiamin
99 mg calcium	0.16 mg riboflavin
76 mg phosphorus	2.2 mg niacin
1.4 mg iron	0 mg vitamin C

NUTRIENT CONTENT OF 1 WHOLE-WHEAT ENGLISH MUFFIN (TOASTED)	
(about 1¾ ounces; 50 grams)	
111 calories	346 mg sodium
5 g protein	114 mg potassium
1 g fat, 0 saturated	4 g dietary fiber
0 mg cholesterol	0 RE vitamin A
22 g carbohydrate	0.13 mg thiamin
144 mg calcium	0.07 mg riboflavin
154 mg phosphorus	1.7 mg niacin
1.3 mg iron	0 mg vitamin C

Enoki, Enokitake: See MUSHROOMS.

Enriched, Enrichment Program: When wheat is milled into white flour or refined into breads and cereals, it loses iron plus three important members of the B-complex—thiamin, riboflavin and niacin. The federal enrichment program, established by the Enrichment Act of 1942 but no longer mandatory, required millers, bakers and cereal makers to restore the lost iron and three B vitamins to their products in amounts that approximated the nutritional content of whole wheat (in truth, riboflavin was restored to double the original amount). In addition, many Southern states, where corn breads were the staple, instituted cornmeal enrichment programs. Today only six states require enrichment of wheat flours and cereals as set forth by the 1942 mandate, many of them the Southern states that also insist upon cornmeal enrichment.

Enriched flours, cereals and breads may be superior to the unenriched, but they're not as healthful as the whole grain. Nutritionists now know that in addition to removing the big four (iron, thiamin, riboflavin and niacin), the milling and refining processes also rob grains of fiber, vitamin B₆, folacin, magnesium and zinc, not to mention other trace minerals. Still, with America mostly white-bread country (at least beyond the major metropolitan areas), it's important that refined flours, cornmeals, breads and cereals be enriched. **NOTE:** With more and more imports finding their way onto American supermarket shelves, you should know that in many foreign countries, *enriched* means the addition not only of vitamins and minerals but also of protein concentrates or amino acids. Read the fine print.

Enteral Nutrition: The taking of food—usually easily digested, amino acid- and carbohydrate-rich liquid formulas—by mouth or gastrointestinal tube. The practice is often called simply **tube feeding.**

Enterotoxin: In certain types of food poisoning, it's the toxin the bug produces that makes you sick, not the bug itself. Two examples of these enterotoxins are those generated by *Staphylococcus aureus* and *Clostridium botulinum*. See BACTERIA.

Environmental Protection Agency: See EPA.

Enzyme: Every body cell contains thousands of different enzymes, protein-based catalysts that speed the complex series of biochemical reactions involved with every stage of metabolism. Some of them require COENZYMES (most of which are vitamins) to do their job efficiently—or, indeed, at all.

EPA (eicosapentaenoic acid): One of the omega-3 fatty acids found in oily fish (anchovies, sardines, salmon, tuna and the like) reputed to reduce not only blood cholesterol levels but also arterial plaque (by making blood platelets less sticky and less likely to clump). For years researchers have pointed to the fact that Eskimos, whose diet is high in oily fish, suffer few strokes and heart attacks. They do, however, bruise easily and, when cut, bleed profusely. Meaning that gobbling omega-3 fish-oil capsules may do more harm than good. Eating oily fish frequently is beneficial, to be sure, but overdosing on fish-oil supplements can cause excessive bleeding and anemia and may even increase the risk of stroke. Buyer, beware.

EPA (Environmental Protection Agency): The federal bureau whose responsibilities include setting and monitoring safe residue levels for the hundreds of agricultural pesticides that show up in our food and drinking water. The EPA has come under fire recently for dragging its heels (notably during the ALAR/apple scare a few years back), also for not recognizing that its pesticide residue allowances, though considered safe for the average adult, do not sufficiently protect children, who are at greater risk. A National Academy of Sciences committee, after evaluating EPA performance, recommended an overhaul of current pesticide regulation allowances and procedures that would pay greater attention to the eating habits of young children and thus better safeguard them against harmful pesticides.

Ephedrine: This upper, sold over the counter in pharmacies, sports shops and health-food stores across the land, masquerades under many names: HerbTrim, Mega Trim, Diet Max and Diet Pep, to name a few. Whatever its form (pill or herbal tea), whatever its name, ephedrine is a best-seller because it's said to boost energy, increase athletic prowess and burn body fat. Related to "speed" or amphetamines, ephedrine was originally used to treat asthma. Today it's become the drug of choice for many teens. Girls pop ephedrine pills to lose weight; jocks swallow them to play longer, harder, better. But make no mistake, ephedrine can be dangerous—make that *deadly*. A seventeen-year-old footballer recently died of a heart attack after taking ephedrine. And in a single year, ephedrine pills caused three strokes, two of them fatal. Although the FDA lacks the manpower to rid the shelves of ephedrine-based diet and pep pills, some states have taken matters into their own hands. New Mexico now bans the sale of ephedrine without a doctor's prescription. And Texas forbids its sale to minors. Still, savvy teens know other ways to get ephedrine. At least one Chinese herbal—MA HUANG—contains it, fortunately in lower doses. See also ENERGY BOOSTERS.

Epinephrine: Better known as **adrenaline,** this stress hormone, which the body synthesizes out of phenylethylamine, recently grabbed gobs of press. Chocolate, it seems, is loaded with phenylethylamine, a major player in emotional arousal. Was chocolate, then, an aphrodisiac? Alas, no. When National Institute of Mental Health researchers went on a chocolate binge to test the theory, they were rewarded with headaches. Nothing more.

Epsom Salts, Magnesium Sulfate (additive): A flavor enhancer and processing aid that the FDA considers safe when used at prescribed levels. It's also a powerful cathartic and TV and movie stars, aiming to drop weight fast, sometimes dose themselves with epsom salts. A dangerous practice.

Ergogenic Aids: Something (often dietary) said to improve athletic performance, to turn athletes into superathletes (see ENERGY BOOSTERS).

Ergosterol: A crystalline white sterol present in molds and yeasts that sunlight activates as vitamin D_2.

Ergot, Ergotism: A rare but deadly disease caused by ergot, a toxin produced when a certain mold—*Claviceps purpurea*—infects rye and other grains. In medieval times, outbreaks of ergotism, then known as St. Anthony's fire, were common, particularly among the poor of cold, damp countries who subsisted upon rye bread. It wasn't until the mid-sixteenth century that Hessian physicians traced the cause to the parasitic fungus *C. purpurea* and to the poison it produced. Like many toxins, ergot in minute quantities is a valuable medication. It raises blood pressure and physicians often prescribe it to women who have suffered miscarriages or hemorrhaged after giving birth.

Erythorbic Acid (additive): This antioxidant used in such cured meats as pastrami, hot dogs and bologna is, believe it or not, thought by some people to consist of earthworms! Not true! Its role is to accelerate and regulate the nitrite curing process, also to help preserve the bright rosy color of cured meats. Though related to ascorbic acid, it's nonnutritive. GRAS; however, when heated, erythorbic acid sends off acrid fumes.

ESADDI: See ESTIMATED SAFE AND ADEQUATE DAILY DIETARY INTAKE.

Escarole: A broad-leafed bright green chicory eaten raw in salads. Also called **Batavia endive;** a bunched variety (**spadona**) is popular in Italy. See SALAD GREENS.

Escherichia coli: A bacterium that's been causing havoc in the fast-food and meat industries. See BACTERIA.

Esophagitis, Reflux Esophagitis: A painful inflammation of the esophagus that's often caused by the backing up of stomach contents. Stomach juices are extremely acidic, burn like fury in the esophagus, which is why esophagitis is also called **heartburn**. Those who are overweight or who have a hiatal hernia (the two often go together) are most likely to suffer from esophagitis. Al-

though antacids ease the burn, they do not correct the problem. **BEST REMEDIES:** Avoid any foods that you know will give you heartburn; shun fatty foods, chocolate, alcohol, coffee, tea, colas and anything else containing caffeine; eat several small meals instead of three whopping squares a day; wear loose clothes, especially while eating; and don't lie down immediately after eating. It's best to stay upright so that gravity pulls food down into the stomach and helps to keep it there. If esophagitis persists, see your doctor or registered dietitian and, if necessary, lose weight.

Essential Amino Acids (EAAs): See AMINO ACIDS.

Essential Fatty Acids: See FAT.

Estimated Safe and Adequate Daily Dietary Intake (ESADDI): RDAs haven't yet been established for all nutrients, and until they are, the Food and Nutrition Board of the National Academy of Science has established tentative recommendations for biotin, pantothenic acid, copper, manganese, fluoride, chromium and molybdenum. These recommendations are called—and it's a mouthful—Estimated Safe and Adequate Daily Dietary Intakes (ESADDI) or, more simply, Estimated Safe and Adequate Amounts (ESAs). The board urges that top levels of the ESA range not be exceeded over time because some trace elements are toxic.

Ethanol Grain Alcohol, Ethyl Alcohol: Alcohol distilled from yeast-fermented grains or other carbohydrates, the form of alcohol present in beer, wine, whiskey and other alcoholic beverages. Some people consider ethanol fattening because drinking *can* pack on the pounds. And in truth, the body metabolizes ethanol at 198 calories per ounce (7 calories per gram). See also ALCOHOL, ALCOHOLIC BEVERAGES.

Ethoxylated Mono- and Diglycerides (additives): Water-soluble emulsifiers made of vegetable fats that food processors use to condition yeast doughs, also to stabilize and smooth peanut butters, ice creams, frostings and whipped toppings. These additives are fairly new and consumer advocates urge further testing. GRAS when used according to federal regulations. When heated, these compounds decompose, emitting acrid fumes.

Ethyl Acetate (additive): A clear, volatile, highly combustible solvent used primarily to decaffeinate coffees and teas. Though a natural compound that apples, bananas and pineapples produce as they ripen, ethyl acetate is mildly toxic when ingested, so the FDA strictly restricts the amounts of it that can be used.

Ethylene: In the old days when fruits were picked at their peak of perfection, they could never be shipped cross-country because they would rot en route. If only apples, berries, cherries, grapes, melons, bananas, tomatoes and other fragile produce could be picked and shipped while they were still hard and green, farmers would save millions of dollars. Early attempts failed because shippers didn't know how to ripen the immature fruits. Now they do. Fruits left to mature naturally in orchards and fields produce ethylene gas, the key, it turns out, to the ripening process. Today shippers can ripen green fruits in warehouses simply by pumping in ethylene gas. The process is not only harmless but also, in some ways, beneficial because ethylene actually increases the vitamin C content (in tomatoes by as much as 16 percent) and leaves the vitamin A unaffected. Fanciers of just-picked fruits loathe the texture and flavor of the warehouse-ripened. And even farmers admit that the ethylene treatment doesn't work for carrots. It makes them bitter.

Ethyl Maltol (additive): A powerful, synthetic flavor enhancer added to wines, chocolate-, vanilla- and fruit-flavored drinks and desserts. Tests conducted by the additive's manufacturers have found it safe. However, watchdog groups demand further testing to prove that ethyl maltol is not only noncarcinogenic but also harmless. At present, the FDA limits its use to 100 milligrams per liter.

Ethyl Vanillin (additive): A perfumy artificial vanilla flavoring that's 3½ times more powerful than the real thing. It's cheaper, too, which explains why manufacturers like to use it in soft drinks, ice creams and baked goods. GRAS.

Evaporated Milk: Canned, unsweetened whole milk with about half the water removed. It's as thick as cream, about the color of cream, too, but diluted 50–50 with water, it can double for whole milk both as a beverage and as a recipe ingredient. Many people object to the slightly caramel taste of evaporated milk (caused by processing at high temperatures), but in fact it's wonderfully compatible with chocolate and butterscotch (try substituting evaporated milk for whole milk in fudge, brownies, chocolate puddings and sauces, also in caramel or brown-sugar pie). Today, evaporated milk is not only fortified with vitamin D, but also available in low-fat and skim-milk versions. **NOTE:** Evaporated milk is not the same as sweetened condensed milk, which is intensely sweet and spoon-up thick.

NUTRIENT CONTENT OF ½ CUP EVAPORATED MILK

(4 fluid ounces; 126 grams)

169 calories	133 mg sodium
9 g protein	382 mg potassium
10 g fat, 6 saturated	0 g dietary fiber
37 mg cholesterol	68 RE vitamin A
13 g carbohydrate	0.06 mg thiamin
329 mg calcium	0.40 mg riboflavin
255 mg phosphorus	0.2 mg niacin
0.2 mg iron	1 mg vitamin C

NUTRIENT CONTENT OF ½ CUP FORTIFIED EVAPORATED LOW-FAT MILK

(4 fluid ounces; 127 grams)

110 calories	140 mg sodium
8 g protein	400 mg potassium
3 g fat, 2 saturated	0 g dietary fiber
10 mg cholesterol	167 RE vitamin A
12 g carbohydrate	0.04 mg thiamin
320 mg calcium	0.40 mg riboflavin
267 mg phosphorus	0.2 mg niacin
0.3 mg iron	1 mg vitamin C

NUTRIENT CONTENT OF ½ CUP FORTIFIED EVAPORATED SKIM MILK

(4 fluid ounces; 128 grams)

99 calories	147 mg sodium
10 g protein	423 mg potassium
0 g fat, 0 saturated	0 g dietary fiber
5 mg cholesterol	150 RE vitamin A
15 g carbohydrate	0.06 mg thiamin
369 mg calcium	0.40 mg riboflavin
248 mg phosphorus	0.2 mg niacin
0.4 mg iron	1 mg vitamin C

Evening-Primrose Oil, Efamol: Some women believe the promise that if they swallow two capsules of evening-primrose oil every day for three months, they can say good-bye to bloating, tender breasts and other symptoms of premenstural syndrome (see PMS). Evening-primrose oil, health-food store catalogs explain, supplies gamma-linolenic acid, which the body needs to produce prostaglandin E-1, which in turn eliminates the symptoms of PMS. The truth? No one's proved that PMS comes from a shortage of gamma-linolenic acid. Indeed, it's linolenic acid—not *gamma*-linolenic acid—that's an essential fatty acid. Researchers now suspect that a diet high in sweets and low in B vitamins, iron and zinc may be responsible for PMS. The jury is still out. Meanwhile, let's just say that evening-primrose oil is no magic bullet.

Exchange List, Exchange System: To simplify menu planning for those who must stick to special diets, a joint American Diabetes Association/American Dietetic Association committee came up with a flexible system of food exchanges. There are six broad food-group lists, each with similar per-portion calorie, fat, carbohydrate and protein counts: (1) Starch/Bread; (2) Meat/Meat Alternate; (3) Vegetable; (4) Fruit; (5) Milk; (6) Fat. In addition, there's a roster of so-called free foods (broths, celery, cucumbers and such) that can be eaten with impunity because none contains more than 20 calories per portion. Finally, there's a list of combination foods—casseroles, pastas, soups and so on—together with their exchange rates, so dieters will know how to fit them into their meal plans.

Exercise (diet and): The soundest, *surest* way to lose weight and keep it off is to adopt a regular, sensible program of exercise. Here's why: If you diet without so much as lifting a finger, you will lose lean muscle mass as well as fat, and the lean will be gone forever. But those hard-lost "fat" pounds will pile back on—*plus* more. If, on the other hand, you exercise half an hour a day while you count calories, you'll not only jump-start your metabolism but also program your body to use fat for fuel instead of glucose. Better yet, the more lean muscle you develop, the more fat you'll burn. Exercise delivers other bonuses, too. You'll feel better and look better. You'll lower your blood pressure and, very possibly, elevate your mood, too.

Expiration Date: See OPEN DATING.

Extrinsic Factor: Before vitamin B_{12} was identified, it was referred to as an extrinsic factor, meaning "something from the outside." Physicians and nutritionists knew that a certain substance found in liver extracts was needed by the body to prevent pernicious anemia. Only in 1948 was this extrinsic factor isolated and named vitamin B_{12}. See B_{12}, VITAMIN.

Extrusion: It's the way cheese and corn puffs, breakfast cereals and potato chips are made. Unfortunately, this new method of extruding doughs and pastes into fancy shapes robs food of such heat-sensitive vitamins as A, C and B_1, also of some amino acids. Intense heat and pressure are often needed to squeeze food pastes through tubes and dies, and when the extruding is also done in the presence of oxygen, nutrients are further sacrificed. The trouble with extruded foods is that kids love to snack on them, then have no room for more nutritious food.

Eyesight (diet and): "Eat your carrots" mothers urge their children, promising the vegetable will make their hair curly or make them see better in the dark. The "see better" part may be true thanks to the high beta-carotene content—or vitamin A potential—of carrots. The link between vitamin A and healthy eyes is stronger than ever; the nutrient is essential for good vision and the ability to see in dim light. Adequate amounts of vitamin A prevent not only night blindness but, in many instances, blindness period. And not just in children. Ophthalmologists now theorize that antioxidants like beta-carotene and vitamins C and E may actually protect older people against macular degeneration and cataracts, two eye diseases common among seniors. In lab studies, rats fed antioxidants were slower to develop either disease, both of which, researchers now believe, develop not only after years of exposure to the sun's ultraviolet rays but also, over time, due to the ravaging effects of oxygen-glutted free radicals. These by-products of metabolism, often called agents of aging, circulate constantly in the body, attacking DNA and possibly initiating cancer and heart disease. Antioxidants seem to depower free radicals before major damage is done—to the eyes or to other parts of the body. There's no proof yet, but studies continue and the results look promising.

Fad Diets: See DIETS.

Failure to Thrive: When babies or children fail to grow at the expected rate for several months, the diagnosis is often failure to thrive. Though a medical problem may be responsible, a third or more of the cases are due to poor nutrition (including too little food), poor feeding techniques, child neglect or incompatibility between mother and child. Some parents make the mistake of feeding their children low-fat, low-cholesterol diets, believing that what's good for the adult is good for the child. What they fail to realize is that children need fat and calories to grow and develop properly.

Falafel: Long a Middle Eastern staple, these small, garlicky, deep-fried burgers made of finely ground dried chickpeas are becoming popular in metropolitan America. They're usually served in pita bread with yogurt, sliced cucumbers, chopped tomatoes and sometimes tahini (sesame-seed paste) sauce, too. Falafel mixes are now sold in top-tier supermarkets (look for them in the ethnic food section). **NOTE:** Nutrient counts are unavailable for falafel, but there's no denying that they're high in protein, carbohydrate and, alas, fat.

Farina: From the Italian word *farina* (meaning "meal" or "flour"), farina can come from any grain, root or tuber. But in the United States it most often means wheat middlings (the small hard bits left in the bolting machine after the flour has been sifted out). Packaged as cereal, farina must be cooked before it's eaten. It contains no fat or cholesterol (that's without cream, of course) and almost no sodium, making farina a good choice for those who must restrict their cholesterol and sodium intake.

NUTRIENT CONTENT OF 1 CUP COOKED FARINA
(about 8⅓ ounces; 233 grams)

116 calories	1 mg sodium
3 g protein	30 mg potassium
0 g fat, 0 saturated	1 g dietary fiber
0 mg cholesterol	0 RE vitamin A
25 g carbohydrate	0.19 mg thiamin
4 mg calcium	0.12 mg riboflavin
28 mg phosphorus	1.3 mg niacin
1.2 mg iron	0 mg vitamin C

Farmer's Cheese: See COTTAGE CHEESE.

Fast Food: A third of the people who eat out do so at fast-food restaurants, which proliferate across the land. Pick your cuisine and you can get it: pizzas in dozens of permutations; tacos, chili and other Tex-Mex specialties; French croissants tricked out with scores of fillings; traditional English fish and chips; Greek gyros and Middle Eastern falafel; curry-in-a-hurry, not to mention any of half a dozen different Chinese cuisines. The latest fast-food fad: sushi bars and Japanese box lunches. Then there are the all-American favorites—burgers and hot dogs with all the trimmings, fried chicken, pancakes, sodas and shakes. All are fast; all are cheap. But they ooze fat and calories. According to *The New England Journal of Medicine,* 40 to 55 percent of the calories in the average fast-food meal come from fat. Ouch! But there *are* ways to eat wisely, even at fast-food restaurants:

- Choose broiled or grilled food over fried or deep-fat-fried.

- Choose burgers and hot dogs minus all the trimmings, especially chili, which is nearly always loaded with fat.

- Choose baked potatoes instead of french fries or hashed browns and top them with a slim pat of butter or, better yet, a spoonful of yogurt. "Hold" the grated cheese, the bacon bits, the creamy toppers.

- Order onion, sweet pepper or mushroom pizzas instead of pepperoni or Italian sausage.

- At the salad bar, concentrate on greens, tomatoes, onions and other vegetables but shun the coleslaw and potato salad. To top a green salad, choose a lean vinaigrette or low-fat dressing; skip the grated Cheddar or Swiss, croutons, bacon bits and all thick gloppy dressings.

- Substitute skim milk or fruit juice for milk shakes.

- Choose fruit desserts, ices or sherbets instead of pies, puddings and ice creams.

- At breakfast, avoid egg- and/or cheese-stuffed croissants, also fancy omelets full of melted cheese. Settle instead for poached or simply scrambled eggs or for pancakes or French toast, omitting the butter and topping with syrup.

Fasting: In the old days, people believed that fasting (going without food) would purge the body of poisons and, indeed, some religions still recommend it as a means of purification. Although fasting for a day or two won't hurt the healthy person, longer fasting not only *doesn't* rid the system of toxins, but it fills the blood with ketones, which can damage the kidneys. In the later stages of fasting, muscles and vital organs begin to surrender their protein. Also lost: calcium, phosphorus, potassium and sodium. Fasting is risky, even the **modified fasting** of some low-calorie diet formulas. These evolved from the **protein-sparing modified fast** (PSMF) prescribed by physicians in the 1970s to grossly overweight patients. These high-protein, nutrient-filled liquids soon landed in drugstores and weight-obsessed Americans began swilling them down three times a day. Five dozen died and with them the diet-formula craze. The high-protein liquids, it turns out, don't protect body muscle as well as a mixture of proteins and carbohydrates. Today's protein-sparing modified fasts use powdered blends of carbohydrates, proteins and other nutrients. They're safer, and when used as directed under medical supervision, they do get dieters off to a quick start. That's the good news. The bad news is that unless dieters adjust their long-term eating habits and adopt a sensible program of exercise, they're likely to regain the lost weight. *Plus* some.

Fat: With so many Americans crazy to be model-thin, is it any wonder that *fat* has become a dirty word? What most Americans don't know is that fat is a nutrient as essential to good health as protein or carbohydrate. It's needed for the regulation of cholesterol metabolism; for the transport and absorption of fat-soluble vitamins (A, D, E and K); for the synthesis of hormonelike chemicals integral to certain biochemical processes; for healthy skin; and for energy. Fat is the body's most efficient source of energy, each gram of it delivering 9 calories (as compared to 4 each for protein and carbohydrate). Fat circulates constantly in the blood but the lion's share of it is stored in adipose tissue. Even this fat is useful: It cushions vital organs, insulates the body from cold and provides a ready source of fuel.

So far we've spoken of fat in the singular. In truth, there are many different fats—in nature, in the human body: solids, semisolids, liquids both thin and viscous. Each is composed of three fatty-acid molecules plus one glycerol molecule, which is why doctors and nutritionists call fats triglycerides. Although all fatty acids are composed of carbon, hydrogen and oxygen, their specific chemical makeup determines whether they are **polyunsaturated** (PUFA), **monounsaturated** (MUFA) or **saturated** (SFA). **NOTE:** The more hydrogen a fatty acid contains, the more saturated it is.

Two polyunsaturated fatty acids—LINOLEIC ACID and LINOLENIC ACID—are further categorized as **essential fatty acids** (EFA) because the body cannot function normally without them. Indeed, a controversial new Boston University study suggests that if your diet lacks EFA, you may be setting yourself up for high blood pressure, hardening of the arteries and cardiovascular disease sometime down the road. It further suggests that 10 percent of all Americans may be deficient in essential fatty acids, which are found in sunflower seeds, walnuts, leafy green vegetables and corn, canola, cottonseed, safflower, soybean, sunflower and walnut oils. *But—make a note—olive oil is not a good source.* The best-known and most widely available monounsaturated fatty acids are OLEIC ACID and palmitoleic acid (of which canola oil and olive oil are superb sources). As for saturated fatty acids, the most common are PALMITIC ACID and STEARIC ACID. They're found not only in animal fats (the marbling in red meat, butter, cream, eggs and cheese, etc.) but also in coconut, chocolate and palm oil. Saturated fatty acids, nutritionists now believe, do more to raise blood levels of "bad" cholesterol (LDL, or low-density lipoprotein) than the cholesterol present in food.

There are also FREE FATTY ACIDS, by-products of fat or triglyceride digestion, which are not attached or bonded to any other substance. They're formed when the fats in butter, lard, margarines or cooking oils turn rancid. Free fatty acids taste and smell terrible, so you should avoid eating them. A quick sniff will tell you whether something is rancid.

Americans have always loved fatty food—prime ribs, fried chicken, doughnuts, french fries, pizza, pound cake, pies, pastries, ice cream. And those who pig out on such fare several times a week—or, horrors! several times a day—are usually unhealthier for it. Of late, however, many Americans are wising up and trying in earnest to eat less fat, particularly saturated fat. For a heart-healthy diet, nutritionists recommend that no more than 30 percent of the day's calories come from fat (although some researchers would like to see that lower still) and only 10 percent of the day's total from saturated fat. (Results of a recent National Cancer Institute study also suggest that nonsmoking women whose diets include 15 percent or more of saturated fat are at six times the risk of developing lung cancer than those whose dietary saturated fat is 10 percent or less. There was a reason for choosing nonsmokers for the study—it would have been difficult, impossible even, to filter out the carcinogenic effects of smoking.) Preliminary results of an ongoing Texas study show that among the six dozen men and women monitored over a two-year period (all of whom had already had skin cancer), those who slashed their daily fat intake (to 20 percent of the total calories) developed two-thirds fewer precancerous lesions. See also individual fats (BUTTER; LARD; MARGARINE; VEGETABLE SHORTENING) and oils (CANOLA OIL; CORN OIL; OLIVE OIL; PEANUT OIL; SAFFLOWER OIL; etc). For information on the omega-3 fatty acids, see FISH OILS.

The latest buzz is about **brown fat,** or, as it's been called, the fat that thins. According to Bradford Lowell, who's been researching brown fat at Boston's Beth Israel Hospital, "White fat is just fat and people who are obese have a lot of it. But brown fat is quite different, and opposite in its function." In studies with mice, Lowell has shown that brown fat actually burns energy and that when mice are deprived of it, they become grossly obese. If ways can be found to stimulate brown fat activity in humans, will fat people become forever thin? Time will tell. Meanwhile, pharmaceutical companies, always eager for new methods of weight control, are exploring the potential of brown fat.

"Fat-Free": What does this mean on a food label? In the past, not much. But with the implementation of strict new food-labeling laws, no food containing more than ½ gram of total fat per serving can be called fat-free. See also FOOD LABELING.

Fat-Soluble Vitamins: There are four of them: A, D, E and K. Because these nutrients do not dissolve in water, fats are needed to carry them to the intestine. Here they're absorbed, then shuttled by plasma lipids (fats) through the bloodstream and delivered wherever they're needed. Unneeded fat-soluble vitamins are deposited in fatty tissue and stored for future use. This means accumulations of them can build up—sometimes to toxic levels—so it's important not to gobble fat-soluble vitamins like popcorn. Unlike the water-soluble B vitamins and C, the excess is not excreted. Each of the fat-soluble vitamins operates independently in the body and each performs vital chores. For example, the body converts vitamin D into a hormone that regulates the absorption of calcium. Vitamin A is involved in the building of cell membranes and the retina. Vitamin K increases the blood's clotting power (the reason it's often prescribed

to surgical patients). And vitamin E is an effective anti-oxidant. For more detailed information, see the individual vitamins: A, D, E and K.

Fat Substitutes: With people aware of the risks of eating too much fat but slow—or unable—to kick the habit, manufacturers have been racing to create "miracle" substitutes blessed with all the lush, creamy richness of the real thing but with none (or few) of the calories. Among the recent discoveries, some now available in commercial foods, some not yet on the market, are:

"Carbohydrate" Fat Substitutes: These water-soluble gums and starches were the first fat substitutes and are basically nothing more than colloidal gels that ape the thickness and creaminess of fat. The newest of these—Oatrim (also called TrimChoice)—is synthesized from oat flour. Because it contains soluble fiber, this fat substitute actually lowers blood levels of "bad" cholesterol (LDL) without affecting the "good" cholesterol (HDL). Or so a recent five-week USDA study of two dozen people with high blood cholesterol suggests. All carbohydrate fat substitutes are effective in salad dressings, puddings, frostings, pie fillings, cake and cookie mixes, not to mention the whole repertoire of frozen desserts. They average about 4 calories per gram versus 9 for fat (Oatrim, however, contains a mere 1 calorie per gram). Although widely used by food manufacturers, none of these carbohydrate fat substitutes is yet available to home cooks.

Combination Fat Substitutes: Several manufacturers have developed fake fats by combining one or more of the substitutes detailed here and adding twists of their own. Four of the more promising are Prolesra, Nutrifat, Finesse and Colestra. All await FDA approval.

"Protein" Fat Substitutes: The best known is Nutra-Sweet's Simplesse, already approved by the FDA (and confirmed as GRAS) for use in ice creams, sherbets and other frozen desserts. It's synthesized from milk whey and/or egg protein, heated, blended and whirred at intense speed so that any rough edges of the protein particles are smoothed. As for calories, 1 gram of Simplesse weighs in at 1⅓ calories compared to almost seven times that for a gram of fat. But there are drawbacks. Simplesse cannot be heated or used in cooking. Kraft

General Foods has come up with a protein-based fat substitute, too—Trailblazer—but has yet to earn FDA approval.

Synthetic Fat Substitutes: Olestra is the name that's known, not a brand name, it turns out, but a generic for a family of sucrose polyester "fats" that are virtually interchangeable with the original. They look the same, taste the same, don't break down when heated, so that they can be used for all manner of cooking and baking, even deep-fat frying. The one difference—and it's a huge one, say Procter & Gamble chemists who developed olestra—is that it passes through the digestive tract and is excreted unchanged. That adds up to zero calories. (Early formulations did cause diarrhea in some people but this has now been corrected.) P&G wants FDA approval to reformulate its vegetable shortenings and oils, substituting olestra for 35 percent of the fat. It's still waiting.

Three other synthetics are in the works, all with ominous chemical names: **esterified propoxylated glycerols,** or EPGs (with clonelike similarity to true fat), **dialkyl dihexadecymalonate,** or DDM (a fatlike alcohol ester synthesized from two organic acids), and **trialkoxytricarballate,** or TATCA (a different organic acid esterified with a variety of fatty alcohols that's being developed by Best Foods for use in its mayos and margarines). None has FDA approval but all are being carefully tested for toxicity and safety. See also APPETIZE; CARPENIN and SALATRIM.

Fatty Acids: The building blocks of FAT.

Fava Beans: See BEANS, FRESH.

Favism: A serious, sometimes fatal illness that afflicts people of Mediterranean descent who have an inherited enzyme deficiency (specifically of glucose-6-phosphate-dehydrogenase). As a result, toxins in the skin of the fava bean destroy their red blood cells. People without this genetic defect aren't harmed by eating fava beans. See also FAVA BEANS under BEANS, FRESH.

Feijoa, Pineapple Guava: The size and shape of an egg, this green- to khaki-colored subtropical fruit is beige of flesh, gritty of texture and its tart flavor suggests a hybridization of eucalyptus, grapes, pineapple and lemons. Although feijoas were grown in California around the turn of the century, they fell from favor with the ascendency of the avocado. Today, most of our supply comes from New Zealand. At their peak of perfection, feijoas can be eaten raw, but make no mistake, they *are* acidic. They're best poached gently in sugar syrup for a few minutes, or cooked to mush and pureed into sauces that can be ladled over ice creams and sherbets or stirred into them. They are also superb slipped, the New Zealand way, into pies, jellies, chutneys and relishes. Feijoas are extremely low in calories and a moderately good source of vitamin C. **SEASON:** Spring and summer with supplies dwindling in fall.

NUTRIENT CONTENT OF 1 MEDIUM-SIZE FEIJOA	
(about 1¾ ounces; 50 grams)	
25 calories	2 mg sodium
1 g protein	78 mg potassium
0 g fat, 0 saturated	2 g dietary fiber
0 mg cholesterol	0 RE vitamin A
5 g carbohydrate	0 mg thiamin
8 mg calcium	0.02 mg riboflavin
10 mg phosphorus	0.1 mg niacin
0 mg iron	10 mg vitamin C

Feingold Diet: Unruly, hyperkinetic children were once said to calm down when certain food additives and salicylates (these are found not only in aspirin but also in many fruits and vegetables, herbs and spices) were withheld from their diets. The theory was advanced in 1975 by Dr. Benjamin Feingold, an allergist with the Kaiser-Permanente medical complex in California and author of *Why Your Child Is Hyperactive*. Several large-scale blind studies underwritten by the National Institutes of Health ultimately proved Feingold wrong. Still, some people remain unconvinced and continue to quote Feingold in their hard sells for their products.

Fenfluramine: A mild appetite suppressant doctors prescribe to help patients win the losing battle. It makes it easier for dieters to keep off the pounds they've lost. See DIET PILLS; DEXFENFLURAMINE.

Fennel, Finocchio: There are several varieties of fennel but the most familiar is Florence fennel, celerylike stalks rising from a bulbous base and terminating in feathery green tops; both stalks and tops have a delicate licorice flavor, which fades on cooking. Finocchio is believed to be native to the Mediterranean basin, perhaps to Italy, which explains why Italians are so fond of it. They prefer the fleshy stalks—raw, cooked, marinated, any way at all. But the French dote upon the tops and team them with fish. They sometimes fuel their grills with fronds of dried fennel so that an even subtler anise flavor wafts up and bathes the fish. **SEASON:** Fall through spring with supplies at their peak in winter.

NUTRIENT CONTENT FOR 1 CUP SLICED RAW FENNEL
(about 3 ounces; 87 grams)

27 calories	45 mg sodium
1 g protein	360 mg potassium
0 g fat, 0 saturated	1 g dietary fiber
0 mg cholesterol	11 RE vitamin A
6 g carbohydrate	0.01 mg thiamin
43 mg calcium	0.03 mg riboflavin
43 mg phosphorus	0.6 mg niacin
0.6 mg iron	11 mg vitamin C

Fennel Seeds: These come not from finocchio but from wild fennels that grow abundantly throughout the Mediterranean, Asia Minor and points east. Fennel seeds taste of licorice, of nuts and, depending upon the species, they may be mild or sharply bitter. The French, Portuguese and Italians mix fennel seeds into a variety of sausages. The Spaniards ferment them with other herbs into *hierba,* a liqueur sipped after dinner. And in India (as well as in many Indian restaurants in this country) saucers of fennel seeds are set out as digestives. And they do seem to make incendiary curries sit more easily.

Fermentation: In the dim, dark days of history man learned—quite by accident—that certain foods, allowed to bubble and froth, to sour, to mold kept better than fresh food. He had no idea why. What mattered was that he could increase the shelf life of staples by turning milk into cheese, grapes into wine, bread and water into beer and cabbage into sauerkraut. We now know that these foods were being fermented and their acidity increased, which kept microbes of spoilage in check. Fermentation, still an effective preserver, is applied to a long roster of foods today: cheeses both soft and hard; cervelats, salami and pepperoni; buttermilk, sour cream and yogurt; sauerkraut,

olives and pickles. Fermented foods don't keep forever, though, so the table below is a guide.

If in doubt about the edibility of any fermented food—if it seems slimy, wrinkled, splodged with mold or scum—throw it out without tasting.

RECOMMENDED STORAGE TIMES

Food	In Refrigerator	In Freezer
Cheddar cheese	4 to 8 weeks	6 months
Gruyère, Emmentaler cheese	4 weeks	6 months
Blue cheese, Roquefort, Gorgonzola, Stilton	2 to 4 weeks	6 months
Brie, Camembert	1 to 1½ weeks	6 months
Buttermilk	1 to 2 weeks	3 months
Sour cream	2 to 3 weeks	Not recommended
Yogurt	1 to 2 weeks	Not recommended
Salami, cervelat, Lebanon bologna	1 to 2 weeks	4 months
Hard salami, Genoa salami, pepperoni	2 to 3 weeks	6 months
Fresh sauerkraut	1 week	Not recommended
Pickles and olives	1 to 2 months	Not recommended

Ferritin: A protein that's the body's storehouse of iron. Found in the liver, spleen, bone marrow and intestinal lining, ferritin can store up to 20 percent of its weight in iron, then release it as needed by the body.

Ferrous Gluconate: (additive; dietary supplement): This form of iron is granular, gray to pale chartreuse in color and emits a burned-sugar smell. Pharmaceutical companies have long made it the iron component of vitamin/mineral supplements. Food processors also use ferrous gluconate to boost the iron content of cornmeal, assorted breakfast cereals, diet foods, soy products and beverages. Finally, canners add it to ripe olives to make them uniformly black. Although moderately toxic, ferrous gluconate is considered GRAS when used within FDA limits.

Ferrous Sulfide: Ever noticed that ugly dark green ring separating the yolk from the white of a hard-cooked egg? It's perfectly harmless, just unsightly. Whenever eggs are cooked too long or at too high a temperature, or when they are not chilled fast enough after they're done, the iron of the yolk will migrate out to meet the sulfur of the white, and presto! the ferrous sulfide ring. To prevent it, cook the eggs gently only until set—18 minutes should do it. Then plunge at once into ice water and quick-chill 3 to 5 minutes.

Feta: A crumbly, salty Greek cheese made from ewe's milk, now widely available in the United States. In the mountains of Greece, shepherds still make feta from unpasteurized milk. It's softer than the pasteurized varieties made for export, spicier, too, and when drizzled with Hymettus honey, it's ambrosial.

NUTRIENT CONTENT OF 1 OUNCE (28 GRAMS) FETA

75 calories	315 mg sodium
4 g protein	18 mg potassium
6 g fat, 4 saturated	0 g dietary fiber
25 mg cholesterol	36 RE vitamin A
1 g carbohydrate	0.04 mg thiamin
139 mg calcium	0.24 mg riboflavin
96 mg phosphorus	0.3 mg niacin
0.2 mg iron	0 mg vitamin C

Fetal Alcohol Syndrome: The babies of alcoholic mothers—or women who drink 3 ounces or more of alcohol a day while pregnant—often suffer low birth weight, cardiovascular defects, stunted mental and physical growth, even deformed arms, legs and heads. The defects are congenital and permanent. Prevention is the only medicine and means swearing off alcohol for the duration of pregnancy.

Fiber, Crude: The old term for **water-insoluble dietary fiber.** See FIBER, DIETARY.

Fiber, Dietary: Given all the media hype about fiber, you'd assume it was a vital nutrient. You'd be wrong. Although classified as a carbohydrate, fiber supplies no vitamins, minerals or even calories. It does, however, play important roles in the body. Basically, there are two types of fibers: those that dissolve in water (**water-soluble** or, more simply, **soluble fiber**) and those that don't (**water-insoluble** or **insoluble fiber**). The water-soluble fibers—**pectins, gums** and **mucilages**—are found mainly in citrus fruits, apples, potatoes, dried peas and beans, oatmeal and oat bran. In the body, they bind bile acids (the liver synthesizes these out of cholesterol), and as the acids are bound, cholesterol is withdrawn from the blood and converted to bile acids to replace the deficit. The cholesterol-lowering effect may be subtle; still, it reduces the risk of heart disease. Water-soluble fiber also lowers—or at least stabilizes—blood sugar (glucose) levels. And that's good news for diabetics. Intricately bound to digestible carbohydrates, which the body breaks down to form glucose, fiber acts like a brake, slowing the digestion of carbohydrates and subsequent release of glucose into the blood.

The two most common water-insoluble fibers, **cellulose** and **lignin,** form the framework of plant cell walls. Neither cellulose (found in wheat bran, whole wheat, whole-grain breakfast cereals, broccoli and carrots) nor lignin (asparagus, wheat bran and pears) will dissolve in water, but both have the ability to absorb it. This means they bulk up stools and speed the passage of waste through the intestines, functions believed to reduce the risk of colon cancer.

If you haven't been eating enough fiber, it's wise to increase your intake slowly. Doing so all at once can cause gas, bloating, diarrhea. It's also important to drink plenty of water when eating lots of fiber. Otherwise, you may irritate, even block your digestive tract.

So how much fiber is enough? There is no RDA for fiber, but most nutritionists recommend 20 to 35 grams of fiber a day (most Americans get no more than 10 to 13 grams). They also recommend that you include both the water-soluble and water-insoluble fiber in your diet. No problem if you regularly eat a wide variety of fruits, vegetables and whole-grain breads and cereals. **NOTE:** Many grains, brans, fruits and vegetables contain both types of fiber. But no animal food (meat, eggs, milk, cheese, etc.) provides any fiber whatsoever.

Fibrocystic Breast Disease (diet and): These benign but painful breast lumps afflict 10 to 20 women in 100 and they tend to wax and wane with the menstrual cycle. One study—controversial—suggests that eliminating caffeine from the diet will ease the symptoms. Other health professionals favor vitamin E therapy—but only under a physician's direction.

Fiddlehead Ferns: The fiddlehead gatherer, like the mushroomer, must know what he is about. Botanically, there is no such thing as a fiddlehead. It's merely the tightly coiled young shoot of a fern—any fern. But the gastronome and botanist know that only the **ostrich fern** is safe to eat. **Bracken,** popular in New England, Canada and Japan, contains not only a toxin that can damage bone marrow but also another compound—possibly QUERCITIN or ptaquiloside—that's a powerful carcinogen. Cattle grazing heavily upon bracken often develop bladder cancer within two to five years. Studies suggest that people are more at risk of developing cancer of the esophagus. Ostrich ferns, however, are considered safe; they're also moderately good sources of vitamins A and C and fiber. Proceed with caution. **Season:** April through early July. **Note:** Specific nutrient counts unavailable.

Figs: The miracle of figs is that so lush, so honeyed a fruit can thrive on hardscrabble ground, but thrive they do on the rocky slopes of Greece and sandy shores of North Africa. Three thousand years before Christ, figs were known in the Middle East. They grew in the Hanging Gardens of Babylon and later were adored by Cleopatra, the Greeks and Romans. That adventurous Roman cook Apicius fed imported Syrian figs to his hogs, the better to fatten their livers. The Elizabethan English, who kept dried figs on hand, preferred to mince them and fold them into sweets. As indeed do we, although we also dote on California's fresh mission figs (so named because they were introduced by the Spanish mission fathers). **Season:** Summer and early fall.

Filberts: See HAZELNUTS.

Finnan Haddie: See HADDOCK.

Fish, Lean White: These fish—COD and scrod, HALIBUT, FLOUNDER, SOLE, HAKE, HADDOCK, PERCH, PIKE, SEA BASS, RED SNAPPER, TURBOT and oh, so many more—have their oils concentrated in the liver. Their flesh is lean and white and their flavor nearly always delicate. Because there isn't space to give detailed nutrient counts for each and every lean white fish and because the counts are reasonably similar, we offer here the nutrient counts for flounder, which can be used as a guide for all other lean white fish.

NUTRIENT CONTENT OF 1 MEDIUM-SIZE FRESH FIG
(about 1¾ ounces; 50 grams)

37 calories	1 mg sodium
0 g protein	116 mg potassium
0 g fat, 0 saturated	2 g dietary fiber
0 mg cholesterol	7 RE vitamin A
10 g carbohydrate	0.03 mg thiamin
18 mg calcium	0.03 mg riboflavin
7 mg phosphorus	0.2 mg niacin
0.2 mg iron	1 mg vitamin C

NUTRIENT CONTENT OF 1 MEDIUM-SIZE DRIED FIG
(about ⅔ ounce; 19 grams)

48 calories	2 mg sodium
1 g protein	133 mg potassium
0 g fat, 0 saturated	2 g dietary fiber
0 mg cholesterol	2 RE vitamin A
12 g carbohydrate	0.01 mg thiamin
27 mg calcium	0.02 mg riboflavin
13 mg phosphorus	0.1 mg niacin
0.4 mg iron	0 mg vitamin C

NUTRIENT CONTENT OF 3 OUNCES (85 GRAMS) POACHED/STEAMED BONED, SKINNED FLOUNDER

97 calories	77 mg sodium
20 g protein	327 mg potassium
1 g fat, 0 saturated	0 g dietary fiber
51 mg cholesterol	9 RE vitamin A
0 g carbohydrate	0.08 mg thiamin
19 mg calcium	0.07 mg riboflavin
176 mg phosphorus	2.6 mg niacin
0.4 mg iron	1 mg vitamin C

NUTRIENT CONTENT OF 3 OUNCES (85 GRAMS) POACHED/STEAMED FLOUNDER
(with skin and bones)

89 calories	79 mg sodium
18 g protein	260 mg potassium
1 g fat, 0 saturated	0 g dietary fiber
51 mg cholesterol	8 RE vitamin A
0 g carbohydrate	0.06 mg thiamin
14 mg calcium	0.08 mg riboflavin
219 mg phosphorus	1.7 mg niacin
0.3 mg iron	0 mg vitamin C

NUTRIENT CONTENT OF 3 OUNCES (85 GRAMS) BROILED/PANBROILED BONED, SKINNED FLOUNDER

100 calories	89 mg sodium
21 g protein	293 mg potassium
1 g fat, 0 saturated	0 g dietary fiber
58 mg cholesterol	9 RE vitamin A
0 g carbohydrate	0.07 mg thiamin
15 mg calcium	0.10 mg riboflavin
245 mg phosphorus	1.9 mg niacin
0.3 mg iron	1 mg vitamin C

NUTRIENT CONTENT OF 3 OUNCES (85 GRAMS) BROILED/PANBROILED FLOUNDER

(with skin and bones)

89 calories	79 mg sodium
18 g protein	260 mg potassium
1 g fat, 0 saturated	0 g dietary fiber
51 mg cholesterol	8 RE vitamin A
0 g carbohydrate	0.06 mg thiamin
14 mg calcium	0.08 mg riboflavin
219 mg phosphorus	1.7 mg niacin
0.3 mg iron	0 mg vitamin C

NUTRIENT CONTENT OF 3 OUNCES (85 GRAMS) FRIED/SAUTÉED BONED, SKINNED FLOUNDER

116 calories	90 mg sodium
21 g protein	293 mg potassium
3 g fat, 1 saturated	0 g dietary fiber
58 mg cholesterol	9 RE vitamin A
0 g carbohydrate	0.07 mg thiamin
16 mg calcium	0.09 mg riboflavin
246 mg phosphorus	1.9 mg niacin
0.3 mg iron	0 mg vitamin C

NUTRIENT CONTENT OF 3 OUNCES (85 GRAMS) FRIED/SAUTÉED FLOUNDER

(with skin and bones)

105 calories	79 mg sodium
18 g protein	260 mg potassium
3 g fat, 1 saturated	0 g dietary fiber
81 mg cholesterol	8 RE vitamin A
0 g carbohydrate	0.06 mg thiamin
14 mg calcium	0.08 mg riboflavin
219 mg phosphorus	1.7 mg niacin
0.3 mg iron	0 mg vitamin C

Fish, Oily: These fish have their oils distributed evenly throughout their flesh, not concentrated in their livers as lean white fish do. Although the family of oily fish isn't as extended as that of lean fish, its numbers are impressive and include everything from ANCHOVIES, EEL and SARDINES to POMPANO, BLUEFISH, SALMON and TROUT to such deep-sea giants as SWORDFISH and TUNA. Oily fish are invariably darker of flesh than lean fish; more strongly flavored, too. Their nutritive value also varies more than it does with lean white fish, so we discuss their nutrient counts in individual entries for various oily fish.

Fish Oils: Before the dawn of handy vitamin supplements, health-conscious mothers force-fed their children a teaspoon or two of vitamin A- and D-rich cod-liver oil every morning before sending them off to school. Cod-liver oil still exists, mostly in more palatable mint-flavored form. The latest buzz, however, is about the **omega-3 fatty acids** in fish oils and their ability to reduce the risk of heart disease. The polyunsaturated omega-3s, **eicosapentaenoic acid** (EPA) and **docosahexaenoic acid** (DHA), function quite differently in the body from the polyunsaturated plant oils. First, they reduce the amount of cholesterol the liver manufactures, and second, they "thin" the blood, making clots less likely to form among the deposits of arterial plaque.

Although cardiologists sometimes prescribe fish-oil capsules, they urge—and nutritionists agree—that they should never be taken without a physician's guidance. Overdosing on fish-oil capsules can cause excessive bleeding, both externally and internally; it can also induce anemia, even strokes. The best policy is simply to eat fish high in the omega-3s: albacore tuna, anchovies, bluefish, cod, halibut, herring (but not kippered or pickled), trout, mackerel, pollack, salmon, fresh sardines, sablefish and sea trout. In addition, these shellfish are excellent sources of omega-3 fatty acids: clams, crab, mussels, scallops and shrimp. And just how often should you eat fish? A new study conducted by the Harvard School of Public Health suggests that five or six times a week is no better than once or twice when it comes to reducing the risk of heart disease. Still, other nutritionists believe that fish, especially those high in omega-3 fatty acids, are "healthy" food and that eating more may still be more healthy. Stay tuned.

And what of the other claims for fish-oil capsules? That they'll ease the pain of arthritis and psoriasis, prevent allergic asthma, migraines, even cancer? And what about their being used to treat diabetes? The only conditions for which they may hold some promise are arthritis and psoriasis. Studies continue.

Fish Roe: The eggs of fish. There are two types, the **hard roe,** or eggs and ovaries of the female, and **soft roe,** the milt of the male (a particular favorite among Native Americans). The roe we prize the most is CAVIAR. But there are two others popular in the United States: salmon roe (sometimes called red caviar) and shad roe. Most of us haven't yet learned to appreciate sea urchin, scallop, mackerel or herring roe although Tidewater Virginians have made a delicacy of the latter. The American shad, a relative of the herring, swims upriver in spring to spawn. Shad season, it's called by those living along the James, the Hudson and other great East Coast rivers where shad roe is considered a great spring delicacy. Polluted waters have taken their toll, but efforts to clean up the rivers are working, and shad are once again swimming upriver to spawn. The best shad roe is delicately flavored, creamy rather than gritty. It is exceptionally fragile and will burst and splatter if cooked

---

NUTRIENT CONTENT OF 3 OUNCES (85 GRAMS) FRIED/SAUTÉED SHAD ROE

166 calories	431 mg sodium
22 g protein	222 mg potassium
10 g fat, 2 saturated	0 g dietary fiber
363 mg cholesterol	113 RE vitamin A
2 g carbohydrate	0.21 mg thiamin
23 mg calcium	0.72 mg riboflavin
372 mg phosphorus	1.7 mg niacin
0.6 mg iron	14 mg vitamin C

NUTRIENT CONTENT OF 1 OUNCE (28 GRAMS) SALMON ROE (RED CAVIAR)

58 calories	NA mg sodium
7 g protein	NA mg potassium
3 g fat, NA saturated	0 g dietary fiber
NA mg cholesterol	NA RE vitamin A
0 g carbohydrate	0.11 mg thiamin
NA mg calcium	0.20 mg riboflavin
NA mg phosphorus	0.6 mg niacin
NA mg iron	5 mg vitamin C

---

over too high a flame. It's best gently browned in butter, then served with a squeeze of fresh lemon. Anything more is lily gilding.

Salmon roe, as glistening, as red as fresh currants, is less seasonal than shad roe because it is salted and put up in little jars (look for it in the refrigerator counters of better groceries). It's so rich, so salty a little of it goes a long way. Most cooks use it to garnish canapés.

Flat-Sour: A form of spoilage that's common among home-canned low-acid vegetables, less so among the commercial. Flat-sour spoilage is not easily detected because the can ends or dome lids remain flat during souring. *Sour* refers to the buildup of acid within the can. Though not harmful, flat-sour foods have lost their palatability and should be discarded.

Flatulence: That gassy, bloated feeling may not come from something you ate. It may simply be air you swallowed *with* your food. Or the bubbles of carbonated drinks—and that includes beer. On the other hand, certain foods do produce carbon dioxide, hydrogen and methane gases in the intestines, which are then "passed." That old childhood chant, "Beans, beans, the musical fruit, the more you eat, the more you poot" isn't far off the mark. Beans contain complex sugars, unassimilable to us, which intestinal bacteria feed upon; the by-product is gas. Other foods apt to cause social (if not medical) grief are onions, cabbage (especially cooked), apples and apple juice, peanuts, radishes, raisins, bananas, even sometimes potatoes. People with a lactose intolerance also suffer from intestinal gas, but lactase supplements, now widely available, usually ease the problem. There is also an over-the-counter enzyme product called Beano that's said to knock the "wind" out of beans (though scientific evidence of its effectiveness is weak). What also helps—with dried beans, at least—is draining and rinsing them well after they've soaked, then cooking them in freshwater.

Flavonoids, Bioflavonoids: A group of colorless or white to yellow pigments concentrated in the skin, rind and outer layers of many fruits and vegetables that are being scrutinized as possible anticarcinogens. Flavonoids are also found in beer, coffee, tea and wine. See also PHYTOCHEMICALS.

Flavor Enhancers (additives): They don't taste like much—sometimes like nothing at all—yet these chemical compounds intensify desirable flavors in meats, fish, poultry, vegetables, fruits, cakes, breads and beverages. They also mask undesirable flavors. MONOSODIUM GLUTAMATE (MSG), sold as Accent and Aji-no-moto, is undoubtedly the best known. But there are other important flavor enhancers, the most widely used being DISODIUM 5'-GUANYLATE, DISODIUM 5'-INOSINATE and ETHYL MALTOL. Each of these enhancers is discussed in an individual entry.

Flavorings (additives): Of the nearly three thousand additives mixed into our food, nearly 70 percent are flavorings. Many are natural—aromatic pods, seeds, barks, rinds, etc., or their volatile oils blended into extracts with alcohol. Other flavorings are synthetic—for good reason. They're usually more potent, more stable than natural flavorings, and they're invariably cheaper. Because flavorings are used in such minute quantities, the government has found it impractical—*make that impossible*—to test each and every one for safety. Still, the FDA rates 69 percent of them GRAS.

Flavor Labeling: It's confusing at best, meaningless at worst. Natural flavors (those derived from vanilla beans, for example, from cloves and other natural substances) can be identified on a label as "natural flavors." Identical flavorings synthesized in the lab, however, must be labeled "artificial." Then there's the mystifying phrase "with other natural flavors" (WONF), which means that the dominant natural flavor has been bolstered with other natural flavors (perhaps lemon or orange or vanilla or all three). To illustrate the nuances of the labeling process, let's look at five different peach pies listed below.

Flax, Flaxseeds: To Americans, flax means linen. Period. But to Europeans, flaxseeds and cold-pressed flaxseed (or linseed) oil are important as food. We would do well to follow their lead because these tiny, shiny, red-brown seeds contain anticarcinogens called lignans. Flaxseeds also contain omega-3 fatty acids, which some medical researchers believe may prove valuable in treating psoriasis and rheumatoid arthritis. This doesn't mean that you should rush out, buy a can of linseed oil and use it to dress salads or sauté fish. Far from it. In the United States, linseed oil is processed specifically for use in paints and varnishes, linoleum and printer's ink and isn't edible. Better to buy flaxseeds from a health-food store, spread them in a pie tin, toast 10 to 12 minutes in a 325°F. oven, then sprinkle into green salads or knead into yeast breads (⅓ to ½ cup toasted flaxseeds per loaf is about right; too many of them can cause diarrhea). They have a pleasant, nutty flavor.

EXAMPLES OF FLAVOR LABELING

	Source of Flavor	Correct Label
Peach Pie 1	Peaches only	"Peach pie"
Peach Pie 2	Peaches plus a bit of natural peach flavoring	"Peach pie" (but scrutiny of ingredients shows peach flavoring was added)
Peach Pie 3	Plenty of added natural peach flavoring because there were too few peaches to do the job	"Natural peach-flavored pie"
Peach Pie 4	Maybe peaches, maybe not; plenty of natural peach flavoring plus assorted other natural flavors to intensify the peach flavor	"Natural peach-flavored pie with other natural flavors"
Peach Pie 5	Pie with artificial flavors added	"Artificially flavored peach pie" (the catch is that the pie may also contain real peaches and natural peach flavor. But as long as it contains any artificial flavor, it must be so labeled)

Fletcherism: At the turn of this century, food faddist Horace Fletcher espoused a new theory: For good health, people should chew every forkful of food thirty-two times. No more, no less. The idea was to bring out the full flavors of food but, more important, to set the digestive juices in motion so that food was more completely digested. Fletcher also believed that by Fletcherizing, people would be more quickly satisfied, eat less and thus maintain a healthful weight. Fletcherism may now sound like quackery, but its proponents included Thomas Edison and John D. Rockefeller. Fletcher died in 1919 at the age of seventy, but some still practice Fletcherism today.

Flounder: This delicate flatfish often masquerades in the United States as sole, but the only true sole is Dover sole from the English Channel and surrounding waters. Flounder isn't so fine or firm of texture as sole; it's a bigger fish, too, so what usually shows up in U.S. markets are fillets.

They are supremely versatile and can be broiled or pan-broiled, steamed, poached, sautéed (either breaded or not), curled into rolls and simmered in wine or court bouillon, even pureed and smoothed into fish loaves, mousses and pâtés. For an indication of nutritive content, see FISH, LEAN WHITE.

Flour: When whole grains are pulverized, the result is flour. To Americans, that means wheat flour and, over much of America, white flour although the move from chemically **bleached,** highly refined flours to the more natural **unbleached** is gaining ground. Both are available as all-purpose and the higher-protein bread flour. The percentage of protein to starch varies not only from one type of flour to another but also from region to region.

Baking needs differ. In the Great Lakes and upper Plains states, settled in large part by Germans, Poles and Scandinavians, yeast breads are the thing. And the chewier the

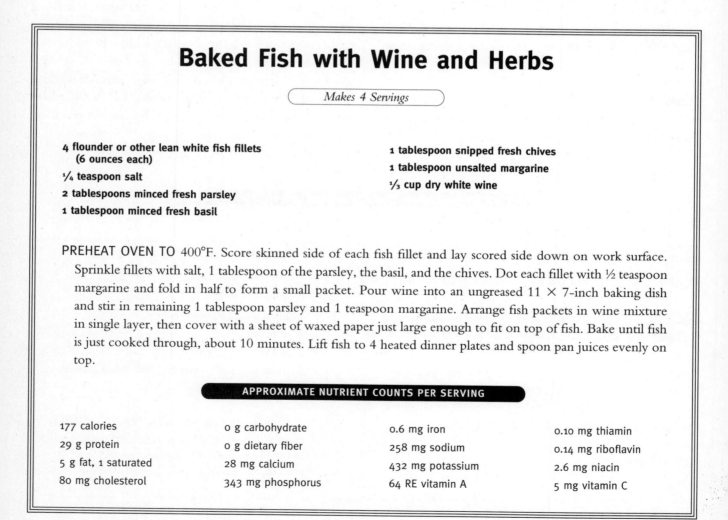

Baked Fish with Wine and Herbs

Makes 4 Servings

4 flounder or other lean white fish fillets
  (6 ounces each)
¼ teaspoon salt
2 tablespoons minced fresh parsley
1 tablespoon minced fresh basil

1 tablespoon snipped fresh chives
1 tablespoon unsalted margarine
⅓ cup dry white wine

PREHEAT OVEN TO 400°F. Score skinned side of each fish fillet and lay scored side down on work surface. Sprinkle fillets with salt, 1 tablespoon of the parsley, the basil, and the chives. Dot each fillet with ½ teaspoon margarine and fold in half to form a small packet. Pour wine into an ungreased 11 × 7-inch baking dish and stir in remaining 1 tablespoon parsley and 1 teaspoon margarine. Arrange fish packets in wine mixture in single layer, then cover with a sheet of waxed paper just large enough to fit on top of fish. Bake until fish is just cooked through, about 10 minutes. Lift fish to 4 heated dinner plates and spoon pan juices evenly on top.

APPROXIMATE NUTRIENT COUNTS PER SERVING

177 calories	0 g carbohydrate	0.6 mg iron	0.10 mg thiamin
29 g protein	0 g dietary fiber	258 mg sodium	0.14 mg riboflavin
5 g fat, 1 saturated	28 mg calcium	432 mg potassium	2.6 mg niacin
80 mg cholesterol	343 mg phosphorus	64 RE vitamin A	5 mg vitamin C

better. So flour blends sold in these areas contain plenty of protein-rich hard wheat (rye flours are also popular there). Down South women like biscuits and cakes so light they levitate. And that calls for flours ground from soft wheat— plenty of starch but maybe only 10 percent of the proteins GLIADIN and GLUTENIN, which combine to form GLUTEN, the tough elastic framework of wheat breads. Southerners also cling to snowy, silky bleached flours, insisting they produce flakier biscuits, featherier cakes than unbleached flours. They're right.

But these flours have been chemically bleached—with benzoyl peroxide, perhaps, or chlorine dioxide, chlorine or acetone peroxide. All are currently recognized as safe by the FDA; still, any flour thus treated must be clearly marked "bleached." (Wheat flour will bleach naturally over time when exposed to air. The chemicals just speed up the process.) Consumer watchdogs are calling for further testing of at least one of these chemical bleaches— acetone peroxide.

Although the federal government doesn't require it, most refined flours have been ENRICHED. This means that important nutrients lost in the milling—iron, thiamin, riboflavin and niacin—have been added in amounts to approximate the nutritional content of whole wheat (actually, enriched flour has twice as much riboflavin as whole wheat). And now for a quick look at the flours widely used across America today:

All-Purpose Flour: This delicate balance of hard and soft wheats contains just enough protein for sturdy yeast breads but not enough to toughen simple butter cakes, cookies and piecrusts. It's not a good choice for angel food. Unbleached all-purpose flours tend to produce cakes and quick breads of lower volume and less tender crumb.

NUTRIENT CONTENT OF 1 CUP UNSIFTED ENRICHED ALL-PURPOSE FLOUR

(about 4½ ounces; 125 grams)

455 calories	2 mg sodium
13 g protein	134 mg potassium
1 g fat, 0 saturated	3 g dietary fiber
0 mg cholesterol	0 RE vitamin A
95 g carbohydrate	0.98 mg thiamin
18 mg calcium	0.62 mg riboflavin
135 mg phosphorus	7.4 mg niacin
5.8 mg iron	0 mg vitamin C

Bread Flour: A high-protein, hard-wheat flour that's a good choice for commercial and home bakers. It's available both bleached and unbleached.

NUTRIENT CONTENT OF 1 CUP UNSIFTED ENRICHED BREAD FLOUR

(about 4¾ ounces; 137 grams)

495 calories	2 mg sodium
16 g protein	136 mg potassium
2 g fat, 0 saturated	5 g dietary fiber
0 mg cholesterol	0 RE vitamin A
99 g carbohydrate	1.11 mg thiamin
21 mg calcium	0.70 mg riboflavin
133 mg phosphorus	10.4 mg niacin
6 mg iron	0 mg vitamin C

Cake Flour: Highly refined, ultrafine, soft-wheat flour, the best choice for angel food and other delicate cakes. It's high in starch, extremely low in protein; thus it doesn't make good bread.

NUTRIENT CONTENT OF 1 CUP UNSIFTED ENRICHED CAKE FLOUR

(about 3¾ ounces; 109 grams)

395 calories	2 mg sodium
9 g protein	115 mg potassium
1 g fat, 0 saturated	0 g dietary fiber
0 mg cholesterol	0 RE vitamin A
85 g carbohydrate	0.97 mg thiamin
16 mg calcium	0.47 mg riboflavin
93 mg phosphorus	7.4 mg niacin
8 mg iron	0 mg vitamin C

Durum Flour: A creamy high-gluten flour milled from hard durum wheat. Food processors use it almost exclusively for pasta because durum doughs are tough and can be extruded into a variety of shapes that won't disintegrate when boiled. **NOTE:** Specific nutrient counts unavailable.

Gluten Flour: With dehydrated gluten added to pump up its protein content to 41 percent protein, this pale tan flour produces too much gluten to be used solo. For best results, use it in pizza doughs, bagels or sturdy, crisp-crusted country loaves, allowing about 1 part gluten flour to 3 or 4 parts all-purpose or bread flour.

NUTRIENT CONTENT OF 1 CUP UNSIFTED GLUTEN FLOUR
(about 5 ounces; 140 grams)

529 calories	3 mg sodium
58 g protein	84 mg potassium
3 g fat, 0 saturated	1 g dietary fiber
0 mg cholesterol	0 RE vitamin A
66 g carbohydrate	0.04 mg thiamin
56 mg calcium	0.04 mg riboflavin
196 mg phosphorus	0.7 mg niacin
0.6 mg iron	0 mg vitamin C

"Instant" Flour: Flour that has been moistened and dried into granules that blend instantly in hot and cold liquids. Though a good choice for cooks who can't get the lumps out of their gravy, instant flour makes lousy cakes, breads, pies and pastries. **NOTE:** Specific nutrient counts unavailable.

Pastry Flour: Mostly the province of professional bakers, pastry flour is not quite as soft or starchy as cake flour but is lower in protein than all-purpose flour. It produces wondrously flaky pastries and meltingly tender cookies. Although specific nutrient counts aren't available, 1 cup pastry flour would be about the same as 1 cup cake flour.

Rye Flour: Milled from rye grains, this tweedy gray to beige flour doesn't lack protein, but its protein isn't the type that builds sturdy loaves. Bakers therefore recommend using anywhere from 25 to 40 percent rye flour and 60 to 75 percent bread flour. Although **medium rye flour** is the most widely available (whole grain minus the husk), there are also **light rye flour** (very pale, very starchy), **dark rye flour** (milled from the part of the grain just beneath the husk) and **rye meal** (pumpernickel flour), a coarse, dark, whole-grain meal that's chock-full of bran. Rye flour may be whole grain, partially or fully refined. The whole grain is an excellent source of dietary fiber, iron, phosphorus, potassium and thiamin, yet it contains almost no sodium.

Self-Rising Flour: The Southerner's choice: cake or all-purpose flour with salt and baking powder added. Those watching their sodium intake should avoid it. But make a note, it is higher in calcium than regular flours because of the calcium salt in the baking powder.

NUTRIENT CONTENT OF 1 CUP UNSIFTED ENRICHED SELF-RISING ALL-PURPOSE FLOUR
(about 4½ ounces; 125 grams)

442 calories	1,587 mg sodium
12 g protein	155 mg potassium
1 g fat, 0 saturated	3 g dietary fiber
0 mg cholesterol	0 RE vitamin A
93 g carbohydrate	0.84 mg thiamin
422 mg calcium	0.52 mg riboflavin
744 mg phosphorus	7.3 mg niacin
5.8 mg iron	0 mg vitamin C

Whole-Wheat Flour: Also called **graham flour** after Sylvester Graham, an early-nineteenth-century minister who championed temperance and wholesome food, this unsifted speckled brown-and-white flour contains the germ and bran of wheat as well as the starchy endosperm. Because of the germ, whole-wheat flour doesn't keep as well as white flour, but it's protein- and fiber-rich. Used by itself, whole-wheat flour yields leaden loaves of poor volume. Experienced bakers use about equal parts whole-wheat and all-purpose or bread flour. **INCIDENTAL INTELLIGENCE:** Sylvester Graham also invented the graham cracker.

NUTRIENT CONTENT OF 1 CUP UNSIFTED MEDIUM RYE FLOUR
(about 3⅔ ounces; 102 grams)

361 calories	3 mg sodium
10 g protein	346 mg potassium
2 g fat, 0 saturated	15 g dietary fiber
0 mg cholesterol	0 RE vitamin A
79 g carbohydrate	0.29 mg thiamin
25 mg calcium	0.12 mg riboflavin
211 mg phosphorus	1.8 mg niacin
2.2 mg iron	0 mg vitamin C

NUTRIENT CONTENT OF 1 CUP UNSIFTED WHOLE-WHEAT FLOUR
(about 4⅓ ounces; 120 grams)

407 calories	6 mg sodium
17 g protein	486 mg potassium
2 g fat, 0 saturated	15 g dietary fiber
0 mg cholesterol	0 RE vitamin A
87 g carbohydrate	0.54 mg thiamin
40 mg calcium	0.26 mg riboflavin
415 mg phosphorus	7.6 mg niacin
4.7 mg iron	0 mg vitamin C

There are specialty flours, too—made from amaranth, arrowroot, buckwheat, chestnuts, corn, oats, millet, potatoes, quinoa (the newly trendy but ancient supergrain of the Andes), soy, tapioca, teff and triticale (a relatively new grain hybridized from wheat and rye). All must be used in combination with wheat flour because they lack the protein needed to give breads, cakes and pastries proper structure. The more unusual flours are usually sold in health-food stores.

Flowers, Edible: Mention edible flowers, and candied rosebuds and violets spring to mind. But that's the short list. Other edible flowers include carnations, chrysanthemums, geraniums, honeysuckle, lavender, marigolds, nasturtiums, pansies, zucchini and other summer squash blossoms (heavenly when stuffed or batter-fried). Savvy cooks are slipping the tarter blossoms into marinades and salads; the sweet, perfumy ones into desserts, confections, jams and jellies. Flowers add interest, color and, yes, vitamins, too. Although no nutrient counts are available for flowers, it's safe to say that the bright orange ones—marigolds, chrysanthemums, nasturtiums and squash blossoms—don't lack for beta-carotene. And that the whole bouquet supplies moderate amounts of vitamin C.

Flowers and Plants, Poisonous: Many of our loveliest flowers are poisonous and should never be used with food—even as a garnish. These include: anemones, autumn crocus, azaleas, buttercups, cardinal flowers, clematis, daffodils, datura, delphiniums, gloriosa lilies, hydrangeas, jasmine, lantana, larkspur, lilies of the valley, lupine, monkshood, narcissus, oleander, poinsettia, rhododendron, star of Bethlehem, sweet peas, tansy and wisteria. In addition, many ornamental plants are poisonous: English ivy, dieffenbachia, mistletoe, pothos and philodendron. Even the dried seeds, bark and wilted leaves of apricot trees, bitter almonds, cherries, peaches, pears and plums contain cyanide. Nothing to be cavalier about.

Fluid Balance: When the amount of liquids consumed equals those excreted and lost through breathing and perspiration, bodily fluids are said to be in equilibrium. When more are taken in than lost, EDEMA results. And when the body loses more liquid than it takes in, cells die. They cannot function—*exist*—without water and electrolytes (ionizable salts, meaning salts with the ability to take on positive or negative electric charges). The proteins in each body cell play a major role in maintaining the body's fluid balance.

Fluid Ounces: A measure of volume; 8 fluid ounces equal 1 cup. The weight will vary from fluid to fluid, however, because some are noticeably heavier than others.

Fluid Retention: See EDEMA.

Fluke: See FISH, LEAN WHITE.

Fluorine, Fluoride: Fluorine is a nonmetallic trace element that activates certain enzymes in the body and suppresses others. It is present in micro amounts in all body tissue, with the greatest concentrations being in the bones, teeth and vital organs. Is fluorine an essential nutrient? Some say yes; others no. There is no denying, however, that fluorine—especially its ionized (salt) form, fluoride—prevents dental cavities. For that reason, many cities have fluoridated their drinking water. Fluorides are readily absorbed by the body and they can also be toxic. Too much fluoride can mottle the teeth and heavy doses of it can be fatal. Good sources of fluorine and fluoride: organ meats, gelatin, saltwater fish and shellfish and—of all things—tea.

Fluoxetine: The generic name for Prozac, an antidepressant that is sometimes used to treat those with anorexia or other eating disorders.

Foie Gras: See LIVER (AS FOOD).

Folacin, Folic Acid, Folate (vitamin): Discovered only in 1945, this B vitamin is used by the body both to synthesize and break down amino acids and to synthesize DNA/RNA–like nucleic acids, which in turn are needed to build new cells, especially new red blood cells. Its role in preventing two devastating birth defects—spina bifida (a condition in which the backbone doesn't envelop and protect the spinal cord) and anencephaly (a fatal malformation of the brain)—is so significant the FDA, to ensure that pregnant women receive sufficient folacin, aims to add it to the list of nutrients now being used to enrich flours, cereals, breads and pastas (140 micrograms folacin per 100 grams [3½ ounces] food is the proposed amount). In addition to preventing these birth defects, folic acid may also protect against certain types of cancer (lung, cervical, colorectal) and CORONARY HEART DISEASE. Even so, nutritionists recommend getting folic acid from food, not vitamin pills. There is some concern, however, that too much folacin masks pernicious anemia and makes it difficult to diagnose. **DEFICIENCY SYMPTOMS:** Anemia, gastrointestinal upsets, impaired brain and nerve function. And, as has already been said, major birth defects. Those most apt to lack folacin are alcoholics, also those who have suffered illnesses or injuries that require the body to manufacture new cells fast—burn or hemorrhage patients, even those with measles and chicken pox. In each case, the body needs to generate new cells and uses up folacin in a hurry. **GOOD SOURCES:** Liver, yeast, nuts, dried beans, whole grains, spinach and other dark leafy greens, oranges, avocados. **PRECAUTIONS:** Cooking destroys about 50 percent of the folacin in vegetables; canning still more. Even storing vegetables at room temperature accelerates the loss of folacin—after three days, most of it's gone (always cover vegetables airtight and store in a cool, dark place).

RDA FOR FOLACIN

Babies:

Birth to 6 months	25 mcg per day
6 months to 1 year	35 mcg per day

Children:

1 to 3 years	50 mcg per day
4 to 6 years	75 mcg per day
7 to 10 years	100 mcg per day
11 to 14 years	150 mcg per day

Men and Boys:

15 to 51+ years	200 mcg per day

Women and Girls:

15 to 51+ years	180 mcg per day

Pregnant Women:

	400 mcg per day

Nursing Mothers:

First 6 months	280 mcg per day
Second 6 months	260 mcg per day

Food, Drug, and Cosmetic Act: In 1938, the U.S. Food and Drug Administration (FDA) limited the amount of toxic chemicals (read additives) that could be present in food. Then in 1954 the Pesticides Chemical Amendment banned the sale of raw agricultural products containing pesticide residues above certain allowed tolerances. See also FOOD ADDITIVES AMENDMENT; FOOD AND DRUG ADMINISTRATION; DELANEY CLAUSE.

Food Additives: See ADDITIVES; the more commonly used ones are listed in individual entries.

Food Additives Amendment: First came the Food and Drug Act of 1906, then the Food, Drug, and Cosmetic Act of 1938, which empowered the federal government to pull adulterated, poisonous or harmful foods off the market. But the laws lacked "teeth" until 1958, when Congress passed the Food Additives Amendment, and two years later, the Color Additive Amendments, which required manufacturers to prove additives and colorings safe before the FDA could authorize them for use. As a result of the 1958 amendment, seven hundred additives, based on their long-term batting averages, were identified as "Generally Recognized as Safe" (GRAS), which absolved the government of testing each for safety. Still, many have been retested (one of the goals set forth at the 1969 White House Conference on Food and Nutrition) and, as a result, a few have been removed from the GRAS list. In addition, another group of additives—prior sanctioned substances—was exempted from testing because they'd already been approved by the USDA or FDA. A further limiting of additives came in 1958 with the adoption of the DELANEY CLAUSE. It banned the use of all carcinogens.

Food and Drug Administration (FDA): An agency of the U.S. Department of Health and Human Services, the FDA tries to ensure that our food and beverages are safe. No small job. It reviews new additives, has them tested for safety before it will approve them for use, then monitors that use to see that it meets federal guidelines. It also watchdogs food labeling. Though concerned with food safety, the FDA is powerless when it comes to limiting the number of additives that can be used or to determining their efficacy. However, because of mounting public concern about the thousands of additives in use, their interactions and long-term effects on health, the FDA is reviewing 450 of those on the GRAS list, both natural and synthetic. It already recommends further study of the preservative BHT, which has damaged the livers of lab rats. The FDA is also scrutinizing 2,100 flavorings, many of them GRAS. As a result of the 1960 Color Additive Amendments bill, 200 colorings were put on a provisional list and 80 have been dropped, either because they were unsafe (the case with Red No. 2) or because their manufacturers voluntarily withdrew them. Many consumer advocates, dissatisfied with FDA performance, are demanding stricter controls on additives, careful testing of many now in use and the banning of others they deem unsafe.

Food-Borne Illnesses: See BACTERIA.

Food Colors: See COLORINGS.

Food Exchange Lists: See EXCHANGE LIST.

Food Fads: *So* many. And so fast they change. It's the old medicine man gone modern, spreading his magical food supplements, diets, pills, potions and promises of "forever thin and fit" in health-food stores, print and electronic infomercials. Most are nothing more than money-making scams aimed at the gullible, the elderly and infirm, who gladly shell out for the latest miracle cure, be it for arthritis, cancer, heart disease, obesity, impotence, baldness or anything else (the annual take is as high as *$10 billion*). The government tries to keep tabs on hucksters, and occasionally the Federal Trade Commission (FTC) shuts someone down for false advertising. But often they're soon back in business with a new product or panacea.

Many health hucksters—"health counselors" they often call themselves, or "nutritionists"—have bought credentials from diploma mills or ordered degrees through the mail. Most have no training or expertise—except for separating innocent victims from their money. Before falling for a pitch, check credentials thoroughly. A registered dietitian, or R.D., for example, is a rigorously trained health professional; a "nutritionist" may or may not be, depending upon whether the degree comes from an accredited college or university. Further, seeing a B.S., M.S. or Ph.D. after a nutritionist's name may not be proof of nutritional training. Some Ph.D. "nutritionists" majored in psychology, communications or other wholly unrelated fields. To check credentials, contact your local hospital, university or county health department. *Also beware of:*

- Foods or nutritional products backed by testimonials. Many testimonials are phony.

- Too-good-to-be-true claims. Any promises of instant cures *are* too good to be true.

- Cures that urge eating certain foods to the exclusion of others—a high-protein diet, for example, to lose weight. Or, conversely, "cures" that urge eliminating

certain foods from the diet—the no-pasta-and-bread reducing diet (what's lost is water, not fat).

- Food supplements or formulas recommended as substitutes for food. The only healthful diet is the well-balanced one.

- Claims that nonorganically grown foods are nutritionally inferior to the organically grown, or that synthesized vitamins are less effective than the natural. Wrong on both counts.

- Pitches that lay on a guilt trip such as "If only you'll eat this food, swallow this elixir or pop these pills, you'll be as beautiful, trim and full of energy as the model in the ad."

SUMMING UP: If fad foods really worked, there wouldn't be a new one a minute. See also DIETS.

Food Groups: In 1943, to educate Americans and encourage them to eat a well-balanced diet, the National Wartime Nutrition Program of the U.S. Department of Agriculture (USDA), following the lead of the Bureau of Home Economics, grouped foods into seven basic categories, suggesting that if you ate a certain number of portions from each group each day, you'd be well nourished. The **Basic Seven,** shown in a pie chart with each food group occupying equal space, were (1) Milk and Milk Products; (2) Meat, Fish, Poultry and Eggs; (3) Green and Yellow Vegetables; (4) Citrus Fruit and Raw Cabbage; (5) Potatoes and Other Fruits and Vegetables; (6) Bread, Flour and Cereal (enriched or whole grain); (7) Butter or Fortified Margarine.

By 1956, with researchers zeroing in on the unhealthfulness of fat and nutritionists revising their opinion on what constituted a healthful diet, the Basic Seven succumbed to the **Basic Four,** with fat being kicked off the list and all fruits and vegetables consolidated. The Basic Four composed a simpler pie chart, with each food group also being given a wedge of equal size: (1) Milk and Milk Products; (2) Meat, Fish, Poultry and Eggs; (3) Fruits and Vegetables; (4) Bread, Flour and Cereals (enriched or whole grain). Variations on the theme appeared in the 1970s and 1980s, but in November 1990 there was a major upheaval: The USDA, cooperating with the Department of Health and Human Services, issued new **Dietary Guidelines for Americans.** Clearly, a new graphic was needed and the one finally adopted, after much controversy and revision, was the FOOD GUIDE PYRAMID.

Food Guide Pyramid: The graphic used to illustrate the new **Dietary Guidelines for Americans,** jointly issued in November 1990 by the USDA and the Department of Health and Human Services. Unlike the pie charts of the **Basic Seven** and **Basic Four,** the pyramid emphasizes the foods we should eat the most of every day for good health. The pyramid's base thus is the Bread, Cereal, Rice and Pasta Group (6 to 11 servings per day). The next two building blocks, identical in size, are the Vegetable Group (3 to 5 servings) and the Fruit Group (2 to 4 servings). Next come two more blocks of equal size: the Milk, Yogurt and Cheese Group (2 to 3 servings) and the Meat, Poultry, Fish, Dry Beans, Eggs and Nuts Group (also 2 to 3 servings). Perched at the very tip of the pyramid is the Fats, Oils and Sweets Group, accompanied by the advice "use sparingly." It took nearly two years for the various government committees to agree on the final form of the pyramid, but the one shown here, adopted in April 1992, seems to have across-the-board support. More important, the Food Guide Pyramid is a classroom hit because it quickly teaches children the fundamentals of good nutrition.

Food Labeling: The Nutrition Labeling and Education Act, passed in 1990, charged the U.S. Department of Health and Human Services with proposing new nutrition labeling by November 8, 1991, and finalizing the regulations a year later. Only with presidential intervention—and compromises all around—did they succeed. The new requirements, in print as hefty as a Manhattan phone book, detail what each of the 257,000 FDA-regulated food products and package sizes must include on their labels, as well as 90 percent of the processed meats and poultry under the aegis of the USDA's Food Safety and Inspection Service. As of the spring of 1994, all food labels must clearly display—in language the consumer can understand—the following:

- Product name.

- Manufacturer's, packer's or distributor's name and address.

- Net contents (count, weight or measure).

- Ingredient list (beginning with the ingredient most abundantly used by weight and ending with the least).

- Serving size and number of servings in the package.

- Nutrition facts. This valuable label addition, designed to educate the public to the benefits of good eating and reduce the risk of cancer, heart disease, osteoporosis, high blood pressure, obesity, etc., looks like this:

Nutrition Facts

Serving Size 1 cup (248g)
Servings Per Container 4

Amount Per Serving	
Calories 150	**Calories from Fat 35**

	% Daily Value*
Total Fat 4 g	**6%**
Saturated Fat 2.5g	**12%**
Cholesterol 20mg	**7%**
Sodium 170mg	**7%**
Total Carbohydrate 17g	**6%**
Dietary Fiber 0g	**0%**
Sugars 17g	
Protein 13g	

Vitamin A 4%	•	Vitamin C 6%
Calcium 40%	•	Iron 0%

*Percent Daily Values are based on a 2,000 calorie diet. Your daily values may be higher or lower depending on your calorie needs:

		Calories:	2,000	2,500
Total Fat	Less than		65g	80g
Sat Fat	Less than		20g	25g
Cholesterol	Less than		300mg	300mg
Sodium	Less than		2,400mg	2,400mg
Total Carbohydrate			300g	375g
Dietary Fiber			25g	30g

Calories per gram:
Fat 9 • Carbohydrate 4 • Protein 4

A few foods are exempted from the new label rulings: raw fish, fresh fruits and vegetables although the FDA wants stores to post labels at points of purchase; spices, coffees and teas whose nutritional content is negligible; nonfood diet supplements; infant formulas (regulated under a separate act); medical foods; boutique (custom-processed) game and fish; food shipped—but not sold—in bulk; meats and poultry products sliced to order at deli counters; minipackages of food weighing less than ½ an ounce. Still, if any of these foods are marketed as healthful or nutritive, they must bear the new nutrition label. There's a further exemption: Food for children less than two years old will list total fat but not saturated fat, cholesterol or calories from fat (baby formulas are still subject to the Infant Formula Act of 1980 [revised 1986], which sets minimum levels for twenty-nine different nutrients and maximum levels for nine).

Food Guide Pyramid

A Guide to Daily Food Choices

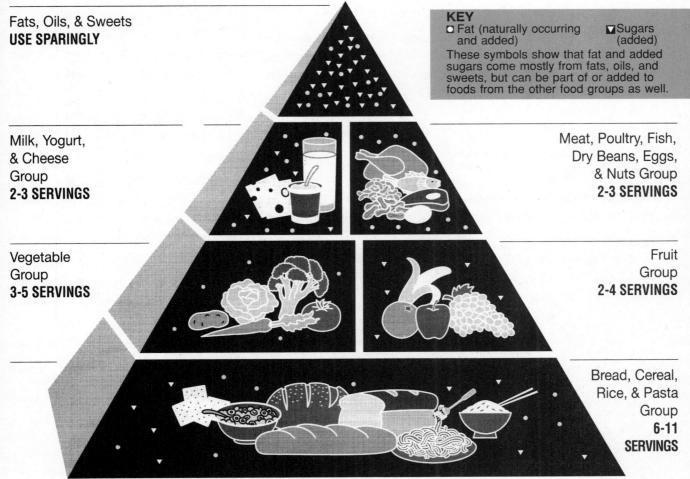

Fats, Oils, & Sweets
USE SPARINGLY

KEY
□ Fat (naturally occurring and added) ▼ Sugars (added)
These symbols show that fat and added sugars come mostly from fats, oils, and sweets, but can be part of or added to foods from the other food groups as well.

Milk, Yogurt, & Cheese Group
2-3 SERVINGS

Meat, Poultry, Fish, Dry Beans, Eggs, & Nuts Group
2-3 SERVINGS

Vegetable Group
3-5 SERVINGS

Fruit Group
2-4 SERVINGS

Bread, Cereal, Rice, & Pasta Group
6-11 SERVINGS

SOURCE: U.S. Department of Agriculture/U.S. Department of Health and Human Services

Use the Food Guide Pyramid to help you eat better every day . . . the Dietary Guidelines way. Start with plenty of Breads, Cereals, Rice, and Pasta; Vegetables; and Fruits. Add two to three servings from the Milk group and two to three servings from the Meat group.

Each of these food groups provides some, but not all, of the nutrients you need. No one food group is more important than another—for good health you need them all. Go easy on fats, oils, and sweets, the foods in the small tip of the Pyramid.

To order a copy of "The Food Guide Pyramid" booklet, send a $1.00 check or money order made out to the Superintendent of Documents to: Consumer Information Center, Department 159-Y, Pueblo, Colorado 81009.

U.S. Department of Agriculture, Human Nutrition Information Service, August 1992, Leaflet No. 572

SOME NEW TERMINOLOGY

"Extra Lean": 100-gram (3½-ounce) portions of meat, game, fowl or seafood may not contain more than 5 grams fat (2 grams saturated) and 95 milligrams cholesterol.

"Free": Examples are "fat-free," "salt-free." Per-serving contents can't exceed 5 calories, 5 milligrams sodium, 2 milligrams cholesterol or ½ gram each sugar, fat and saturated fat.

"Fresh": Preservative-free raw food that's never been heated, frozen or pasteurized. **NOTE:** Food irradiated at low levels can still be called fresh, as can frozen poultry as long as it was never chilled to 0°F. The USDA hopes to change that, allowing no bird to be labeled "fresh" if it has been chilled below 26°F.

"Fresh-Frozen": Flash-frozen fresh food that may or may not have been blanched.

"Good Source": One serving provides 10 to 19 percent of the Daily Value of a specific nutrient.

"Healthy": Processed food that contains, per serving, no more than 3 grams fat (1 gram saturated), 60 milligrams cholesterol and 480 milligrams sodium (in January 1998 this will drop to 360 milligrams). In addition, extra-lean meat and poultry that contain, per 100 grams or 3½ ounces, fewer than 5 grams total fat (2 grams saturated) and 95 milligrams cholesterol can also be called "healthy." Finally, "healthy" food must supply at least 10 percent of the Daily Value for vitamin A, vitamin C, calcium, fiber or protein.

"High": One serving contains at least 20 percent of the Daily Value of a particular nutrient—vitamin C, for example, or dietary fiber.

"Lean": 100-gram (3½-ounce) portions of meat, game, fowl or seafood may not contain more than 10 grams fat (4 grams saturated) and 95 milligrams cholesterol.

"Less": Contains 25 percent fewer calories or 25 percent less of a particular nutrient than the standard reference food.

"Light," "Lite": Food in which the calories have been reduced by a third and the fat by half. Also, if a low-calorie, low-fat food is 50 percent lower in salt than the standard version, it can be labeled "low in sodium." Finally, "light" has long been used to describe color ("light brown sugar") or texture ("light and fluffy") and these terms are still valid.

"Low": Examples are "low calorie," "low sodium," "low fat," "low cholesterol." Per-serving contents or 50-gram (1¾-ounce) amounts can't exceed 40 calories, 140 milligrams sodium, or 3 grams fat (1 gram saturated), or put another way, no more than 15 percent of the calories may come from saturated fat. Further, these same quantities of "low-cholesterol" foods cannot contain more than 20 milligrams cholesterol and 2 grams of saturated fat. Limits are not spelled out for sugar.

"More": One serving exceeds the Daily Value of a specific nutrient in the standard version by 10 percent. "More" can also be used to describe enriched or fortified foods—flours and milks, for example.

"Percent Fat-Free": The food in question must first be low in fat or fat free, and the percentage of fat present in 100 grams (3½ ounces) must be accurately stated. For example, 2 percent milk is 98 percent fat free.

"Reduced": A food in which the calories or a particular nutrient have been reduced by 25 percent. **NOTE:** If the food is already low in calories or the nutrient in question, the term *reduced* cannot be used.

"Very Low Sodium": 35 milligrams of sodium or fewer per serving or 50 grams (1¾ ounces).

Food Phytochemicals: See PHYTOCHEMICALS.

Food Poisoning: See BACTERIA.

Food Preservation:

Canning: This technique dates back to the days of Napoleon. In an effort to find better ways of provisioning his troops, the French emperor offered a prize of twenty thousand francs to anyone who came up with a way to preserve military rations. Nicolas Appert succeeded in 1810 by heating sealed jars of food in boiling water. This unofficial "father of canned food" didn't know why sealed food didn't spoil, however. Only fifty years later would Louis Pasteur link microbes to spoilage. Canning revolutionized eating—and cooking—on a global scale, putting seasonal foods (to say nothing of regional exotics) on market shelves twelve months of the year. Only with the arrival of frozen food did canned foods lose some of their luster. Today, certain foods still can better than they freeze, tomatoes being a prime example. The biggest shortcoming of canned foods (apart from their often high sodium content) is that they lose some of their vitamins B_1 (thiamin) and C because of the high processing temperatures. And if the can liquid is thrown out, a number of water-soluble vitamins and minerals will go down the drain. **NOTE:** If food is packed in glass, some riboflavin will also be lost because it's sensitive to light.

Cryogenic Freezing: A method of flash-freezing food with liquid gas at temperatures as low as $-315°F$. The liquid gas of choice is nitrogen although nitrous oxide (laughing gas) and carbon dioxide are also used. Here's how it works: The food to be frozen is conveyor-belted through a chamber where it's sprayed with liquid gas; sometimes, however, it's mixed with crushed dry ice (frozen carbon dioxide). Either way, the food freezes almost instantly and the ice crystals inside it are minute. As a result, there's little damage to meat tissues or plant cell walls, meaning that cryogenically frozen foods are virtually indistinguishable from the fresh (there's less nutrient loss, too). Mushrooms, for example, which go mushy under ordinary freezing methods, emerge almost unchanged after cryogenic freezing. Shrimp, another fragile food, is now often cryogenically flash-frozen, as are some meats and poultry. The only drawback? Cost. Cryogenic freezing is more expensive than conventional methods of freezing.

Drying: As old as man himself, drying is still an effective, inexpensive way to preserve food, even fish—as the Portuguese, who make a specialty of dried salt cod, have long known. The reason that drying is so successful is that life—and that means the bacteria, molds and yeasts that spoil food—cannot live in the absence of water. So as long as dried foods are kept dry, they won't spoil. For that reason, and because there are now powerful, carefully regulated dehydrators, the list of dried or dehydrated foods now includes such specialty items as wild mushrooms, celery, parsley, onions, garlic and citrus rinds. The disadvantages are that dried foods often discolor, lose some of their nutrients (especially vitamin C) and must usually be soaked before they can be eaten.

Freeze-drying: This new method of preserving food is also the priciest. The process involves freezing food in a vacuum, all the while vaporizing the ice crystals until, after ten to twenty-four hours, the food contains only 1 to 8 percent of its original moisture. Almost anything can be freeze-dried—chops, steaks, fruits, vegetables. The advantages are obvious: compactness, lightness, extraordinary shelf life under stressful conditions (astronauts feed on freeze-dried foods, and Sir Edmund Hillary took pounds of it up Mount Everest) and, not least, good flavor, texture and nutrient content when reconstituted although such easily oxidized vitamins as vitamin C may be lost. Because of cost, however, freeze-drying is pretty much limited to coffee, fresh herbs (notably chives) and camp rations.

Freezing: Freezing isn't as new as it may seem. Eskimos, Laplanders and others in polar climates have always known that solidly frozen fish and meat would keep for months, even years. Brooklynite Clarence Birdseye, the father of the frozen-food industry, was the first to apply this method of food preservation to other foods—and in warmer climes. While on an expedition in Labrador for the U.S. Fish and Wildlife Service in 1914, Birdseye was interested to see that fish froze the instant it was pulled from the water but, more important, that when cooked, this flash-frozen fish was a match in every way for the fresh.

Birdseye returned to the United States and, at the close of World War I, went into the fish business in Gloucester, Massachusetts. Birdseye also did a bit of moonlighting, tinkering around, trying to invent a machine that would freeze—preserve—all a food's freshness and flavor. He succeeded in the 1920s but commercially frozen foods didn't catch on until after World War II. It took that long for problems of packaging, shipping and distribution to be licked.

Miraculous as freezing is, it isn't suited to all food. Many vegetables—cucumbers, summer squash, onions, potatoes, sweet peppers, cabbage, tomatoes and fragile lettuces—go all mushy. There are vitamin C losses, too, especially when fruits or vegetables have been cut into small pieces and exposed to the air (oxygen destroys vitamin C faster than anything).

The foods that freeze best (aside from the standard repertoire of frozen desserts) are meat, fish and fowl;

breads, pastas and pasta sauces; cakes, cookies and pastries; also such vegetables as green peas and beans, whole-kernel corn, and purees of winter squash, rutabagas or sweet potatoes. Good fruit candidates for the freezer are cranberries, blueberries, strawberries, raspberries, sliced peaches and all manner of purees and juices.

For safety's sake (not to mention top quality), all frozen foods should be held at 0°F. Supermarkets are often quite cavalier about monitoring their frozen-food bins and keeping the temperatures within the safety range. Always reject any squishy "frozen" foods, also any packages that are misshapen (dead giveaways that the contents have thawed and refrozen).

Salting, Brining: These ancient methods of preserving food are still widely used, especially for meat, fish, pickles and sauerkraut. The downside? They raise the sodium content of food at a time when most people are trying to cut back. And the sodium nitrates, so popular for ham and bacon, will, when overheated, combine with the amino acids in protein and produce carcinogens called NITROSAMINES.

Food Safety:
Monitoring America's food supply for wholesomeness and safety is a job so gargantuan the responsibility is shared by eight federal agencies. Agriculture, as the USDA is nicknamed, not only inspects and grades eggs, meat and poultry sold in interstate commerce but is also active in nutrition research and education; the Bureau of Alcohol, Tobacco and Firearms ensures the purity of alcoholic beverages; the CDC strive to prevent and control food-borne illnesses; the Department of Justice tries those alleged to have violated food safety laws; the EPA determines pesticide safety, residue tolerance levels in food and safety standards for drinking water; the Federal Trade Commission (FTC) cracks down on those making false claims for food or food supplements; the FDA assures wholesomeness of all food shipped across state lines (except for eggs, meat and poultry, the province of USDA); and the National Marine Fisheries Service, an arm of the Department of Commerce, safeguards the quality of fish and shellfish.

In addition, most state governments regularly spot-check homegrown foods sold within their borders for wholesomeness and enforce strict standards of sanitation in restaurants, delis, supermarkets, specialty food shops, even granaries, mills and dairies. Some states, moreover, monitor locally caught, locally sold fish.

Since improperly cooked fast-food-chain hamburgers were shown to have caused the recent, serious outbreaks of *E. coli* food poisoning in the Pacific Northwest, the U.S. government has been beefing up its inspection system. First, it's commissioned scientists to learn why certain farm animals carry harmful germs and how these bugs can be kept out of the food chain. Second, it's developing quicker methods of IDing harmful bacteria not only at slaughterhouses but also at every pivotal stage of meat and poultry production. Specifically, the more foolproof Hazard Analysis and Critical Control Points program (see HACCP) used by NASA to ensure the purity of astronaut food is expected to be added as an extra safeguard in the inspection of meat, poultry and seafood.

Finally, all packages of raw or partially cooked meat and poultry must carry new safe-food-handling labels with this information:

> Some animal products may contain bacteria that could cause illness if the product is mishandled or cooked improperly. For your protection, follow these safe-handling instructions:
>
> - Keep refrigerated or frozen. Thaw in refrigerator or microwave.
>
> - Keep raw meats or poultry separate from other foods. Wash work surfaces (including cutting boards), utensils and hands after touching raw meat or poultry.
>
> - Cook thoroughly.
>
> - Refrigerate leftovers within two hours.

Consumer advocates are now urging clarification of "Cook thoroughly" and suggest that the safety labels specify an internal meat temperature of 160°F.

Food Spoilage:
The digestive upsets many people attribute to stomach flu can often be traced to spoiled food. There's not much we can do about restaurant food other than to be fussy about the restaurants and foods we choose. But we are in charge at home. Needless to say, all perishables—meats, fish, poultry, dairy, eggs, deli salads and so forth—should be rushed home from the supermarket and refrigerated or frozen straightaway. Meats, poultry and fish should also be rewrapped. For refrigerator storage, the safest policy is to transfer the food to a large plate or tray, cover *loosely* with plastic food wrap, then store in the coldest part of the refrigerator—that means between 32°F. and 40°F. Foods to be frozen should be snugly rewrapped

in foil or freezer wrap, labeled, dated and placed directly on the freezing surface of a 0°F. freezer. The greatest danger is in letting food languish at room temperature (60°F. and up) for more than two hours because microbes multiply at great speed and the production of toxins is accelerated. It's also important to cook food thoroughly so molds and bacteria are destroyed. **NOTE:** If you question the accuracy of your refrigerator or freezer, keep refrigerator/freezer thermometers on hand (they're available at housewares stores). And if the freezer or refrigerator isn't functioning properly, have it serviced. See also BACTERIA.

Formulas:

It may not seem that babies, "fatties" desperately trying to shed pounds and postoperative patients have anything in common. Yet they do. All are given nutrient-balanced formulas or liquid diets (as are those with advanced kidney and liver disease). To be sure, the nutritional breakdown varies from group to group. Dieters are put on **very low-calorie diets** of 400 to 800 calories a day, often in the form of an egg- or milk-protein-based liquid formula; the standard proportion is 30 to 45 grams carbohydrate, 33 to 70 grams protein, a smidgeon of fat plus assorted vitamins and minerals. The **liquid formulas for tube-fed patients** (enteral feeding) vary according to the medical problem, with recipes often being formulated by registered dietitians and doctors. All, however, contain carbohydrate, protein, fat, water, vitamins and minerals. **Baby formulas** were standardized by the Infant Formula Act of 1980, which mandated that all formulas meet the nutrient recommendations set forth by the American Academy of Pediatrics. Then in 1982, the FDA began monitoring baby formulas for safety and wholesomeness. The standard infant formula begins with cow's milk, but the amount of protein, carbohydrate, linoleic acid (an essential fatty acid) and important minerals have been pumped up to approximate the nutritive value of breast milk.

Fortified, Fortified Foods, Fortification:

When vitamins and minerals are lost in processing, then those same nutrients put back in to restore food to its original nutritive level, that food is, by government definition, ENRICHED. But when the added vitamins and minerals boost the nutritive value beyond that of the original, the food is fortified. Prime examples: milks and margarines fortified with vitamins A and D, fruit drinks with vitamin C, soy milk with calcium and vitamin B_{12}, even salt with iodine. The most highly fortified foods now available are breakfast cereals, some of which supply a day's quota of certain vitamins and minerals. **NOTE:** If the nutrients have been pumped up so much they're 50 percent more than the Daily Value (DV), the food must be sold as a "supplement."

Framingham Heart Study:

No study has done more to link high blood cholesterol levels to coronary heart disease than this long-range study of 5,209 Framingham, Massachusetts, men (aged thirty to sixty-two) begun in 1949. Cholesterol, however, wasn't the only heart-disease risk identified. Others were high blood pressure, cigarette smoking, obesity and lack of exercise. Although diet wasn't a part of the original study, it is integral to a companion study begun in 1972. What's interesting is that its 5,000 participants, some of them relatives of the original 5,209, were already more health conscious. They smoked less and had lower blood pressure and lower cholesterol levels.

Frankfurters:

The original franks came from Frankfurt, Germany, where quality controls are rigid. Genuine frankfurters must be made in the Frankfurt area; they must be 100 percent pork and free of fat, fillers and chemical additives. They must be stuffed into sheep casings, smoked by traditional methods and sold in linked pairs. Unrestricted by court edict, our meatpackers make hot dogs of beef, of beef and pork, even of chicken and turkey. They may or may not use fillers, may or may not pump their "dogs" full of water, but most rely on sodium nitrate or nitrite as a preservative. The casings on their franks are usually synthetic, but worse, the franks themselves are apt to drip with fat—make that *saturated fat*. The latest hot-dog scare, detonated by the results of a study conducted among 232 Los Angeles children by the University of

NUTRIENT CONTENT OF 1 MEDIUM-SIZE BOILED/STEAMED PORK AND BEEF FRANKFURTER	
(about 2 ounces; 57 grams)	
182 calories	638 mg sodium
6 g protein	95 mg potassium
17 g fat, 6 saturated	0 g dietary fiber
29 mg cholesterol	0 RE vitamin A
1 g carbohydrate	0.11 mg thiamin
6 mg calcium	0.07 mg riboflavin
49 mg phosphorus	1.5 mg niacin
0.7 mg iron	15 mg vitamin C

Southern California School of Medicine, suggests that youngsters who eat more than a dozen franks a month are more likely to develop leukemia than those who eat fewer hot dogs or none at all. The culprit? The nitrites used to cure the hot dogs, which, when exposed to the amines found in many foods, bond to form cancer-causing NI-TROSAMINES. Scientists who've reviewed the California study admit that while it's far from definitive or conclusive, it raises worrisome questions.

NUTRIENT CONTENT OF 1 MEDIUM-SIZE BOILED/STEAMED ALL-BEEF FRANKFURTER

(about 2 ounces; 57 grams)

180 calories	585 mg sodium
9 g protein	95 mg potassium
16 g fat, 7 saturated	0 g dietary fiber
35 mg cholesterol	0 RE vitamin A
1 g carbohydrate	0.03 mg thiamin
11 mg calcium	0.06 mg riboflavin
50 mg phosphorus	1.4 mg niacin
0.8 mg iron	14 mg vitamin C

NUTRIENT CONTENT OF 1 MEDIUM-SIZE BOILED/STEAMED TURKEY FRANKFURTER

(about 2 ounces; 57 grams)

129 calories	813 mg sodium
8 g protein	102 mg potassium
10 g fat, 3 saturated	0 g dietary fiber
61 mg cholesterol	0 RE vitamin A
1 g carbohydrate	0.02 mg thiamin
60 mg calcium	0.10 mg riboflavin
76 mg phosphorus	2.4 mg niacin
1.1 mg iron	0 mg vitamin C

Free Fatty Acids: When triglycerides are broken down in the stomach and intestine, free fatty acids are formed. Absorbed into the body through the intestinal walls, they may be (1) used immediately for energy; (2) stored as a future source of energy; (3) used to build essential body compounds; or (4) integrated into body cells. Free fatty acids occur naturally in food, too, as triglycerides decompose—especially in nuts and seeds, butters and margarines. Indeed, they are the "agents of rancidity."

Free Radicals: Scavenging by-products of metabolism that circulate in the blood, damaging cells. Biomedical researchers have recently fingered free radicals as possible causes of cancer as well as of breakdowns in the body's immune system. Antioxidants like beta-carotene, vitamins C and E are mopper-uppers of free radicals and help keep them from zapping body cells.

Free-Range Poultry and Other Animals: There's a notion that poultry and animals that have been allowed to roam, to scratch about in the dirt for bugs and worms, to forage are superior to the pen or battery raised. They may be more flavorful—depending on what they ate—although recent blindfold taste tests refute that. They may or may not be free of pesticides, herbicides, insecticides, even antibiotics—once again, diet determines. Now comes evidence that free-range chickens are twice as apt to be infected with salmonella as battery-raised fowl. The reason, researchers explain, is that these chickens are exposed to bacteria in the soil, in the droppings of wild birds, even those carried by insects. All free-range animals will unquestionably be tougher than the battery or pen raised because exercise develops sinew. They will also be pricier (up to 2½ times so) because they are the province of health-food stores and boutique butchers.

Freeze-drying: See FOOD PRESERVATION.

Freezer Burn: Hoary, dry patches that occur whenever frozen foods are poorly wrapped and exposed to the air. Though they're unsightly (and may have lost some flavor and nutritive value), freezer-burned foods are safe to eat.

Freezing, Frozen Foods: See FOOD PRESERVATION.

French Paradox: The fact that the French, who don't stint on high-fat, high-cholesterol foods, have a far lower incidence of heart disease than Americans, who curb dietary fat and cholesterol. Responsible, some researchers believe, are one or more chemicals in the red wines the French sip with meals (see QUERCITIN; RESVERATROL). An even newer study, comparing fifty middle-class Parisians with fifty middle-class Bostonians, theorizes that the reason the French suffer fewer heart attacks is that they take their main meal at noon and do not snack before dinner, which comes at least five hours later.

Fresh Start: To upgrade the nutritional quality of school lunches across America, the USDA launched a long-term program at the end of 1993. Called Fresh Start, it aims to strip fat from fat-clogged school menus by buying twice as many fruits and vegetables and substituting low-fat foods for standard versions (skim milk for whole, low-fat or non-fat yogurt for regular and so forth). At present, the National School Lunch Program operates in all but 5 percent of the nation's schools. So if Fresh Start works, twenty-five million schoolchildren will be better fed. Scarcely small potatoes.

Fromage Blanc: French for *cottage cheese*. However, *fromage blanc* is a little softer than our cottage cheese and a little more finely curded. Boutique cheese makers in the United States are now producing *fromage blanc,* upscale food shops stock it and trendy cooks are finding it a good substitute for fatter cheeses in such perennial favorites as cheesecake. **NOTE:** Specific nutrient counts are unavailable for *fromage blanc* but they would approximate those of COTTAGE CHEESE.

Frozen Desserts: See ICE CREAM; ICE MILK; ICES, GRANITÉS, SORBETS.

Frozen Yogurt: See YOGURT.

Fructose, Fruit Sugar: Also called **levulose,** this simple sugar (monosaccharide) occurs naturally in honey and fresh fruits. Because it's twice as sweet as table sugar (sucrose), commercial bakers use fructose in cakes, breads and cookies to make them brown better. And dieters trying to shave calories substitute it for regular sugar in sweets because they need use only half as much. But make a note, fructose can't be subtituted measure for measure for sugar in baked goods because its chemical and physical properties are different. Instead, use it to sweeten puddings, fruits, sauces and ice creams. It's available in many health-food stores. See also CARBOHYDRATES.

Fruit Cocktail: The canned variety, which most of us know from school lunch, hasn't changed much over the years. There are bits of pear, pineapple, grapefruit, cherries and maraschino cherries. Some people still make a meal of fruit cocktail, ladling it over a scoop of cottage cheese. Others suspend it in fancy gelatin molds, then serve it as salad or dessert. Nutritionally or otherwise, canned fruit cocktail is no match for the fresh. But because fresh fruit cocktails vary so, the only accurate food values are for the canned.

NUTRIENT CONTENT OF 1 CUP CANNED FRUIT COCKTAIL (PACKED IN HEAVY SYRUP)

(about 9 ounces; 255 grams)

186 calories	15 mg sodium
1 g protein	224 mg potassium
0 g fat, 0 saturated	3 g dietary fiber
0 mg cholesterol	51 RE vitamin A
48 g carbohydrate	0.05 mg thiamin
15 mg calcium	0.05 mg riboflavin
28 mg phosphorus	1.0 mg niacin
0.7 mg iron	5 mg vitamin C

NUTRIENT CONTENT OF 1 CUP CANNED FRUIT COCKTAIL (PACKED IN WATER)

(about 8³/₄ ounces; 245 grams)

78 calories	10 mg sodium
1 g protein	230 mg potassium
0 g fat, 0 saturated	3 g dietary fiber
0 mg cholesterol	61 RE vitamin A
21 g carbohydrate	0.04 mg thiamin
12 mg calcium	0.03 mg riboflavin
27 mg phosphorus	0.9 mg niacin
0.6 mg iron	5 mg vitamin C

Fruit Juices, Fruit Drinks: Fresh squeezed is definitely best from a nutritional standpoint, but even here valuable fiber is lost—and if the juice is strained, the amount is considerable. Next best are the **frozen juice concentrates,** but these should be reconstituted just before serving and no sooner, or some of the vitamin C will be sacrificed. The trouble with many **bottled** and **canned fruit beverages** is that although many are unsweetened, undiluted fruit juices, others are 90 percent flavored, sweetened colored water and only 10 percent real juice. Anything labeled "fruit juice cocktail" or "fruit drink" will *not* be 100 percent juice. And don't confuse "100 percent juice" (just what it says) with "100 percent *natural*" (*not* what it implies; these fruit drinks are *not* pure juice. Although to be fair, it should be said that some of these fruit drinks have been fortified with vitamin C. And that's a plus). **NOTE:** Under the new food-labeling laws, the percentage of fruit juice must be listed for all fruit drinks. And what about the new **bottled fruit sparklers**? They're nothing more than carbonated water blended with a small amount of fruit juice. Some are sweetened; some not. The labels tell the story.

Fruit Juices as Sweeteners: Playing upon a public misconception—and with their eyes firmly on the bottom line—some food manufacturers are producing cookies and spreads "sweetened with concentrated fruit juices," the implication being that they're more nutritious than those made with sugar. Some food writers have fallen for the pitch, too, and are busily developing "better-for-you sweets," subbing concentrated fruit juices for sugar. *The facts?* Reducing fruit juice to syrup not only concentrates the fruit sugar (fructose) but also destroys vitamin C and other heat-perishable nutrients. Don't be misled. Fruit syrups *are* sugar syrups, which, like granulated sugar, brown sugar, corn syrup and honey, will be converted by the body to glucose.

Fruits: Because of their carbohydrate, fiber, vitamin and mineral content, fruits should be eaten several times a day (the FOOD GUIDE PYRAMID recommends two to four servings daily). To be sure, not all fruits are created equal. Strawberries, for example, are sky high in vitamin C, as are citrus fruits and melons. Orange-fleshed fruits—apricots, mangoes and papayas, to name three—are loaded with beta-carotene; bananas, cantaloupes and honeydew melons are stellar sources of potassium. For more detail, look up the fruits that interest you in this book.

Fruit Sugar: See FRUCTOSE; also CARBOHYDRATES.

Frying, Deep-Fat Frying: America's love affair with the deep-fat fryer shows no signs of waning although we now know perfectly well that Southern fried chicken, french fries, fish sticks, doughnuts, fritters and such contain more fat than is good for us. At home we can opt for vegetable oils, heat them to the proper temperature (in the 350°F. to 360°F. range) to minimize the amount of fat absorbed by the batter or breading. Fast-food restaurants, on the other hand, sometimes use cheap animal fats like tallow (from sheep or cattle) for frying and don't regulate the deep-fat temperatures as carefully as they should. Pushed to the smoke point, they emit noxious ACROLEIN; too cold and the food in the fryer sucks up fat like a sponge. A no-win situation. Frying, shallow-frying, even stir-frying can load food with unwanted fat, too—ever watched a Chinese chef upend a bottle of oil over his sizzling wok? Home cooks, however, can control the amount of fat used, the kind and the temperature. And if we use the bare minimum of oil or margarine (possible if the skillet is first coated with nonstick vegetable cooking spray), then rush the food in and out of the skillet, we can turn out heart-healthy meals. *Sauté,* by the way—which *sounds* healthful—is merely the French word for "fry."

Fudge: This chocolate candy will never make it as "health food," but because people love it so, we include nutrient counts here. Properly made, fudge is as smooth as country cream, with no sugar grains discernible on the tongue. If nuts are folded in, fudge has a bit more food value. But, alas, more calories, too.

NUTRIENT CONTENT OF 1 OUNCE (28 GRAMS) HOMEMADE CHOCOLATE FUDGE

108 calories	18 mg sodium
0 g protein	29 mg potassium
2 g fat, 1 saturated	1 g dietary fiber
4 mg cholesterol	13 RE vitamin A
23 g carbohydrate	0 mg thiamin
12 mg calcium	0.02 mg riboflavin
16 mg phosphorus	0 mg niacin
0.1 mg iron	0 mg vitamin C

NUTRIENT CONTENT OF 1 OUNCE (28 GRAMS) HOMEMADE CHOCOLATE FUDGE WITH NUTS

121 calories	17 mg sodium
1 g protein	45 mg potassium
5 g fat, 2 saturated	1 g dietary fiber
4 mg cholesterol	13 RE vitamin A
21 g carbohydrate	0.02 mg thiamin
14 mg calcium	0.02 mg riboflavin
26 mg phosphorus	0.1 mg niacin
0.2 mg iron	0 mg vitamin C

Fumaric Acid (additive): White, odorless crystals used to stabilize the flavors and increase the shelf life of dessert and drink mixes, candies and pie fillings. In fat- or oil-based foods, processors frequently team fumaric acid with BHA and BHT (see BHA) to boost their antioxidant powers. GRAS.

Functional Foods: Just when we were adding DESIGNER FOODS, NUTRACEUTICALS and PHYTOCHEMICALS to our lexicon of nutrition, the Food and Nutrition Board of the Institute of Medicine decreed (and the American Dietetic Association agreed) that these terms should be lumped together as *functional foods,* meaning "foods with ingredients thought to prevent disease." Though you'll be reading more about functional foods in years to come, no nutritionist, physician or food pro expects the terms *designer foods, nutraceuticals* and *phytochemicals* to vanish from our vocabulary anytime soon, if ever. They all refer to functional foods, yet their definitions are more specific. So we continue to use *designer foods, nutraceuticals* and *phytochemicals* in *The Nutrition Bible.* Each is discussed in an individual entry.

Furcelleran (additive): Also called **Danish agar,** this gum obtained from a cold-water red alga is used to stabilize, thicken and/or emulsify commercial ice creams, custards, puddings, jams and jellies. It's on the FDA's "must evaluate" list.

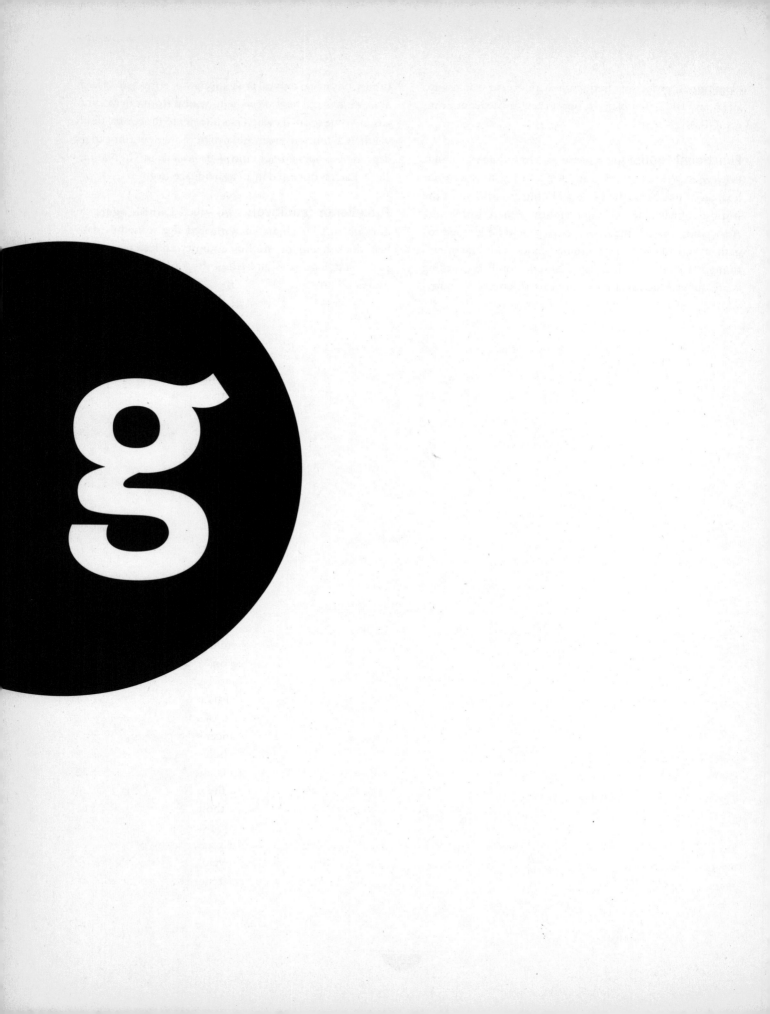

Galactose: When you drink milk, your body splits the milk sugar (LACTOSE) into two simpler sugars—galactose and GLUCOSE. Then the galactose itself is converted to glucose to fuel the body. See also CARBOHYDRATES.

Galactosemia: Some few people are born without one or more of the enzymes needed to turn GALACTOSE into GLUCOSE. The result is toxic blood levels of galactose, which trigger a roster of frightening symptoms, among them jaundice, diarrhea, vomiting, anorexia, cataract formation, even mental retardation. Galactosemia is hereditary and, though serious, treatable if treatment is begun immediately after birth. The only "medicine"? A lifelong galactose-restricted diet, which is free of milk and anything made with milk, as well as brain, liver and other organ meats that store galactose. As with most restrictive diets, processed foods are the bugaboo because they often contain milk, dry milk solids and such milk components as casein, curd, lactose and whey. Lactose or milk sugar, which contains galactose, is the filler used in some artificial sweeteners. Read labels carefully.

Gallbladder, Gallstones (diet and): Think of the gallbladder as a tiny reservoir nestled at the bottom of the liver. Its job is to store the bitter green bile that the liver manufactures to assist in the digestion and absorption of fats as well as in the absorption of fat-soluble vitamins (A, D, E and K) and of the minerals iron and calcium. Whenever bile is needed, the gallbladder shuttles it to the intestines via the bile duct. If the chemical balance of bile is upset, stones may develop. When these lodge in the bile duct, there's searing pain in the upper right abdomen, sometimes accompanied by vomiting. (The fancy name for an inflamed gallbladder, whether chronic or acute, is CHO-LECYSTITIS; for gallstones, it's cholelithiasis.) Often the flow of bile forces the stones along out of harm's way. If not, you should see your doctor at once. Those at risk of gallstones—the elderly and overweight, especially women—should watch what they eat. This means a diet low in fat (it should supply no more than 25 percent of the day's calories) and also, if necessary, avoiding foods that cause gas or other digestive discomfort. With dietary fat thus reduced, the fat-soluble vitamins may be poorly absorbed. No problem. Water-soluble forms of them can be taken as supplements.

Galvanized Utensils: Pots and pans prone to rusting, even water pipes are often galvanized, meaning they're coated with zinc in an electrolytic process developed more than two hundred years ago by Italian chemist Luigi Galvani. Although space age materials are more common in cookware today, enough of the old galvanized stuff remains to issue this warning: Never let acid food or drink stand in galvanized containers for more than a few minutes. You risk making people violently (but not chronically) ill, because the acid in the food reacts with the galvanized coating, leaching out toxic levels of zinc.

Game: Wild animals used as meat. Venison and buffalo, two American favorites, are leaner than beef, veal or lamb. Tougher, too, and for that reason many are being ranch raised. Small game—squirrel, rabbit, raccoon, muskrat and opossum—is popular down South. All are gamy, and the last three disagreeably fat. There's an additional problem. Rabies now afflicts many small game animals, as does tularemia, a prolonged, intermittent fever that can be passed along to man. See also RABBIT; VENISON.

Gamma Rays: The ionizing rays used to zap foods undergoing IRRADIATION.

Garbanzo Beans: See BEANS, DRIED.

Garlic: Garlic's pungency is what has won it so many fans (from Aristotle to Eleanor Roosevelt) and foes (from Shakespeare to Louis XV). The Egyptians grew vast beds of garlic beside the Nile, believing it would hone the minds and bodies of the pyramid builders. And ancient Greeks thought so highly of this "onion" that they roasted it and ate it as we do potatoes. Not a bad idea. Garlic contains powerful anticarcinogens (see PHYTOCHEMICALS). Recent studies of the medicinal value of this "lily of the field" show that in addition to its cancer-fighting prowess, garlic can lower blood glucose *and* cholesterol levels (good news for diabetics and heart patients alike). In other lab tests, garlic seems not only to boost the immune system but also to thwart viruses (particularly those of colds, flu and herpes), bacteria (specifically TB) and fungi (mainly *Candida albicans,* a yeast infection that plagues many women). Finally, it turns out that the pyramid builders were right about garlic's ability to boost strength and fight fatigue. All

Roasted Garlic

Makes About ¼ Cup

BUNDLE A LARGE, firm head of garlic in a double thickness of aluminum foil, set on the middle rack of a preheated 300°F. oven, and roast about 1 hour until soft. Cool until easy to handle, then, working directly over small food processor, pinch the pointed end of each clove, squirting roasted garlic into work bowl. Or even easier, slice off the root end of the garlic and squeeze the entire bulb to extract the flesh. Churn until smooth. Spread on bread lightly brushed with olive oil, or smooth a tablespoon or two into potato or dried bean soups, chilis, or stews. Mix with mayonnaise for a quick aioli sauce, or blend 50-50 with pureed black olives or very ripe Brie for a sensational cocktail spread. The more you use roasted garlic, the more ways you'll find to use it.

APPROXIMATE NUTRIENT COUNTS PER TABLESPOON

42 calories	9 g carbohydrate	0.5 mg iron	0.06 mg thiamin
2 g protein	2 g fiber	5 mg sodium	0.03 mg riboflavin
0 g fat, 0 saturated	51 mg calcium	114 mg potassium	0.2 mg niacin
0 mg cholesterol	44 mg phosphorus	0 RE vitamin A	5 mg vitamin C

of which make this lowly bulb seem like some sort of miracle food.

Not so fast. There are downsides apart from "garlic breath." In high doses, garlic can be quite toxic, so garlic extracts, pills and powders should be taken only on a full stomach. And for all its "healing powers," garlic isn't very nutritious (maybe because such a little of it goes such a long way). A single clove weighs in at 2 calories, contains no cholesterol and has only traces of sodium. With fresh garlic so widely available, there's no reason to substitute the ersatz garlic powder or, worse, sodium-laden garlic salt. Beware, too, of jars of minced garlic in oil. *Clostridium botulinum,* the "bug" that causes a deadly form of food poisoning, has been found in some of these preparations.

Garlic Oil (additive): A smelly amber oil extracted from crushed garlic that's used to flavor everything from chewing gum to ice cream to fruit drinks. Thanks to the alchemy of food processing, the finished products neither taste nor smell like garlic. GRAS.

Gas: See FLATULENCE.

Gastric Balloon: A nonsurgical way to treat obesity that involves inflating a balloon inside the stomach. The balloon reduces appetite, also the amount of food that can be eaten comfortably. But the balloon can't be left in place indefinitely. After three months (the FDA time limit on gastric balloon use), there's a risk of ulcers, intestinal blockage and internal bruising.

Gastric Juice: The mix of liquids and enzymes (lipase, pepsin and rennin) that the gastric gland releases into the stomach to help digest food. The key ingredient is hydrochloric acid, which, as every chemistry student (and ulcer sufferer) knows, is powerful stuff. Even so, carbohydrates, proteins and fats are only partially broken down in the stomach. The intermediate products of digestion are then shunted into the intestines, which finish the job.

Gastric Stapling: The grossly obese who can't lose weight may, as a last resort, have their stomachs stapled into two pouches, a small one to receive food and a larger one to sit idly by. With reduced stomach capacity, patients do lose weight. But that's not all. Because of frequent vomiting, they may become dehydrated. They may get insufficient iron and vitamin B_{12} and suffer liver dysfunction. Then, too, there's the risk of damaging stomach tissue, of staples' popping loose and of scar formation. Eating patterns must change dramatically, with many small meals replacing breakfast, lunch and dinner, and food supplements correcting any vitamin/mineral shortfall. Gastric stapling is not an operation to be undertaken lightly.

Gastrointestinal Diseases and Disorders: The following are brief looks at the more common problems on a long, long list. (See also CONSTIPATION; DIARRHEA.)

Gastric Ulcers: See PEPTIC ULCERS.

Gastritis: Inflammation of the stomach lining, which may be chronic or acute. **CAUSES:** Everything from food allergies to overeating to cancer. **BEST DIET:** For chronic gastritis, soft, bland foods taken six times a day plus daily iron/B_{12} supplements. For acute attacks, a twenty-four-hour fast may be prescribed (to give the stomach a rest), then twenty-four hours of clear liquids, then nutritionally balanced liquid formulas and, finally, soft, bland solids.

Gastroenteritis: The "trots" or "throw-ups," usually virus-driven and short-lived. Sometimes there's fever, sometimes not. **BEST DIET:** The same as for acute gastritis.

Gefilte Fish: You might call these fish dumplings Jewish quenelles. Believed to have originated in Central or Eastern Europe, gefilte fish is now popular across America. Authentic recipes call for the dumplings to be made with equal parts carp and pike or whitefish, bound with matzo

meal and eggs, flavored with onion and poached in vegetable broth. Many women still make gefilte fish the Old World way, stuffing the forcemeat into the fish skins—*gefilte fish* means "stuffed fish."

Gelatin: In the old days, women spent hours boiling calves' feet, bones and sinew to obtain gelatin. Among them was Mrs. Charles B. Knox of Johnstown, New York. Dismayed at the work involved, her salesman husband figured there must be an easier way. He'd heard about dried sheets of gelatin, which surely could be pulverized and packaged. Mrs. Knox, delighted to be sprung from the drudge of boiling calves' feet, began working with her husband's powdered gelatin, developing recipes for his give-away leaflets, even teaching his door-to-door salesmen how to demonstrate the marvels of this new convenience food. That happened in 1890 and the rest is history. Except for this footnote: Fifty years earlier, Peter Cooper, inventor of the Tom Thumb steam engine,

NUTRIENT CONTENT OF 1 ENVELOPE PLAIN GELATIN
(about ¼ ounce; 7 grams)

23 calories	14 mg sodium
6 g protein	1 mg potassium
0 g fat, 0 saturated	0 g dietary fiber
0 mg cholesterol	0 RE vitamin A
0 g carbohydrate	0 mg thiamin
4 mg calcium	0.02 mg riboflavin
3 mg phosphorus	0 mg niacin
0.1 mg iron	0 mg vitamin C

NUTRIENT CONTENT OF 3 OUNCES (85 GRAMS) GEFILTE FISH

70 calories	440 mg sodium
8 g protein	76 mg potassium
2 g fat, 0 saturated	0 g dietary fiber
25 mg cholesterol	22 RE vitamin A
6 g carbohydrate	0.06 mg thiamin
20 mg calcium	0.06 mg riboflavin
62 mg phosphorus	0.8 mg niacin
2.1 mg iron	1 mg vitamin C

NUTRIENT CONTENT OF 1 CUP SUGAR-SWEETENED FRUIT-FLAVORED GELATIN
(about 9½ ounces; 270 grams)

159 calories	113 mg sodium
3 g protein	3 mg potassium
0 g fat, 0 saturated	0 g dietary fiber
0 mg cholesterol	0 RE vitamin A
38 g carbohydrate	0 mg thiamin
5 mg calcium	0.01 mg riboflavin
59 mg phosphorus	0 mg niacin
0.1 mg iron	0 mg vitamin C

mixed powdered gelatin with artificial fruit flavors and sugar, and presto! the precursor of Jell-O. But Cooper was a man ahead of his time. Jell-O didn't gel with the public until the early 1900s.

NUTRIENT CONTENT OF 1 CUP SUGAR-FREE FRUIT-FLAVORED GELATIN (ARTIFICIALLY SWEETENED)

(about 8²/₃ ounces; 242 grams)

17 calories	116 mg sodium
3 g protein	0 mg potassium
0 g fat, 0 saturated	0 g dietary fiber
0 mg cholesterol	0 RE vitamin A
2 g carbohydrate	0 mg thiamin
5 mg calcium	0.01 mg riboflavin
65 mg phosphorus	0 mg niacin
0 mg iron	0 mg vitamin C

Genes: See HEREDITY.

Genetic Engineering, Gene Splicing: It's the buzz of the food world. A big concern, too. Will altering the DNA or genetic blueprint of plant foods to create insect- and disease-resistant species be hazardous to our health? Will developing varieties that taste "garden fresh" even though they were picked green and shipped thousands of miles? Will pumping up the nutritive value of fruits and vegetables? Alarmists worry that "mad scientists" might loose chain reactions that could devastate the environment and perhaps even do us all in.

Not so fast. There are legitimate concerns about genetic engineering, true. If, for example, genes from peanuts or fish, two highly allergenic foods, are inserted into the DNA of corn or tomatoes, two fairly "safe" foods, will people allergic to peanuts or fish then also be allergic to the altered corn and tomatoes? So far no one knows. If such proves to be the case, the FDA demands that the genetically altered foods be so labeled. And if vitamin C should be "bio-teched" out of normally vitamin C–rich tomatoes, labels must declare that fact, too. Despite public uneasiness, plant breeders believe that genetic engineering will provide us all with more abundant, more healthful, more delicious food at lower cost (first to debut was the Flavr Savr Tomato but coming soon are two more "wonder foods," a virus-resistant squash and a pest-resistant potato).

Through gene-splicing, scientists hope, among other things, to increase the amino acids in vegetables, reduce the caffeine in coffee beans, eradicate the natural carcinogens present in food and increase the anticarcinogens. Can they do it? Time will tell. See also BIOTECHNOLOGY.

Genistein: A powerful isoflavone (anticarcinogen) found in concentrated form in soybeans and soybean products. Isoflavones seem to diminish estrogen production in pre-menopausal women, and genistein, scientists suspect, prevents new blood vessel formation. Since estrogen is linked to breast cancer and since tumors can't grow without blood vessels, the value of genistein is becoming clear. This may also explain why Japanese women, who eat soybeans in one form or another every day, have 75 percent less breast cancer than Western women. See also PHYTOCHEMICALS.

Gentian (flavoring): A bitter extract of the gentian root of southern Europe. It's used in everything from Angostura bitters to chocolate to vermouth and vanilla flavorings. Gentian even shows up in candies and ice creams. Safe.

Geophagia: Another term for PICA or clay eating.

Geraniol (flavoring): This oily compound, aromatic of roses, exists naturally in plants as disparate as apples, bay leaves, grapefruit and tea. It's used to scent perfumes, also to flavor a huge variety of beverages, baked goods, candies, ice creams and chewing gums. GRAS when used within FDA limits.

Geranium (GE-132): Health faddists hype these capsules, lozenges and powders as a way to flush toxic metals from the system and elixirs of health. The truth? They have caused irreversible kidney damage.

Geriatric Nutrition: See ELDERLY PERSONS.

Germ: Although wheat germ is the best known, this is the oil- and nutrient-rich heart of all grain kernels, the part that germinates or initiates new life. Because the germ quickly turns rancid, whole-grain flours have a far shorter shelf life than refined flours (cooks with refrigerator space to spare often store their whole-grain flours in the refrigerator; good practice, too, for wheat germ). *Germ* is also, of course, another word for BACTERIA.

Gestational Diabetes Mellitus (GDM): Some pregnant women, usually those who are overweight and/or have DIABETES in their families, develop abnormally high levels of blood glucose. The cause? The placenta secretes hormones that block the action of insulin, the hormone that regulates carbohydrate metabolism. Gestational diabetes usually disappears after childbirth, but it may recur with subsequent pregnancies. Women who've suffered GDM, by the way, are likely to develop non-insulin-dependent diabetes (NIDDM or Type II) later on. GDM can usually be controlled by diet alone, and a doctor will have a dietitian rework the patient's diet. What works best is limiting breakfast carbohydrates to 10 percent of the day's total, lunch and dinner carbs to 30 percent each and dividing the remaining 30 percent equally among three between-meals snacks. In addition, the dietitian will stress the value of milk, lean meat, fish, eggs and cheese and recommend that 20 to 25 percent of the day's calories come from top-quality protein. Finally, GDM patients will be urged to choose complex carbohydrates over simple sugars, to drink plenty of liquids and to exercise regularly. If this regimen doesn't stabilize blood sugar at acceptable levels, doctors may prescribe medication and monitor the blood sugar levels carefully.

Ghee: Butter from which all the milk solids have been removed. It is the preferred cooking fat in India, but it contains slightly more cholesterol and calories than butter because it is pure fat.

Giardiasis: A serious gastrointestinal disease caused by protozoa-infested water and raw food. **SYMPTOMS:** Diarrhea (but occasionally the exact opposite), abdominal cramps, gas and bloating; nausea and vomiting. **PREVENTIVES:** Don't drink the water (this also means no ice and brushing your teeth with mouthwash). While traveling abroad, especially in the Third World, skip salads and other raw food. At home, keep perishables properly refrigerated and cook food thoroughly.

Giblets: The gizzard, heart and liver of poultry. Most are moderately low in fat and calories but high in top-quality protein and iron. Unfortunately, giblets are loaded with cholesterol. Being tender, poultry livers are endlessly versatile. But the tough as Old Nick hearts and gizzards are best poached slowly, then minced into gravies and stuffings.

Gin: Grain alcohol steeped with juniper berries, the foundation of martinis, rickeys and tonics. See also ALCOHOL, ALCOHOLIC BEVERAGES.

Ginger: This pungent rhizome has been used in Asia almost since the beginning of time to treat everything from bubonic plague to seasickness to dyspepsia. Like cinnamon and cloves, ginger has preservative powers, the reason it's abundantly used in steamy climates. The fawn-skinned "hands" of ginger now available in supermarkets are from Hawaii. **Preserved** or **stem ginger** is stocked by most upscale groceries, as is **candied** or **Canton ginger.** These are more or less interchangeable in cooking, although the sugar and syrup should be rinsed off preserved and Canton ginger before they're used in savory dishes. **Powdered ginger** is something else again, the dried rhizome ground

NUTRIENT CONTENT OF 1 OUNCE (28 GRAMS) FRESH GINGER	
20 calories	4 mg sodium
1 g protein	118 mg potassium
0 g fat, 0 saturated	1 g dietary fiber
0 mg cholesterol	0 RE vitamin A
4 g carbohydrate	0.01 mg thiamin
5 mg calcium	0.01 mg riboflavin
8 mg phosphorus	0.2 mg niacin
0.1 mg iron	1 mg vitamin C

NUTRIENT CONTENT OF 1 OUNCE (28 GRAMS) CRYSTALLIZED GINGER	
96 calories	17 mg sodium
0 g protein	747 mg potassium
0 g fat, 0 saturated	1 g dietary fiber
0 mg cholesterol	NA RE vitamin A
25 g carbohydrate	0.06 mg thiamin
65 mg calcium	0.11 mg riboflavin
102 mg phosphorus	2.0 mg niacin
5.9 mg iron	11 mg vitamin C

until as fine as flour. Biting, bitter almost, it's lost all the lovely lemony fragrance of fresh ginger, even the lushness of preserved or candied ginger. For that reason, powdered ginger fares best in cakes and cookies. **SEASON:** Year-round but at their peak in February.

Ginger Ale, Ginger Beer: They aren't the same. Ginger ale is a carbonated drink with biting ginger flavor. Some ginger ales are sweetened with sugar; others with such sugar substitutes as aspartame. Sipped slowly, ginger ale is a good stomach settler. Ginger beer, which owes its bubbles to fermentation, is snappier than ginger ale—but it contains no alcohol.

NUTRIENT CONTENT OF 12 FLUID OUNCES (366 GRAMS) SUGAR-SWEETENED GINGER ALE

124 calories	25 mg sodium
0 g protein	5 mg potassium
0 g fat, 0 saturated	0 g dietary fiber
0 mg cholesterol	0 RE vitamin A
32 g carbohydrate	0 mg thiamin
12 mg calcium	0 mg riboflavin
1 mg phosphorus	0 mg niacin
0.7 mg iron	0 mg vitamin C

Note: The nutrient content of artificially sweetened ginger ale is about the same except that the calories and carbohydrates will plummet to around zero.

Practically Fat-Free Fresh Gingerbread

Makes 24 Servings

With carrots substituting for butter, this recipe is not only low in fat but also high in beta-carotene. Its nippiness comes from freshly minced ginger.

Zest of 1 navel orange, removed in strips with a vegetable peeler

1 cup firmly packed light brown sugar

3½ cups sifted all-purpose flour

1 teaspoon baking soda

½ teaspoon baking powder

1 teaspoon ground cinnamon

½ teaspoon grated nutmeg

1 cup buttermilk

1 cup pureed cooked or canned carrots

½ cup molasses

1 tablespoon fresh lemon juice

¾ cup frozen fat-free egg product, thawed

½ cup finely minced fresh ginger

PREHEAT OVEN TO 350°F. Spray a 13 × 9 × 2-inch baking pan with nonstick vegetable spray; set aside. Churn orange zest and brown sugar in a food processor 30 seconds, scrape bowl down, and churn 30 seconds more until zest is finely grated. Add flour, baking soda, baking powder, cinnamon, and nutmeg, and pulse 10 to 12 times. Transfer to a large mixing bowl and make a well in center. Buzz buttermilk, carrots, molasses, and lemon juice in processor 5 seconds. Add egg product and ginger, and pulse 3 or 4 times. Pour carrot mixture into well in dry ingredients, and with large rubber spatula, fold in gently. Batter should be lumpy; no matter if a few dry flecks show. *Don't overmix; cake will be tough.* Spoon batter into prepared pan, smoothing to corners. Bake 35 to 40 minutes or until a toothpick inserted in center of gingerbread comes out clean. Cool to room temperature in pan on wire rack, then cut into 24 bars.

APPROXIMATE NUTRIENT COUNTS PER BAR

123 calories	25 g carbohydrate	1.5 mg iron	0.12 mg thiamin
3 g protein	1 g dietary fiber	99 mg sodium	0.12 mg riboflavin
1 g fat, 0 saturated	50 mg calcium	198 mg potassium	1.1 mg niacin
1 mg cholesterol	41 mg phosphorus	141 RE vitamin A	2 mg vitamin C

Ginger Tea

Makes 6 Servings

Nothing could be more welcome on a wintry day. Some even go so far as to say that this tea does more for a cold than chicken soup.

3 ounces fresh ginger, peeled and diced

2 strips lemon zest, 3 inches × ½ inch long

6 cups cold water

3 tablespoons honey

BRING GINGER, LEMON zest, and water to a simmer in a medium heavy nonmetallic saucepan over moderate heat. Reduce heat to lowest point and steep, uncovered, 30 minutes. Strain, stir in honey, and serve steaming hot in mugs.

APPROXIMATE NUTRIENT COUNTS PER SERVING

42 calories	11 g carbohydrate	0.1 mg iron	0 mg thiamin
0 g protein	0 g dietary fiber	2 mg sodium	0.01 mg riboflavin
0 g fat, 0 saturated	6 mg calcium	66 mg potassium	0.1 mg niacin
0 mg cholesterol	4 mg phosphorus	0 RE vitamin A	2 mg vitamin C

Gingivitis: Inflamed, bleeding gums that may be caused by a vitamin C deficiency—or at least, partly so. Untreated, it can lead to tooth loss.

Ginkgo Biloba: This is merely the botanical name for the ornamental tree that graces so many American streets and gardens. It's an ancient Chinese plant and the Chinese have long prized its fruits and nuts, which they believe to be blessed with medicinal properties. The *Ginkgo biloba* sold in liquid and tablet form by American health-food stores is a dried extract obtained from ginkgo leaves (it is often called simply GBE, meaning "*Ginkgo biloba* extract"). Extensive pharmacological studies in Germany suggest that it is a vasodilator that increases blood flow to the brain and that it may be effective in treating such geriatric problems as depression, headache, ringing in the ears and short-term memory loss. There is also some evidence that *Ginkgo biloba* may mop up free radicals, those by-products of the metabolism that circulate through the blood, savaging cells, lowering immunity and very possibly raising the risk of cancer. The trouble with the *Ginkgo biloba* sold in the United States is that is has not been ap-

proved for medicinal use and can thus be sold only as a food supplement or health food. Nearly all of the German studies on the efficacy of *Ginkgo biloba* were conducted using a standardized German product manufactured and marketed by Willmar Schwabe. American *Ginkgo biloba* or GBE supplements, depending upon their concentration and formulation, may or may not be as effective.

Ginkgo Nuts: The oily nuts of the ginkgo tree that taste a little like pine nuts. The Japanese, who dote on ginkgo nuts, use them in recipes sweet and savory. The nuts are

NUTRIENT CONTENT OF 1 CUP CANNED GINKGO NUTS
(about 5½ ounces; 155 grams)

173 calories	476 mg sodium
4 g protein	278 mg potassium
3 g fat, 0 saturated	3 g dietary fiber
0 mg cholesterol	NA RE vitamin A
34 g carbohydrate	NA mg thiamin
6 mg calcium	NA mg riboflavin
83 mg phosphorus	NA mg niacin
0.5 mg iron	NA mg vitamin C

actually the seeds of small round fruits so foul smelling that many cities ban the growing of the female ginkgo trees. Roasted, ginkgo nuts are delicious eaten out of hand.

Ginseng: Some herbalists swear that ginseng cures (or at least alleviates) impotence, high blood pressure, diabetes, chest colds and congestion, even the pain of cocaine withdrawal. Also that it's an energizer, a booster of the immune system, a protector against radiation. The truth? This licoricy parsnip-shaped root, one species of which grows wild over much of America, has been used by the Chinese as a sort of fountain of youth for more than five thousand years. Marco Polo made note of ginseng in his diaries, and many centuries later Louis XIV used it to pump up his virility and energy. Medical researchers admit that ginseng is a stimulant, like coffee and tea, but few are willing to raise it to wonder-drug status.

Gizzard: Also called the **crop,** this lean, muscular organ pulverizes whatever a bird eats so it's more digestible. In oven-ready turkeys, chickens, ducks, geese and Rock Cornish hens, the gizzards are packaged along with the other giblets (heart and liver) and tucked inside the body cavity. Gizzards are so tough only slow simmering and mincing will tenderize them. They impart slightly gamy flavor and are best mixed into stuffings and gravies.

NUTRIENT CONTENT OF 3 OUNCES (85 GRAMS) SIMMERED CHICKEN GIZZARD	
133 calories	58 mg sodium
23 g protein	155 mg potassium
3 g fat, 1 saturated	0 g dietary fiber
169 mg cholesterol	49 RE vitamin A
1 g carbohydrate	0.02 mg thiamin
8 mg calcium	0.21 mg riboflavin
135 mg phosphorus	3.5 mg niacin
3.6 mg iron	1 mg vitamin C

Glass: The beauty of glass cookware, preserving jars and storage containers is that they're inert and don't react in any way with what's put into them. Their disadvantages, apart from breakability, are heft (glass is heavy) and inability to conduct heat as smoothly or quickly as metal. Finally, glass jars let the light in, so anything canned (or even stored) in glass will lose light-sensitive riboflavin (vitamin B$_2$).

Gliadin: An incomplete protein found in barley, oats, rye and wheat that lacks the essential amino acid LYSINE. When wheat flour is moistened, then kneaded hard, gliadin combines with GLUTENIN, a second protein, forming GLUTEN, a third protein that's sturdy and pliable enough to serve as the framework of breads, cakes and pastries.

Globe Artichokes: See ARTICHOKES, GLOBE OR FRENCH.

Glossitis: A painfully inflamed tongue. The cause may be something as simple as biting or burning your tongue. Or it may be something more serious. Acute niacin deficiencies trigger glossitis (it's a symptom of pellagra), as can lack of riboflavin (vitamin B$_2$), cobalamin (vitamin B$_{12}$), folacin and iron. Many people with glossitis have trouble eating. In addition to being sore, their tongues are swollen, deeply fissured, sometimes ulcerated and almost always an angry purple-red. When the cause of glossitis is a nutritional inadequacy, correcting the deficiency is the cure.

Glucomannon: A fibrous substance used as an appetite suppressant (see DIET PILLS).

Gluconic Acid (additive): A water-soluble acidulant, antioxidant and clarifier used in wines, syrups and soft drinks. In cake and quick bread mixes, gluconic acid functions as a leavener and, in powdered drink and dessert mixes, as the acid ingredient. Obtained from fermented dextrose (a simple sugar), it has no known toxicity. GRAS.

Glucono-Delta-Lactone (additive): This sweet, white acid salt combines with water to form GLUCONIC ACID. It's used primarily to acidify dry dessert mixes and to fix the color of hot dogs, sausages, salamis and other cured meats. GRAS when used within FDA limits.

Glucose, Dextrose: Glucose is to the human body what gasoline is to the car: *fuel.* Glucose drives our bodies, providing energy for 1,001 physiological processes. The aim and end result of digestion are to break the food we eat down into glucose and other simple chemicals the body can put to good use. Glucose circulates constantly in the blood, delivering instant energy to the brain (it needs 140 grams, or nearly 5 ounces, of glucose a day to function properly) as well as to every other living cell. Whatever glucose the body can't use right away is stored as glycogen or fat, then tapped and recycled as glucose whenever and wherever it's needed.

Glucose Tolerance Test: The way doctors determine the body's ability to use a measured amount of glucose. First comes a twelve-hour fast, then a "glucose cocktail" (50 to 100 grams glucose based on body weight). Half an hour later, a blood sample is analyzed for glucose, then additional samples are taken and tested every hour thereafter for the next four or five hours, the better to plot a glucose tolerance curve. Normally, there will be an initial rise in blood sugar levels that will taper off after two hours. In diabetics, the blood sugar rises more dramatically the first half hour, continues to rise for the next two, and even after four hours remains higher than it should be—or would be in nondiabetics.

Glutamic Acid: One of the nonessential AMINO ACIDS. What few people realize is that glutamic acid is a component of folic acid, a B vitamin the body uses to break down amino acids. Or that one of its salts is MONOSODIUM GLUTAMATE.

Glutamine: In the brain, kidneys and liver, GLUTAMIC ACID, one nonessential amino acid, combines with ammonia to form glutamine, another nonessential acid. Glutamine is a major player in the healing of wounds.

Gluten: A protein in wheat. In wheat flour it forms the structure of breads, cakes and pastries. Actually, gluten is formed only when flour is moistened, then kneaded, forcing two insoluble proteins, GLIADIN and GLUTENIN, to cohere in a sticky, elastic mass. Gliadin alone is syrupy; glutenin, rubbery.

Gluten Flour: See FLOUR.

Glutenin: A tough, elastic protein found in abundance in wheat flour (especially hard-wheat flour) that combines with the softer GLIADIN to form GLUTEN.

Gluten Intolerance: Also called **gluten-sensitive enteropathy, celiac disease, celiac sprue** or simply **sprue,** this malfunction of the small intestine is caused by the in-

ability to tolerate gluten or gliadin, proteins found in barley, oats, rye and wheat. No one knows what causes it although some researchers believe it's the lack of a particular enzyme. Both children and adults can suffer the discomfort of celiac disease—weight loss, diarrhea, nausea, vomiting and malnutrition because the body can't digest or absorb carbohydrate, fat, protein, vitamins and minerals properly. The usual treatment is to ban grains, flours and other foods containing gluten or gliadin from the diet (see GLUTEN- OR GLIADIN-FREE DIET).

Gluten- or Gliadin-Free Diet: An eating program designed for those sensitive to gluten (see GLUTEN INTOLERANCE). All foods containing gluten or gliadin are eliminated from the diet, and that means barley, oats, rye and wheat as well as anything made from them. Because they contain no gluten, corn, potatoes, soybeans, tapioca, arrowroot and rice are allowed, as is gluten-free wheat starch. A gluten-free diet is difficult enough to control when foods are cooked to order. But when processed, foods so integral to the American diet can spell even bigger *trouble.* Cocoa mixes, malted milk, even Ovaltine and cold cuts, for example, contain the taboo grains masquerading as emulsifiers, fillers and stabilizers, as do many other processed foods. Scrutinize labels.

Glutinous Rice: See RICE.

Glycemic Index: To help diabetics and hypoglycemics (those with low blood sugar) eat more wisely (not to mention safely), doctors and dietitians must know how fast specific foods raise blood sugar levels—and how high. In other words, their glycemic effect. A common misconception is that all simple sugars (candies, etc.) send blood glucose levels soaring. It's not that cut and dried. There are too many variables and interactions of one food on another. How digestible, for example, is the starch in a particular food—potatoes, say, or lima beans? Is protein also present, and do the protein and starch interact? What about other molecules that might bind the starch? Is the food liquid or dry? In a single piece, finely minced or mashed? Is it cooked or raw? How much fat does it contain, how much fiber? All determine how fast and how precipitously a specific starch will elevate blood sugar levels. Those starches creating slow, moderate rises of blood sugar are said to have a low glycemic index, among them lentils, dried peas and beans. These are the best choices for diabetics and hypoglycemics. Ice cream, believe it or not, has a lower glycemic index than pasta (36 versus 50), and carrots, at 92, a higher one than cornflakes, at 80. At the top of the list is glucose, with a glycemic index of 100.

Glycerides: When a molecule of glycerol bonds with three fatty acid molecules, glycerides are formed. Or to be more specific, **triglycerides.** These circulate constantly in the blood, ferrying fat-soluble vitamins (A, D, E and K) to locations where they're needed. Glycerides are also involved in the synthesis of hormonelike chemicals integral to certain biochemical processes; they are essential for healthy skin, and, not least, for energy. Mono- and diglycerides (a molecule of glycerol bonded with one or two fatty acid molecules, respectively) are used in the food industry as emulsifiers.

Glycerin, Glycerol (additive): A viscous, crystalline liquid formed when fat molecules split, forming free fatty acids and glycerin. About half as sweet as sugar, glycerin is used to keep baked goods, jelly beans, marshmallows and even tobacco moist, to plasticize cheese, gelatin desserts, processed meats, hot fudge sauces and chewing gums. GRAS when used according to FDA standards.

Glycine: The simplest amino acid; a nonessential one. See AMINO ACIDS.

Glycogen: Before glucose can be stored in the body, it must be converted to a complex sugar (polysaccharide) called glycogen. This animal starch is warehoused in the muscles and liver, then withdrawn whenever the body needs energy. Nothing depletes it quicker than fasting or vigorous exercise.

Goat Cheese: Goat's milk cheeses are made in nearly every country but the French are the masters. Depending on whether they're cured or aged, goat cheeses may be mild or biting. Textures range from firm to chalky to creamy, but color is confined to a palette of whites (except for the caramel-sweet Norwegian **gjetost,** which looks like Fels Naptha soap). Most **chèvres** (the French word for "goats") are shaped into small rounds, drums, logs or pyramids. Seemingly rich, goat cheeses are sometimes

lower in butterfat than cow's milk cheeses. They weigh in the 25 to 30 percent range. Compare that with 50 percent for a Bleu d'Auvergne.

NUTRIENT CONTENT OF 1 OUNCE (28 GRAMS) SEMISOFT GOAT CHEESE	
103 calories	146 mg sodium
6 g protein	45 mg potassium
9 g fat, 6 saturated	0 g dietary fiber
22 mg cholesterol	162 RE vitamin A
1 g carbohydrate	0.02 mg thiamin
84 mg calcium	0.19 mg riboflavin
106 mg phosphorus	0.3 mg niacin
0.5 mg iron	0 mg vitamin C

NUTRIENT CONTENT OF 1 OUNCE (28 GRAMS) SOFT GOAT CHEESE	
76 calories	104 mg sodium
5 g protein	7 mg potassium
6 g fat, 4 saturated	0 g dietary fiber
13 mg cholesterol	130 RE vitamin A
0 g carbohydrate	0.02 mg thiamin
40 mg calcium	0.11 mg riboflavin
73 mg phosphorus	0.1 mg niacin
0.5 mg iron	0 mg vitamin C

NUTRIENT CONTENT OF 1 OUNCE (28 GRAMS) HARD GOAT CHEESE (GJETOST)	
132 calories	170 mg sodium
3 g protein	399 mg potassium
8 g fat, 5 saturated	0 g dietary fiber
27 mg cholesterol	78 RE vitamin A
12 g carbohydrate	0.09 mg thiamin
113 mg calcium	0.39 mg riboflavin
126 mg phosphorus	0.2 mg niacin
0.1 mg iron	0 mg vitamin C

Goat's Milk: The raising of goats is once again fashionable in the United States, but nearly all the milk goes into cheese. The nutritional value of goat's milk varies from species to species and, to some extent, from animal to animal and from season to season because diets vary. As a rule, however, goat's milk averages a little over 4 percent butterfat as compared to 3.8 percent for cow's milk. It's slightly higher in protein and minerals, too.

NUTRIENT CONTENT OF 1 CUP GOAT'S MILK
(8 fluid ounces, 244 grams)

168 calories	122 mg sodium
9 g protein	499 mg potassium
10 g fat, 7 saturated	0 g dietary fiber
28 mg cholesterol	137 RE vitamin A
11 g carbohydrate	0.12 mg thiamin
326 mg calcium	0.34 mg riboflavin
270 mg phosphorus	0.7 mg niacin
0.1 mg iron	3 mg vitamin C

Goiter (diet and): Five thousand years ago the Chinese began treating enlarged thyroid glands—goiters—with food supplements made of seaweed. They were on target, but America didn't catch up until the early twentieth century. Only then did U.S. researchers test the Chinese theory that something in seaweed cured goiter, despite the fact that an 1820 Swiss study identified that something as IODINE. In 1917, with goiter widespread in inland America, American scientists finally put the Swiss and Chinese cures to the test. What they learned was that people living within the sound of the surf, people eating plenty of iodine-rich saltwater fish were far less likely to develop goiter than those in the Great Lakes and Great Plains states. In the 1930s, when iodized salt went on the market, goiter virtually disappeared from the American heartland. Today nutritionists know that although iodine deficiencies cause 96 percent of the goiters, the rest may come from eating too many cruciferous vegetables. The whole huge cabbage family, it turns out, contains goitrogens—compounds that block the thyroid's ability to use iodine. What's needed to prevent goiter is a delicate balance of dietary iodine and cruciferous vegetables.

Goitrogens: Chemical substances present in broccoli, brussels sprouts, cabbage, cauliflower, collards and kale, which by thwarting the body's ability to absorb and utilize iodine, cause GOITER. All cruciferous vegetables contain goitrogens, and these include—in addition to the more obvious family members already named—horseradish, kohlrabi, mustard, radishes, rutabaga, turnips and turnip greens.

Goldenseal (Hydrastis): It was the Cherokee who taught the American colonists how to make infusions of goldenseal and use it to treat skin diseases and also as a wash for sore eyes. Years later, this bitter tonic became a general remedy for a variety of gastric and genitourinary disorders. Around the turn of the century, goldenseal was the major ingredient in many patent medicines, among them Dr. Pierce's Golden Medical Discovery. The active ingredients in this herb are alkaloids, which when brewed into tea are marginally effective as a treatment for mouth sores and cracked and bleeding lips. But what has made goldenseal a hot ticket today is its rumored ability to "beat" urine tests for the detection of cocaine and marijuana use. *Those rumors are false.* See below.

Golden Syrup: A mellow, amber cane syrup long popular in Great Britain that has only recently become popular in the United States. First developed by Abram Lyle, a nineteenth-century Scottish sugar refiner, the recipe for golden syrup remains a trade secret. Although Britons drizzle golden syrup over suet pudding, it can be used interchangeably in recipes with light corn syrup, honey or molasses. **NOTE:** Specific nutrient counts unavailable but they would not be so very different from those given for MOLASSES.

Goose: Pharaonic murals tell us the Egyptians fancied geese and historians that the Greeks fattened them on gruel. Still, these geese were no match for those Marco Polo found in China (one gander weighed 24 pounds!).

Type of Tea	Health Claims	The Facts
Goldenseal	Eases pain of sore mouth, relieves gastric distress, helps cure genitourinary disorders; renders urine tests for cocoaine and marijuana use ineffective.	Mildly effective in treating sore mouth; ineffective as a remedy for gastric and genitourinary problems; has no effect on urine drug tests.

Because geese could be put out to graze like sheep, Europeans, from the Middle Ages on, considered them poor man's pheasant, yet Elizabeth I doted on them, stuffed with sage and apples, roasted crisp and caramel brown. Geese are served that way in England today at Christmastime, also in Germany and parts of France. Geese have always been more popular abroad than in the United States, perhaps because turkey is the centerpiece of major American feasts. Still, geese are widely available here, frozen or fresh and ready to cook. They are considerably fatter than turkey or chicken, but pricked and roasted at high temperature, they lose much of their fat as drippings.

NUTRIENT CONTENT OF 3 OUNCES (85 GRAMS) ROASTED GOOSE (WITHOUT SKIN)

202 calories	65 mg sodium
25 g protein	330 mg potassium
11 g fat, 4 saturated	0 g dietary fiber
82 mg cholesterol	11 RE vitamin A
0 g carbohydrate	0.08 mg thiamin
12 mg calcium	0.33 mg riboflavin
263 mg phosphorus	3.5 mg niacin
2.5 mg iron	0 mg vitamin C

Gooseberries: The Scandinavians, Germans and British are mad for these pale green, puckeringly tart "marbles." Many New Englanders, like their British ancestors, grow gooseberry bushes in their yards, the better to have fresh fruit for jams and foods. They know that the sour green berry will soon show blushes of pink, then purple, and that it will soften and sweeten. Other Americans couldn't care less about gooseberries. **SEASON:** Summer.

NUTRIENT CONTENT OF 1 CUP GOOSEBERRIES CANNED IN LIGHT SYRUP

(about 9 ounces; 252 grams)

184 calories	5 mg sodium
2 g protein	194 mg potassium
1 g fat, 0 saturated	6 g dietary fiber
0 mg cholesterol	35 RE vitamin A
47 g carbohydrate	0.05 mg thiamin
40 mg calcium	0.13 mg riboflavin
18 mg phosphorus	0.4 mg niacin
0.8 mg iron	25 mg vitamin C

Goose Liver, Foie Gras: When geese are force-fed, their livers double or triple in size and turn the color of lard. What most of us know is canned goose-liver pâté, studded with bits of truffle, but it can't compare with the top-quality foie gras served in France. It takes three to six weeks to fatten a goose liver and a good one weighs 2 to 3 pounds. Two French provinces claim to produce the best *foie gras*—Alsace and Perigord. The demand for Alsatian *foie gras* is now such that fattened goose livers must be imported from Hungary, the Czech Republic, Poland and Israel. Once the livers arrive in Alsace, they are cooked, lightly seasoned and pressed into blocks. Or they are sliced thin, then browned zip-quick so they remain pink and quivery inside. A great delicacy.

NUTRIENT CONTENT OF 1 OUNCE (28 GRAMS) CANNED GOOSE-LIVER PÂTÉ

131 calories	198 mg sodium
3 g protein	39 mg potassium
12 g fat, 4 saturated	0 g dietary fiber
43 mg cholesterol	284 RE vitamin A
1 g carbohydrate	0.02 mg thiamin
20 mg calcium	0.09 mg riboflavin
57 mg phosphorus	0.7 mg niacin
1.6 mg iron	1 mg vitamin C

Gorgonzola: This biting Italian blue cheese has been made in the village of Gorgonzola near Milan ever since the eleventh century. It is a cow's milk cheese, butter soft, pale ivory but profusely marbled with blue-green *Penicillium glaucum* mold. In the old days, Gorgonzola was made by farmers and aged in caves, but most of the production is now big time, with warehouses replacing caves and fac-

NUTRIENT CONTENT OF 1 OUNCE (28 GRAMS) GORGONZOLA

111 calories	512 mg sodium
7 g protein	26 mg potassium
9 g fat, 6 saturated	0 g dietary fiber
25 mg cholesterol	103 RE vitamin A
0 g carbohydrate	0.01 mg thiamin
149 mg calcium	0.09 mg riboflavin
121 mg phosphorus	0.2 mg niacin
0.1 mg iron	0 mg vitamin C

tories, farmhouses. Still, to be certified as a Gorgonzola, the cheese must be made and cured in one of these northern Italian provinces—Bergamo, Brescia, Como, Cremona, Cuneo, Milan, Novara, Pavia or Vercelli. It takes about two months to produce good Gorgonzola.

Gouda: The second of Holland's "cannonball cheeses" (the first is EDAM), this semihard pale yellow cow's milk cheese comes from Gouda, a quaint old town near Rotterdam. Young Goudas are nutty and mild; aged ones sharp.

NUTRIENT CONTENT OF 1 OUNCE (28 GRAMS) GOUDA	
101 calories	232 mg sodium
7 g protein	34 mg potassium
8 g fat, 5 saturated	0 g dietary fiber
32 mg cholesterol	49 RE vitamin A
1 g carbohydrate	0.01 mg thiamin
198 mg calcium	0.10 mg riboflavin
155 mg phosphorus	0 mg niacin
0.1 mg iron	0 mg vitamin C

Gout (diet and): Doctors used to believe that high blood levels of uric acid (a result of faulty metabolism of purines, which are by-products of nucleic acid—read *protein*—breakdown) caused this excruciating inflammation of the joints. Today they suspect it's the other way around, that gout raises uric acid levels. Even though physicians now treat this metabolic disorder with medication, most of them still tell their gout patients to swear off foods rich in purines (anchovies, caviar and other fish roe, mussels, organ meats and sardines). They also prescribe plenty of water. Unchecked, gout can mean a buildup of uric acid crystals in the kidneys, heart and other vital organs. Serious business. **NOTE:** Men are ninety-five times more likely to get gout than women.

Grading of Food: A voluntary grading offered by the USDA to packers and processors of food—mainly meats, poultry, eggs, milk, butter and cheese but also fruits and vegetables, both fresh and canned—that's an indication of size and quality. Don't assume that foods of high grade are nutritionally superior to those of lower grades. They aren't. Nor, with the exception of milk, are they more wholesome (Grade A milk has a lower bacterial count than Grade B or C although these are perfectly safe). INSPECTION OF FOOD attempts to certify that food is safe to eat. The trouble with grading is that the government has yet to standardize the terms. Below, starting with the top grades and working downward, are a few of the USDA grades.

All grades, preceded by *USDA* or *U.S.,* are shown inside badge- or shield-shaped emblems. In addition, the U.S. Department of Commerce's National Marine Fisheries Service, through its Fishery Products Inspection Program, offers fish processors the option of having their products inspected and graded (at their own expense). Those meeting the standards set for plant sanitation, for fish wholesomeness and quality can label their seafood "U.S. Grade A."

Beef	Veal	Lamb	Eggs	Poultry, Milk	Cheddar	Fresh Fruit
Prime	Prime	Prime	AA	A	AA	Fancy
Choice	Choice	Choice	A	B	A	1
Select	Good	Good	B	C	B	2
Standard	Standard	Utility			C	3
Commercial	Utility	Cull				
Utility	Cull					
Cutter						
Canner						

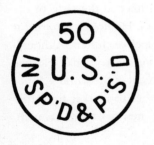

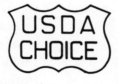

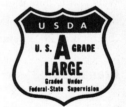

Graham Crackers: One of America's early health foods, these crisp, sweet crackers made of whole-wheat (graham) flour are named for nineteenth-century vegetarian Sylvester Graham, who championed the eating of whole grains and bran. Graham crackers were first mass-produced in 1882.

NUTRIENT CONTENT OF 2 SQUARE GRAHAM CRACKERS	
(about ½ ounce; 14 grams)	
60 calories	66 mg sodium
1 g protein	23 mg potassium
1 g fat, 0 saturated	0 g dietary fiber
0 mg cholesterol	0 RE vitamin A
11 g carbohydrate	0.05 mg thiamin
5 mg calcium	0.04 mg riboflavin
17 mg phosphorus	0.4 mg niacin
0.4 mg iron	0 mg vitamin C

Graham Flour: Another term for whole-wheat flour, named for Sylvester Graham, who first pushed its use. See FLOUR.

Grain Alcohol: See ETHANOL.

Grains: Maybe Sylvester Graham, of graham cracker fame, was on to something after all. One hundred fifty years ago, he urged organizing the diet around a variety of whole grains, much as builders of today's FOOD GUIDE PYRAMID do. The pyramid's base is the Bread, Cereal, Rice and Pasta Group, from which we're told to eat at least six helpings a day. Small wonder. Whole grains are rich in bran, B vitamins, iron and other minerals, all of which do us a world of good. Grains are also low in saturated fats and devoid of cholesterol. See also individual grains—BARLEY; CORN; RICE; RYE; WHEAT; etc.—listed alphabetically elsewhere.

Gram: A metric unit of weight used everywhere in the civilized world except the United States. Even home cooks weigh out their ingredients in grams instead of using the more cumbersome, less precise measuring cup method. For the record, 28.35 grams = 1 ounce.

Granadilla: See PASSION FRUIT.

Granités: See ICES, GRANITÉS, SORBETS.

Granola: The "hippie health food" of the 1960s has gone mainstream. Recipes vary hugely, but all granolas are crunchy mixes of rolled oats and other whole-grain cereals, toasted coconut, assorted dried fruits, nuts and seeds, the lot usually sweetened with honey or brown sugar and spiced with cinnamon. There are plenty of B vitamins, fiber and minerals in granola, but no shortage of calories or fat.

NUTRIENT CONTENT OF ½ CUP HOMEMADE GRANOLA	
(about 2 ounces; 61 grams)	
297 calories	6 mg sodium
8 g protein	306 mg potassium
17 g fat, 3 saturated	6 g dietary fiber
0 mg cholesterol	2 RE vitamin A
34 g carbohydrate	0.37 mg thiamin
38 mg calcium	0.15 mg riboflavin
247 mg phosphorus	1.1 mg niacin
2.4 mg iron	1 mg vitamin C

Grapefruit: Most citrus fruits are as old as man. And all of them originated in the Old World. *Except* grapefruit. "After some hesitation," Waverley Root writes in *Food*, "the grapefruit was accepted in 1830 as a genuine species and gratified with the name *Citrus paradisi*." He adds that Jamaica is the grapefruit's probable place of origin, then points out that its beginnings are swirled about in mystery. Food historians believe that the grapefruit is a natural cross between citrus fruits brought to the Indies by Europeans or—and Root subscribes to this theory—that it's a natural mutation of the PUMMELO (or pomelo). It is known that an East Indian trader, a Captain Shaddock, brought pummelo seeds to Barbados toward the turn of the seventeenth century (in the Indies, grapefruits are still sometimes called **shaddocks**). So how did the pummelo make the west-by-northwest journey to Jamaica? More than likely its seeds traveled in the bellies of gulls or other wide-ranging seabirds. The name *grapefruit* was apparently coined by John Lunan; the first mention of it appears in his *Hortus Jamaicensis,* published in 1814. Lunan likened the taste of the plump yellow citrus fruit to grapes. He noted, too, that it grew on the tree's branches in grapelike clusters. Although neither is true, the name *grapefruit* stuck. Today Florida, Texas and California grow 90 percent of the world's grapefruit but only half of the crop goes to market fresh (the balance is juiced or segmented, then frozen or canned).

The two basic types of grapefruit grown today are the tart and biting **white** and the bland, honey-sweet **pink** or **red**. (Note that the pink or red contain significantly more vitamin A than the white.) **SEASON:** Year-round, with supplies peaking in winter.

NUTRIENT CONTENT OF ½ WHITE GRAPEFRUIT
(about 4¼ ounces; 120 grams)

38 calories	0 mg sodium
1 g protein	167 mg potassium
0 g fat, 0 saturated	2 g dietary fiber
0 mg cholesterol	1 RE vitamin A*
10 g carbohydrate	0.04 mg thiamin
14 mg calcium	0.02 mg riboflavin
10 mg phosphorus	0.3 mg niacin
0.1 mg iron	41 mg vitamin C

*For ½ pink grapefruit, 32 RE vitamin A.

NUTRIENT CONTENT OF 1 CUP CANNED GRAPEFRUIT (PACKED IN JUICE)
(about 9 ounces; 249 grams)

93 calories	19 mg sodium
2 g protein	420 mg potassium
0 g fat, 0 saturated	3 g dietary fiber
0 mg cholesterol	0 RE vitamin A
23 g carbohydrate	0.07 mg thiamin
38 mg calcium	0.04 mg riboflavin
30 mg phosphorus	0.6 mg niacin
0.5 mg iron	84 mg vitamin C

NUTRIENT CONTENT OF 1 CUP CANNED GRAPEFRUIT (PACKED IN LIGHT SYRUP)
(about 9 ounces; 254 grams)

152 calories	4 mg sodium
1 g protein	328 mg potassium
0 g fat, 0 saturated	3 g dietary fiber
0 mg cholesterol	0 RE vitamin A
39 g carbohydrate	0.10 mg thiamin
36 mg calcium	0.05 mg riboflavin
25 mg phosphorus	0.6 mg niacin
1.0 mg iron	54 mg vitamin C

Grapefruit Juice: Fresh squeezed is best because the vitamin C hasn't had a chance to oxidize—unless, of course, the canned or frozen juices have been fortified with vita-min C. What's sacrificed most, especially if the juice is strained, is the fiber.

NUTRIENT CONTENT OF 1 CUP FRESH GRAPEFRUIT JUICE
(8 fluid ounces; 247 grams)

96 calories	2 mg sodium
1 g protein	400 mg potassium
0 g fat, 0 saturated	0 g dietary fiber
0 mg cholesterol	2 RE vitamin A
23 g carbohydrate	0.10 mg thiamin
22 mg calcium	0.05 mg riboflavin
37 mg phosphorus	0.5 mg niacin
0.5 mg iron	94 mg vitamin C

NUTRIENT CONTENT OF 1 CUP CANNED UNSWEETENED GRAPEFRUIT JUICE
(8 fluid ounces; 247 grams)

93 calories	3 mg sodium
1 g protein	378 mg potassium
0 g fat, 0 saturated	0 g dietary fiber
0 mg cholesterol	2 RE vitamin A
22 g carbohydrate	0.10 mg thiamin
18 mg calcium	0.05 mg riboflavin
27 mg phosphorus	0.6 mg niacin
0.5 mg iron	72 mg vitamin C

Grape Juice: Both the red and the white juices are now available and neither is particularly nutritious. Most grape juices have a "foxy" or Concord grape flavor, and some brands are so acidic they are don't "set easy" on delicate stomachs. The best you can say about grape juice is that it's fat and cholesterol free, extremely low in sodium and, at the same time, a splendid source of potassium, and, if fortified with vitamin C, a good source of that valuable nutrient. Read labels.

NUTRIENT CONTENT OF 1 CUP BOTTLED RED GRAPE JUICE
(8 fluid ounces; 253 grams)

155 calories	7 mg sodium
1 g protein	334 mg potassium
0 g fat, 0 saturated	0 g dietary fiber
0 mg cholesterol	2 RE vitamin A
38 g carbohydrate	0.07 mg thiamin
22 mg calcium	0.09 mg riboflavin
27 mg phosphorus	0.7 mg niacin
0.6 mg iron	0 mg vitamin C

NUTRIENT CONTENT OF 1 CUP RECONSTITUTED FROZEN GRAPE JUICE (FORTIFIED WITH VITAMIN C)
(8 fluid ounces; 250 grams)

128 calories	5 mg sodium
1 g protein	53 mg potassium
0 g fat, 0 saturated	2 g dietary fiber
0 mg cholesterol	3 RE vitamin A
32 g carbohydrate	0.04 mg thiamin
9 mg calcium	0.07 mg riboflavin
11 mg phosphorus	0.3 mg niacin
0.3 mg iron	60 mg vitamin C

Grapes: When offered grapes as dessert, a dining companion of Brillat-Savarin, the eighteenth-century French food writer, grumbled, "I am not accustomed to taking my wine as pills." A rude remark, and an ignorant one, too. Thousands of years earlier, the Persians, Egyptians, Greeks and Romans had already recognized that there were two distinct types of grapes: those for eating out of hand and those for fermenting into wine. One of the first fruits to be cultivated, the grape probably originated in Sumeria; there are cuneiform references to them. Those early Old World vines, crossed and hybridized down the centuries, gave rise to the eight thousand European species and cultivars known today. But there were ancient American varieties, too—plumper, slip-skinned grapes, some of which grew singly rather than in clusters. Excavations of Native American middens have turned up grape seeds nearly four thousand years old. Strangely, the native American grapes—the muscadines and scuppernongs—won't grow west of the Rockies, and the imported European varieties do less well east of them, which explains why America's top wines come from the West Coast. The grapes that concern us here, however, are "table grapes"—

the **green** (Thompson Seedless and Muscat), the **red** (Flame Seedless, Tokay and Emperor) and the **black** (Concord; Black Corinth, Zante or Champagne Grape; Exotic and Ribier). **SEASON:** One or more of these grapes are available year-round, but supplies are at their peak in late summer and early autumn.

Grape-Seed Oil: Primarily a drying oil used to improve the looks of seeded raisins and keep them from clumping, grape-seed oil is now also being used by innovative chefs for cooking and dressing salads. Specific nutrient counts are unavailable, but it's safe to say that grape-seed oil contains no cholesterol and about the same number of calories (120 per tablespoon) as other vegetable oils. Also not known: the fatty acid breakdown of grape-seed oil—i.e., the percentage of saturated, monounsaturated and polyunsaturated. Grape-seed oil has a faint raisiny flavor and should be used with discretion.

Grape Sugar: Another name for GLUCOSE.

GRAS (Generally Recognized as Safe): This category of food additives was established in 1958 by the Food and Drug Administration as part of the revised Food, Drug, and Cosmetic Act of 1938. The original GRAS list included around 700 food additives that had stood the test of time and were believed to be harmless. However, grumbles—then shouts—from consumer advocates insisted that an overhaul of the GRAS list was long overdue. As a result, the FDA has been reevaluating and reclassifying all GRAS additives and banning any deemed hazardous. In addition, it's scrutinizing some 200 food dyes and 2,100 flavorings. See also DELANEY CLAUSE.

Gravy: A hot sauce, either thickened or not, made of meat or poultry drippings. Some gravies are made with milk,

NUTRIENT CONTENT OF 1 CUP FRESH CONCORD GRAPES
(about 3⅓ ounces; 92 grams)

58 calories	2 mg sodium
1 g protein	176 mg potassium
0 g fat, 0 saturated	1 g dietary fiber
0 mg cholesterol	9 RE vitamin A
16 g carbohydrate	0.09 mg thiamin
13 mg calcium	0.05 mg riboflavin
9 mg phosphorus	0.3 mg niacin
0.3 mg iron	4 mg vitamin C

NUTRIENT CONTENT OF 1 CUP CANNED BEEF GRAVY
(8 fluid ounces; 233 grams)

124 calories	1,305 mg sodium
9 g protein	189 mg potassium
6 g fat, 3 saturated	0 g dietary fiber
7 mg cholesterol	0 RE vitamin A
11 g carbohydrate	0.07 mg thiamin
14 mg calcium	0.08 mg riboflavin
70 mg phosphorus	1.5 mg niacin
1.6 mg iron	0 mg vitamin C

others with water and still others with stock. The gravies lowest in fat, calories and cholesterol will be natural meat juices, skimmed of as much fat as possible.

"Grazing": This snacking throughout the day instead of sitting down to three squares may actually be good for you. You're less likely to overload your body with calories at any one time and send blood sugar levels soaring. Hypoglycemics (those with low blood sugar) are actually encouraged to graze to hold their blood sugar levels within the normal range. It's important, however, that you graze on a variety of foods, getting—*each day*—two to four helpings of fruit, three to five of vegetables and six to eleven of grains plus a couple of helpings of meat (or other protein food) and milk. The worst thing you can do is nosh on chips, puffs and other deep-fried crunchies to the exclusion of everything else.

Green Beans: See BEANS, FRESH.

Green Bell Peppers: See SWEET PEPPERS under PEPPERS, CAPSICUMS.

Greengage Plums: See PLUMS.

Green Peas: See PEAS.

"Green Pills": Many health-food stores push these dehydrated vegetable tablets as cancer cures, but scrutiny of a green pill label proves the lie. By law, a *label* cannot make false claims.

Greens: We're not talking lettuce here but dark leafy vegetables that brim with beta-carotene, vitamin C, iron and other minerals: BEET GREENS; BROCCOLI RABE; COLLARDS; DANDELION GREENS; KALE; MUSTARD GREENS; SPINACH; TURNIP GREENS. They are all low in calories, contain zero cholesterol and, some of them, when young and tender, can be slipped raw into salads. Most greens are more versatile than we think—superb when stir-fried zip-quick in a little olive oil with garlic and onion, when steamed in nothing more than their own rinse water and then dressed with a nippy vinaigrette, when shredded raw and tossed just before serving into a steaming kettle of potato soup—it's a Portuguese specialty called *caldo verde*. Most of these greens can be substituted for one another in recipes. Each green is discussed individually elsewere.

Green Tea: Unlike black tea, green tea is not fermented, which explains its fresh, herby flavor. The leaves are plucked, dried, rolled into tiny balls ("gunpowder"), then carefully steeped to extract their essence. In China and Japan, where green tea is drunk many times a day, the incidence of gastrointestinal cancer is very low. Biomedical researchers now believe that the catechins in green tea are powerful anticarcinogens, also that they lower blood cholesterol levels and bolster the immune system. Studies continue. Meanwhile, more than a few of those researching catechins are so convinced of their medicinal powers they sip several cups of green tea a day.

Griddle Cakes: See PANCAKES.

Grilling: See BROILING, GRILLING.

Grissini: Crisp Italian breadsticks, some of them as slim as pencils.

NUTRIENT CONTENT OF 2 UNSALTED GRISSINI	
(about ¾ ounce; 20 grams)	
77 calories	140 mg sodium
2 g protein	18 mg potassium
1 g fat, 0 saturated	0 g dietary fiber
1 mg cholesterol	0 RE vitamin A
15 g carbohydrate	0.13 mg thiamin
6 mg calcium	0.10 mg riboflavin
20 mg phosphorus	1.3 mg niacin
0.9 mg iron	0 mg vitamin C

Grits: You might call this the Southern polenta. *Except* that grits is white (yes, grits *is* singular), a meal made from dried hominy. And hominy? It is white field corn puffed

NUTRIENT CONTENT OF 1 CUP COOKED ENRICHED GRITS	
(about 8½ ounces; 242 grams)	
146 calories	0 mg sodium
4 g protein	54 mg potassium
1 g fat, 0 saturated	5 g dietary fiber
0 mg cholesterol	0 RE vitamin A
31 g carbohydrate	0.24 mg thiamin
1 mg calcium	0.15 mg riboflavin
29 mg phosphorus	2.0 mg niacin
1.6 mg iron	0 mg vitamin C

in a lye bath, then frozen, canned or dried. Although most Southerners are weaned on gruels of grits, others find grits as appealing as library paste. The classic Southern breakfast is fried eggs and country ham plus a hillock of grits puddled with "red-eye," a coffee-spiked gravy made from the ham's skillet drippings. Any leftover grits is spread in a pan, hardened, then cut in squares and browned in butter. Or it's baked, gnocchilike, with sprinklings of cheese.

Groats: Although the dictionary defines *groats* as the broken fragments of whole grains—barley, rye, wheat, etc.—in cooking, it almost always means BUCKWHEAT.

Grouper: A huge family of lean white-fleshed fish numbering four hundred species. Most groupers are huge; indeed, some of them—the jewfish—tip the scales at 700 pounds. Because of their size and because they are most at home in tropical or temperate waters, groupers top the list of fish likely to cause CIGUATERA POISONING. See also FISH, LEAN WHITE.

Grouse, Partridge: A small game bird, lighter-meated than some, but stronger-flavored, too, depending upon diet. The finest grouse—those reserved for the queen's first shoot—are the red grouse of Scotland, which feed upon berries, seeds and shoots. The British have a particular fondness for grouse, especially birds that have been hung until quite "high" (very smelly). The best way to cook young grouse is to grill or roast them simply in a quick oven. One bird will serve one person nicely.

NUTRIENT CONTENT OF 3 OUNCES (85 GRAMS) GRILLED GROUSE	
219 calories	82 mg sodium
26 g protein	326 mg potassium
13 g fat, 4 saturated	0 g dietary fiber
76 mg cholesterol	44 RE vitamin A
0 g carbohydrate	0.03 mg thiamin
40 mg calcium	0.13 mg riboflavin
248 mg phosphorus	5.0 mg niacin
6.5 mg iron	2 mg vitamin C

Gruyère: Switzerland's second most important cheese (after EMMENTALER), Gruyère is made from the raw, whole milk of two breeds of cows (the Fribourg and Simmenthal) that graze flowery Alpine meadows. Curded, pressed, dry salted, molded into wheels about 2 feet across, cured, then aged from for ten months, Gruyère emerges firm but smooth, pale yellow, shot full of holes and with a flavor that's at once sweet and nutty.

NUTRIENT CONTENT OF 1 OUNCE (28 GRAMS) GRUYÈRE CHEESE	
117 calories	95 mg sodium
9 g protein	23 mg potassium
9 g fat, 5 saturated	0 g dietary fiber
31 mg cholesterol	85 RE vitamin A
0 g carbohydrate	0.02 mg thiamin
287 mg calcium	0.08 mg riboflavin
172 mg phosphorus	0 mg niacin
0 mg iron	0 mg vitamin C

Guar Gum (additive): Extracted from the seeds of an East Indian plant, dried and ground to powder, guar has about eight times the thickening power of cornstarch. It's used to stabilize frozen fruits and fruit drinks, to bind everything from dressings to soft drinks to meats to baked goods. It's even a component of pills (it keeps them from disintegrating), laxatives, toothpastes and cosmetics. GRAS if used according to FDA guidelines. What is *not* within FDA guidelines is an over-the-counter guar gum diet pill called Cal-Ban 3000 that has been hawked as a way to lose up to 30 pounds in thirty days. The idea is this: When wet, the pill swells in the stomach—to many times its original size—making you feel full. Unfortunately, it can also swell in the throat, the esophagus, the intestines and do serious harm. In the nine years Cal-Ban 3000 has been on the market, it has caused seventeen throat blockages, ten hospitalizations and one death, albeit indirectly.

Guava: Native to Brazil, this plumlike cousin of cloves, eucalyptus and allspice now grows around the world but mostly—with the exception of the Caribbean, Florida, California, Hawaii, Arizona and India—in the Southern Hemisphere. Most of us know guava as canned nectar or paste although fresh fruits sometimes put in an appearance in fancy food stores. In *Uncommon Fruits & Vegetables,* the definitive work on edible exotics, Elizabeth Schneider writes that guava flesh "may be sweet to sour, may taste like strawberries or pineapple or banana, or all three or none of the above, and may be colored white to yellow to salmon to red." She adds that green fruits smell like a gym, properly ripe ones like "the garden of Eden." Clearly, ripe guavas are the ones to go for. If you should spot plump, sweet-smelling guavas in the store, by all means buy them and try them. They're low in calories and sodium, powerhouses of vitamin C and best when pureed and smoothed into puddings, ice creams and sherbets. **IN-CIDENTAL INTELLIGENCE:** Guava extracts are also used to flavor commercial jellies. **SEASON:** Late spring through early fall.

NUTRIENT CONTENT OF 1 RIPE GUAVA	
(about 3¼ ounces; 90 grams)	
46 calories	3 mg sodium
1 g protein	255 mg potassium
1 g fat, 0 saturated	5 g dietary fiber
0 mg cholesterol	71 RE vitamin A
11 g carbohydrate	0.05 mg thiamin
18 mg calcium	0.05 mg riboflavin
23 mg phosphorus	1.1 mg niacin
0.3 mg iron	165 mg vitamin C

Gum Arabic (additive): This water-soluble gum extracted from acacia trees does many jobs for the food processor. It prevents candies from crystallizing, it enhances the flavor of fruit drinks, smooths ice creams, even stabilizes the foam in ales and beers. **INCIDENTAL INTELLIGENCE:** Gum arabic is also integral to many hair sprays and setting lotions. GRAS.

Gum Ghatti, Ghatti Gum (additive): The stems of an East Indian plant exude a viscous liquid that's invaluable as an emulsifier. If you read the fine print, you'll find ghatti gum in many salad dressings and "butterized" syrups. GRAS when used within FDA limits.

Gum Guaiac (additive): Another important vegetable gum widely used in the food industry. Extracted from the resin of a West Indian wood, gum guaiac is a preservative and antioxidant that helps keep fats and oils from turning rancid. GRAS.

Gum Karaya (additive): As essential to cosmetics and pharmaceuticals as it is to processed foods, gum karaya is the dried sap of an East Indian tree. Mixed with water or alcohol, this particular gum swells, forming a soft, stable gel, a property not lost on frozen-food manufacturers who use it to keep frozen sauces and gravies from breaking down. GRAS.

Gums, Vegetable: Down the years man has learned that certain plant saps, resins and extracts can improve the quality of processed foods. Some come from trees, others from seeds or roots, still others from seaweed. Usually these saps, resins and extracts are dried, then powdered so that when mixed with liquid they swell into viscous gels or gums that don't easily disintegrate. For that reason, vegetable gums are major players in the food industry, serving as thickeners, emulsifiers and stabilizers. The most important of them are discussed in entries beginning with GUM. See also AGAR; CARRAGEENAN; FURCELLARAN; GUAR GUM.

Gum Tragacanth (additive): Indigenous to the Fertile Crescent, the plants that exude this clear, odorless "glue" have been known since the beginning of time. So, too, has the value of their "glue"—early healers used it to blend potions. Today, food manufacturers use gum tragacanth to stabilize and thicken everything from candies and jellies to salad dressings and sherbets. GRAS.

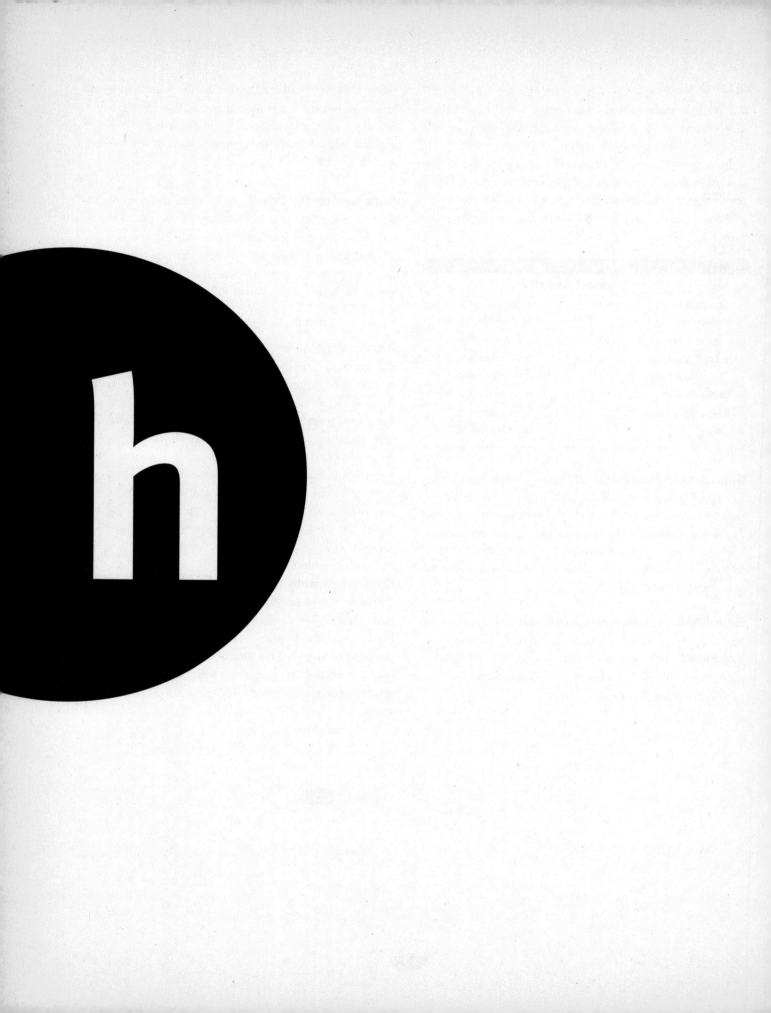

HAAs (Heterocyclic Aromatic Amines): Potentially harmful compounds that form in meats, fish and fowl baked, broiled, fried, grilled or roasted at intense temperatures. HAAs are suspected of being carcinogenic. See also PAHs.

Habaneros: See HOT PEPPERS under PEPPERS, CAPSICUMS.

HACCP (Hazard Analysis and Critical Control Points): A highly scientific, highly effective way of testing the purity and wholesomeness of food—mainly meat, fish and fowl—at a series of checkpoints that's used by many major food purveyors. One of the first was NASA, to ensure the safety of astronaut meals. This technique is expected to be incorporated into—and to improve—current federal methods of food inspection. HACCP's approach is five-pronged: (1) Study the hazards; (2) identify where they occur; (3) tighten controls to eliminate problems or potential problems; (4) monitor all controls; (5) keep meticulous records. See also FOOD SAFETY.

Haddock: Averaging only 2 to 3 pounds apiece, this small first cousin to cod is one of America's biggest sellers. Finer fleshed than cod, more fragile, too, haddock is best when eaten fresh, although plenty of it comes to market frozen. **Finnan haddie** (smoked haddock) originated more than two hundred years ago in Findon, Scotland, where **haddie,** as the Scots call haddock, were split, dried on racks and smoked over peat fires. The making of finnan haddie remained a cottage industry until the nineteenth-century Factory Act threw the business to the more hygienic fish

---

Fish in the Style of the Greek Islands

Makes 4 Servings

Any fillets of lean white fish can be prepared this way as long as they're cut ½ inch thick.

- 4 cod or haddock fillets (6 ounces each), thawed if frozen
- ½ teaspoon salt
- ⅛ teaspoon freshly ground black pepper
- 2 tablespoons olive oil
- 1 medium yellow onion, thinly sliced

- 2 garlic cloves, minced
- 2½ cups chopped low-sodium canned tomatoes
- 2 tablespoons minced fresh parsley
- 2 tablespoons minced fresh mint
- ½ teaspoon dried oregano
- 4 thin lemon slices

PREHEAT OVEN TO 400°F. Sprinkle fish with ¼ teaspoon of the salt and all the pepper. Arrange in a single layer in an ungreased 11 × 7-inch baking dish pretty enough to take to the table; then set aside. Heat olive oil 1 minute in a large, heavy nonstick skillet over moderate heat. Add onion and garlic, and cook, stirring occasionally, until limp and golden, about 7 minutes. Add tomatoes, parsley, mint, oregano, and remaining ¼ teaspoon salt, and cook, stirring occasionally, until sauce is lightly thickened and flavors meld, about 8 minutes. Spoon over fish, top with lemon slices, and bake until fish barely flakes, about 12 minutes. Serve at once.

APPROXIMATE NUTRIENT COUNTS PER SERVING

228 calories	10 g carbohydrate	1.7 mg iron	0.11 mg thiamin
29 g protein	3 g dietary fiber	396 mg sodium	0.12 mg riboflavin
8 g fat, 1 saturated	66 mg calcium	1,008 mg potassium	4.1 mg niacin
55 mg cholesterol	304 mg phosphorus	123 RE vitamin A	33 mg vitamin C

houses of towns like Aberdeen. In the United States, finnan haddie has never become popular outside New England. For approximate nutrient counts, see FISH, LEAN WHITE.

Hair Analysis: Although analysis of hair may be of limited use in determining the general nutritional status of broad segments of the population of a particular area, the send-us-a-sample-of-your-hair-and-we-will-tell-you-what's-wrong-with-you offers are scams. First, your hair grows too slowly to give a true picture of your nutritional health at a given moment. Second, there are no vitamins in your hair (except at the very root) and third, too many external factors affect the mineral content of your hair—the shampoo or dye you use, the comb, even the air you breathe. To test the accuracy of hair analysis, the *Journal of the American Medical Association* sent hair samples from two healthy teenagers to a dozen different laboratories and received wildly divergent results. Most labs cited dire deficiencies of one sort or another, which, they hastened to point out, their vitamin and mineral supplements would correct. Enough said!

Hake: Another popular member of the cod family that's often marketed as **whiting.** Coarser of texture than either cod or haddock, stronger flavored, too, hake is delicious when cooked the Portuguese way—with plenty of onions, garlic and fresh tomatoes. The Portuguese like their *pescada* (hake) small enough to cook whole (1 to 2 pounds) and scoop them up by the thousands in offshore waters. For approximate nutrient counts, see FISH, LEAN WHITE.

Halal: The Islamic term applied to meat animals slaughtered by certified Muslims according to the guidelines set forth by the Koran. See also ISLAMIC DIETARY LAWS.

Half-and-Half: See CREAM.

Halibut: There are many halibuts—**Atlantic, Greenland, California, Pacific**—and all are flatfish of the flounder family. The most abundant is probably the Atlantic halibut, a cold-water, deep-water giant that sometimes weighs an awesome 600 pounds. Although those that come to market are much smaller, they are usually sold as chunks, steaks or fillets. Halibut is white, lean and dense of flesh yet, despite its size, surprisingly delicate. It is also unusually versatile, ideal for broiling, grilling, baking, braising, sautéing, even stewing. And because halibut holds

together when ground, it's perfect for fish dumplings and puddings. For approximate nutrient counts, see FISH, LEAN WHITE.

Halogenated Compounds: To halogenate is to treat or bond an organic compound with a halogen such as chlorine, fluorine, iodine or bromine. Much of the seaweed eaten by Hawaiians and the Japanese contains high levels of halogenated compounds that are believed to be carcinogenic. Studies have shown that Hawaiians have more cancer than any other American ethnic minority; the incidence of liver cancer is particularly high.

Ham: Technically, the hind leg of a hog, cured and/or smoked. But that definition doesn't begin to describe all the different hams available or the nuances of color, texture and flavor. There is, first off, **pink ham,** the mass-produced packing-house special familiar to every American cook.

The choicest American ham, most people would agree, is **Smithfield ham,** which by Virginia statute must be "cut from carcasses of peanut-fed hogs raised in the peanut belt of the State of Virginia or the State of North Carolina, and cured, treated, smoked and processed in the town of Smithfield in the State of Virginia." Smithfield ham is known for firm flesh the color of mahogany and for a deep smoky-salty flavor. Although some ready-to-eat Smithfield hams are now being sold, no proper Southern cook would dream of shortcutting the soaking/simmering process.

Virginia ham is not quite the same because it isn't "cured, treated, smoked and processed in the town of Smithfield." But only connoisseurs can tell the two apart. Kentucky and Vermont have their own methods of curing and aging hams, as indeed does North Carolina.

As for European hams, the finest are the French **Bayonne,** the German **Black Forest** and **Westphalian,** the English **York,** the **Irish,** the Italian **prosciutto,** the Spanish **serrano** and the Portuguese **presunto.** Their color, texture and flavor vary according to how the hogs were fed and how the hams were cured or smoked and aged.

The trouble with most hams, both the domestic and the imported, is that they are extremely high in sodium—bad news for anyone keeping an eye on his blood pressure. They are also apt to have been cured with sodium nitrate or nitrite, which not only gives hams their bright rosy color but also discourages the growth of *C. botulinum,* the bacterial cause of botulism, a deadly form of food poisoning.

Unfortunately, with improper cooking at intense heat nitrites can be converted into NITROSAMINES, particularly powerful carcinogens.

Meat packers, responding to the bad press on the nitrates and nitrites in hams, bacons and other cured meats, have begun using much less of them and sometimes none at all. To help guard against botulism, they've been adding sodium ascorbate, which also injects a healthy dose of vitamin C. This doesn't make hams health food, however, so they should be eaten in moderation.

NUTRIENT CONTENT OF 3 OUNCES (85 GRAMS) SLICED REGULAR BOILED HAM

(about 11 percent fat)

155 calories	1,119 mg sodium
15 g protein	282 mg potassium
9 g fat, 3 saturated	0 g dietary fiber
49 mg cholesterol	0 RE vitamin A
3 g carbohydrate	0.73 mg thiamin
6 mg calcium	0.22 mg riboflavin
210 mg phosphorus	4.5 mg niacin
0.9 mg iron	24 mg vitamin C

NUTRIENT CONTENT OF 3 OUNCES (85 GRAMS) EXTRA-LEAN SLICED BOILED HAM

(about 5 percent fat)

111 calories	1,215 mg sodium
16 g protein	297 mg potassium
4 g fat, 1 saturated	0 g dietary fiber
40 mg cholesterol	0 RE vitamin A
1 g carbohydrate	0.79 mg thiamin
6 mg calcium	0.19 mg riboflavin
186 mg phosphorus	4.1 mg niacin
0.6 mg iron	22 mg vitamin C

Hamburger: A catchall term for ground beef. What supermarkets label "hamburger" is usually composed of ground scraps and trimmings of different beef cuts and often these are 30 percent fat, much of it saturated. **TIP:** The paler the meat or the more heavily flecked with white, the fatter it is. **Ground chuck,** depending on how carefully it's trimmed, may be somewhat less fatty (20 to 25 percent). If lean ground beef is what you're after, go for **ground sirloin** or, better yet, **ground round** (17 percent fat or, if sharply trimmed, 15 percent). Today many butchers and

supermarkets mark fat percentages on packages of ground beef (15 percent fat, for example) or note the percentage of lean (85 percent), leaving the arithmetic to you. Alas, fat is what makes hamburgers so flavorful and juicy. Ground round makes a dry burger, although mixing in finely chopped onion, garlic and/or celery, even a bit of beef broth and a few soft bread crumbs to bind everything together will create the illusion of succulence.

Hamburgers have hit the headlines recently because major outbreaks of E. coli food poisoning in the northwest and northeast have been traced to contaminated ground meat. In the northwest the "bugged" burgers were those served by a fast-food chain. But in upstate New York, sixteen teenagers got sick on home-cooked burgers. The culprit? Supermarket ground beef processed in a single plant. The reason hamburger—make that all ground meat—presents such a problem is that it may come not only from different parts of one animal but from several animals. One bad bit can contaminate a huge batch because all the trimmings that go into ground meat are so thoroughly mixed as they're ground.

Though federal meat inspectors have promised to heighten their vigilance, microbiologists agree that their present "see, touch, smell" technique is useless when it comes to detecting E. coli. There is pressure for the USDA to develop a vaccine that will keep meat animals free of E. coli; pressure, too, for all ground meat to be irradiated before it's sold, which will certainly eliminate any harmful bacteria. But that in itself is highly controversial (see IRRADIATION).

Meanwhile, the USDA is mounting a publicity campaign to teach every consumer (and that includes schoolchildren and the elderly, those most susceptible to E. coli illness) not only how to handle raw ground meat but also how to recognize a "safe" burger. In addition to posting safe-handling instructions on all packages of ground meat, the USDA is spreading the word via open letters, press releases and classroom demos. Here are the safety guidelines it recommends for ground meat:

1. Refrigerate or freeze ground meat the minute you get home from the store.
2. Thaw ground meat in the refrigerator, never on the counter. And never leave any raw meat at room temperature for more than two hours.
3. Wash your hands, cutting boards, counters, knives and other utensils in hot sudsy water after handling raw meat to keep bacteria from spreading.

4. Check all cooked hamburgers with a fork before tasting—both at home and in a restaurant. To be safe, they must be brown in the middle (160°F.). And their juices must run clear, not red, not pink.

5. Never serve burgers on an unwashed platter that held raw meat, poultry or fish.

6. When eating out, send all undercooked meat back to the kitchen before tasting and demand that it be cooked well done.

NUTRIENT CONTENT OF 3 OUNCES (85 GRAMS) BROILED (WELL-DONE) EXTRA-LEAN HAMBURGER

(about 17 percent fat)

225 calories	70 mg sodium
25 g protein	314 mg potassium
14 g fat, 5 saturated	0 g dietary fiber
84 mg cholesterol	0 RE vitamin A
0 g carbohydrate	0.06 mg thiamin
8 mg calcium	0.21 mg riboflavin
161 mg phosphorus	5.0 mg niacin
2.4 mg iron	0 mg vitamin C

NUTRIENT CONTENT OF 3 OUNCES (85 GRAMS) BROILED (WELL-DONE) LEAN HAMBURGER

(about 21 percent fat)

238 calories	76 mg sodium
24 g protein	297 mg potassium
15 g fat, 6 saturated	0 g dietary fiber
86 mg cholesterol	0 RE vitamin A
0 g carbohydrate	0.05 mg thiamin
10 mg calcium	0.20 mg riboflavin
155 mg phosphorus	5.1 mg niacin
2.1 mg iron	0 mg vitamin C

NUTRIENT CONTENT OF 3 OUNCES (85 GRAMS) BROILED REGULAR (WELL-DONE) HAMBURGER

(about 27 percent fat)

243 calories	51 mg sodium
20 g protein	187 mg potassium
18 g fat, 7 saturated	0 g dietary fiber
74 mg cholesterol	0 RE vitamin A
0 g carbohydrate	0.03 mg thiamin
9 mg calcium	0.14 mg riboflavin
116 mg phosphorus	4.0 mg niacin
2.1 mg iron	0 mg vitamin C

Hangover: There are no magic cures, no ways to shake off the effects of a night on the town, or even, alas, to speed recovery. The body can rid itself of alcohol only at its own pace (an average-size man needs two hours to metabolize one drink). Prevention is definitely the best medicine. Never, for example, drink on an empty stomach. Take highballs instead of on-the-rocks drinks and use plain water or fruit juices as mixers, not "bubblies," which send alcohol into the bloodstream and to the brain faster. Pace yourself, nursing a drink as long as possible or alternating drinks with plain water or fruit juice. Finally, choose your tipple carefully. Brandy causes the worst hangovers, then red wine, rum, whiskey, white wine, gin and vodka—in that order. The drinks at the top of the list are loaded with congeners, by-products of fermentation and distillation that exacerbate the effects of alcohol.

Hard Swell Spoilage: Hydrogen buildup inside a can is what makes its ends bulge and the cause may be either chemical (an acid food reacting with the metal of the can, for example) or bacteriological (due to a faulty can or canning methods). Whatever the reason, discard any bulging cans, depositing them where neither people nor animals will find them.

Hare: A large, long-eared, furry rodent similar to the RABBIT but of a different genus. Hares have dark meat; rabbits white meat.

Haricot Beans: See GREEN BEANS under BEANS, FRESH.

Hazard Analysis and Critical Control Points: See HACCP.

Hazelnut Oil: A particularly mellow amber oil that's good for dressing salads, for shortening cakes and cookies (when substituted for about a fourth of the butter or shortening called for), for flavoring pastries and fillings. Specific nutrient counts are unavailable, but it's safe to say that hazelnut oil is cholesterol free and contains about the same number of calories (120 per tablespoon) as other vegetable oils. It's also very low in saturated fatty acids.

Hazelnuts, Filberts: These sweet, round, brown-skinned nuts are believed to be older than man (but who can say for sure?). What is known is that they originated somewhere in Asia (or Middle Asia) and that they've been popular since the Stone Age (among the Swiss Lake Dwellers, they were second only to acorns). Pastry cooks have always prized hazelnuts for cakes, cookies and candies and love to team them with chocolate. Their flavor is elusive. Some liken it to browned butter (in French, *noisette* means both "browned butter" and "hazelnut"). Others say hazelnuts taste like morels with hints of truffle. Not bad. Today chopped toasted hazelnuts are trendy among American chefs, who sprinkle them into salads, fold them into scones and shortbreads or use them as breading for fillets of turkey, veal or salmon. There's no end to the possibilities. Most of this country's commercial crop comes from the Pacific Northwest but wild hazelnuts grow across much of America. **TIP:** To skin hazelnuts, spread the nuts in a pie tin and toast 25 to 30 minutes in a 350°F. oven. Cool 10 minutes, bundle in a clean dish towel and rub hard to remove the skins. Don't worry about any recalcitrant bits. They'll add color.

NUTRIENT CONTENT OF 1 OUNCE (28 GRAMS) HAZELNUTS

179 calories	1 mg sodium
4 g protein	126 mg potassium
18 g fat, 1 saturated	2 g dietary fiber
0 mg cholesterol	2 RE vitamin A
4 g carbohydrate	0.14 mg thiamin
53 mg calcium	0.03 mg riboflavin
88 mg phosphorus	0.3 mg niacin
0.9 mg iron	0 mg vitamin C

HDL: The abbreviation for high-density lipoprotein, or the so-called "good" cholesterol, which helps prevent the buildup of arterial plaque by decreasing the amount of LDL, or "bad" cholesterol, in the blood.

Headaches (diet and): We're not talking about the intense fleeting pain that comes from eating ice cream too fast, but about full-blown migraines. In a recent British study of migraine-prone children, 93 percent became headache free when put on an elimination diet (one free of suspect foods). There were more than fifty foods on the "guilty" list, with cow's milk, eggs, chocolate, oranges and wheat (but *not* highly refined wheat flours) being the major culprits. Additional troublemakers: cheese, tomatoes and rye. The study also showed that children crave the very foods that cause them pain.

Other substances may sometimes bring on headaches, too (although not necessarily migraines): TYRAMINE (an amino acid found in overripe avocados and bananas, also in aged cheeses, chicken livers, fava beans and red wines like Chianti); the sugar substitute ASPARTAME (sold as Equal or NutraSweet); MONOSODIUM GLUTAMATE (MSG, a flavor enhancer beloved by Asian chefs); sodium nitrites (preservatives found in bacon, hot dogs, ham and other cured meats); CONGENERS (by-products of fermentation and distillation found in brandy, rum, Scotch and other whiskeys).

Then there's CAFFEINE, specifically caffeine withdrawal. Heavy coffee, tea and/or cola drinkers sometimes suffer weekend headaches because they're getting far less caffeine than they do during the workweek.

All of this said, most researchers believe that headaches are more likely to be induced by stress or emotional problems than by food allergies, intolerances or sensitivities. Especially among adults. See also ALLERGY; ELIMINATION DIET.

Headcheese: A gelatinous, coarsely textured loaf made of the odds and ends of pork (or other meat). Originally parts of the head were used (and still are in many parts of the Deep South). Headcheese is sliced and eaten cold. The British call it **brawn.**

NUTRIENT CONTENT OF 1 OUNCE (28 GRAMS) HEADCHEESE

60 calories	356 mg sodium
5 g protein	9 mg potassium
5 g fat, 1 saturated	0 g dietary fiber
23 mg cholesterol	0 RE vitamin A
0 g carbohydrate	0.01 mg thiamin
5 mg calcium	0.05 mg riboflavin
17 mg phosphorus	0.3 mg niacin
0.3 mg iron	6 mg vitamin C*

*From the sodium ascorbate added during processing.

Head Start: A federal aid program begun in the mid-1960s to give poverty-line preschoolers a leg up before entering the first grade. Meals prepared by Head Start centers are as integral to the program as is mental and physical development.

Healing Process (and diet): Persons deficient in certain nutrients—vitamin C and zinc, for example—may not heal from injuries or surgery as fast as persons with no nutritional deficit. Ironically, you can't speed healing by taking vitamin C and/or zinc supplements.

Health and Human Services, U.S. Department of (USDHHS):

This huge arm of the government advises the president on national matters of health, on welfare and Social Security (from the cradle to the grave). Among its units directly concerned with health and nutrition are the Administration on Aging (AOA), the Administration for Children, Youth and Families (ACYF), the Administration for Native Americans (ANA), the Centers for Disease Control (CDC), the Food and Drug Administration (FDA), the Public Health Service (PHS), the National Institutes of Health (NIH), which include the National Cancer Institute (NCI) and the National Heart, Lung and Blood Institute (NHLBI). Also under its broad umbrella are the Alcohol, Drug Abuse and Mental Health Administration and the President's Council on Physical Fitness and Sports.

Health Foods:

If ever the buyer should beware, it's in the matter of health foods, a multibillion-dollar business that too often preys on the elderly and infirm, guaranteeing quick fixes for everything that ails them. Even healthy persons sometimes fall for "magic" pills, potions and powders that promise the impossible—dramatic weight loss, greater sexual prowess, eternal youth. It's the old-medicine-man-gone-modern with a slick vocabulary of pseudoscientific mumbo jumbo. No matter how convincing his claims, just remember that there is no legal definition of *health food*. See also FOOD FADS; ORGANIC FOODS.

"Healthy":

In order for a food to be labeled "healthy," no serving can contain more than 3 grams fat (1 gram saturated), 60 milligrams cholesterol and 480 milligrams sodium. This, of course, would apply to many candies, so the requirements also stipulate that "healthy" food must supply at least 10 percent of the Daily Value for vitamin A, vitamin C, calcium, fiber or protein. See also FOOD LABELING.

Heart (as food):

Americans have always been squeamish about eating certain organ meats and heart is one of them. Too bad, because it's economical and fairly nutritious. NOTE: Because heart is loaded with cholesterol, the American Heart Association lists it among the foods to avoid for those at risk of coronary heart disease. Heart isn't difficult to cook, but being highly muscular, it requires long, slow simmering if it's to be tender enough to enjoy. Or it can be ground, combined with minced onion and parsley and oatmeal, shaped into patties and browned like burgers (a Scottish favorite). The tenderest, most delicately flavored hearts come from young lamb or veal.

NUTRIENT CONTENT OF 3 OUNCES (85 GRAMS) SIMMERED BEEF HEART	
148 calories	54 mg sodium
22 g protein	198 mg potassium
5 g fat, 1 saturated	0 g dietary fiber
164 mg cholesterol	0 RE vitamin A
0 g carbohydrate	0.12 mg thiamin
5 mg calcium	1.31 mg riboflavin
212 mg phosphorus	3.5 mg niacin
6.4 mg iron	1 mg vitamin C

Heartburn:

See ESOPHAGITIS.

Heart Health (diet and):

The one message the government seems to have hammered through to the American public: "Cut down on fat. . . . Cut down on fat. . . . Cut down on fat." Most of us now know that no more than 30 percent of the day's calories should come from fat, and no more than 10 percent of the total from saturated fat. We also know we should cut down on cholesterol. So we're eating fewer eggs, cooking with vegetable oils instead of lard, butter and solid shortening, trimming our steaks more closely and insisting on extra-lean hamburger. But this is only part of an extremely complicated picture.

Coronary heart disease (CHD) remains America's number-one killer and many of us, it seems, are quite literally "digging our graves with our teeth." But according to the American Heart Association (AHA), it's never too late to switch from bad eating habits to good. Toward that end, it has drawn up *The American Heart Association Diet: An Eating Plan for Healthy Americans,* copies of which are available through local chapters of the AHA, also through many physicians, public health services and hospitals that provide special consumer education courses.

To summarize as briefly as possible, the AHA Diet divides the daily menu into six major food groups, suggests number of servings, then lists foods within each group to avoid:

1. Meat, poultry and fish (for complete protein, B-complex, iron and other minerals): two 3-ounce servings per day (no more) of fat-trimmed lean meat, poultry (without skin) or fish. Limit high-cholesterol organ meats to one 3-ounce serving per month. **BEST CHOICE:** Liver, with its high-iron bonus.

2. Eggs (for complete protein, B-complex, iron and other minerals): unlimited egg whites but no more than 3 to 4 yolks per week.

3. Vegetables and fruits (for vitamins, minerals, fiber): five or more servings per day, either cooked or raw. A serving may be a medium-size fruit, ½ cup fruit juice or ½ to 1 cup cooked or raw vegetable. Olives and avocados count as fat, below, and starchy vegetables are grouped with breads and cereals. **NO-NO:** Coconut; it's full of saturated fat.

4. Milk products (for complete protein, calcium, phosphorus, niacin, riboflavin, vitamins A and D): Children two to ten and adults from twenty-five onward should get two servings per day. Pregnant women, nursing mothers and those aged eleven through twenty-four should get three to four servings a day. And what exactly is a serving? It may be 1 cup (8 ounces) skim or low-fat (1 percent) milk, 1 cup nonfat or low-fat yogurt, 1 ounce low-fat cheese or ½ cup low-fat cottage cheese.

5. Breads, cereals, pasta and starchy vegetables (for fiber, iron and B vitamins): six or more servings per day; for example, 1 cup dry cereal (flakes) or cooked rice or pasta; ½ cup cooked cereal; ½ to ¼ cup starchy vegetable; ¼ cup dry granular cereal; 1 slice bread or 1 roll or English muffin or pita bread.

6. Fats and oils (for vitamins A and/or E): depending on calorie needs, five to eight servings per day, no more. What constitutes a serving? 1 teaspoon vegetable oil or regular margarine; 2 teaspoons diet margarine, mayonnaise or peanut butter; 1 tablespoon salad dressing, seeds or nuts; 5 large olives (or 10 small); ⅛ medium-size avocado.

It is also wise to avoid highly salty foods, to use salt sparingly and, if you drink, to do so in moderation (that means no more than two drinks a day, be they beer, wine *or* whiskey).

There's been a flurry of interest recently about the power of certain nutrients—notably folic acid, vitamin B_6 and such antioxidants as beta-carotene, vitamins C and E—to reduce the risk of heart disease. Research is intensive and ongoing, and although some of the scientists involved in these very studies take vitamin supplements "just in case," they aren't willing to recommend them to others. There are plenty of promising data about the role of these nutrients in promoting good health, most recently the role

of folic acid (and possibly vitamin B_6) in lowering blood levels of the amino acid HOMOCYSTEINE. If it builds up in the blood, blood vessels may be damaged, leading, some medical researchers believe, to hardening of the arteries and also perhaps to heart attacks or strokes.

Hearts of Palm: The tender young shoots of the cabbage palm or palmetto, stripped of their fibrous outer sheath. Hearts of palm, like leeks, are chunky, many-layered stalks as pale as ivory. Unlike leeks, they have little flavor other than the faintest suggestion of nuts. The only hearts of palm widely available are the canned, both whole or sliced. Either way, they are best in tartly dressed salads. Notwithstanding their anemic color, hearts of palm are deceptively rich in iron, phosphorus and potassium. At the same time, they are extremely low in sodium and contain zero fat and cholesterol.

NUTRIENT CONTENT OF 3 OUNCES (85 GRAMS) SLICED COOKED OR CANNED HEARTS OF PALM	
87 calories	12 mg sodium
2 g protein	1,536 mg potassium
0 g fat, 0 saturated	1 g dietary fiber
0 mg cholesterol	6 RE vitamin A
23 g carbohydrate	0.04 mg thiamin
15 mg calcium	0.15 mg riboflavin
119 mg phosphorus	0.7 mg niacin
1.4 mg iron	6 mg vitamin C

Heat (effect on vitamins): Improper cooking can destroy three important vitamins—C, thiamin (B_1) and folic acid, another member of the B-complex. For maximum vitamin content, use fresh or frozen vegetables instead of canned (the heat of processing has already destroyed some of the vitamins), then (1) cook quickly in a minimum of water in a covered pan; (2) steam in a vegetable steamer; (3) stir-fry; or (4) microwave (you may need no additional liquid because the rinse water clinging to the vegetable is sufficient). Finally, serve vegetables the minute they're done. Those that languish at the back of the stove suffer even more vitamin loss.

Heavy-Metal Toxicity: We're alarmed by reports of mercury in fish, of lead in canned foods, of arsenic in drinking water. But these are only three of the heavy metals that may find their way into our food and drink and cause serious bodily harm, even death, if ingested in large quantities. These toxic chemicals are becoming an increasing problem because of their industrial use. From A to Z, they are:

Aluminum: It not only goes into cookware, deodorants, antacids and other medications but is also used to process certain foods and purify water. **POTENTIAL DAMAGE OF TOXIC LEVELS:** Brain and spinal cord disease, skeletal aches. Aluminum also binds (renders unavailable) phosphate, a salt of phosphoric acid, which is essential to the body.

Antimony: A hardener for lead, antimony shows up most often in batteries. **POTENTIAL DAMAGE OF TOXIC LEVELS:** Lung disease and possibly skin cancer. Smokers are at the greatest risk.

Arsenic: Once used to treat syphilis, arsenic is still integral to many pesticides and its gaseous form, arsine, is sometimes released into the air from sewage treatment plants. **POTENTIAL DAMAGE OF TOXIC LEVELS:** Impaired kidney and brain function, cancer.

Bismuth: An ingredient in many medications (for treating everything from ear infections to hemorrhoids to stomach disorders). **POTENTIAL DAMAGE OF TOXIC LEVELS:** Anorexia, headaches, rashes, neurological disorders, impaired kidney function, ulcers of the stomach, mouth and lips.

Cadmium: Used in batteries and in electroplating. **POTENTIAL DAMAGE OF TOXIC LEVELS:** Anemia, fatigue, headache, emphysema, kidney failure, faulty mineral metabolism.

Chromium: Used in plumbing fixtures, fancy automobile trims. **POTENTIAL DAMAGE OF TOXIC LEVELS:** Kidney damage, lung or other respiratory tract cancer. **NOTE:** One of the heavy metals essential to good health; the body can't manufacture chromium and depends on outside sources for the minute amount it needs.

Cobalt: Used in paints and glazes, also to treat cancer. **POTENTIAL DAMAGE OF TOXIC LEVELS:** Anorexia, nausea and vomiting, goiter, heart, nerve or kidney damage. **NOTE:** One of the heavy metals essential to good health (it's a component of vitamin B_{12}). The body can't manufacture cobalt and depends on outside sources for the traces it needs.

Copper: Pipes are made of it, also wires, pots and pans and oh, so many other items we have around the house. **POTENTIAL DAMAGE OF TOXIC LEVELS:** Blood disorders and flulike symptoms. **NOTE:** Copper is another of the trace elements the body needs for good health but cannot manufacture.

Gold: It is everywhere around us—in our jewelry, our teeth—and most of us would like more of it. But too much of it in the body is bad, something rheumatoid arthritics being treated with gold salts should be especially aware of. **POTENTIAL DAMAGE OF TOXIC LEVELS:** Headache, vomiting, stomach and intestinal bleeding, jaundice, skin rashes, depressed bone marrow activity.

Lead: Ever since leaded gasolines, lead solder and lead paints were phased out, the rate of lead poisoning in this country has dropped by about a third. And according to the CDC, the number of Americans with elevated lead levels has plummeted more than 70 percent since the late 1970s. Still, there's no lack of lead in our lives. Old house paints are loaded with it and those most apt to suffer lead poisoning are children who eat the paint slaking off walls of antiquated apartments and houses. Recent surveys show that more than two million American children now suffer from chronic lead poisoning, which apes many of the symptoms of ATTENTION DEFICIT HYPERACTIVITY DISORDER (ADHD): inability to concentrate, impulsive behavior. To exacerbate the problem, lead has been showing up in crayons imported from China. The government now tests every shipment at point of entry and has ordered massive recalls. It can't stop children from chewing crayons but it does aim to keep all lead-based colors out of the country.

Some years back, the problem was lead-based pottery glazes and American tourists bringing home potentially dangerous pots and place settings from Mexico and elsewhere. The solution then was to drill holes in the bottoms of all leaded pottery to prevent its use with food. **ALSO HAZARDOUS:** Lead pipes (many old houses have them), old pewter, the metal wrappers atop wine bottles, the solder in imported cans of food (tomatoes, tomato sauces and pastes are especially hazardous because their acid erodes lead).

Lead is still integral to the making of fine crystal but the alarm has been sounded. Unfortunately, lead leaches into food and drink and that plus industrial contamination of soil and water can mean lead poisoning.

There's another source of lead poisoning, too: dolomite and bonemeal taken as calcium supplements. In the 1980s, the FDA assayed samples of both and found excess levels of lead. As a result, it warned physicians to discourage the use of these two "natural" calcium supplements, especially for babies, children, pregnant women and nursing mothers. **THE LESSONS HERE:** Never store wine or whiskey in lead-crystal decanters; never use pewter, lead-glazed china or pottery for storing, cooking or serving food; avoid dolomite and bonemeal supplements. And most of all, buyer beware. **NOTE:** To learn how to have your tap water tested for lead or, for that matter, any suspicious ceramics or metal, contact your local health department or Environmental Protection Agency office.

Lithium: Its prime use is in stabilizing the mood swings of manic-depressives. **POTENTIAL DAMAGE OF TOXIC LEVELS:** Diseases of the stomach and digestive tract, the kidneys and the central nervous system.

Manganese: This metal is used in the manufacture of other metals. **POTENTIAL DAMAGE OF TOXIC LEVELS:** "Silly giggles" (honest!), pneumonia, damage to the central nervous system. **NOTE:** Manganese is another of the trace elements the body needs for good health but cannot manufacture.

Mercury: It goes into thermometers of all types, but it's also used by the ton in major manufacturing. Mercury, especially the highly dangerous methylmercury, has been a major polluter of rivers and streams. **POTENTIAL DAMAGE OF TOXIC LEVELS:** Hot tempers, extreme excitability, inability to concentrate, memory loss and permanent brain damage, headache, fatigue, muscular weakness, digestive upsets, dehydration, kidney damage.

Molybdenum: Integral to the hardening of steel. **POTENTIAL DAMAGE OF TOXIC LEVELS:** It depletes the body's supply of copper, minute amounts of which are essential to good health. **NOTE:** Here again is a heavy metal that the body needs as a trace element yet is unable to synthesize.

Nickel: Nickels don't contain much nickel anymore, but the metal is used in electroplating and in the manufacture of alloys. In a recent series of weekly analyses of the Mississippi done by a New Orleans lab, the Greenpeace environmental watchdog group reported that 732,973 pounds of nickel were dumped into the river in a single year (along with plenty of aluminum, cadmium, chromium and copper). **POTENTIAL DAMAGE OF TOXIC LEVELS:** Damage to the central nervous system; also assorted respiratory diseases and that includes cancer. **NOTE:** One of the heavy metals essential to good health; the body can't manufacture nickel and depends on outside sources for the traces it needs.

Silver: We eat with it, we wear it and our burns are sometimes treated with it. **POTENTIAL DAMAGE OF TOXIC LEVELS:** Nausea, vomiting, diarrhea, also a condition called argyria, which is a silvery gray cast to the skin and hair.

Vanadium: This silvery gray metal is used primarily to harden steel. **POTENTIAL DAMAGE OF TOXIC LEVELS:** Throat and nasal irritation, acute bronchitis accompanied by a racking cough, anorexia. **NOTE:** Vanadium is another of the heavy metals essential to good health; the body can't manufacture it and depends on outside sources for the traces it needs.

Zinc: It's used in galvanizing iron, in such alloys as brass, and in many medications. **POTENTIAL DAMAGE OF TOXIC LEVELS:** Digestive disturbances, impaired liver function and flulike symptoms known collectively as metal fume disease. **NOTE:** Here again is a heavy metal that the body needs as a trace element yet is unable to synthesize.

Fortunately, most cases of heavy-metal poisoning are treatable, but they require immediate medical assistance.

Hematocrit: The volume ratio of blood cells to plasma. Whenever there's fluid loss without cell loss, the hematocrit is high. On the other hand, hemorrhage and anemia can thin the blood, producing a low hematocrit. Hematocrit readings are a way to diagnose anemia.

Heme: The iron-rich component of hemoglobin that absorbs oxygen from the blood and carries it to the cells.

Heme Iron: A form of iron found in meat and poultry that's more easily and completely absorbed by the body than the nonheme iron in plant foods.

Hemicelluloses: Polysaccharides (complex carbohydrates) enmeshed in plant cellulose. They absorb water, increase stool bulk and are broken down by microbial action in the colon. Think of them as dietary fiber.

Hemochromatosis: A bronzy cast to the skin caused by faulty iron metabolism and subsequent buildup of iron in the body. More serious problems associated with hemochromatosis are diabetes (called bronzed diabetes) and liver and pancreas damage. The condition may be inherited; indeed, some million Americans suffer from an intestinal defect that makes them absorb far more iron than the average person (the excess is usually deposited in the bone marrow, liver, spleen and other organs). Some reserve of iron is good, but too much of it can be devastating, even deadly. Good ways to avoid iron overload are to donate blood regularly and to avoid iron-rich foods.

Hemoglobin: The principal protein in red blood cells and the one with the highest concentration of iron (one molecule of hemoglobin can piggyback four molecules of iron). Hemoglobin's job is to absorb oxygen and ferry it to cells throughout the body, then to pick up and remove carbon dioxide. A normal hemoglobin count for men is 14 to 18 percent (14 to 18 grams per 100 milliliters of blood); for women, 12 to 16 percent; for children, 12 to 14 percent; and for newborns, 14½ to 24½ percent.

Hemorrhoids (diet and): Also called **piles,** these are varicose veins of the rectum. Those occurring below the anal sphincter are classified as **external,** those above it **internal.** Toward the end of their pregnancies, many women become constipated and, in straining to evacuate, develop hemorrhoids. Eating high-fiber foods and drinking plenty of liquid will help most hemorrhoid sufferers because they soften the stool, making bowel movements less difficult and painful.

Hen: See CHICKEN.

Hepatitis: Travelers to the Third World should take every precaution to avoid hepatitis A and E, two food- and waterborne diseases characterized by serious inflammation of the liver. Both are caused by viruses and are rampant in areas of poor sanitation. Gamma globulin shots are short-lived, but a more effective hepatitis A vaccine, already in use abroad, has at long last been given FDA approval for use in the United States. When the full course of shots is taken, immunity to hepatitis A lasts ten years. **VIRAL SOURCE:** Feces of infected persons, which can contaminate water and crops in the field. The viruses can also be carried on the hands, tainting food, beverages and kitchen utensils. **SYMPTOMS OF HEPATITIS:** Nausea, vomiting, fever, headache and the sort of general malaise usually associated with flu; then, as the disease progresses, light stools, dark urine and jaundice. **HOW SOON SYMPTOMS OCCUR:** Unfortunately, it takes about six weeks, but if you've been traveling in developing countries and suspect you may have hepatitis, see your doctor at once. **PREVENTIVES:** Drink bottled water only (veteran travelers insist on carbonated water, which is less likely to have been tampered with) and take all drinks neat (without ice). Pass on all raw shellfish (no oysters or clams on the half shell), all raw vegetables, and eat only thick-skinned fruits that you peel yourself. Insist that all meats, fish and fowl be cooked well done, and avoid buffet spreads like the plague (many of them have languished under the sun—or in hot rooms—for hours).

Herbal Teas: See TEA.

Herbicides, Pesticides: Farmers insist they need them; environmentalists say they're poisoning our food and water, the very air we breathe. Both are right. The use of herbicides, pesticides and, yes, fertilizers, too, has become a catch-22 of global significance. **FACT:** According to USDA estimates, weeds destroy 12 percent of the U.S. agricultural crop (a loss of $12 billion) despite the fact that another $18 billion is spent to eradicate them. **FACT:** Much of the broccoli we eat contains 100 times the amount of pesticide needed to produce it, all because we demand picture-perfect vegetables. How have we gotten ourselves into this mess? And is there any solution? The greatest culprits appear to be specialization (one- or two-crop farms that quickly deplete the soil) and high-tech agribusiness.

This corporate takeover of vast swatches of farmland means that eyes are firmly fixed on the bottom line. The goal of agribusiness: greater production, greater production, greater production at whatever cost to the environment. Even government subsidies (for herbicides, pesticides, fertilizers, etc.) have favored agribusiness over small independent farmers, often driving them out of business because they can't compete, pricewise, with the agricultural giants.

After intensive study, the National Research Council (NRC) of the National Academy of Sciences recently reported that agricultural runoff is this country's major polluter of surface water. The NRC also concluded that if we are to survive over the long haul, we must change our methods of farming. "Alternative Agriculture," which sounds very much like "the good old days," the way our great-grandfathers farmed, is what the NRC advocates. In a word, *diversification,* which can mean less reliance on herbicides, pesticides and fertilizers. Federal policies, the council points out, must change to favor diversification, and an all-out effort must be made to teach farmers how to grow a variety of crops successfully.

Still, diversification alone won't solve the problem. Population growth must be strictly controlled—on a global scale. And Americans must learn to eat foods nearer the bottom of the food chain—for example, grains, fruits and vegetables instead of meats, which cost us—and the earth—dear. As it is, meat animals eat ten times the grain that we do. Our appetite for meat means vast acreages must be devoted to fodder, not to mention tons of herbicides, pesticides, fertilizers, even fuel (tractors don't run on air).

Herbs:
The great advantage of herbs is that a judicious use of them makes it possible to cut down on salt and, yes, even fat, because their pungency does so much to enrich sweets and savories without upping the calories, cholesterol or fat. No home arsenal of herbs should be without basil, bay leaves, coriander, cumin, dill, marjoram, oregano, rosemary, sage and thyme. Needless to add, fresh herbs are preferable to dried.

Heredity:
Genes predispose us to certain illnesses (diabetes, heart disease and cancer, to name three) as well as a few metabolic disorders like phenylketonuria (PKU), an inability of the body to metabolize phenylalanine, an amino acid. But do they also program us to be fat or thin? The old saying that a man can tell what his fiancée will look like twenty or thirty years down the line by looking at her mother isn't far off the mark. The rate at which we burn calories, it seems, *is* inherited. So if both parents were fat, chances are you will be, too. But if only one parent was overweight, your chances of being heavy plummet to 40 percent. By eating wisely and in moderation, you may be able to lower the odds further still, not only for obesity

but for other inherited illnesses as well. Good nutrition is the key to lowering your risk of disease and to maximizing the good in your genetic makeup. See also FOOD GUIDE PYRAMID; HEART HEALTH.

Hero Sandwiches:
Also called **submarines, hoagies, bombers** and **grinders,** these rib-sticking sandwiches—chunks of Italian or French bread piled high with an assortment of meats, cheeses, roasted peppers, condiments and lettuces—have become almost as popular as pizza. And like pizza, most of them are freighted with fat, calories and cholesterol. As Clementine Paddleford, food editor of the old *New York Herald Tribune,* once observed, "You have to be a hero to eat such a sandwich." **NOTE:** Because the composition of heroes varies so, giving an accurate nutrient count is impossible.

Herring:
These oily little fish, which have nourished nations for thousands of years, were responsible for the rise and fall of the Hanseatic League, and even today they remain king throughout most of northern Europe. There herring are salted, cured, smoked or pickled according to time-honored methods. They are also, for the most part,

NUTRIENT CONTENT OF 1 KIPPERED HERRING FILLET	
(about 1½ ounces; 40 grams)	
87 calories	367 mg sodium
10 g protein	179 mg potassium
5 g fat, 1 saturated	0 g dietary fiber
33 mg cholesterol	16 RE vitamin A
0 g carbohydrate	0.05 mg thiamin
33 mg calcium	0.13 mg riboflavin
130 mg phosphorus	1.8 mg niacin
0.6 mg iron	0 mg vitamin C

NUTRIENT CONTENT OF 1 PIECE PICKLED HERRING	
(about ½ ounce; 15 grams)	
39 calories	131 mg sodium
2 g protein	10 mg potassium
3 g fat, 0 saturated	0 g dietary fiber
2 mg cholesterol	39 RE vitamin A
2 g carbohydrate	0.01 mg thiamin
12 mg calcium	0.02 mg riboflavin
13 mg phosphorus	0.5 mg niacin
0.2 mg iron	0 mg vitamin C

eaten cold, usually as an appetizer or in salads (Germans also swear that nothing cures a hangover quicker than herring). **Matjes** are the choicest herring—young, plump and tender because they haven't yet spawned. In the north of Germany, June is *Matjes* month, a time of feasting and celebration. Although the British don't honor herring with merrymaking, they dote upon **kippers** (smoked herring) and like them hot for breakfast. **NOTE:** Much of the herring being brined today is much less salty than it once was and needs only the briefest rinse or milk bath before it's eaten.

Heterocyclic Aromatic Amines: See HAAs.

Hexose: A type of simple sugar. GLUCOSE is a hexose, as are FRUCTOSE and GALACTOSE. The name comes from the fact that these sugars each contain six (*hex*) carbon atoms.

Hiatal Hernia (diet and): Those with a hiatal hernia (a weakening of the diaphragm at the point where the esophagus joins the stomach) sometimes suffer painful heartburn or esophagitis. Proper diet can help alleviate the problem. Usually it's better to eat five or six small meals a day instead of three big ones, also to remain upright for about an hour after eating. Finally, it makes good sense to avoid food and drink that might cause distress. These include alcohol, chocolate, coffee, colas, tea (and everything else containing caffeine), also food that is overly spicy, rich or fatty. The people most likely to develop hiatal hernias are those who are overweight and/or elderly, especially if they are also smokers. So both losing weight and giving up tobacco will help. See also ESOPHAGITIS.

Hickory Nuts: These American natives, wild nuts related to the pecan, are supremely sweet and an excellent keeper. The best of them come from the shagbark hickory, which

NUTRIENT CONTENT OF 1 OUNCE (28 GRAMS) SHELLED HICKORY NUTS	
186 calories	0 mg sodium
4 g protein	124 mg potassium
18 g fat, 2 saturated	2 g dietary fiber
0 mg cholesterol	4 RE vitamin A
5 g carbohydrate	0.25 mg thiamin
17 mg calcium	0.04 mg riboflavin
95 mg phosphorus	0.3 mg niacin
0.6 mg iron	1 mg vitamin C

grows over much of the eastern United States. Use hickory nuts wherever you would pecans or walnuts.

High Blood Pressure: See HYPERTENSION.

High-Fructose Corn Syrup: A corn-syrup-based sweetener used in fizzy soft drinks, milk drinks, canned fruits and frozen desserts. It's sweeter than sugar and dissolves more completely.

High-Protein Diet: Also called the **low-carbohydrate diet,** this has been touted as a way to drop 5 to 10 pounds practically overnight. But it's risky. Once the body has exhausted its own reserves of glycogen (starch warehoused in the muscles and liver as a ready source of energy), it begins to feed upon itself, just as it does during a fast. So what's lost isn't fat but protein, water and valuable minerals. And make a note, the pounds pile back on as soon as you resume normal eating.

High-Quality Protein: A COMPLETE PROTEIN contains all the amino acids the body needs and adequate amounts of each. A high-quality protein is not only complete but also highly digestible, meaning the body gets all the amino acids it needs in a single, immediately usable dose.

Histamine: A by-product of HISTIDINE metabolism. As a powerful dilator of blood vessels, histamine can lower blood pressure. It's also used to treat some allergies because it opens the airways and increases nasal secretion.

Histidine: One of the essential AMINO ACIDS; this one promotes growth and also, it's believed, the repair of body tissues.

Hives (and diet): **Acute urticaria,** to give the medical name for these pale, irregular, intensely itchy skin patches, can be triggered by a food allergy—to shellfish, for example, to peanuts, to the sulfites used in many wines and processed foods, to the salicylates naturally present in everything from almonds and apples to peaches and potatoes (salicylates are also a major component of aspirin). These are common troublemakers.

Holistic Medicine: The idea is that the *whole person,* not just the afflicted area, is treated. Unfortunately, many practitioners of holistic medicine use unorthodox, unproved diagnostic techniques and treatments. In recent years, however, many reputable M.D.s are embracing the idea of treating the whole person.

Homeopathy: Another pseudomedicine. The theory is that if hefty doses of a substance induce symptoms in healthy individuals—headaches, for example, or diarrhea—small amounts of those same substances will cure people suffering the identical symptoms. Although homeopathy is of questionable value, many homeopathic remedies remain on the market and enjoy brisk sales.

Hominy: Corn kernels (usually white) boiled in a weak lye bath until they're twice their original size, then degermed, hulled, washed and dried. Hominy may be cooked and canned. Or it may be sold in the dried form, either whole (like Mexican **pozole**) or ground into the beloved **grits** of the South. Needless to say, hominy isn't as nutritious as fresh corn, but it is a good source of complex carbohydrate.

NUTRIENT CONTENT OF 1 CUP CANNED WHITE HOMINY
(about 5½ ounces; 160 grams)

115 calories	336 mg sodium
2 g protein	14 mg potassium
1 g fat, 0 saturated	2 g dietary fiber
0 mg cholesterol	0 RE vitamin A
23 g carbohydrate	0.01 mg thiamin
16 mg calcium	0.01 mg riboflavin
56 mg phosphorus	0.1 mg niacin
1.0 mg iron	0 mg vitamin C

Note: Nutrient counts for canned yellow hominy are identical except that it contains 18 RE vitamin A.

NUTRIENT CONTENT OF ½ CUP COOKED WHITE GRITS
(about 4⅓ ounces; 121 grams)

73 calories	0 mg sodium
2 g protein	27 mg potassium
0 g fat, 0 saturated	2 g dietary fiber
0 mg cholesterol	0 RE vitamin A
16 g carbohydrate	0.12 mg thiamin
0 mg calcium	0.07 mg riboflavin
15 mg phosphorus	1.0 mg niacin
0.8 mg iron	0 mg vitamin C

Note: Nutrient counts for cooked yellow grits are identical except that these contain 7 RE vitamin A.

Homocysteine: For years doctors have considered high blood levels of this amino acid a warning of future heart disease, because the buildup injured blood vessels. Researchers have now linked high blood levels of homocysteine with vitamin B_6 and folic acid deficiencies. Studies continue, but it appears that getting adequate daily amounts of these two B vitamins may indeed reduce the risk of heart attacks.

Homogenize: To whirl an oil and nonoily liquid at intense speed until the two are homogeneous—smooth and creamy. Many of the salad dressings we use have been homogenized, as indeed has much of the milk. But the process for homogenizing MILK is different: Under 2,000 to 2,500 pounds pressure, milk is forced through grids of tiny holes so its fat particles are reduced to uniform fineness. The technique stabilizes the milk and keeps the fat from separating out.

Honey: A sweetener of biblical antiquity and practically the only one in wide use until sugar was mass-produced in the New World. There are dozens of different honeys, named for the flowers the bees feed on: **clover** (the most common), **alfalfa, acacia** (the cherished honey of Greece), **locust, sourwood** (Southerners consider this the finest honey in all creation), **heather, lavender, rosemary, pine** (a German favorite) and so on. Honeys vary in color from the pale, pale yellow to a deep, warm amber, and in viscosity from syrupy to spoon-up thick, the stiffest of all being those still in the comb. People have the notion that honey is nutritionally superior to sugar, that something magical happens as bees metamorphose flower nectar into liquid gold. The truth is that apart from traces of calcium, phosphorus, iron and potassium honey, like sugar, is pure carbohydrate. But make a note, it contains 18 more calories

NUTRIENT CONTENT OF 1 TABLESPOON HONEY
(about ¾ ounce; 21 grams)

64 calories	1 mg sodium
0 g protein	11 mg potassium
0 g fat, 0 saturated	0 g dietary fiber
0 mg cholesterol	0 RE vitamin A
17 g carbohydrate	0 mg thiamin
1 mg calcium	0 mg riboflavin
1 mg phosphorus	0 mg niacin
0.1 mg iron	0 mg vitamin C

Honeyed Vinaigrette

(*Makes About 1 Pint*)

A useful salad dressing to have on hand. Stored tightly covered in the refrigerator, it will keep for about a week. It's best with mixed green salads.

1⅓ cups fruity olive oil

⅓ cup balsamic vinegar

⅓ cup red wine vinegar or tarragon vinegar

⅓ cup honey (any type)

1 tablespoon Dijon mustard

1 tablespoon paprika

1 teaspoon salt

¼ teaspoon freshly ground black pepper

PLACE ALL INGREDIENTS in a 1-quart preserving jar, screw the lid on tight, and shake well to combine. Store, tightly covered, in the refrigerator and shake well before using.

APPROXIMATE NUTRIENT COUNTS PER TABLESPOON

92 calories	3 g carbohydrate	0.1 mg iron	0 mg thiamin
0 g protein	0 g dietary fiber	73 mg sodium	0.01 mg riboflavin
9 g fat, 1 saturated	1 mg calcium	13 mg potassium	0 mg niacin
0 mg cholesterol	2 mg phosphorus	13 RE vitamin A	0 mg vitamin C

per tablespoon than refined sugar. **CAUTION:** Honey may contain *Clostridium botulinum* spores, to which infants have little resistance. Once swallowed, the spores may germinate, giving off deadly toxins. To be safe, never daub honey on pacifiers of babies less than one year old and don't use it in preparing baby foods. By the time they can walk, most babies have developed some resistance to the *botulinum* spores that may lurk in honey. **TIP:** To liquefy crystallized honey, warm the jar of honey on a rack in a pan of barely simmering water three to five minutes—no longer, or the honey will taste "cooked."

Honeydew Melon: See MELONS.

Hordein: The protein in barley. It is incomplete protein and lacks the elasticity needed to make good bread.

Hormone: An organic compound manufactured by the body (usually the endocrine glands) that is released directly into the bloodstream to regulate the action of the body's different organs. Insulin is a hormone and so are estrogens and androgens.

Hormones (in meat production): Since 1989, American beef has been banned by the European Community (EC) because it contains hormones the EC considers harmful. EC nations aren't alone. Many Americans are eating less meat lest its residual hormones increase their risk of cancer. Are such fears justified? How safe are U.S. beef, veal, lamb and pork? At present, the FDA permits livestock growers to use nine brand-name anabolic agents (hormones) to fatten and finish their animals faster with less feed. These fall into four generic categories: **natural steroid hormones** (estradiol, testosterone and progesterone), **synthetic steroid hormones** (melengestrol acetate [MGA] and trenbolone acetate), **natural xenobiotic hormones** of plant origin (zeranol) and **growth-promoting compounds** (genetically engineered bovine somatotropin, now approved for use in dairy cows, and porcine somatotropin). Eight of the "allowed" hormones come in time-release pellets, which, when slipped under the skin of the ear, release a slow but steady dose of hormones for about four months. When the animals are slaughtered, the pellets are discarded. The ninth hormone—MGA—is mixed with the feed.

If denied these hormones, meat producers insist, they stand to lose billions of dollars (that's *billions,* with a *b*). Is the bottom line endangering our health? After much study, FDA and World Health Organization (WHO) scientists have concluded that these hormones, if administered within FDA limits, pose no threat. Only 10 percent of the residue actually gets into our bodies. Small, indeed, given the fact that the amount of hormone residue the FDA allows in meat is just 1 percent of that produced in a day by a prepubertal boy (his endocrines are far less active than those of men, women or even girls of the same age). The FDA began monitoring hormone residue levels in slaughterhouse meat in 1978 and has yet to uncover any signs of abuse or misuse.

Hormones (used by athletes): See STEROIDS.

Horseradish: Since the beginning of time, this pungent root, like cabbage a member of the cruciferous family of vegetables, has been used as food and medicine. In his splendid book *Food,* Waverley Root writes that the Delphic Oracle told Apollo that the "radish was worth its weight in lead, the beet its weight in silver, the horseradish its weight in gold." He also writes that horseradish "(probably its leaves, which when young and tender are usable in salads) was one of the five bitter herbs which the Jews were enjoined to eat at Passover" to commemorate their Exodus from Egypt in 1500 B.C. Horseradish is so ancient no one knows for sure where it originated. Some say Asia, some the Mediterranean basin, but Root is inclined to think it might have been Germany because the Germans, more than anyone else, know how to glorify it. To Americans, horseradish is merely something to heighten the nip of shrimp cocktail sauce or to put a little fire in bloody

---

NUTRIENT CONTENT OF 1 TABLESPOON PRESERVED HORSERADISH

(about ²/₃ ounce; 18 grams)

7 calories	17 mg sodium
0 g protein	52 mg potassium
0 g fat, 0 saturated	0 g dietary fiber
0 mg cholesterol	0 RE vitamin A
2 g carbohydrate	0 mg thiamin
11 mg calcium	0 mg riboflavin
6 mg phosphorus	0 mg niacin
0.2 mg iron	0 mg vitamin C

Marys. Although fresh horseradish is available in some areas, most of us must settle for preserved horseradish, either the red (colored with beet juice) or the white. Unfortunately, preserved horseradish quickly loses its bite, so the best plan is to buy it in small jars, then replenish it as needed.

"Hot-Dog Headache": People sensitive to the nitrates/nitrites used in assorted cold cuts and cured meats sometimes get headaches after eating hot dogs containing one of these preservatives. See also HEADACHES.

Hot Dogs: See FRANKFURTERS.

Hot Flashes (diet and): Unfortunately, no diet or food or vitamin is known to relieve these symptoms of menopause, these sudden flushes and sweats and feelings of exhaustion. And that includes vitamin E, which some health-food stores push as a cure for hot flashes.

Hubbard Squash: See SQUASH.

Huckleberries: See BLUEBERRIES.

Humectants (additives): A group of moisturizers added to grated coconut, marshmallows and other candies to keep them soft and fresh. Among them are glycerol (also called GLYCERIN), PROPYLENE GLYCOL and SORBITOL, which is also used as an artificial sweetener.

Hummus: A creamy Middle Eastern dip made with chickpeas, garlic and tahini (sesame-seed paste). Because its principal ingredient is a vegetable, hummus is more nutritious than many other cocktail dips.

Hunger: People used to think that you were hungry whenever your stomach was empty. It's not that simple. Sensations of hunger are intricately tied up with many factors, some psychological, some physiological. The sight and scent of food, for example, get the digestive juices going. But more powerful are the "feed me" signals sent to the hypothalamus in the brain whenever blood sugar levels drop. A number of brain and body chemicals also play roles. Among them are endorphins, morphinelike compounds that trigger responses of pain and pleasure; insulin; and, to a lesser degree, adrenaline. Too much adrenaline, in fact, acts like an amphetamine and depresses the

Low-Fat Hummus

Makes 1½ Cups

Authentic Middle Eastern hummus contains plenty of fat and calories. This slimmed–down version packs plenty of flavor.

2 garlic cloves, peeled

1½ cups cooked chickpeas, or 1 can (15 ounces) chickpeas, rinsed and drained

⅓ cup plain nonfat yogurt

2 teaspoons fresh lemon juice

1½ teaspoons Asian sesame oil

½ teaspoon salt

⅛ teaspoon cayenne pepper

2 tablespoons chopped fresh cilantro or flat-leaf parsley

BLANCH THE GARLIC for 2 minutes in a small pan of boiling water and drain. Transfer to a food processor fitted with the metal chopping blade, add all remaining ingredients except cilantro, and churn 30 seconds. Scrape down work bowl and churn 60 seconds longer, until smooth. Add cilantro and pulse to combine. Serve as a cocktail spread or dip with pita bread or sesame crackers.

APPROXIMATE NUTRIENT COUNTS PER TABLESPOON

22 calories	3 g carbohydrate	0.3 mg iron	0.01 mg thiamin
1 g protein	1 g dietary fiber	48 mg sodium	0.02 mg riboflavin
1 g fat, 0 saturated	13 mg calcium	42 mg potassium	0.7 mg niacin
0 mg cholesterol	23 mg phosphorus	2 RE vitamin A	1 mg vitamin C

appetite. Medical researchers now believe that the chemicals that stimulate appetite and those that depress it constitute a delicate system of checks and balances. Put simply, they tell you to eat when you need food and to stop when you've had enough. Sadly, many people suffer from psychological eating disorders so serious they no longer can hear what their bodies are telling them and either starve themselves to death or go on eating binges. See also AN-OREXIA NERVOSA, BULIMIA.

Husk: The coarse outer coat of grain kernels and a major source of bran and fiber. When flours are highly refined, the husk is removed.

Hydration: If you've ever watched marathoners, you know that they often grab cool drinks on the run. What they're doing is hydrating their bodies, restoring fluids lost through perspiration. You also know that those who fail to take regular drinks suffer muscle cramps and severe disorientation. Keeping the body hydrated isn't just for cham-

pion runners, however. It's for anyone who exercises strenuously, particularly in hot weather. And there are right ways to go about it:

1. Drink 2 cups cool water two hours before exercising, then another 2½ cups fifteen minutes before setting out.

2. While exercising, drink ½ to ¾ cup cool water every fifteen minutes, and if you are exercising for an hour or more, switch to watered-down fruit juices, which will help keep your energy up. Avoid full-strength fruit juices; they may cause bloating and cramping.

3. Weigh yourself after exercising, then for each pound lost, drink 2 cups water, undiluted fruit juice or fruit drink.

Hydrazines: Carcinogens present in many raw mushrooms, including *shiitake* and cultivated white mushrooms, which have caused tumors in mice. But the news isn't all bad. Cooking destroys a third of the hydrazines, as does a week in the fridge. Canning destroys them completely.

Hydrocarbons: When meats are charcoal grilled and their fatty drippings sputter down among the coals, hydrocarbons, chains of hydrogen and carbon atoms, are formed. Unfortunately, they are carcinogenic. This doesn't mean you should put the barbecue in cold storage. But it does suggest that charcoal grilling should be a sometime thing. Even in summer.

Hydrochloric Acid: One of the main components of gastric juice. It is manufactured by the gastric glands, then released into the stomach, where it helps to break up proteins, stimulates duodenal secretions and inhibits bacterial growth.

Hydrogen: The H in H_2O is hydrogen. But that's not all. This chemical element is an essential part of the air we breathe, the food we eat; indeed, our bodies are 10 percent hydrogen.

Hydrogenation: The chemical definition is the addition of hydrogen atoms to unsaturated bonds of carbon. What has that got to do with food? Or nutrition? Plenty. To stiffen margarine to the consistency of butter, to make shortenings fluffy, vegetable oils are pumped full of hydrogen or, in a word, hydrogenated. Unfortunately, the process not only saturates the fat but also produces TRANS FATTY ACIDS, which are believed to increase the risk of heart disease. In the body, trans fatty acids perform a sort of double whammy, lowering the amount of "good" cholesterol (HDL) and raising the "bad" (LDL). The firmer a margarine or vegetable shortening, the more hydrogen and trans fatty acids it contains. Reason enough to use liquid oils and squeeze margarines.

Hydrogen Cyanide: A lethal gas that's been used to execute prisoners on death row (30 to 250 milligrams are all it takes to kill a grown man). What few of us realize is that many of the foods we eat contain compounds (cyanogenic glycosides, to give their proper name) that stomach acid can convert to hydrogen cyanide. Cassava, upon which much of the Third World subsists, contains a cyanogen so powerful the cassava must be shredded, then washed and washed and washed to rid it of all poison. Lima beans, black beans and pinto beans also contain cyanogens, and a steady diet of them can be hazardous to your health. Indeed, people have been made very sick by eating dried beans cooked slowly in tightly covered crockpots. Other foods with hydrogen cyanide potential are almonds and bitter almonds (peach pits), bamboo shoots, sorghum, chokecherries, wild black cherries, also the seeds and pits of apples, apricots, cherries, plums and quinces. There have been problems, too, in some parts of the world with almond paste and marzipan (Australia recently slashed the allowable limits of cyanide in them to a tenth). Even watercress has proved deadly to mice. Clearly it pays to know what you're eating, to choose your food with care and to eat everything in moderation.

Hydrogen Sulfide: The stuff of high school stink bombs. But it is also the gas rotten eggs and onions give off.

Hydrolysis: When a chemical compound is split into smaller units in the presence of water, the reaction is called hydrolysis. Many of the chemical processes going on in the body are hydrolytic. During digestion, for example, sucrose is hydrolized into glucose and fructose, two simpler sugars.

Hydrolyzed Vegetable Protein (HVP) (additive): This flavor enhancer comes from wheat and corn gluten, defatted soy flour and cottonseeds. Actually there are two types: the **light,** which is used primarily in cream soups and sauces, and the **dark,** which goes into meaty soups, stews and broths. Both are high in monosodium glutamate and both improve the "mouth feel" not only of sauces, soups and stews but also of processed meats, snacks and crackers. GRAS.

Hydroponics: Fruits and vegetables grown under glass in insectproof greenhouses. They are rooted in gravel troughs through which nutrient-rich water flows. Hydroponic farming is cleaner than dirt farming, and a lot more expensive, too. Many people complain that foods grown this way cost too much and have no flavor.

Hyperacidity: See ESOPHAGITIS.

Hyperactivity: Not so long ago children who fidgeted constantly, couldn't sit still or couldn't concentrate were called hyperactive. The modern medical term for such behavior is ATTENTION DEFICIT HYPERACTIVITY DISORDER (ADHD), and there are several theories as to what causes it and what doesn't. See also FEINGOLD DIET.

Hypercalcemia: Unusually high calcium levels in the blood, which may be caused by an overactive parathyroid gland; by breast, lung or ovarian tumors; even by overdoses of vitamins A and D. Certain medications—calcium-based antacids, lithium, chlorthalidone and thiazide diuretics—can also elevate blood levels of calcium. The condition isn't pleasant. There may be nausea and vomiting, high blood pressure, kidney stones and general muscular weakness. Treatment? A low-calcium diet.

Hyperchlorhydria: A fancy medical term for **acid stomach.** The acid is hydrochloric acid, the principal component of gastric juice, and it's powerful stuff.

Hypercholesterolemia: Elevated blood levels of cholesterol, a condition associated mainly with hardening of the arteries and cardiovascular disease. It may be genetic, hormonal or dietary. Those with hypercholesterolemia are told to limit their cholesterol intake to 200 milligrams a day, to cut down on fat (especially saturated fat) and, if obese, to lose weight.

Hyperemesis Gravidarum: Severe, often uncontrollable vomiting that sometimes occurs in early pregnancy and usually requires hospitalization to prevent dehydration.

Hyperglycemia: Blood sugar (glucose) levels above 140 milligrams per 100 milliters of blood. DIABETES is a common culprit, but a very high carbohydrate diet can do it, too, as can an overactive thyroid, a brain tumor, cerebral hemorrhage or skull fracture. The treatment depends on the cause.

Hyperkalemia: Too much potassium in the blood, which can be quite toxic. Kidney shutdown can lead to hyperkalemia, as can Addison's disease, severe dehydration and a sudden release of cellular potassium that sometimes accompanies such traumas as car crash injuries, major surgery or gastrointestinal hemorrhage. Symptoms include numbness, even paralysis of the extremities, mental confusion, very slow heartbeat and cardiac arrest. The cause determines the treatment.

Hyperkinesis, Hyperactivity: See ATTENTION DEFICIT HYPERACTIVITY DISORDER.

Hypertension: The medical term for **high blood pressure,** which has been called the silent killer because it often shows no symptoms. Unless detected in a medical exam and treated, high blood pressure can result in strokes, heart attacks and kidney failure. What causes high blood pressure? In some cases, it may be hereditary. Obesity is often to blame, as are too little exercise, high-sodium diets, smoking and immoderate drinking. Now comes word of a Johns Hopkins study suggesting that ongoing adolescent stress may lead to chronic hypertension early in life.

When checking blood pressure, two numerical readings are taken and written down, one on top of the other—like a fraction. A normal reading will be written 120/80, the first (or top) number being the **systolic** (heart-pumping) **pressure** and the second (or bottom) being the **diastolic** (between-heartbeats or "resting") **pressure.** Until recently, the diastolic reading was what doctors used as an indicator of hypertension. But new findings in the famous FRAMINGHAM HEART STUDY suggest that high systolic readings (even borderline-high readings of 140 to 159) may portend coronary heart disease and should be brought down, too. Losing weight is perhaps the single most effective way to lower both systolic and diastolic blood pressure and that includes eating a heart-healthy diet (see HEART HEALTH). Also beneficial: adopting a regular but sane program of exercise, stopping smoking and limiting alcoholic drinks to two per day—beer, wine or whiskey, *not* two of each.

Hyperthyroidism: An overactive thyroid gland. Too much thyroid hormone in the body can mean "pop eyes," goiter (thyroid enlargement), fast pulse, extreme nervousness, muscle tremors and weight loss because of a hopped-up metabolism. Once the condition is corrected, the diet must be reworked to compensate for lost weight, exhausted body reserves of energy, depleted vitamins and minerals. That usually calls for a high-calorie/protein/carbohydrate diet plus supplemental calcium, phosphorus, B-complex and D vitamins.

Hypervitaminosis: A toxicity caused by ODing on vitamins, especially on the oil-soluble A and D, which the body stores instead of excretes. This is serious business. Symptoms of hypervitaminosis include excruciating headaches, kidney stones, painful swelling in the arms and legs, rough skin (from excesses of vitamin A), anemia and jaundice. The list is long and grim. The lesson here: Megadoses of vitamins can be deadly.

Hypoglycemia: Abnormally low blood sugar (glucose). Too much insulin can cause hypoglycemia, as can impaired liver or pituitary function, or Addison's disease. The symptoms? Extreme nervousness and hunger, flushed skin, profuse sweating, dizziness, heart palpitations and general feelings of malaise. There are many different types of hypoglycemia, which require different treatments and diets.

Hypokalemia: A potassium deficiency in the blood plasma. Prolonged diarrhea or vomiting can bring it on. So can surgical trauma or something as simple as not eating enough potassium-rich foods. Hypokalemia can reduce your insulin output and thus your tolerance for sugar. It can mean extreme muscular weakness, even heart failure. The cure may involve IV drips of potassium in solution or, in less acute cases, a diet full of such high-potassium foods as bananas, milk, potatoes and orange juice.

Hypothalamus: The part of the brain that controls appetite, among other things.

Hypothyroidism: A sluggish thyroid gland. With too little thyroid hormone, you feel bone-tired; your hands, face and, especially, eyelids may puff up; and because your metabolism kicks into low gear, you may gain weight. On the other hand, children with underactive thyroid glands may not grow properly and actually be stunted. To correct the condition, thyroid hormone is usually prescribed and, if the patient is overweight, a diet low in calories.

Hyssop: A bushy dark-leaved herb with bright blue flowers native to the Mediterranean basin, the Middle East and Ukraine. Both its leaves and flowers are brewed into teas that do seem to ease the congestion of colds. Hyssop is used in cordials and liqueurs, and many herb gardeners insist that it adds a nice minty tang to soups and salads. Hyssop is easy enough to grow; indeed, it's escaped the garden and now runs wild over much of the United States.

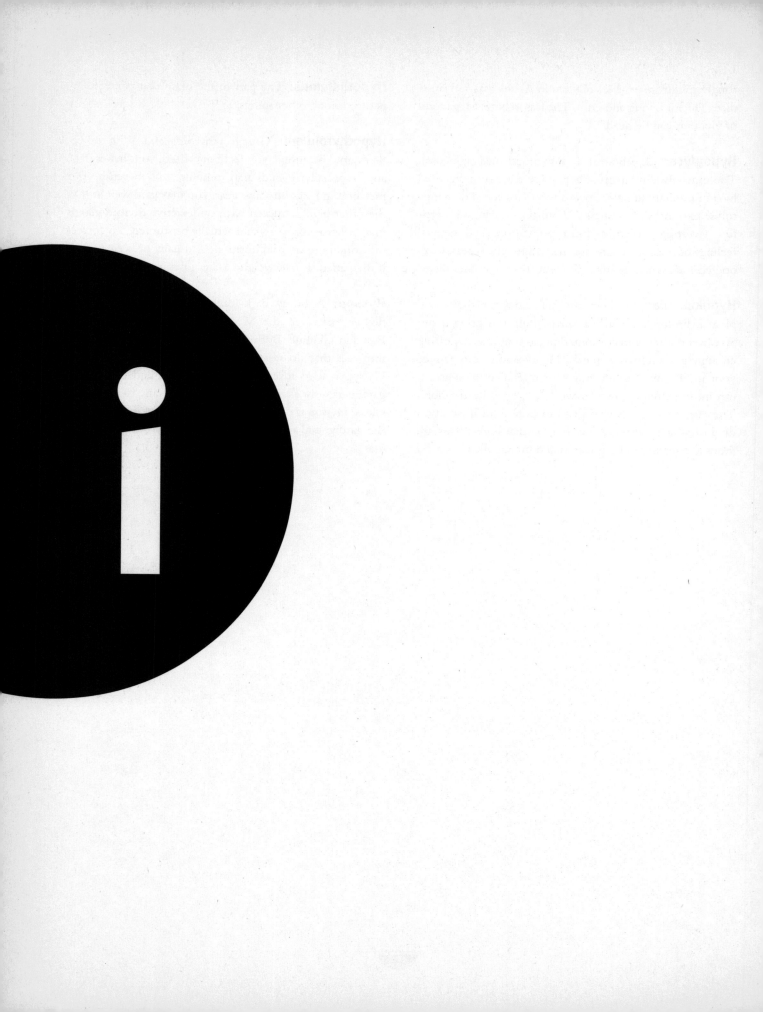

Ibuprofen: A relatively new nonsteroid painkiller that those sensitive to aspirin may be able to tolerate (Advil, Motrin and Nuprin are major brands). For some, it's kinder to the stomach than aspirin; and because it reduces inflammation, it has proved particularly helpful to those with arthritis. But there is a downside. Ibuprofen can upset the stomach and cause gastrointestinal bleeding, blurred vision, skin rashes, water retention and weight gain. To minimize side effects, take ibuprofen on a full stomach. Or wash it down with milk.

Iceberg Lettuce: See SALAD GREENS.

Ice Cream: Americans are so passionate about this smooth, frozen dessert that it's easy to assume ice cream was an American invention. Not so. Marco Polo came home from Asia with a recipe for sweet frozen milk. The Italians went on to glorify ice cream, and when Catherine de Médicis married Henry II of France, her Florentine chefs created a different flavor for each day of the wedding festivities. George Washington doted on ice cream, but Thomas Jefferson did him one better by serving it at the White House—*inside* hot pastries! By the mid-nineteenth century, there were fancy ice cream parlors across the eastern half of the country, and during the next fifty years, Americans came up with the soda, the sundae, the shake and the ice cream cone. Soon ice cream was being mass-produced—and losing much of its character as bottom-liners found ways to cut costs by faking the rich "mouth feel" of heavy cream with a variety of emulsifiers and stabilizers. Only recently, with the arrival of boutique ice creameries, have things come full circle. And, alas, the percentage of milk fat is edging ever upward.

Today, ½ cup of superpremium ice cream weighs in at 17 grams of mostly saturated fat—about the same as 1½ tablespoons of butter. Even ordinary ice creams, which owe their voluptuousness more to the air and stabilizers pumped into them than to milk fat, average 8 grams of fat per ½ cup.

Until recently, law decreed that the milk fat content of any frozen dairy product sold as ice cream had to amount to 10 percent of its weight at the very least. Today, aiming to encourage healthier eating patterns, the FDA has lightened up on its restrictions and now allows the following terminology (in order of fat content) to apply to commercial ice creams, provided they meet certain qualifications (in the past, these all had to be labeled "ice milk," a decided turnoff):

Nonfat Ice Cream: Must contain less than 0.5 gram milk fat per ½-cup portion.

Light or Low-Fat Ice Cream: Cannot exceed 3 grams milk fat per ½-cup portion.

Reduced-Fat Ice Cream: Must contain 25 percent less milk fat than regular ice cream, which is 10 percent milk fat.

To give low-fat ice creams superpremium sensuality, commercial manufacturers use a variety of stabilizers (guar and cellulose, to name two), which bind some of the water in the ice cream mix. It's a simple equation: Less liquid equals fewer ice crystals. Then, too, there's the powerful pulverizing, fluffing action of industrial ice cream machines.

NUTRIENT CONTENT OF 1 CUP PREMIUM VANILLA ICE CREAM (16 PERCENT FAT)

(about 5¼ ounces; 148 grams)

356 calories	83 mg sodium
5 g protein	236 mg potassium
24 g fat, 15 saturated	0 g dietary fiber
90 mg cholesterol	272 RE vitamin A
33 g carbohydrate	0.06 mg thiamin
173 mg calcium	0.24 mg riboflavin
141 mg phosphorus	0.1 mg niacin
0.7 mg iron	1 mg vitamin C

NUTRIENT CONTENT OF 1 CUP STANDARD VANILLA ICE CREAM (11 PERCENT FAT)

(about 4½ ounces; 132 grams)

266 calories	106 mg sodium
5 g protein	262 mg potassium
15 g fat, 9 saturated	0 g dietary fiber
58 mg cholesterol	154 RE vitamin A
31 g carbohydrate	0.50 mg thiamin
169 mg calcium	0.32 mg riboflavin
139 mg phosphorus	0.2 mg niacin
0.1 mg iron	1 mg vitamin C

Ice Cream Headache: If you gobble ice cream or any hard-frozen dessert, you may suffer an excruciating headache. Mercifully, the pain is fleeting. What causes it? Blood vessel spasms triggered by the intense cold. These interrupt the flow of blood and the vessels swell much as they do during a migraine. To prevent ice cream headache, eat slowly.

Ice Milk: Fast becoming obsolete, this term used to apply to a frozen dessert, usually a flavor other than fruit, made with milk instead of cream. The "nutritionally correct" new terms for ice milk are "reduced-fat ice cream," "light" or "low-fat ice cream" and "nonfat ice cream." Needless to say, the calorie, fat and cholesterol counts of these are significantly lower than in ice cream. To prove the point, compare the following nutrient counts with those for premium and standard ICE CREAM. See also SHERBET.

NUTRIENT CONTENT OF 1 CUP VANILLA ICE MILK OR LIGHT ICE CREAM (3 PERCENT FAT)

(about 4½ ounces; 132 grams)

183 calories	112 mg sodium
5 g protein	278 mg potassium
6 g fat, 3 saturated	0 g dietary fiber
19 mg cholesterol	62 RE vitamin A
30 g carbohydrate	0.08 mg thiamin
183 mg calcium	0.35 mg riboflavin
144 mg phosphorus	0.2 mg niacin
0.1 mg iron	1 mg vitamin C

Ices, Granités, Sorbets: Frozen desserts, often fruit based, that contain neither milk nor cream. Ices often are granular—hence their French and Italian names, *granité* and

NUTRIENT CONTENT OF 1 CUP NONCITRUS ICE OR SORBET

(about 7 ounces; 200 grams)

188 calories	28 mg sodium
1 g protein	156 mg potassium
0 g fat, 0 saturated	0 g dietary fiber
0 mg cholesterol	6 RE vitamin A
47 g carbohydrate	0.02 mg thiamin
10 mg calcium	0.06 mg riboflavin
16 mg phosphorus	0 mg niacin
0.5 mg iron	0 mg vitamin C

granita. They are, for the most part, fat and cholesterol free and, if made with fresh fruit, rich enough in vitamins and minerals to matter. The fluffier, more finely grained ices are called sorbets.

NUTRIENT CONTENT OF 1 CUP CITRUS ICE OR SORBET

(about 7 ounces; 200 grams)

184 calories	16 mg sodium
1 g protein	200 mg potassium
0 g fat, 0 saturated	0 g dietary fiber
0 mg cholesterol	54 RE vitamin A
46 g carbohydrate	0.02 mg thiamin
18 mg calcium	0.06 mg riboflavin
26 mg phosphorus	0.3 mg niacin
0.9 mg iron	51 mg vitamin C

Icing: The "icing on the cake," alas, adds calories and, if made with butter or cream, plenty of fat and cholesterol, too. Calorie counters as well as anyone trying to trim fat and cholesterol would do well do settle for unfrosted cakes or those dusted with confectioners' sugar. If they must have frosting, they should settle for the snowy fat-free classic Seven-Minute, which is made with egg whites, sugar, water and lots of air.

IDDM (Insulin-Dependent Diabetes Mellitus): See DIABETES.

Ileitis (diet and): Inflammation, either chronic or acute, of the lower reaches of the small intestine or ileum. There may be abdominal cramping, bloody diarrhea, anemia, weight loss. The first order of treatment is to stop the diarrhea and reduce pain. Next, to reverse the anemia and weight loss, the doctor or registered dietitian will prescribe a high-protein and -carbohydrate diet with supplemental vitamins and minerals. For ongoing or recurrent bouts, the dietitian may check for lactose and/or fat intolerance. See also CROHN'S DISEASE.

Ileum: The lower part of the small intestine and the area from which most digested foods are absorbed into the bloodstream.

Imitation Foods: Apart from flavor, it doesn't matter if you use "imitation vanilla"; it has no nutritive value. But if it's "imitation chocolate milk" you're drinking, you may

Berry Sorbet with Lime

Makes 8 Servings

This good basic recipe lends itself to improvisation. Use any combination of berries you fancy, substitute orange or lemon juice for lime, and increase the sugar and/or corn syrup as needed.

½ cup superfine sugar

1 envelope (¼ ounce) unflavored gelatin

1 cup water

1 cup light corn syrup

¼ cup fresh lime juice

1 teaspoon very finely grated lime zest

2 packages (10 ounces each) frozen raspberries, thawed slightly

1 package (10 ounces) frozen strawberries, thawed slightly

COMBINE SUGAR AND gelatin in a small heavy saucepan, pressing out lumps. Blend in water and corn syrup, and cook, stirring often, 3 to 5 minutes over moderate heat until sugar and gelatin dissolve. Off the heat, mix in lime juice and zest; then cool.

MEANWHILE, PUREE THE two berries in a food processor fitted with the metal chopping blade, then force puree through a fine sieve. Stir gelatin mixture into sieved puree, pour into a large shallow pan (13 × 9 × 2 inches is about right), and freeze until mushy. Quickly beat mush until fluffy in an electric mixer at high speed or in a food processor. Again freeze until mushy, beat as before, then freeze until mushy-firm. Scoop out and serve.

APPROXIMATE NUTRIENT COUNTS PER SERVING

255 calories	66 g carbohydrate	0.8 mg iron	0.03 mg thiamin
1 g protein	4 g dietary fiber*	53 mg sodium	0.05 mg riboflavin
0 g fat, 0 saturated	19 mg calcium	144 mg potassium	0.3 mg niacin
0 mg cholesterol	19 mg phosphorus	6 RE vitamin A	29 mg vitamin C

*If made with unsieved berries; sieved berry sorbet contains 1 gram dietary fiber.

be sure it is nutritionally inferior to the real thing. In fact, it may contain little or no milk. The label will tell the truth, so read the fine print before buying anything called imitation.

Immune System (diet and): The body's immune system is a chain of defenses of stunning intricacy. The skin, mucous membranes, bodily secretions, lymph nodes and white blood cells are all major players in the fight against infection. Where, then, does diet fit in? And can pumping up on vitamins and minerals boost the immune system, as so many health-food stores would have you believe? What's fact? What's fiction?

Fact: Severely malnourished persons do suffer more colds, flu and other infections than healthy individuals. Fact: Certain nutrients do seem to bolster the immune system—the whole family of antioxidants (beta-carotene and vitamins C and E, which depower scavenging free radicals before they can damage body cells), four of the B-complex (B_6, folic acid, pantothenic acid and B_{12}) and the minerals iron and zinc. In addition, new studies suggest that allicin, a sulfurous compound in garlic, may strengthen the body's natural resistance, in particular to stomach cancer. This doesn't mean you should gobble megadoses of vitamins, minerals and garlic tablets, which may indeed be harmful. What it does mean is that you should eat wisely and well every day of your life (see FOOD GUIDE PYRAMID). Now comes evidence to suggest that stress may weaken the immune system and simple pleasures (cheerful outings with family or friends) may help toughen it. This research, however, is both preliminary and ongoing.

Fiction: **Astragalus** (an old Chinese remedy), **chlorella, shark–liver oil** and **spirulina** all fortify the immune system. Health-food stores are busy hawking them, targeting AIDS patients in particular. The truth is that no reputable scientific study has ever shown them to strengthen the body's natural defenses. Fact: The New York City Department of Consumer Affairs recently lowered the boom on four supplement manufacturers making just such false claims. According to one physician, the only benefit of these so-called immunity-boosting supplements is to the companies that sell them.

Immunoglobulin E (IgE):
Antibodies manufactured by the body's immune system. These, in turn, release chemicals that subdue allergens, the substances that trigger allergic reactions. Ironically, chemicals produced by IgE can themselves set off major allergic responses—swollen lips and tongue, difficulty in breathing. Not many foods trigger such violent allergies, but shellfish, peanuts and sulfites used as food and wine preservatives have all been guilty.

Inborn Error of Metabolism:
The inability to digest certain sugars or amino acids is sometimes hereditary, usually because the body lacks the enzyme needed to do the job. Three of the most common inborn metabolic errors are GALACTOSEMIA, PHENYLKETONURIA and tyrosinemia, incapacities to handle, respectively, GALACTOSE (a sugar), PHENYLALANINE and TYROSINE (two amino acids). Careful monitoring of the diet, restricting or eliminating troublesome foods, can ease or eliminate the symptoms but does not correct the genetic error.

Incomplete Proteins:
Proteins, most often plant proteins, that lack one or more of the essential amino acids. Vegetarians must build their diets carefully, making sure they receive their full complement of essential amino acids.

Index of Nutrient Quality (INQ):
An equation that enables nutritionists to determine the nutrient density of individual foods. Higher INQs mean a food is more nutrient dense—i.e., a better source of the particular nutrient.

Indigestion:
Partial or faulty digestion of food accompanied by gas, heartburn or abdominal pain. Many cases of **dyspepsia,** as indigestion is also called, are brought on by stress, by eating overly fatty or highly spiced food or by poor eating habits in general.

Indoles:
Cancer-fighting compounds (anticarcinogens) that exist naturally in many foods, among them such cruciferous vegetables as broccoli, cabbage, brussels sprouts, kale and collards. See PHYTOCHEMICALS.

Infant Nutrition:
For most babies, mother's milk is best, and although it is low in iron and vitamin D, it contains particularly digestible forms of them, which seem to be sufficient for most newborns. Breast milk also contains antibodies that help build the baby's immune system. If a mother's milk supply runs short, or if for some reason it doesn't agree with the baby, a commercial formula is second best. Over time these have been perfected until their nutrient content now closely parallels that of breast milk, especially when it comes to fatty acids and lipids—crucial to a newborn's growth.

Today, commercial baby formulas are the most carefully regulated foods in the United States because the FDA considers them special diet foods. Based on recommendations of the American Academy of Pediatrics Committee on Nutrition, the FDA specifies exactly what nutrients must go into infant formulas and in what amounts. At present, those based on cow's milk must contain twenty-six different nutrients, from vitamin A to zinc. Non-cow's milk formulas must also include INOSITOL plus two additional members of the B-complex—biotin and choline.

When should a baby begin taking solid or semisolid food? Usually between the age of four and six months, when the suckling reflex begins to diminish. Although commercial baby foods and junior foods now contain no salt and little or no sugar, many parents prefer to prepare their own, believing them to be more healthful and wholesome. Not necessarily. Making baby food means knowing what foods are suitable for infants and working in kitchens of almost antiseptic cleanliness. Here's a quick guide to making safe, nutritious baby food.

1. Use top-quality fresh meats, poultry, milk and dairy products, fruits and vegetables, grains and grain products.

2. Make certain that all work surfaces, all implements, utensils, pots and pans are scrupulously clean (pay special attention to cutting boards; sieves; blender, grinder and food processor parts). The same goes for your hands. Wash them well in hot sudsy water before preparing baby food and, if necessary, wash them again as you work.

3. Cook food in a minimum of water and only until tender. Heat destroys vitamin C, thiamin (vitamin B_1) and folic acid, another important member of the B-complex. These same vitamins, plus a good many more, are water soluble. They will leach out into the cooking water and be lost, unless the water is used in the pureeing.

4. Hold the salt and pepper. And whatever you do, do not use honey. It may harbor spores of *Clostridium botulinum,* the bug that causes a fatal form of food poisoning called botulism. Babies less than one year old have little resistance to it, so if the spores are swallowed, they may germinate in the baby's body, producing potentially deadly toxins.

5. Puree foods in a pristine blender, food processor or baby-food grinder, adding only enough liquid to make the job easy. Or force the food through a food mill or sieve.

6. Quick freeze the purees in ice cube trays by setting them directly on the freezing surface of a 0°F. freezer. When solid, pop out of the ice cube trays, bundle in freezer bags, label and date and store in the freezer.

7. Thaw only what amounts you will need for a single feeding and heat in a water bath just to serving temperature. **CAUTION:** Avoid using the microwave because there tend to be "hot spots" in the food that may scald the baby's hands or mouth.

8. Never refreeze baby food once it has thawed.

Infection (diet and): See IMMUNE SYSTEM.

Inflammatory Bowel Disease (IBD): An umbrella term that includes regional enteritis or CROHN'S DISEASE and ULCERATIVE COLITIS.

Infrared Broiling: Many hotel and restaurant chefs use powerful infrared units to speed-broil meat, fish, fowl and vegetables. They also keep plated food hot under batteries of infrared bulbs until waiters can rush them to the table. Until now, no one has known how infrared rays affect the nutrient value of food. At long last, tests are being conducted in several university labs to determine if infrared broiling is any more destructive of nutrients than the hot forced air of convection ovens. So far results are inconclusive. In some foods, heat-sensitive vitamins like C and thiamin appear to suffer more from infrared broiling than from convection baking. Yet in others just the opposite holds true. Stay tuned.

Inositol, Myoinositol: Inositol is a glucoselike compound that's essential to good health. There are in fact nine different forms of inositol, but the one involved with human nutrition is myoinositol. All animal cells contain it in large measure. It's found in plant cells, too, although here it's part of phytic acid, which can block the absorption of calcium, iron and zinc. Body cells actually manufacture inositol, so deficiencies are unknown.

Insoluble Fiber: See FIBER, DIETARY.

Insomnia (diet and): *When* you eat may have more to do with a good night's sleep than *what* you eat. Studies have shown that people prone to churning stomachs, heartburn and gas rest more comfortably if they eat early in the evening. And not just because their stomachs have a chance to settle. According to new Swiss research, healthy men and women fed ham and cheese sandwiches at 9 P.M. had stomach acid levels 20 percent higher than those who dined on ham and cheese sandwiches at 6. And their higher stomach acid levels lasted all night long.

What about the bedtime glass of warm milk? Does that induce sleep? Not really, researchers say. Milk does contain TRYPTOPHAN, an amino acid that can make you drowsy. Unfortunately, it would take 2 quarts of milk to send you into the arms of Morpheus. As for the tryptophan supplements touted by health-food stores as "nature's own sleeping pill," they are dangerous. Tryptophan megadoses have been linked to eosinophilia myalgia syndrome (EMS), a serious blood disorder that not only causes runaway fevers and intense muscular pain but may also kill you. Of the more than three dozen people who died recently of EMS, almost all had been on tryptophan. It isn't clear whether tryptophan itself was the culprit or the supplements were contaminated. Whatever the reason, the FDA yanked all tryptophan supplements off the market.

Inspection of Food: All meat and poultry shipped across state lines must be checked and passed by government inspectors before it can be sold. In the best of times, this meant our beef, veal, mutton, lamb, pork, chickens, turkeys, Cornish hens, ducks, geese, pheasants and so on were disease free and that the slaughterhouses handling them

were sanitary enough to pass federal muster. But recent outbreaks of food poisoning traced to salmonella-contaminated meat and poultry have left America wary. And sent journalists scurrying, camcorders in hand, to investigate every episode of illness and document every abattoir infraction. As a result, the USDA aims to clean up its act by tightening safeguards. This will mean incorporating the Hazard Analysis and Critical Control Points program (see HACCP) into its present program of inspection and increasing its jurisdiction, perhaps, to seafood. Or at least working closely with the proper federal bureau to ensure the safety of our fish and shellfish. HACCP was developed for NASA as a sort of high-tech taster of astronaut food to make sure no spaceman got *turista* while orbiting earth. See also FOOD SAFETY.

Instant Flour, Instantized Flour: A blend-on-contact, fine, granular flour that delivers lump-free sauces and gravies every time. Instantized flour (or other starch) is what food processors use in pudding, gravy and sauce mixes. Although instantized flour can be used for dredging, it should never be substituted for regular flour in baking.

Instant Foods: These are the package mixes that make life so easy, the boxed cakes and quick breads, the ready-to-spread frostings, the just-add-water-and-heat soups, the instant gourmet sauces and rice combos. The list is long and lengthening, as a stroll down any supermarket aisle quickly proves. But a glance at the ingredient lists of most of these time-savers reveals a chemical feast of artificial flavorings and colorings, stabilizers, emulsifiers, preservatives, antioxidants, humectants (moisteners), softeners and hardeners. And let's not forget sugar and salt. Suffice it to say, the nearer food is to the source, the more nutritious and wholesome it's likely to be. In other words, support your local farmer and greenmarket. Better yet, grow your own (or at least some of it).

Insulin: A hormone secreted by the pancreas that's integral to the maintenance of normal blood sugar (glucose) levels. Here's how: Insulin blocks the conversion of glycogen (stored energy) into blood sugar (glucose) but hastens the reverse (the transformation of glucose into glycogen). It promotes muscle development by preventing the breakdown of protein into glucose. Finally, it speeds the manufacture of fat from glucose. An insulin deficiency is serious and can lead to diabetes.

Insulin-Dependent Diabetes Mellitus (IDDM): See DIABETES.

Integrated Pest Management: See IPM.

International Unit (IU): The unit formerly used to measure such fat-soluble vitamins as A, D, E and K. It still appears on the labels of some vitamin supplements.

Intestinal Bypass Surgery: Once used as a desperate measure to bring down the weight of grossly obese individuals, this technique of removing part of the small intestine to reduce absorption is rarely used today. It's too risky.

Intestinal Juice: An enzyme-rich fluid secreted by the walls of the small intestine, primarily its uppermost portion, the duodenum, which adjoins the stomach. The main job of this alkaline pale yellow liquid is to combine with and complete the digestion of partially digested food.

Intestine, Large; Colon: This muscular five-foot tube links the small intestine and rectum. As the small intestine deposits undigested material (waste) in the large intestine, the colon shuttles the mass along, absorbing water and returning it to body tissues. If too much water is absorbed, there's constipation; if too little, diarrhea.

Intestine, Small: Four times the length of the large intestine but half its diameter, the small intestine connects stomach and colon. It is divided into three parts: the **duodenum,** which adjoins the stomach; the middle portion (**jejunum**); and the lower end (**ileum**). The role of the small intestine is to receive partially digested food from the stomach, then, with the help of digestive juices from the intestine, gallbladder and pancreas, to turn it into body fuel as well as substances needed for the growth and repair of tissue.

Intrinsic Factor: A protein synthesized by the stomach that's necessary for the absorption of EXTRINSIC FACTOR or vitamin B_{12} (cobalamin). Those unable to produce intrinsic factor develop pernicious anemia. See also B_{12}, VITAMIN.

Inulin: A complex carbohydrate found in Jerusalem artichokes, and to a lesser degree in garlic and onions, that the body can only partially digest and that can cause gas and bloating. A bit of alchemy occurs when inulin-rich foods are put into storage, however. Their inulin is broken down into units of fructose, which the body most definitely can use. Thus the fresher the Jerusalem artichoke, garlic and onion, the less usable sugar and calories they contain. See also ARTICHOKES, JERUSALEM.

Invertases: Enzymes that in the presence of water turn sucrose, a double sugar, into two simpler ones, GLUCOSE and FRUCTOSE. Invertases and the invert sugars they form (see INVERT SUGAR) are important to confectioners because they keep fondants and fudges from going gritty. They also make it possible to produce candies with supremely soft centers. The centers are hard when dipped in chocolate, then—as if by magic—turn creamy on standing. Food companies add invertases to corn syrups and honeys to keep them clear and free flowing; without them, they'd be full of sugar crystals in no time.

Invert Sugar: The sugar formed, a 50-50 mix of GLUCOSE and FRUCTOSE, when enzymes go to work on SUCROSE (table sugar) solutions. Invert sugar is sweeter, more quickly dissolved than sucrose, which makes it important to candy makers, also to commercial bakers, who find that using some invert sugar in their cakes and cookies keeps them fresh and moist longer than baked goods made with sucrose alone. See also INVERTASES.

Iodine: No mineral, no nutrient is more of a specialist than iodine. Its sole role is to become part of the thyroid hormone that regulates the speed of bodily functions, body temperatures, blood cell production, nerve and muscle function, even reproduction and growth. **DEFICIENCY SYMPTOMS:** Enlarged thyroid gland (see GOITER); also, if it occurs during pregnancy, a condition in infants known as CRETINISM. When a fetus's thyroid glands are deprived of sufficient iodine, the child is dwarfed and mentally retarded. **GOOD SOURCES:** Saltwater fish and shellfish, iodized salt, eggs, cheeses (Cheddar, cottage, cream, feta and mozzarella), milk (whole, evaporated, buttermilk). Depending on the soil in which they were grown, dried beans, potatoes, broccoli, spinach may also contain iodine. Finally, because iodine is present in some of the dough conditioners and disinfectants used by food processors, you may get a bit of it from these. **PRECAUTIONS:** Too much iodine, like too little, can decrease thyroid function.

RDA FOR IODINE	
Babies:	
Birth to 6 months	40 mcg per day
6 months to 1 year	50 mcg per day
Children:	
1 to 3 years	70 mcg per day
4 to 6 years	90 mcg per day
7 to 10 years	120 mcg per day
Men and Boys:	
11 to 24 years	150 mcg per day
25 to 51+ years	150 mcg per day
Women and Girls:	
11 to 24 years	150 mcg per day
25 to 51+ years	150 mcg per day
Pregnant Women:	175 mcg per day
Nursing Mothers:	200 mcg per day

Iodine (as water purifier): Boiling water for ten minutes is safer. But that's not always possible. Both tincture of iodine and iodine tablets (the kind sold by drugstores and sporting goods shops) can be used to purify water. But always follow the manufacturer's directions to the letter. Iodine, remember, is poisonous.

Iodized Salt: Table salt enriched with sodium or potassium iodide (1 part per 5,000 to 10,000 parts salt). Iodized salt was developed in the 1920s as a way of reducing the incidence of goiter in America's landlocked heartland, where diets were short on saltwater fish and iodine. After iodized salt became widely available in the 1930s, goiters were virtually eliminated (scientists now know that 96 percent of them are caused by iodine deficiencies). Today federal labeling laws require that all table salt be labeled either as **iodized salt** ("This salt contains added iodine, an essential nutrient") or as **noniodized salt** ("This product does not contain iodine, an essential nutrient"). Health faddists swear by sea salt, but in truth its iodine content is rather low because iodine vaporizes as the salt dries.

IPM (Integrated Pest Management): With more and more Americans freaking out about pesticide residues in their food and drinking water, this ecologically correct method of farming, begun in the 1970s and partially underwritten by the federal government, is gaining ground. In a nutshell, its purpose is to minimize the use of synthetic pesticides (petrochemicals) in favor of methods that are safer, cheaper and equally effective. Among these: resorting to pesticides only when pests get the upper hand (threaten economic damage); using biological controls (letting the pests' natural enemies—parasites, bacteria, viruses and predators—do them in); and making the most of bio-degradable botanical pesticides extracted from plants. Other IPM ways to control pests include crop rotation, mechanical cultivation, irrigation and pruning. First applied to cotton and soybeans, IPM techniques have proved so successful they are now being widely used by fruit and vegetable growers across the country. See also HERBI-CIDES, PESTICIDES.

Irish Moss: The seaweed from which CARRAGEENAN is obtained. This gelatinous material is used by food companies to emulsify and stabilize everything from salad dressings to ice creams to chocolates.

Iron: A mineral that is essential not only to good health but also to life itself. The bulk of the iron in the human body is in the red blood cells' hemoglobin; in fact, it is what makes blood red. Hemoglobin shuttles oxygen from the lungs to every body cell, and without iron, hemoglobin cannot do its job. Another compound, myoglobin, grabs iron from hemoglobin and stores it in muscles where it's crucial to proper muscle function. On hemoglobin's trip to the lungs, its iron carries carbon dioxide, which we then expel as we exhale. And that's not all. Iron is part of the chemical makeup of several vital enzymes and proteins and plays a major role in energy metabolism.

All dietary iron, however, is not created equal. There are two basic types: **heme iron,** the easily absorbable form that accounts for 40 percent of the iron in meats, and **non-heme iron,** the not so easily assimilable form present in vegetables. How well the body absorbs it depends on many things—whether there's sufficient vitamin C, whether antacids, high-fiber or oxalate-rich foods, or coffee or tea are also present. Each of them can thwart the body's ability to absorb iron. **DEFICIENCY SYMPTOMS:** Children deficient in iron often display many of the symptoms of ATTENTION DEFICIT HYPERACTIVITY DISORDER—restlessness, disruptiveness, inability to concentrate—and these may appear long before blood tests show any lack of iron. The reason is that a child's brain reacts to an iron deficit early on. Adults deficient in iron, on the other hand, tire easily, become apathetic, unmotivated—and usually before anemia develops.

An **iron deficiency** is usually defined as dwindling reserves of iron in the body in general. **Anemia,** on the other hand, refers specifically to reduced levels of hemoglobin. With less iron present, the blood cells can't ferry sufficient oxygen from the lungs to body tissues. Symptoms of anemia include extreme fatigue, overall weakness, headaches, apathy and pallor. **GOOD SOURCES OF IRON:** Molasses (especially blackstrap), calf's liver, dried beans, dried prunes and prune juice, iron-fortified cereals, whole-wheat and enriched bread, meat and poultry, broccoli, beet greens, kale and, yes, Popeye's spinach. **PRECAUTIONS:** If the body is to absorb iron properly, it needs vitamin C. Certain other compounds block the body's ability to absorb iron: antacids, dietary fiber, coffee, tea, phosphate salts such as calcium phosphate, and phytates (substances found in whole grains and soy products).

Is it possible to OD on iron? Absolutely! In fact, several new studies (among them ones conducted at Harvard and in Finland) suggest that most normal adults are more likely to get too much iron than too little. This iron overload, they further suggest, increases the risk of both cardiovascular disease and cancer, particularly of the colon. The excess iron bonds with free radicals, scavenging by-products of metabolism that damage cells and increase the risk of cancer (studies with mice show that the more iron they eat, the faster their cancers grow). Most nutritionists agree that if you're healthy and eating a well-balanced diet, there's no need for iron supplements (unless you're pregnant and your doctor prescribes them). Some biomedical researchers go even further, suggesting that you eat less red meat (be guided by the FOOD GUIDE PYRAMID), exercise regularly and become a blood donor. The blood letting of early medicine, they believe, wasn't such a bad idea after all because it does lower iron levels.

RDA FOR IRON

Babies:		
	Birth to 6 months	6 mg per day
	6 months to 1 year	10 mg per day
Children:		
	1 to 10 years	10 mg per day
Men and Boys:		
	11 to 18 years	12 mg per day
	19 to 51+ years	10 mg per day
Women and Girls:		
	11 to 50 years	15 mg per day
	51+ years	10 mg per day
Pregnant Women:		30 mg per day
Nursing Mothers:		15 mg per day

Some two thousand American children suffer from iron poisoning every year, mostly because they've gobbled powerful iron supplements that were carelessly left within their reach (all it takes to kill a 22-pound toddler are five 110-milligram iron pills).

Sometimes HEMOCHROMATOSIS, a possibly inherited inability to metabolize iron, is responsible for an iron buildup. Overloads of iron can damage the liver and pancreas, leading in some cases to diabetes.

Iron Cooking Utensils: Cooking in iron pans does add to the body's supply of iron, although only marginally. Few people use cast-iron cookware these days except for frying because it rusts and it's heavy. **NOTE:** There are no nutritional benefits from cooking in enameled cast iron because the iron is clad with an inert porcelain glaze.

Irradiation: It's not as new as you think. A hundred years ago scientists discovered that irradiation (the zapping of food with gamma or X rays or radioactive cobalt) killed bacteria, yeasts, molds and parasites in food, prolonging shelf life. And in the 1920s, the idea of irradiating pork to kill the microscopic parasites that cause trichinosis was actually patented. But the idea didn't leave the lab for sixty years. And only recently has irradiation become a hot (no pun intended) topic.

Many people believe that irradiation makes food radioactive (they once thought that about microwaving, too). It doesn't. Low doses don't change the color, flavor, texture or nutritive value of food although high doses do (another fusilade aimed by antiirradiationists). It does create radiolytic compounds (which alarmists quickly point out) but in amounts experts consider too small to be harmful (which alarmists *don't* admit).

What also hasn't been publicized is that *nonirradiated foods also contain radiolytic compounds*. Or that doctors have been sterilizing their instruments via irradiation for years. Or that manufacturers have been doing the same with many popular nonfood items—cotton swabs, contact lenses, teethers and tampons, to name a few.

The reason for irradiating food is to destroy insects, bacteria, yeasts, molds and parasites that cause spoilage, illness and death. Thirty-five countries do it today and the United States is among them. **NOW APPROVED BY THE FDA FOR IRRADIATION:** Wheat and wheat flours; white potatoes; herbs, spices, aromatic seeds and dry vegetable seasonings; pork (both carcasses and fresh uncut processed

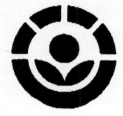

meat); fresh fruits and vegetables; and poultry (none too soon given the fact that 60 percent of our poultry is contaminated with salmonella).

The FDA requires that all irradiated foods be labeled, also that they bear the internationally adopted pictograph (see above), which shows, at a glance, which foods have been zapped.

Given the controversial nature of irradiation and people's fear of it, many major food companies refuse to zap any of their products. And are being quite vocal about it. Researchers, on the other hand, know that disease-bearing organisms in food cause millions of people to sicken every year and that thousands of them die. Researchers know, too, that enormous amounts of food are lost every year because of insects and other pests.

Among scientists, the consensus is that once the American public understands that irradiation is not only safe but also the surest way to ensure an adequate supply of safe food, their resistance to it will pass. Just as it did with microwaving. That's why Vindicator, a Florida company, is forging ahead and busily irradiating a wide variety of food, some of which is already on supermarket shelves and in hospital kitchens.

Irritable Bowel Syndrome (IBS) (diet and): Irregular bowel patterns with alternate bouts of constipation and diarrhea. Sometimes there is pain, gas and the feeling after a bowel movement that there's more to come. No one knows exactly what causes IBS. Many physicians believe it may be stress related, also that laxatives, caffeine, antibiotics, too little sleep and not drinking enough liquid can trigger it. Because many IBS sufferers are underweight, edgy and upset, eating a nutritious diet patterned along the lines of the FOOD GUIDE PYRAMID may help. Needless to add, foods that cause gastric distress should be avoided.

Islamic Dietary Laws: According to the Islamic Food and Nutrition Council of America, founded in the 1980s, no pork or pork by-products are allowed in the Muslim diet, and no alcohol (not even fermented vegetables). Further, in order for meat to be HALAL, animals must be slaughtered by certified Muslims, who may be either religious or technical professionals. Also taboo: birds of prey and four-footed animals that down their kill with their mouths. But there are no forbidden food combinations as there are in kosher law, only forbidden foods.

Isoflavones: Natural compounds found in soybeans and soy products, which National Cancer Institute researchers report have cancer-fighting properties. See PHYTOCHEMICALS.

Isoleucine: One of the nine essential AMINO ACIDS. It's found in all foods that contain complete protein (meat, poultry, fish, eggs, milk and dairy products). The body's inability to metabolize isoleucine (as well as leucine and valine, two other amino acids) causes MAPLE SYRUP URINE DISEASE, so named because of the sweet smell of the urine. It is a genetic disease showing up in newborns, with symptoms appearing within four or five days. The babies refuse to feed, become lethargic and may vomit. Failure to treat the condition can lead to seizures, coma and death. Although this rare metabolic defect isn't fully understood, doctors are able to treat it.

Isopropyl Citrate (additive): An antioxidant used by food processors to retard the staling of margarines and vegetable oils. GRAS.

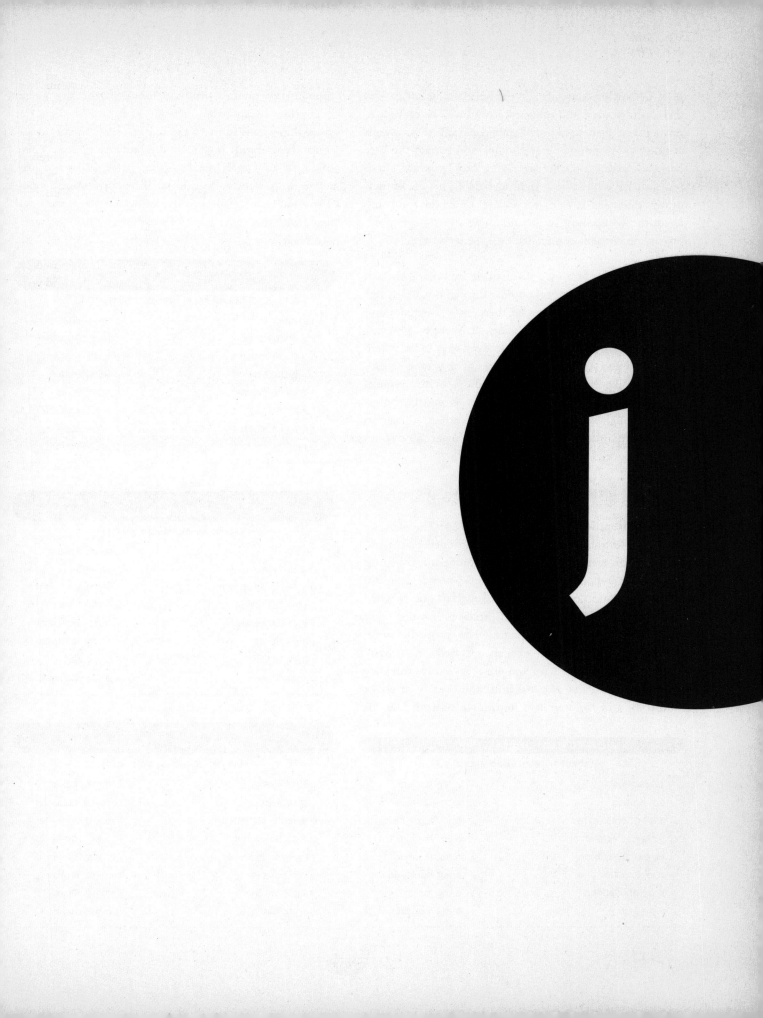

Jack Crevalle: A member of the huge family of jack fish that swim tropical and subtropical waters. The crevalle is smaller than the better known amberjack; still, it can weigh as much as 40 pounds. For cooking and eating, the best crevalles are much smaller, averaging 2 to 3 pounds. These lean fish have meat both light and dark, but the dark is usually discarded as being too coarse. Once the fish is filleted, the white meat broils and sautés superbly. For approximate nutrient counts, see FISH, LEAN WHITE.

Jaggary: A crude brown sugar made by boiling the sap of the date palm. Jaggary is popular throughout India, also among the British once posted there, as a sweetener and as a mellower of vegetarian curries. It is shaped into coconut-size balls and shipped to bazaars all over India, where it's hacked into smaller pieces and sold by the gram. Jaggary tastes a bit like dark brown sugar, although there are vinous undertones. Like other sugars, jaggary is pure carbohydrate. Though its calorie count is not known, it's safe to say it approximates that of dark brown sugar: 52 calories per tablespoon.

Jalapeño: See HOT PEPPERS under PEPPERS, CAPSICUMS.

Jams, Jellies, Marmalades, Preserves: The old song that went "It must be jelly 'cause jam don't shake like that" was right on target. Perfect jellies—compounded of fruit juice, sugar and pectin—are jewel bright, crystal clear, stiff enough to stand alone yet tender enough to quiver when nudged with a spoon. Jams and preserves, on the other hand, contain bits of fruit and, when properly made, should just slide—not run—off an upended spoon. Marmalades are much like jams and preserves except that they are usually made out of citrus fruits and contain shreds of rind. None of the four is a nutritional powerhouse, although jams, preserves and marmalades have a slight edge over jellies because they're made of fruits *and* juice, not juice alone. And some of the newer ones contain no additional sugar, only highly concentrated fruit juices. These of course are largely sugar, so these jams, jellies and preserves are no lower in calories than conventional ones. Those labeled "diabetic" are artificially sweetened and made with methoxypectin, a form of pectin that gels without sugar.

NUTRIENT CONTENT OF 1 TABLESPOON REDUCED-SUGAR JELLY

(about 3/4 ounce; 20 grams)

34 calories	0 mg sodium
1 g protein	13 mg potassium
0 g fat, 0 saturated	0 g dietary fiber
0 mg cholesterol	0 RE vitamin A
9 g carbohydrate	0 mg thiamin
1 mg calcium	0 mg riboflavin
1 mg phosphorus	0 mg niacin
0 mg iron	0 mg vitamin C

NUTRIENT CONTENT OF 1 TABLESPOON ARTIFICIALLY SWEETENED JELLY

(about 3/4 ounce; 20 grams)

6 calories	0 mg sodium
0 g protein	12 mg potassium
0 g fat, 0 saturated	0 g dietary fiber
0 mg cholesterol	0 RE vitamin A
1 g carbohydrate	0 mg thiamin
1 mg calcium	0 mg riboflavin
1 mg phosphorus	0 mg niacin
0 mg iron	0 mg vitamin C

NUTRIENT CONTENT OF 1 TABLESPOON JELLY

(about 3/4 ounce; 20 grams)

52 calories	7 mg sodium
0 g protein	12 mg potassium
0 g fat, 0 saturated	0 g dietary fiber
0 mg cholesterol	0 RE vitamin A
14 g carbohydrate	0 mg thiamin
2 mg calcium	0 mg riboflavin
1 mg phosphorus	0 mg niacin
0 mg iron	0 mg vitamin C

NUTRIENT CONTENT OF 1 TABLESPOON JAM/PRESERVE/MARMALADE

(about 3/4 ounce; 20 grams)

48 calories	8 mg sodium
0 g protein	15 mg potassium
0 g fat, 0 saturated	0 g dietary fiber
0 mg cholesterol	0 RE vitamin A
13 g carbohydrate	0 mg thiamin
4 mg calcium	0 mg riboflavin
2 mg phosphorus	0 mg niacin
0.1 mg iron	0 mg vitamin C

NUTRIENT CONTENT OF 1 TABLESPOON REDUCED-SUGAR JAM/PRESERVE/MARMALADE
(about ¾ ounce; 20 grams)

29 calories	3 mg sodium
0 g protein	12 mg potassium
0 g fat, 0 saturated	0 g dietary fiber
0 mg cholesterol	0 RE vitamin A
7 g carbohydrate	0 mg thiamin
1 mg calcium	0 mg riboflavin
1 mg phosphorus	0 mg niacin
0 mg iron	0 mg vitamin C

NUTRIENT CONTENT OF 1 TABLESPOON ARTIFICIALLY SWEETENED JAM/PRESERVE/MARMALADE
(about ¾ ounce; 20 grams)

2 calories	0 mg sodium
0 g protein	14 mg potassium
0 g fat, 0 saturated	1 g dietary fiber
0 mg cholesterol	0 RE vitamin A
1 g carbohydrate	0 mg thiamin
2 mg calcium	0 mg riboflavin
2 mg phosphorus	0 mg niacin
0.1 mg iron	0 mg vitamin C

Jarlsberg: A pale nut-sweet Emmentaler-type cow's milk cheese imported from Norway. It's a good substitute for Swiss cheese and, though slightly lower in fat, melts beautifully.

NUTRIENT CONTENT OF 1 OUNCE (28 GRAMS) JARLSBERG

85 calories	239 mg sodium
6 g protein	53 mg potassium
7 g fat, 4 saturated	0 g dietary fiber
20 mg cholesterol	72 RE vitamin A
0 g carbohydrate	0.01 mg thiamin
110 mg calcium	0.14 mg riboflavin
98 mg phosphorus	0.2 mg niacin
0.1 mg iron	0 mg vitamin C

Jasmine Tea: A perfumy tea popular in Asia made by blending dried jasmine blossoms with tea. Apart from flavor, jasmine tea has no known benefits although some people find it soothing.

Jaundice: A yellowing of the skin and eyeballs associated with hepatitis or other liver disease. Responsible for the yellowing is bilirubin, an ocher pigment in bile. Even in healthy people, there is always a bit of bilirubin circulating in the blood. It's a by-product of hemoglobin breakdown and is usually disposed of by the liver. But when the liver is diseased, its ability to handle bilirubin falters and there's a buildup of it in the blood. Jaundice itself is not a disease, merely a symptom of it.

Jaw Wiring: Some people are so desperate to lose weight they have their jaws wired so all they can handle are liquid formulas. Such drastic measures produce dramatic weight loss. But usually only temporarily. Once patients are unwired, they begin eating solid food and regaining all the lost pounds.

Jejunum: The middle portion of the small intestine and a major site of digestion and absorption of food, especially of fats and proteins.

Jellies: See JAMS, JELLIES, MARMALADES, PRESERVES.

Jell-O: The brand name for powdered fruit-flavored sweetened GELATIN mixes first patented in 1865 by New Yorker Peter Cooper. Women's magazines did much to popularize Jell-O by dreaming up dozens of "congealed" fruit salads. So did the Jack Benny radio show, which Jell-O sponsored for years. Today General Foods manufactures Jell-O in both sugar and sugar-free versions. Together they sell more than two million boxes—*every day*.

Jelly Beans: Chewy, lollipop-bright candies the size and shape of kidney beans. President Ronald Reagan gave jelly beans a certain cachet by keeping a jar of them on his desk in the Oval Office. First manufactured around the turn of the century, jelly beans might have been made with real fruit juices in the beginning. Today they're more likely to be compounded of artificial flavors and colors, sugar and just enough pectin or gelatin to firm them up. In the revised edition of *The Dictionary of American Food and Drink,* John Mariani writes, "Jelly beans were first advertised in the July 5, 1905, edition of the *Chicago Daily News* at nine cents a pound." Other than providing hefty doses of sugar, today's jelly beans are nutritional ciphers. They weigh in at 104 calories per ounce.

Jerky: Air- or sun-dried strips of beef once carried by Native Americans and cowboys. Jerky kept well, provided lots of protein, minerals and energy and could be chewed or simmered into soup. It is now being sold as snack food, but make a note, it is extremely high in sodium.

NUTRIENT CONTENT OF 1 OUNCE (28 GRAMS) JERKY	
96 calories	814 mg sodium
11 g protein	173 mg potassium
3 g fat, 3 saturated	0 g dietary fiber
31 mg cholesterol	28 RE vitamin A
6 g carbohydrate	0.06 mg thiamin
11 mg calcium	0.26 mg riboflavin
108 mg phosphorus	2.5 mg niacin
1.7 mg iron	3 mg vitamin C

Jerusalem Artichoke Pasta: Health-food stores, even some supermarkets, sell drab gray-green pastas made from artichoke flour, which claim to be safe for diabetics. The truth is, regular pastas are safe for diabetics, too.

Jerusalem Artichokes: See ARTICHOKES, JERUSALEM.

Jet Lag (diet and): Anyone who's jetted across four time zones or more knows what jet lag is—a fuzzy-headed, bone-tired, I'd-give-anything-to-sleep-but-can't feeling. It's said that eastbound travel (from the United States to Europe, for example) is worse than the return trip. That depends on whether you're a night owl or a lark. As a rule, owls welcome the gained westbound hours as a way to sleep off jet lag. Not so early birds, who, with their biological clocks still on European time, wake at midnight raring to begin the day. For their internal clocks to readjust to U.S. time, larks usually need one day for each hour's difference in time. On eastbound trips, however, larks fare better because they can tumble into bed and when it's their normal U.S. wake-up time, it's already 10 A.M. abroad. Night owls, on the other hand, are just winding down when it's time to rise and shine. Every frequent flier has pet ways to lick jet lag. Whatever works. For most travelers, that means drinking plenty of fluids (not alcoholic) en route, eating lightly with an emphasis on high-fiber fruits and vegetables, and sticking to decaf coffees and teas. The latest "preventive" is TRYPTOPHAN, an amino acid formerly available in over-the-counter pills, which seems to lessen and shorten the symptoms of jet lag. It boosts the production of serotonin, a brain chemical that encourages sleep. But physicians and nutritionists caution against taking tryptophan. Doing so can be risky.

Jewfish: The giant among groupers, weighing in sometimes at 700 pounds. They're shallow feeders that swim the warm Florida and Gulf of Mexico waters. Despite their size, jewfish are tender, lean, white and sweet. Unfortunately, they are also one of the fish apt to be contaminated with ciguatoxin (see CIGUATERA POISONING). For approximate nutrient counts, see FISH, LEAN WHITE.

Jicama: The crisp-fleshed, turnip-shaped tuber of a subtropical legume. Pronounced *HEE-kama,* it is showing up in supermarkets across the country. With flesh the color and texture of water chestnuts, with a sweet, nutty flavor, jicama is delicious sliced raw into salads or slipped into stir-fries (it doesn't lose its crunch). Jicama is low in calories and sodium, contains zero fat or cholesterol, yet is a moderate source of fiber and potassium and an excellent one of vitamin C. **SEASON:** Year-round.

NUTRIENT CONTENT OF 1 CUP SLICED RAW JICAMA (about 4½ ounces; 130 grams)	
50 calories	6 mg sodium
1 g protein	195 mg potassium
0 g fat, 0 saturated	2 g dietary fiber
0 mg cholesterol	3 RE vitamin A
12 g carbohydrate	0.03 mg thiamin
16 mg calcium	0.04 mg riboflavin
23 mg phosphorus	0.3 mg niacin
0.8 mg iron	26 mg vitamin C

Jin Bu Huan: A Chinese herbal used as a painkiller. But when three Colorado preschoolers accidentally swallowed it, they had to be rushed to the hospital and put in intensive care. *Jin bu huan* triggered severe breathing problems, depressed their central nervous systems and slowed their heartbeats to a life-threatening pace. P.S.: They all recovered, but not without quick and accurate medical intervention.

Juice, Juicing: Quick to believe that fruit and vegetable juices cure (or prevent) everything from colds to cancer, people rush out to buy expensive juicers. Many juicers extract the fiber-rich pulp, which is tossed out, and some of the vitamin C may be sacrificed, too. On the other hand, the pulverizing action of juicers is believed to make beta-carotene more easily absorbed by the body. The juicers that don't extract pulp produce juices so sludgy and sharp they must be watered down or, worse yet, sweetened before they can be drunk. There's no denying that juiced fruits and vegetables are preferable to soft drinks; still, they shouldn't be touted as "energizers," "detoxifiers," "preventives" or "cures" for this and that. They aren't.

Junior Foods: Lumpy baby food as opposed to silken purees. The time to begin introducing cooked, soft, fork-mashed fruits and vegetables—either commercial or homemade—to infants is between the ages of six and seven months. Older babies are more difficult to wean off purees.

Junket: Powder or tablets made from RENNIN, an enzyme secreted by the lining of a calf's stomach, also a milk custard set with junket. Cheese makers use junket to curdle milk at the beginning of the cheese-making process.

Junk Food: All the fat- and/or sugar-rich chips, cookies, crackers and snacks people love to munch between meals. Apart from their lack of nutritive value and their load of calories, they may kill the appetite so there's no room for healthful food come mealtime.

Juvenile-Onset Diabetes: The preferred name is now **insulin-dependent diabetes mellitus** (IDDM). See DIABETES.

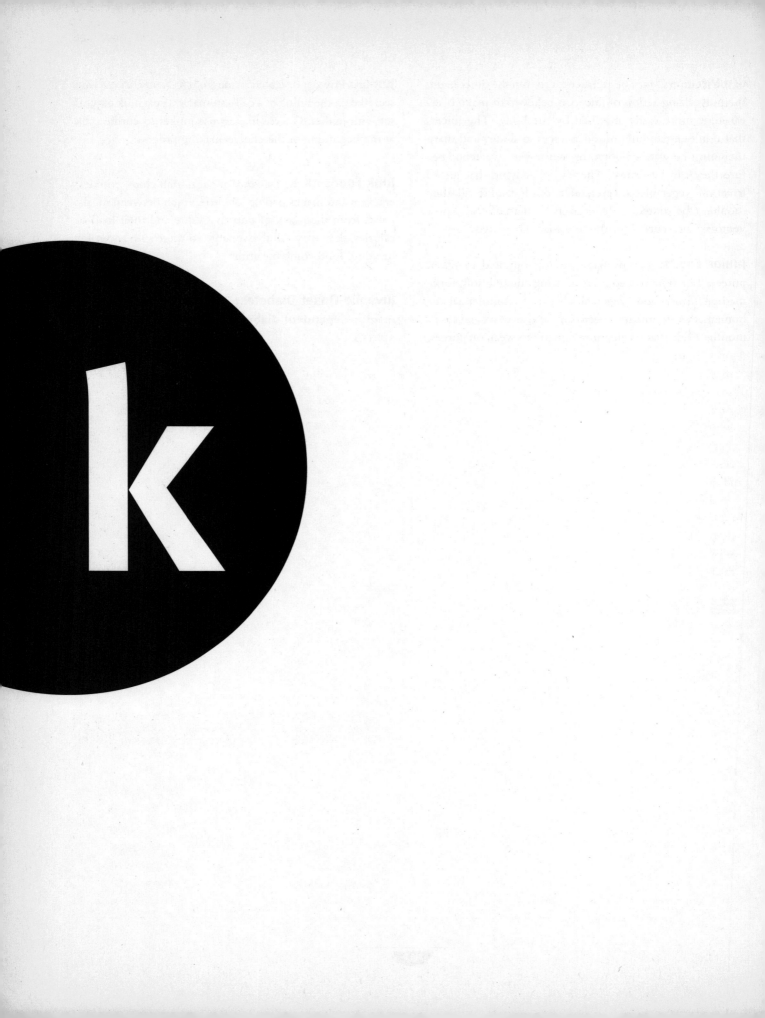

K, Vitamin: Known as the blood-clotting vitamin, K helps the body synthesize at least four of the proteins integral to clot formation, which is why so many surgeons prescribe it to patients before surgery. But vitamin K also cooperates with vitamins A and D in helping to build bone protein. What makes vitamin K a unique fat-soluble vitamin is that bacteria in the gastrointestinal tract synthesize it, albeit in amounts too small to supply daily needs. **DEFICIENCY SYMPTOMS:** Blood that's slow to clot, which can be fatal during surgery; indeed, any time a vein or artery is cut. An ongoing deficiency leads to hemorrhagic disease. Newborns are at particular risk because their digestive tracts contain no vitamin K-producing bacteria and their plasma levels of prothrombin, a major clotting protein, are low (the body's way of reducing the risk of fatal blood clotting in the baby during birth). One shot of vitamin K is usually all that's needed to avoid hemorrhagic disease in new babies. Sadly, for all its ability to "thicken" blood, vitamin K does not cure hemophilia, an inherited disease. **GOOD SOURCES:** Collards, kale, spinach and other dark leafy greens, cabbage, brussels sprouts, broccoli, liver, milk and eggs. **PRECAUTIONS:** Like vitamins A, D and E, vitamin K is fat soluble, meaning that it can be stored in the body and that it's possible to OD on powerful supplements. The worst case scenario: brain or liver damage, jaundice, the destruction of red blood cells. But there are problems of a different sort, too. Patients on anticoagulants (a standard medication for those with heart dis-ease) should cut down on high vitamin K foods and avoid multivitamin pills containing vitamin K because these cancel out the effects of the medication.

Kaiser Roll: A crisp-crusted white roll the size of a burger bun with a petaled or crownlike top. It's also called a **Vienna roll** because that's where it was first made—in honor, some say, of the Emperor Franz Josef. Sometimes kaiser rolls are topped with poppy seeds, sometimes not. Although the kaiser roll is often simply called **hard roll,** its insides are puffy soft. At least in American versions.

NUTRIENT CONTENT OF 1 MEDIUM-SIZE KAISER ROLL	
(about 1¾ ounces; 50 grams)	
156 calories	312 mg sodium
5 g protein	48 mg potassium
2 g fat, 0 saturated	2 g dietary fiber
0 mg cholesterol	0 RE vitamin A
30 g carbohydrate	0.20 mg thiamin
23 mg calcium	0.12 mg riboflavin
46 mg phosphorus	1.7 mg niacin
1.4 mg iron	0 mg vitamin C

Kale: A dark green, loose-leafed member of the cabbage family that's a particularly good source of vitamins A, C and K. Some kale is "curly" with intricately ruffed leaves; some is plain. Both are leathery and require careful cooking: Germans chop it, simmer it and toss it with glazed chestnuts; Scots cream it with potatoes and call it "Kailkenny"; and Southerners let it bubble away most of the day with a piece of side meat. No one knows for sure where kale originated, but botanists think it's closely related to the wild cabbage of Europe. This "farmer's cabbage" thrives in cool, moist cli-

NUTRIENT CONTENT OF 1 CUP BOILED/SIMMERED CHOPPED KALE	
(about 4½ ounces; 130 grams)	
41 calories	30 mg sodium
3 g protein	296 mg potassium
1 g fat, 0 saturated	1 g dietary fiber
0 mg cholesterol	962 RE vitamin A
7 g carbohydrate	0.07 mg thiamin
94 mg calcium	0.09 mg riboflavin
36 mg phosphorus	0.7 mg niacin
1.2 mg iron	53 mg vitamin C

RDA FOR VITAMIN K	
Babies:	
Birth to 6 months	5 mcg per day
6 months to 1 year	10 mcg per day
Children:	
1 to 3 years	15 mcg per day
4 to 6 years	20 mcg per day
7 to 10 years	30 mcg per day
Men and Boys:	
11 to 14 years	45 mcg per day
15 to 18 years	65 mcg per day
19 to 24 years	70 mcg per day
25 to 51+ years	80 mcg per day
Women and Girls:	
11 to 14 years	45 mcg per day
15 to 18 years	55 mcg per day
19 to 24 years	60 mcg per day
25 to 51+ years	65 mcg per day
Pregnant Women:	65 mcg per day
Nursing Mothers:	65 mcg per day

mates, even on poor soil, and has nourished the poor of northern Europe for centuries. **SEASON:** Year-round with supplies peaking in winter.

Karaya Gum (additive): The dried and powdered sap of an East Indian tree. When reconstituted in water, karaya puffs into a soft gel—a property not lost on food processors, who use it as a binder in baked goods, candies, toppings, ice creams and sherbets. Because of its stickiness, karaya gum also makes a dandy denture adhesive. GRAS when used within FDA guidelines.

Kasha: Roasted buckwheat groats, which are as popular as potatoes in Eastern Europe. Indeed, many of the Russians, Hungarians and Poles who emigrated to this country

years ago continue to use kasha in Old World ways—simmered in beef broth with browned onions, tossed with bow-tie pasta or served as a gravy sop for braised oxtails. Many Americans dislike the faintly iodiny flavor of kasha.

NUTRIENT CONTENT OF 1 CUP BOILED KASHA
(about 7 ounces; 199 grams)

178 calories	7 mg sodium
6 g protein	165 mg potassium
1 g fat, 0 saturated	3 g dietary fiber
0 mg cholesterol	0 RE vitamin A
39 g carbohydrate	0.11 mg thiamin
13 mg calcium	0.14 mg riboflavin
164 mg phosphorus	2.6 mg niacin
1.3 mg iron	0 mg vitamin C

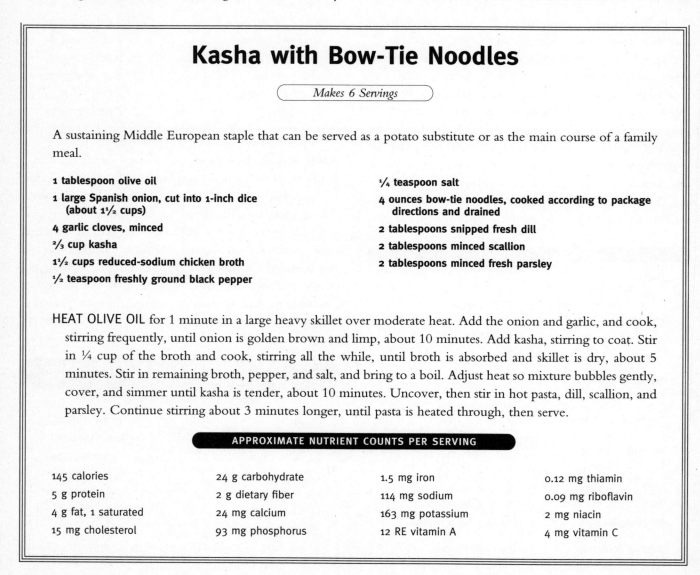

Kasha with Bow-Tie Noodles

Makes 6 Servings

A sustaining Middle European staple that can be served as a potato substitute or as the main course of a family meal.

1 tablespoon olive oil

1 large Spanish onion, cut into 1-inch dice (about 1½ cups)

4 garlic cloves, minced

⅔ cup kasha

1½ cups reduced-sodium chicken broth

½ teaspoon freshly ground black pepper

¼ teaspoon salt

4 ounces bow-tie noodles, cooked according to package directions and drained

2 tablespoons snipped fresh dill

2 tablespoons minced scallion

2 tablespoons minced fresh parsley

HEAT OLIVE OIL for 1 minute in a large heavy skillet over moderate heat. Add the onion and garlic, and cook, stirring frequently, until onion is golden brown and limp, about 10 minutes. Add kasha, stirring to coat. Stir in ¼ cup of the broth and cook, stirring all the while, until broth is absorbed and skillet is dry, about 5 minutes. Stir in remaining broth, pepper, and salt, and bring to a boil. Adjust heat so mixture bubbles gently, cover, and simmer until kasha is tender, about 10 minutes. Uncover, then stir in hot pasta, dill, scallion, and parsley. Continue stirring about 3 minutes longer, until pasta is heated through, then serve.

APPROXIMATE NUTRIENT COUNTS PER SERVING

145 calories	24 g carbohydrate	1.5 mg iron	0.12 mg thiamin
5 g protein	2 g dietary fiber	114 mg sodium	0.09 mg riboflavin
4 g fat, 1 saturated	24 mg calcium	163 mg potassium	2 mg niacin
15 mg cholesterol	93 mg phosphorus	12 RE vitamin A	4 mg vitamin C

Still, it's a grain with great potential and, with the new FOOD GUIDE PYRAMID urging everyone to eat six to eleven servings a day from the Bread, Cereal, Rice and Pasta Group, a grain well worth trying. Kasha is available whole or ground three ways—coarse, medium or fine.

Kashruth, Kashrut, Kashrus: The Jewish dietary laws used to make foods KOSHER. There are hundreds of kashruth rules, but in the main they govern how meats and poultry are slaughtered and how foods are cleaned, prepared and cooked.

Kefir, Kafir: A creamy, mildly alcoholic fermented cow's milk popular in the Caucasus. To get the milk bubbling and souring, the kefir maker drops in grains of kefir, a type of sorghum. Because people of the Caucasus often live into their nineties and beyond, health faddists have snatched upon kefir as the reason. It *is* an excellent source of vitamin A, also of calcium, phosphorus and potassium. But unless made with skim milk, it is hardly fat free.

NUTRIENT CONTENT OF 1 CUP KEFIR (2 PERCENT MILK FAT)
(8 fluid ounces; 233 grams)

122 calories	50 mg sodium
9 g protein	205 mg potassium
5 g fat, 3 saturated	0 g dietary fiber
10 mg cholesterol	155 RE vitamin A
8 g carbohydrate	0.45 mg thiamin
350 mg calcium	0.44 mg riboflavin
319 mg phosphorus	0.3 mg niacin
0.5 mg iron	0 mg vitamin C

Kelp: The Japanese are fond of this giant brown seaweed. They dry it, boil it, compress it or powder it and call it **kombu,** an ingredient absolutely essential to a variety of soups and fish dishes. Tons of kelp are harvested in California waters and although health-food stores (with a shocking disregard for truth) push kelp powders as a way to combat everything from hair loss to goiter to ulcers to obesity, most of it is processed into a jellylike stabilizer that's used in commercial ice creams, pudding mixes and salad dressings.

Keratin: The principal protein in skin, hair, nails and tooth enamel. A lack of vitamin A can lead to keratinization—rough, hardened scaly patches on the skin or in the respiratory, gastrointestinal and genitourinary tracts.

Keratomalacia: An ulceration or dryness of the cornea caused by a vitamin A deficiency.

Ketchup, Catsup, Catchup: The original was pickled Chinese fish sauce—*ket-tsiap*. British sailors took the word (if not the recipe) home to England where it was Anglicized and applied to a variety of spicy condiments. Enter the Americans and a bottled sauce by the Heinz Company of Pittsburgh. Tomato ketchup, they called it. Today we slosh it on fries, burgers, hot dogs—Richard Nixon even liked it on cottage cheese. We mix ketchup into meat loaves, cocktail sauces, bloody Marys; indeed, it's hard to imagine life without it. Its first cousin, chili sauce, is a bit spicier but not so smooth.

NUTRIENT CONTENT OF 1 TABLESPOON TOMATO KETCHUP
(about ½ ounce; 15 grams)

16 calories	156 mg sodium
0 g protein	54 mg potassium
0 g fat, 0 saturated	0 g dietary fiber
0 mg cholesterol	16 RE vitamin A
4 g carbohydrate	0.01 mg thiamin
3 mg calcium	0.01 mg riboflavin
8 mg phosphorus	0.2 mg niacin
0.1 mg iron	2 mg vitamin C

Ketoacidosis: This excessive acidity in the body is due to the accumulation of ketones. A complication of DIABETES, it can, if untreated, lead to diabetic coma. **SYMPTOMS:** Nausea, vomiting, difficulty breathing, mental confusion, "fruity breath."

Ketone Bodies: Three toxic compounds—**acetone, acetoacetic acid** and **beta hydroxybutyric acid**—that appear in the blood when fatty acids are not fully oxidized.

Ketosis: A buildup of ketone bodies in the blood. It happens most often in semistarvation or strict reducing diets when the body begins to oxidize excessive amounts of its own fat. It also occurs in uncontrolled DIABETES mellitus. Uncontrolled ketosis can lead to KETOACIDOSIS.

Kidney Beans: See BEANS, DRIED.

Kidneys (as food): Beef, veal, mutton, lamb and pork kidneys are all edible, but the choicest are veal and lamb because they are often young, sweet and tender enough to slice and sauté. Not so the kidneys of older animals, which must always be braised, simmered or stewed to succulence. Often they're chopped (another effective tenderizer) and teamed with another meat, as in the beloved steak and kidney pie of Britain. Kidneys are stellar sources of vitamin A, riboflavin, niacin and iron. They are low in fat but, alas, loaded with cholesterol. Just ounces contain the day's quota.

NUTRIENT CONTENT OF 3 OUNCES (85 GRAMS) SIMMERED BEEF KIDNEY

122 calories	114 mg sodium
22 g protein	152 mg potassium
3 g fat, 1 saturated	0 g dietary fiber
329 mg cholesterol	317 RE vitamin A
1 g carbohydrate	0.16 mg thiamin
15 mg calcium	3.45 mg riboflavin
260 mg phosphorus	5.1 mg niacin
6.2 mg iron	1 mg vitamin C

NUTRIENT CONTENT OF 3 OUNCES (85 GRAMS) BRAISED VEAL KIDNEY

139 calories	93 mg sodium
22 g protein	135 mg potassium
5 g fat, 1 saturated	0 g dietary fiber
672 mg cholesterol	171 RE vitamin A
0 g carbohydrate	0.16 mg thiamin
25 mg calcium	1.69 mg riboflavin
316 mg phosphorus	3.9 mg niacin
2.6 mg iron	7 mg vitamin C

NUTRIENT CONTENT OF 3 OUNCES (85 GRAMS) BRAISED LAMB KIDNEY

117 calories	128 mg sodium
20 g protein	151 mg potassium
3 g fat, 1 saturated	0 g dietary fiber
481 mg cholesterol	116 RE vitamin A
1 g carbohydrate	0.30 mg thiamin
15 mg calcium	1.76 mg riboflavin
246 mg phosphorus	5.1 mg niacin
10.5 mg iron	10 mg vitamin C

NUTRIENT CONTENT OF 3 OUNCES (85 GRAMS) BRAISED PORK KIDNEY

128 calories	68 mg sodium
22 g protein	121 mg potassium
4 g fat, 1 saturated	0 g dietary fiber
408 mg cholesterol	66 RE vitamin A
0 g carbohydrate	0.34 mg thiamin
11 mg calcium	1.35 mg riboflavin
204 mg phosphorus	4.9 mg niacin
4.5 mg iron	9 mg vitamin C

Kidneys (diet and): These two vital organs bracketing the spinal column are essential to life. They filter the blood and, by removing wastes, keep blood volume and composition constant, they maintain the pH of body fluids at normal levels and they excrete wastes via urine. Diabetics are at particular risk of kidney shutdown, reason alone to sustain safe blood sugar levels. Some medications stress the kidneys (the cholesterol-lowering lovastatin, to name one) and patients on them may be advised to cut down on protein, which is also hard on the kidneys. Heavy meat eaters and those who consume lots of food high in oxalates (beets, rhubarb, spinach, etc.) are prime candidates for KIDNEY STONES.

Kidney Stones: When there's an overload of certain compounds in the urine—oxalates, for example; magnesium and/or ammonium phosphate or carbonate; uric acid or cystine, a semiessential amino acid—these tend to precipitate forming stones. Kidney stones may be no bigger than grains of sand or they may be big enough to block the flow of urine. Large stones must be surgically removed or broken up via sound waves into particles small enough to excrete. Persons at greatest risk of kidney stones are those with overactive parathyroid glands or chronic kidney infections. Until recently, calcium was considered the major culprit and those with kidney stones were told to avoid calcium supplements, antacids containing calcium, milk and dairy products. Now a study of more than forty-five thousand men (with no history of kidney stones) conducted by the Harvard School of Public Health disputes that once-conventional wisdom. Indeed, Harvard researchers were startled to learn that the men in the study who ate the most calcium got a third fewer kidney stones.

How come? They theorize that calcium helps flush the real culprit—oxalates—from the body. So what's one to eat to avoid kidney stones? Or *not* eat? The latest advice: Don't worry about calcium but *do* cut down on high-oxalate foods (beets, chocolate, nuts, rhubarb, spinach, strawberries, tea and wheat bran). Also avoid vitamin C supplements (oxalate is a by-product of C metabolism) and cut down on protein (especially meat). Finally, bulk up on potassium-rich fruits and vegetables (potassium protects against kidney stones), eat plenty of complex carbohydrates and drink loads of water (or other liquids).

Kielbasa: A garlicky Polish pork sausage. Smoked or cured, kielbasa is moderately hard and dry, moderately fatty, and a single link is long enough to loop into a horseshoe, which is how it's usually sold. A few slices of kielbasa do wonders for baked beans and vegetable soups, even for boiled collards or kale.

NUTRIENT CONTENT OF 1 OUNCE (28 GRAMS) KIELBASA	
88 calories	305 mg sodium
4 g protein	77 mg potassium
8 g fat, 3 saturated	0 g dietary fiber
19 mg cholesterol	0 RE vitamin A
1 g carbohydrate	0.07 mg thiamin
12 mg calcium	0.06 mg riboflavin
42 mg phosphorus	0.8 mg niacin
0.4 mg iron	6 mg vitamin C

Kilocalorie, K Calorie: Usually shortened to *calorie,* this is a unit of heat used to measure the energy value of food. Specifically, it is the amount of heat needed to raise 1,000 grams of water through 1 degree of temperature Celsius—from 10.5°C. to 11.5°C., for example.

Kimchi: A crisp and peppery pickled vegetable slaw from Korea that's becoming popular in the United States. NOTE: Recipes vary, so specific nutrient counts are unavailable. Still, it's safe to say that *kimchi* is loaded with vitamin C and, if made with plenty of carrots, with beta-carotene, too.

Kingfish: Small members of the drum family, barely a foot long, that swim off the Atlantic shore and along the Gulf Coast. Of the four species, the **gulf kingfish** and the **southern kingfish** are choicest. They are lean, white meated and tender, but they don't often come to market except in areas where they're caught. The **corbina** is a California cousin. For approximate nutrient counts, see FISH, LEAN WHITE.

Kippers: A form of smoked herring popular in Great Britain. See HERRING.

Kiwanos: Also called **horned melons,** these New Zealand fruits look like overgrown lemons that have suddenly turned orange and grown spikes. Inside, *kiwanos (kee-WAH-nos)* are lime green and soft. Their flavor has been described as part banana, part lime. According to Frieda's, Inc., of Los Angeles, which imports *kiwanos* and sells them to supermarkets across the country, these exotic little fruits are a new best-seller. Stored at room temperature, they keep well for many weeks. Never, ever store *kiwanos* in the refrigerator because these tropical fruits deteriorate quickly in the cold. NOTE: Specific nutrient counts are unavailable for *kiwanos,* but they probably supply some vitamin C and, because of their orange color, beta-carotene. SEASON: Late winter–early spring.

Kiwifruit: A fuzzy khaki-skinned fruit about the size of a jumbo egg. Kiwis are Chinese gooseberries (no relation to the real thing) and a major New Zealand crop. California farmers grow plenty of kiwis, too, but connoisseurs prefer the imported ones because they are superior in taste and texture. Kiwi flesh, aside from an ivory core ringed with edible seeds as small and dark as pepper grains, is lime green, one reason it's such a popular garnish. Kiwis are good eating, too, buttery and sweet with just enough acid

NUTRIENT CONTENT OF 1 MEDIUM-SIZE KIWI	
(about 2¾ ounces; 76 grams)	
46 calories	4 mg sodium
1 g protein	252 mg potassium
0 g fat, 0 saturated	1 g dietary fiber
0 mg cholesterol	13 RE vitamin A
11 g carbohydrate	0.02 mg thiamin
20 mg calcium	0.04 mg riboflavin
31 mg phosphorus	0.4 mg niacin
0.3 mg iron	75 mg vitamin C

to make them interesting. High in vitamin C, low in calories, they contain zero fat and cholesterol. **SEASON:** Year-round.

Knackwurst, Knockwurst: Chunky, crisp-skinned little links that *knack* (crunch) and spurt at each bite. They look like baby frankfurters, taste a bit like them, too, except that they're spicier, more garlicky and, unlike true German frankfurters (always 100 percent beef), made with a mix of beef and pork. German cooks like to warm knackwursts in simmering water, then split them and grill them. Or slice them into dried pea soup. Unfortunately, knackwursts don't lack for fat, saturated fat, cholesterol or sodium, but they do offer moderate doses of thiamin, potassium and niacin, too. The surprise is that some of them contain a bit of vitamin C, which is added during processing in the form of sodium ascorbate.

NUTRIENT CONTENT OF 1 KNACKWURST

(about 2½ ounces; 68 grams)

209 calories	687 mg sodium
8 g protein	136 mg potassium
19 g fat, 7 saturated	0 g dietary fiber
39 mg cholesterol	0 RE vitamin A
1 g carbohydrate	0.23 mg thiamin
7 mg calcium	0.09 mg riboflavin
67 mg phosphorus	1.9 mg niacin
0.6 mg iron	18 mg vitamin C

Knob Celery: See CELERY ROOT.

Kohlrabi: Could Charlemagne have known the nutritional power of kohlrabi when he ordered that it be planted throughout his domain? Probably not. It's more likely he knew it would grow well in the cool damp climate of medieval Europe and feed millions of peasants. *Kohlrabi* is German for "turnip cabbage" and, indeed, this bulbous root looks like a turnip (albeit an apple green one) and tastes like cabbage, the family to which it belongs. Nowhere is kohlrabi more popular today than in Germany, "the kingdom of cabbage," although American supermarkets are beginning to sell it. A good thing, too, because kohlrabi is an excellent source of vitamin C and potassium. Like most members of the cabbage family, it is very low in calories and is fat and cholesterol free. **SEASON:** Hit or miss, year-round with supplies peaking in spring.

NUTRIENT CONTENT OF 1 CUP COOKED KOHLRABI

(about 6 ounces; 165 grams)

48 calories	34 mg sodium
3 g protein	561 mg potassium
0 g fat, 0 saturated	2 g dietary fiber
0 mg cholesterol	6 RE vitamin A
11 g carbohydrate	0.07 mg thiamin
41 mg calcium	0.03 mg riboflavin
74 mg phosphorus	0.6 mg niacin
0.7 mg iron	89 mg vitamin C

Kola Nut Extract (additive): A bittersweet flavoring used in commercial caramels, chocolates, ice creams, icings, baked goods and soft drinks; it was also once used as a treatment for epilepsy. Extracted from the big red-brown seeds of the kola tree, it contains both caffeine and kolanin, a heart stimulant. In tropical West Africa, Jamaica, Brazil and India, where kola trees grow, natives chew the nuts to stave off fatigue and hunger. GRAS.

Kombucha: It's all the rage just now, this ancient Manchurian (or Japanese or Egyptian) herbal, this "magic mushroom tea." Those into alternative medicine swear that it can cure everything from acne to impotence to cancer and swallow 4 ounces of it three times a day. Actually, *kombucha* is not a mushroom but a slimy yeast/fungal/bacterial growth that's left to ferment in water spiked with a bit of sugar and tea. After ten days the "tea" is ready, a brownish liquid as sour as vinegar. Despite all the "miracles" attributed to *kombucha,* there's no hard scientific evidence that it cures cancer—or anything else. The FDA has yet to pass judgment on *kombucha,* but bona fide physicians urge caution. Indeed, one Iowa woman died after sipping *kombucha* and another became very sick. As a result, the Iowa Department of Public Health has ordered an investigation of the death and illness, which may or may not be linked to *kombucha.* They have also warned Iowans about the possible dangers of drinking *kombucha.*

Konjac Root: The source of a fibrous filler called glucomannan used in diet pills that's supposed to make you feel full and eat less. Health-food companies have seized upon it and packaged it as Super-Mannan, "the weight-loss secret that has been in the Orient for five thousand years." No scientific study has proved *konjac* effective (or

Creamed Kohlrabi

Makes 6 Servings

2 pounds tender young kohlrabi, trimmed, peeled, and
  coarsely shredded
1 cup rich beef broth, diluted with ¾ cup water
1 cup coarsely chopped yellow onion
1½ tablespoons vegetable oil
3 tablespoons all-purpose flour

¼ teaspoon grated nutmeg
⅓ cup milk
½ teaspoon salt
¼ teaspoon freshly ground black pepper
¼ cup minced fresh parsley

BOIL KOHLRABI IN broth mixture for 5 minutes in a covered large heavy saucepan over moderate heat. Drain kohlrabi in a fine sieve over a heatproof bowl, pressing dry. In same pan, sauté onion in oil for 3 minutes, until golden. Turn heat to lowest point, cover, and steam 10 minutes, stirring often. Blend flour and nutmeg into onion mixture, then add reserved broth mixture and milk. Cook, stirring constantly, over moderately low heat 3 to 5 minutes, until thickened and smooth. Return kohlrabi to pan, then add salt, pepper, and parsley. Toss well, warm 2 to 3 minutes, and serve.

APPROXIMATE NUTRIENT COUNTS PER SERVING

84 calories	10 g carbohydrate	0.8 mg iron	0.08 mg thiamin
3 g protein	3 g dietary fiber	331 mg sodium	0.07 mg riboflavin
4 g fat, 1 saturated	45 mg calcium	341 mg potassium	0.9 mg niacin
2 mg cholesterol	63 mg phosphorus	20 RE vitamin A	48 mg vitamin C

harmful); still, nutritionists believe too much of it can cause bloating and diarrhea. They further suspect that such fillers may block (or at least thwart) the absorption of vital nutrients.

Kosher: A Yiddish variation of the Hebrew word *kasher,* meaning "proper." When applied to food, it means that meat and milk must at all times be kept separate. They cannot be eaten together, cooked in the same pans, served on the same dishes. Thus kosher cooks keep two sets of pans and implements, two sets of china, two sets of flatware. The Old Testament defines "clean" or kosher animals as cud chewers with cloven hooves (beef, lamb, etc.) and the unclean as cud chewers with uncloven hooves (pork). Scaled finfish are kosher; scavengers (lobster, shrimp, crabs, etc.) are taboo, as are birds of prey. Even today kosher meats come only from animals slaughtered according to rabbinical law. Although few non-Jews realize it, thousands of the packaged foods they buy are kosher—look for a *K,* or for a *K* or a *U* in a circle or the word PAREVE. *Pareve* means that the product contains neither milk nor meat and thus can be used with either one (but of course not both at the same time).

Kosher Salt: See SALT.

Kudzu: An Asian legume originally imported to the United States to control erosion on spent soil down South. It makes good animal forage; indeed, the Japanese eat tons of the starchy kudzu pods themselves, steaming the tender young leaves, and only recently have nutritionists begun to take note. Studies with hamsters have shown that kudzu contains an Antabuse-like substance that may become useful in treating alcoholics. At least, the hamsters that ate kudzu lost their appetite for alcohol. (Antabuse is the brand name for disulfiram, which is often prescribed to alcoholics to discourage further drinking; if they drink while on Antabuse, they will vomit.)

Kumquats: Averaging only an inch in diameter, these little golden ovals are the world's smallest citrus fruits. Cultivated throughout the citrus belt mostly as ornamental evergreen shrubs, kumquats grow in grapelike clusters. Though plenty tart, they can be eaten raw, skin and all. They also make splendid marmalades and preserves.

Kwashiorkor: A severe protein-energy deficiency disease common throughout the Third World, particularly among children. **SYMPTOMS:** Stunted growth, anemia, edema, diarrhea, changes in hair and skin color plus a general wasting of muscles. Luckily, many cases can be cured. The first task is to reverse dehydration and restore electrolyte imbalance in body fluids. Next, a gradual introduction of a high-protein diet based on soy and/or skim milk powders with supplementary vitamins and minerals.

NUTRIENT CONTENT OF 1 KUMQUAT	
(about ¾ ounce; 19 grams)	
12 calories	1 mg sodium
0 g protein	37 mg potassium
0 g fat, 0 saturated	1 g dietary fiber
0 mg cholesterol	6 RE vitamin A
3 g carbohydrate	0.02 mg thiamin
8 mg calcium	0.02 mg riboflavin
4 mg phosphorus	0.1 mg niacin
0.1 mg iron	7 mg vitamin C

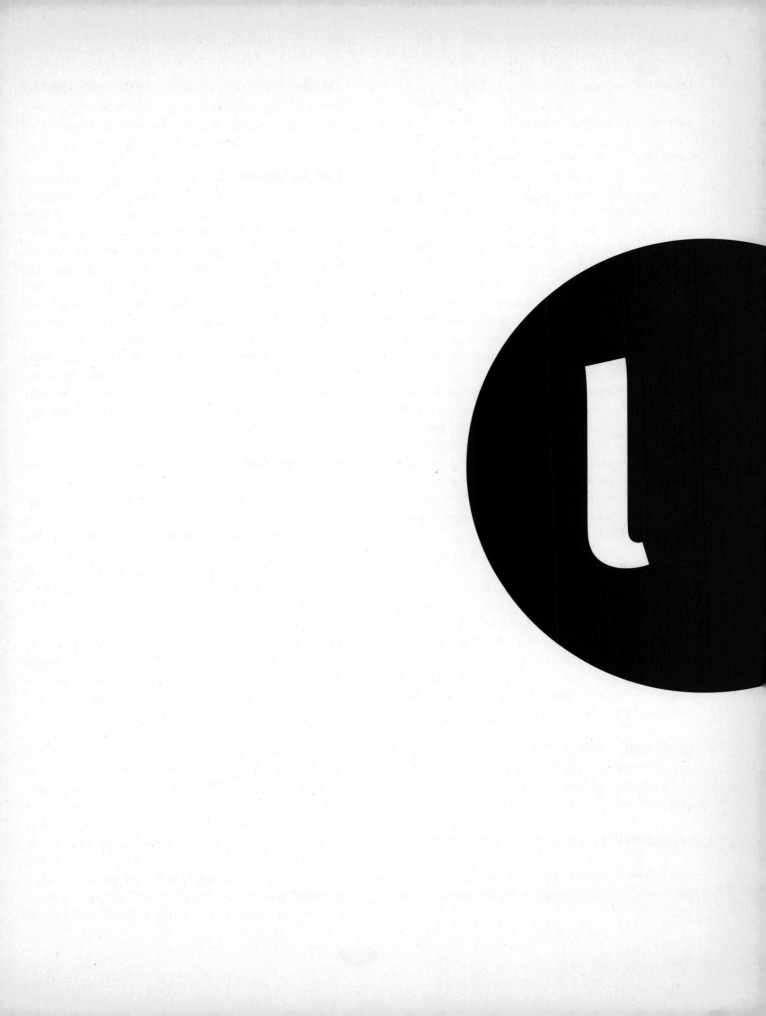

Labeling: See FOOD LABELING.

Labna: See YOGURT.

Lactaid: The brand name of a supplementary form of LACTASE manufactured for those whose own bodies lack this vital enzyme and cannot digest the sugar in milk and milk products. The liquid form, added to milk twenty-four hours ahead of use, can reduce milk's lactose content by 70 percent. Also available: tablets that can be swallowed right along with high-lactose foods.

Lactalbumin: A soft, easily digested milk protein. About half the protein in breast milk is lactalbumin; most of the rest is the hard-curded, less digestible casein. Cow's milk contains five times as much casein as lactalbumin.

Lactase: An enzyme in the intestines that breaks LACTOSE (a double sugar) into two simple ones, GLUCOSE and GALACTOSE. When the supply of lactase dwindles—as happens in blacks and Asians and in certain diseases, as well as in old age—you may suffer from diarrhea, gas and abdominal cramps. It's estimated that 70 percent of the world's adults suffer some degree of lactose intolerance. Fortunately, there are now lactase supplements that alleviate the problem (see LACTAID).

Lactation: See BREAST FEEDING.

Lactic Acid: An acid produced during the fermentation of milk sugar (LACTOSE). To make cheese and yogurt, to sour cabbage into sauerkraut, even to leaven sourdough bread, food processors capitalize on the lactic-acid-forming capabilities of certain bacteria (lactobacilli) to break down a variety of different sugars, among them lactose, sucrose (table sugar), GLUCOSE and MALTOSE.

Lactobacillus bifidus Factor: An element in breast milk that promotes the development of "good" bacteria in the intestines of newborns. These produce an "acid climate" that inhibits the growth of harmful bacteria.

Lactoglobulin: A protein found in milk whey.

Lacto-Ovo-Vegetarians: Vegetarians who will eat eggs, milk and other dairy products but no meat, poultry or seafood.

Lactose: The compound sugar found in milk. Before the body can use "milk sugar," it must be broken down into two simpler sugars—GLUCOSE and GALACTOSE. And that requires an intestinal enzyme called LACTASE.

Lactose Intolerance: Certain people lack LACTASE, an intestinal enzyme needed to digest milk sugar (LACTOSE). Without it, lactose remains in the small intestine, pulling water from bodily fluids into the gut (result: bloating). Bacteria ferment the undigested sugar, producing lots of gas and causing painful cramping and diarrhea. Such people are said to have a lactose intolerance and are put on a lactose-restricted diet in which high-lactose dairy foods (milk, fresh cheeses, cream, ice cream and so on) are curtailed and/or replaced by more easily digested milk products (yogurts and aged cheeses). In addition, any foods containing lactose are taken with meals, not on an empty stomach. There are other options, too: to use lactose-reduced milk and other dairy products or to take lactase supplements (see LACTAID).

Lactovegetarians: Vegetarians who include milk and milk products in their diets but ban all other animal protein—and that includes eggs as well as meat, fish and fowl.

Lactylic Stearate (additive): Commercial bakers use this dough conditioner to keep breads, cakes and cookies moist. It's the salt of a fatty acid that exists naturally in vegetable oils and animal fats and it's as widely used in the cosmetic industry as it is in the food business. GRAS.

Laetrile: A cyanide-containing compound obtained from peach and apricot pits that health hucksters push among the sick and elderly as a cure for cancer. Misnamed vitamin B_{17}, laetrile is pooh-poohed by reputable nutritionists and physicians.

Lamb: A sheep less than a year old; also the meat from it. Was lamb man's first meat? Some food historians think so. Certainly it was *one* of the earliest; a cache of charred nine-thousand-year-old lamb bones found in Iraq proves that prehistoric man not only had advanced from hunter to shepherd but was also civilized enough to prefer succulent young lamb to strong and sinewy mutton. Today, lamb is categorized this way: **Baby lamb** (also sometimes called **milk-fed lamb**) is six to eight weeks old, **spring lamb** three to five months and **lamb** anything between six

NUTRIENT CONTENT OF 3 OUNCES (85 GRAMS) BRAISED LAMB ARM (SHOULDER) CHOP

235 calories

30 g protein

12 g fat, 4 saturated

103 mg cholesterol

0 g carbohydrate

22 mg calcium

196 mg phosphorus

2.3 mg iron

65 mg sodium

288 mg potassium

0 g dietary fiber

0 RE vitamin A

0.06 mg thiamin

0.23 mg riboflavin

5.4 mg niacin

0 mg vitamin C

NUTRIENT CONTENT OF 3 OUNCES (85 GRAMS) BROILED LAMB LOIN CHOP (LEAN ONLY)

185 calories

26 g protein

8 g fat, 3 saturated

81 mg cholesterol

0 g carbohydrate

16 mg calcium

194 mg phosphorus

1.7 mg iron

72 mg sodium

320 mg potassium

0 g dietary fiber

0 RE vitamin A

0.09 mg thiamin

0.24 mg riboflavin

5.9 mg niacin

0 mg vitamin C

Lamb with Green Beans, Chickpeas, and Tomatoes

Makes 6 Servings

Here lamb is more of a seasoning than a principal ingredient. Still, there's no shortage of protein—vitamins or minerals, either. When served over bulgur or brown rice, this stew exemplifies the new FOOD GUIDE PYRAMID's definition of a healthy meal.

1 tablespoon olive oil

¾ pound lean, boneless lamb shoulder, trimmed of all fat and cut into ½-inch cubes

1 large yellow onion, chopped

3 garlic cloves, minced

2 cans (14½ ounces each) no-salt-added stewed tomatoes, chopped with their juices

1 teaspoon dried rosemary, crumbled

¾ teaspoon salt

½ teaspoon freshly ground black pepper

2 tablespoons minced fresh parsley

1 pound green beans, tipped and cut into 2-inch lengths

1 cup rinsed and drained canned chickpeas

PREHEAT OVEN TO 350°F. Coat a large heavy nonstick skillet well with nonstick cooking spray, add the olive oil, and heat 1 minute over moderate heat. Add the lamb and brown 5 minutes. Remove with a slotted spoon and transfer to a small Dutch oven. Reduce heat to low, add onion and garlic to skillet, and cook, stirring occasionally, until onion has softened, about 7 minutes. Transfer onion mixture to Dutch oven and set oven over moderate heat. Stir in tomatoes, rosemary, salt, pepper, and parsley. As soon as mixture boils, cover and set in oven. Bake, stirring occasionally, until lamb is almost tender, about 30 minutes. Mix in green beans, re-cover, and cook until beans are nearly tender, about 15 minutes. Stir in chickpeas and heat gently on top of the stove just until chickpeas are heated through and green beans are tender, about 5 minutes. Serve over bulgur, brown rice, rice, or couscous.

APPROXIMATE NUTRIENT COUNTS PER SERVING

231 calories

20 g protein

7 g fat, 2 saturated

46 mg cholesterol

25 g carbohydrate

6 g dietary fiber

107 mg calcium

197 mg phosphorus

4.1 mg iron

323 mg sodium

764 mg potassium

128 RE vitamin A

0.19 mg thiamin

0.24 mg riboflavin

4.1 mg niacin

28 mg vitamin C

months and a year. There's also something called **yearling mutton,** adolescents that are neither as tender nor as delicate as lamb, yet not as muscular as **mutton** (adult sheep). One nutritional advantage of lamb is that it's somewhat less marbled with fat than beef; also that its outer layer of fat is hard and easy to remove. Loin is leaner than shoulder and leg leanest of all. **NOTE:** All nutrients given here are for well-trimmed lamb.

NUTRIENT CONTENT OF 3 OUNCES (85 GRAMS) ROAST LEG OF LAMB

162 calories	58 mg sodium
24 g protein	287 mg potassium
7 g fat, 2 saturated	0 g dietary fiber
76 mg cholesterol	0 RE vitamin A
0 g carbohydrate	0.09 mg thiamin
7 mg calcium	0.25 mg riboflavin
175 mg phosphorus	5.4 mg niacin
1.8 mg iron	0 mg vitamin C

NUTRIENT CONTENT OF 3 OUNCES (85 GRAMS) BROILED LAMB PATTY

240 calories	69 mg sodium
21 g protein	288 mg potassium
17 g fat, 7 saturated	0 g dietary fiber
83 mg cholesterol	0 RE vitamin A
0 g carbohydrate	0.09 mg thiamin
19 mg calcium	0.21 mg riboflavin
170 mg phosphorus	5.7 mg niacin
1.5 mg iron	0 mg vitamin C

Lamb's-quarter, Mâche: See SALAD GREENS.

Lanolin: The waxy secretion of the oil glands of sheep that softens and waterproofs the wool. Lanolin is used in everything from chewing gum to wrinkle creams to lipsticks to shampoos. Despite advertisers' hard-sell claims that lanolin smooths away wrinkles, moistens skin and restores dry, brittle hair to its original luster, there's no proof of it. Indeed, some people are allergic to lanolin.

Lard: Rendered hog fat, once the Deep South's shortening of choice. It makes superbly flaky biscuits and pastries, but it's pure fat (much of it saturated) and calorie

laden. To be specific, 1 tablespoon lard contains 116 calories, 13 grams fat and 12 milligrams cholesterol. Hardly health food.

Lasagne: Next to pizza, lasagne is probably America's favorite Italian dish. But, alas, it can—and usually does—ooze fat. Next time you make lasagne, substitute low-fat or nonfat ricotta for the regular. That will help bring the counts down. So will using part-skim mozzarella and greasing the pan with nonstick vegetable cooking spray instead of oiling it.

NUTRIENT CONTENT OF 1 PORTION CLASSIC LASAGNE
(about 7½ ounces; 213 grams)

338 calories	647 mg sodium
20 g protein	443 mg potassium
13 g fat, 7 saturated	3 g dietary fiber
49 mg cholesterol	137 RE vitamin A
35 g carbohydrate	0.19 mg thiamin
227 mg calcium	0.29 mg riboflavin
261 mg phosphorus	3.2 mg niacin
3.0 mg iron	14 mg vitamin C

Lassi: A refreshing, nutritious East Indian drink in which yogurt is buzzed up with rosewater, sugar and ice cubes or instead sometimes just with fresh mango, papaya or other fruit.

Lathyrogens: Leg spasms and paralysis caused by the toxins in certain legumes. Chickpeas are a major culprit, but it would take a steady diet of them to cause trouble.

Lauric Acid (additive): A highly saturated fatty acid found in butter, coconut oil and palm oil as well as in the seeds of the spice bush. Food manufacturers use lauric acid as a lubricant and defoaming agent, mostly in vegetable shortenings but also to some extent in candies, ice creams, baked goods and assorted drinks, gelatin and pudding mixes. A mild irritant, lauric acid is nonetheless considered GRAS when used within government guidelines.

Laxatives: There are four basic types: **softeners and lubricants** (mineral oil, for example); milk of magnesia and other **osmotic agents,** which increase the amount of water and thus the pressure in the bowel; high-fiber **bulking**

agents that pump up stool mass and activate peristalsis (intestinal contractions); and finally, **stimulants,** among them castor oil and senna (other stimulants to look for on a label are bisacodyl, danthron and phenolphthalein). These act like a sort of double whammy by increasing bowel liquid *and* speeding intestinal contractions. Anyone plagued by constipation should avoid (or kick) the laxative habit, as should bulimics and dieters trying to drop weight overnight. Laxative dependencies can permanently damage the colon and upset the body's fragile fluid and electrolyte balances. Long-term mineral oil use was once believed to hinder the absorption of four fat-soluble vitamins—A, D, E and K—however, new studies refute this. Still, habitual laxative use can exhaust the body's potassium reserves and weaken both heart and muscles. Clearly, laxatives aren't harmless. For that reason, most physicians urge patients to exercise more, eat more high-fiber foods and drink more liquids before resorting to laxatives. Often nothing more is needed.

L-Cysteine (additive): An amino acid used in commercial yeast breads to prevent oxidation. It's on the FDA "further-study" list. GRAS when used within FDA guidelines.

Lead: See HEAVY-METAL TOXICITY.

Lead Crystal (and lead poisoning): See LEAD under HEAVY-METAL TOXICITY.

Leafy Vegetables: Chard, collards, kale, spinach, turnip greens, even beet tops. All are powerhouses of fiber, beta-carotene and vitamin C, and most are also good sources of folic acid, riboflavin, calcium and iron. **TIP:** The darker green the leaf, the greater the supply of beta-carotene. See also the individual vegetables.

Leavening Agents: The oldest of all is **yeast,** discovered in some dim, dark long ago when crude bread doughs began to ferment and bubble. Of more concern from a health standpoint because many of them contain sodium, and some of them aluminum, are the chemical leaveners—**baking soda** (sodium bicarbonate) and **baking powders,** all of which release carbon dioxide gas and send it bubbling through batters and doughs. Baking powders are of three

basic types: **tartrate** (the active ingredient is tartaric acid, obtained from grapes, and all that's needed to set it bubbling is liquid); **phosphate** (calcium-acid-phosphate-based powders that release most of their gas when mixed with liquid, then a smaller amount when heated); and **double-acting,** blends of calcium acid phosphate and sodium aluminum sulfate. These powders also react twice, weakly when mixed with liquid, then powerfully when heated. **NOTE:** Those on low-sodium diets should know that many baked goods contain high-sodium leaveners.

Lecithin: Derived from *lekithos* (Greek for "egg yolk"), this phospholipid (fat/glycerol/phosphoric acid combo) is a prime source of choline, a B vitamin relative. It exists naturally in plants and animals—egg yolks, to be sure, but also corn and soybeans. Our own livers synthesize it and our bodies use it to strengthen cell membranes. Lecithin is an effective emulsifier, a fact not lost on food processors, who use it to produce smooth and silky chocolates, ice creams and margarines. Or on unscrupulous "medicine men," who sell quarts of the stuff, claiming it will dissolve cholesterol and unclog arteries. What they don't say—and probably don't know—is that ingested lecithin never reaches the bloodstream intact. It's broken down during digestion. Furthermore, lecithin deficiencies are unheard of. Not so lecithin overdoses, which can upset the stomach, kill the appetite and cause profuse sweating.

Lectins: Toxic compounds found in many seeds, grains and legumes. Castor beans are so loaded with a particularly deadly lectin they're inedible; even raw black beans contain enough lectins to kill rats in less than a week. In humans, lectins can damage the heart, kidneys and liver; lower the blood's clotting ability; destroy the lining of the gastrointestinal tract; and inhibit cell division. Fortunately, cooking detoxes lectins, and digestive juices further neutralize them. Besides, most of them are poorly absorbed and reach the colon intact. There lectins seem to become anticarcinogenic, exactly how no one knows. Some medical researchers theorize that lectin toxins attack tumor cells directly; others that the lectins themselves stimulate an oversecretion of intestinal juices, which in turn reduce the risk of cancer. **NOTE:** People living at high altitudes where water boils at temperatures well below 212°F. should cook lectin-containing foods in pressure saucepans; otherwise their toxins may not be sufficiently depowered.

Leeks: Although botanists point to the Mediterranean basin as the probable place of origin for leeks, food historian Waverley Root thinks it might be Celtic Britain. Legend has it that St. Patrick saved a dying Irishwoman by turning rushes into leeks and commanding her to eat them. And to this day, the leek is the national emblem of Wales. Whatever their origin, leeks are the sweetest of all the onions, indispensable throughout Europe to soups, stews, side dishes and salads. And they're gaining ground in the United States, too. Leeks are a good source of iron and dietary fiber; they are low in calories and sodium and contain no fat or cholesterol. **SEASON:** Year-round.

NUTRIENT CONTENT OF 1 MEDIUM-SIZE BOILED/STEAMED LEEK

(about 4½ ounces; 124 grams)

38 calories	13 mg sodium
1 g protein	108 mg potassium
0 g fat, 0 saturated	4 g dietary fiber
0 mg cholesterol	6 RE vitamin A
10 g carbohydrate	0.03 mg thiamin
37 mg calcium	0.03 mg riboflavin
21 mg phosphorus	0.3 mg niacin
1.4 mg iron	5 mg vitamin C

Left-handed Sugars, L-Sugars: Mirror images of conventional sugars that exist in tiny amounts in certain algae, sugar beets, plantains and seaweed. They look, taste and bake like normal sugars but are calorie free because we're able to only metabolize right-handed sugars. Great news for dieters. One L-sugar has already been patented and, if given a clean bill of health by the FDA, is expected to be snapped up by food processors. One day it may even hit supermarket shelves. Lev-O-Cal is the name to look for.

Legionnaires' Disease: Not usually associated with food or drink, this pneumonialike bacterial infection has been transmitted via contaminated water systems aboard cruise ships, even by the misters supermarkets use to keep produce fresh. Legionnaires' bacteria thrive in poorly maintained water systems. Though serious (and sometimes fatal), Legionnaires' disease, if caught early, responds quickly to antibiotics (especially erythromycin). **SYMPTOMS OF LEGIONNAIRES' DISEASE:** Headache, chest pains, coughs, diarrhea and, if fever is very high, delirium.

HOW SOON SYMPTOMS OCCUR: From two to ten days after infection. **PREVENTIVES:** Drink bottled water while traveling; also avoid public Jacuzzis and take tub baths instead of showers where you're more likely to inhale droplets of contaminated water.

Legumes: Peas, beans, lentils, peanuts and other podded plants used as food. We eat more than two dozen different legumes, most of them good sources of dietary fiber, carbohydrate, incomplete protein, certain vitamins and minerals. They are listed in individual entries.

Lemongrass: A lemon-scented, fleshy-stemmed grass integral to Thai cooking. Now grown in the United States, it pumps up the flavor of soups, main dishes and desserts, and makes it possible to use less salt.

Lemon Oil (additive): The intensely aromatic oil extracted from lemon rind. It is widely used in the food industry to flavor candies, baked goods, ices, ice creams, gelatins, puddings, pies and dozens of beverages, even reconstituted lemon juice.

Lemons: Although lemons' origin is clouded with mystery, botanists believe that they are native to Southeast Asia and that they gradually made their way west into the Mediterranean basin, probably in the hands of Arab traders. They also believe that the Crusaders, homeward bound from the holy wars, carried lemons into northern Europe and place the date at about A.D. 1200. Today no citrus fruit is more important, not even the orange. There are actually three types of lemons: the hugely commercial **acid lemon,** a rootstock variety called a **rough lemon** and the **sweet lemon,** the Meyer of California being the best known. What would we do without "a squeeze of lemon," a lemon meringue pie, a frosty lemonade on a hot day? Although frozen lemonade concentrates are widely available, nothing tops the fresh. And bottled lemon juice is a poor substitute for the just-squeezed because it's lost all fruity bouquet. Most people use lemons for the juice alone when in fact the zest (colored part of the rind rich in aromatic oils) is a splendid seasoner for savories as well as sweets. Indeed, lemon zest lends a mellow tang that makes it easy to cut down on salt. All that's needed to flavor a soup, stew or pot of vegetables is a sliver or two. **SEASON:** Year-round.

NUTRIENT CONTENT OF 1 MEDIUM-SIZE LEMON
(about 2 ounces; 58 grams)

17 calories	1 mg sodium
1 g protein	80 mg potassium
0 g fat, 0 saturated	1 g dietary fiber
0 mg cholesterol	2 RE vitamin A
5 g carbohydrate	0.02 mg thiamin
15 mg calcium	0.01 mg riboflavin
9 mg phosphorus	0.1 mg niacin
0.3 mg iron	31 mg vitamin C

NUTRIENT CONTENT OF 1 TABLESPOON FRESH LEMON JUICE
(about ½ ounce; 15 grams)

4 calories	0 mg sodium
0 g protein	19 mg potassium
0 g fat, 0 saturated	0 g dietary fiber
0 mg cholesterol	0 RE vitamin A
1 g carbohydrate	0.01 mg thiamin
1 mg calcium	0 mg riboflavin
1 mg phosphorus	0 mg niacin
0 mg iron	7 mg vitamin C

NUTRIENT CONTENT OF 1 TABLESPOON BOTTLED LEMON JUICE
(about ½ ounce; 15 grams)

3 calories	3 mg sodium
0 g protein	15 mg potassium
0 g fat, 0 saturated	0 g dietary fiber
0 mg cholesterol	0 RE vitamin A
1 g carbohydrate	0.01 mg thiamin
2 mg calcium	0 mg riboflavin
1 mg phosphorus	0 mg niacin
0 mg iron	4 mg vitamin C

NUTRIENT CONTENT OF 1 TABLESPOON FROZEN RECONSTITUTED LEMON JUICE
(about ½ ounce; 15 grams)

3 calories	0 mg sodium
0 g protein	14 mg potassium
0 g fat, 0 saturated	0 g dietary fiber
0 mg cholesterol	0 RE vitamin A
1 g carbohydrate	0.01 mg thiamin
1 mg calcium	0 mg riboflavin
1 mg phosphorus	0 mg niacin
0 mg iron	5 mg vitamin C

NUTRIENT CONTENT OF 1 CUP FROZEN RECONSTITUTED LEMONADE
(8 fluid ounces; 248 grams)

100 calories	8 mg sodium
0 g protein	37 mg potassium
0 g fat, 0 saturated	0 g dietary fiber
0 mg cholesterol	5 RE vitamin A
26 g carbohydrate	0.02 mg thiamin
8 mg calcium	0.05 mg riboflavin
5 mg phosphorus	0 mg niacin
0.4 mg iron	10 mg vitamin C

NUTRIENT CONTENT OF 1 TEASPOON GRATED LEMON ZEST
(0.1 ounce; 2 grams)

1 calorie	0 mg sodium
0 g protein	0 mg potassium
0 g fat, 0 saturated	0 g dietary fiber
0 mg cholesterol	0 RE vitamin A
Trace carbohydrate	0 mg thiamin
3 mg calcium	0 mg riboflavin
0 mg phosphorus	0 mg niacin
0 mg iron	3 mg vitamin C

Lemon Sole: See FLOUNDER.

Lentils: The dried, shelled-out seeds of a bushy, podding pulse of biblical antiquity. Those most familiar to us are khaki brown. But there are other varieties, too: the red lentils for which Esau sold his birthright, the golden lentils of India and lentils as green as garden peas (the French favorite). All of them supply hefty doses of dietary fiber, protein, complex carbohydrate and impressive complements of iron, thiamin, niacin, phosphorus and potassium

NUTRIENT CONTENT OF 1 CUP BOILED BROWN LENTILS
(about 7 ounces; 198 grams)

231 calories	4 mg sodium
18 g protein	731 mg potassium
1 g fat, 0 saturated	10 g dietary fiber
0 mg cholesterol	2 RE vitamin A
40 g carbohydrate	0.34 mg thiamin
38 mg calcium	0.15 mg riboflavin
356 mg phosphorus	2.1 mg niacin
6.6 mg iron	3 mg vitamin C

(not for nothing have lentils been a Lenten favorite throughout much of the world). Unlike dried beans, lentils should not be soaked; they'll cook down to mush.

Leptin: A newly discovered hormone produced by the body's so-called fat gene (OB-GENE) that may revolutionize the way physicians treat obesity. Leptin, isolated in 1995 by a team of researchers led by Dr. Jeffrey Friedman, a molecular geneticist at the Howard Hughes Medical Institute at New York's Rockefeller University who also identifed the ob-gene, is believed to act as an appetite switch that tells the brain the body's had enough food. In other words, it signals the body to stop eating. In the overweight and grossly overweight, the signal fails somewhere down the line; the message doesn't get through. In the Rockefeller tests, obese laboratoy mice injected with leptin lost 30 percent of their body weight in just two weeks. Their blood sugar levels lowered (suggesting that leptin may also be helpful for people with diabetes) and their energy levels soared—all without any adverse side effects.

Sour Lentils

Makes 8 Servings

Just the thing for a cold winter day.

2 cups brown lentils, washed and picked over
4½ cups low-sodium beef broth
¼ teaspoon dried thyme
1 large bay leaf
2 tablespoons fruity olive oil
2 medium yellow onions, coarsely chopped
2 tablespoons all-purpose flour

2 tablespoons minced drained capers
1 teaspoon finely grated lemon zest
½ teaspoon finely grated orange zest
2 tablespoons red wine vinegar
2 tablespoons fresh lemon juice
½ teaspoon salt, or to taste
¼ teaspoon freshly ground black pepper, or to taste

SIMMER THE LENTILS in 3½ cups of the beef broth along with the thyme and bay leaf in a covered saucepan over moderately low heat 1 to 1¼ hours, until firm-tender and all broth is absorbed. Meanwhile, coat a medium heavy saucepan with nonstick spray, add the olive oil, and heat 1 minute over moderate heat. Add the onions and cook, stirring often, 10 to 15 minutes, until limp and richly browned. Blend in the flour and cook 2 to 3 minutes. Mix in the capers and lemon and orange zests. Combine the remaining 1 cup beef broth with the vinegar and lemon juice, pour into the flour mixture, and heat, stirring constantly, about 3 minutes, until thickened and smooth. Reduce the heat to its lowest point and simmer the sauce about 5 minutes longer; set aside. As soon as the lentils are firm-tender, remove and discard the bay leaf. Pour in the reserved sauce and stir well to mix. Season to taste with salt and pepper, and serve as the main course of an informal lunch or supper.

APPROXIMATE NUTRIENT COUNTS PER SERVING

222 calories	30 g carbohydrate	5.0 mg iron	0.24 mg thiamin
16 g protein	6 g dietary fiber	179 mg sodium	0.17 mg riboflavin
5 g fat, 1 saturated	38 mg calcium	635 mg potassium	3.4 mg niacin
9 mg cholesterol	284 mg phosphorus	2 RE vitamin A	5 mg vitamin C

Because humans have an ob-gene nearly identical to that in mice, researchers believe that leptin may be a major player in the body's weight-control mechanism. If so, it may be the "magic bullet" fatties have long sought. Amgen, a southern California pharmaceutical company, is banking on it. It recently paid Rockefeller University twenty million dollars for the commercial rights to leptin and aims to begin testing it on human beings in 1996. If leptin fulfills its early promise, Amgen hopes to make it available by the turn of the century. So far, leptin must be administered daily by injection. But one day biomedical researchers may be able to produce it in pill form. Or perhaps in time-release implants that can be slipped just beneath the skin. Tests to date indicate that once on leptin therapy, always on leptin therapy. That is, the mice no longer given leptin quickly regained all the pounds they'd lost.

Lettuce: See SALAD GREENS.

Leucine: An essential amino acid found in milk, meat and other high-protein foods. It's needed not only for protein synthesis but also for a sound immune system. Some infants can't metabolize leucine (or isoleucine or valine), which causes a condition known as MAPLE SYRUP URINE DISEASE (see ISOLEUCINE). See also AMINO ACIDS.

Levulose: A simple sugar also known as **fruit sugar.** See FRUCTOSE.

Lichee Nuts, Litchi Nuts, Lychee Nuts: Pulpy, perfumy white fruits popular in China for thousands of years. They look rather like peeled white cherries and, like cherries, have a single bitter pit. Although fresh lichees are available in America, most of us settle for the canned. They are superb poached in a light ginger syrup or sliced into a fruit compote. Lichees are a prime source of vitamin C and potassium, yet they are very low in calories, fat and sodium. **SEASON:** July to mid-September.

NUTRIENT CONTENT OF 1 CUP CANNED SWEETENED LICHEE NUTS
(about 9 ounces; 255 grams)

230 calories	4 mg sodium
1 g protein	254 mg potassium
1 g fat, 0 saturated	1 g dietary fiber
0 mg cholesterol	0 RE vitamin A
59 g carbohydrate	0.02 mg thiamin
9 mg calcium	0.10 mg riboflavin
51 mg phosphorus	0.9 mg niacin
0.5 mg iron	82 mg vitamin C

Licorice (additive): A flavoring extracted from the licorice plant, a perennial herb that thrives across Mediterranean Europe and eastward into the Middle East. For years licorice has been used in pharmacology as an expectorant, as well as to mask the taste of bitter medicines. It was also once used to make candy and, in some countries, still is. In the United States, however, almost all licorice candies are artificially flavored. A good thing, too, for in heavy doses, real licorice depletes the body's store of potassium and raises blood pressure. But here's a trade-off: A researcher at Case Western Reserve University recently discovered, in tests with lab mice, that glycyrrhizin, an acid present in black licorice, reduced the risk of skin cancer.

NUTRIENT CONTENT OF 1 OUNCE (28 GRAMS) LICORICE CANDY

104 calories	7 mg sodium
0 g protein	11 mg potassium
0 g fat, 0 saturated	0 g dietary fiber
0 mg cholesterol	0 RE vitamin A
26 g carbohydrate	0 mg thiamin
1 mg calcium	0 mg riboflavin
1 mg phosphorus	0 mg niacin
0.3 mg iron	0 mg vitamin C

Liederkranz: A cow's milk cheese developed in this country by a German immigrant at the turn of the century. It's pale, soft and plenty pungent.

NUTRIENT CONTENT OF 1 CUP FRESH LICHEE NUTS
(about 6¾ ounces; 190 grams)

125 calories	2 mg sodium
2 g protein	325 mg potassium
1 g fat, 0 saturated	1 g dietary fiber
0 mg cholesterol	0 RE vitamin A
32 g carbohydrate	0.02 mg thiamin
10 mg calcium	0.12 mg riboflavin
59 mg phosphorus	1.2 mg niacin
0.6 mg iron	136 mg vitamin C

NUTRIENT CONTENT OF 1 OUNCE (28 GRAMS) LIEDERKRANZ

87 calories	389 mg sodium
5 g protein	68 mg potassium
8 g fat, 5 saturated	0 g dietary fiber
21 mg cholesterol	91 RE vitamin A
0 g carbohydrate	0.01 mg thiamin
110 mg calcium	0.18 mg riboflavin
100 mg phosphorus	0.1 mg niacin
0.1 mg iron	0 mg vitamin C

Life Choice Program: See ORNISH DIET.

Light (effect on vitamins): The vitamin most easily destroyed by light is riboflavin or B$_2$—a major concern back when glass bottles of milk were left on sunny doorsteps. Two hours was all it took for the sun's ultraviolet rays to dispatch half the riboflavin. The problem, however, hasn't gone the way of door-to-door milk deliveries. According to Cornell and Penn State researchers, low-fat milks stored in transparent bottles under fluorescent lights also lose some of their riboflavin. It should be added, however, that acute riboflavin deficiencies are rare in this country. See also B$_2$, VITAMIN.

Lignans: See PHYTOESTROGENS.

Lignin: An insoluble, indigestible fiber found in plants.

Lima Beans: See BEANS, DRIED; BEANS, FRESH.

Limburger: An intensely aromatic yeast- and bacteria-ripened cheese developed in the Limburg Province of Belgium. Its base is cow's milk and the finished cheese is crusted with a reddish bloom of mold. Inside, however, Limburger is as pale as ivory and as soft as Brie. Today, Germany probably makes more of it than Belgium.

NUTRIENT CONTENT OF 1 OUNCE (28 GRAMS) LIMBURGER

93 calories	226 mg sodium
6 g protein	36 mg potassium
8 g fat, 5 saturated	0 g dietary fiber
26 mg cholesterol	90 RE vitamin A
0 g carbohydrate	0.02 mg thiamin
141 mg calcium	0.14 mg riboflavin
111 mg phosphorus	0 mg niacin
0 mg iron	0 mg vitamin C

Lime: A distinctly tropical citrus fruit native to Southeast Asia. Like lemons, limes were brought westward into Mediterranean Europe and Africa by Arabs. Or so food historians believe. Lime juice was once put into the grog of British sailors ("limeys") to ward off scurvy, a sometimes fatal disease caused by vitamin C deficiency. Yet limes are 75 percent lower in vitamin C than oranges or grapefruits (the reason for their use was that they were generally more available and thus cheaper). In the United States two commercial varieties of lime are grown. The common supermarket lime is the fine-fleshed, mild **Persian.** The other, produced on a limited scale, is the smaller, yellower **Mex-**

NUTRIENT CONTENT OF 1 MEDIUM-SIZE LIME
(about 2½ ounces; 67 grams)

20 calories	1 mg sodium
1 g protein	68 mg potassium
0 g fat, 0 saturated	1 g dietary fiber
0 mg cholesterol	1 RE vitamin A
7 g carbohydrate	0.02 mg thiamin
22 mg calcium	0.01 mg riboflavin
12 mg phosphorus	0.1 mg niacin
0.4 mg iron	20 mg vitamin C

NUTRIENT CONTENT OF 1 TABLESPOON FRESH LIME JUICE
(about ½ ounce; 15 grams)

4 calories	0 mg sodium
0 g protein	17 mg potassium
0 g fat, 0 saturated	0 g dietary fiber
0 mg cholesterol	0 RE vitamin A
1 g carbohydrate	0 mg thiamin
1 mg calcium	0 mg riboflavin
1 mg phosphorus	0 mg niacin
0 mg iron	5 mg vitamin C

NUTRIENT CONTENT OF 1 TABLESPOON BOTTLED LIME JUICE
(about ½ ounce; 15 grams)

3 calories	2 mg sodium
0 g protein	12 mg potassium
0 g fat, 0 saturated	0 g dietary fiber
0 mg cholesterol	0 RE vitamin A
1 g carbohydrate	0.01 mg thiamin
2 mg calcium	0 mg riboflavin
1 mg phosphorus	0 mg niacin
0 mg iron	1 mg vitamin C

ican or **Key lime,** which is tart enough to "set" the sweetened condensed milk in a Key lime pie. Although fresh lime juice is always best, it is available bottled and frozen into limeade concentrates. Lime zest, by the way, is as aromatic, as useful in cooking as lemon or orange zest. **SEASON:** Year-round with supplies peaking in summer.

NUTRIENT CONTENT OF 1 CUP RECONSTITUTED FROZEN LIMEADE

(8 fluid ounces; 247 grams)

102 calories	6 mg sodium
0 g protein	33 mg potassium
0 g fat, 0 saturated	0 g dietary fiber
0 mg cholesterol	0 RE vitamin A
27 g carbohydrate	0.01 mg thiamin
7 mg calcium	0.01 mg riboflavin
3 mg phosphorus	0.1 mg niacin
0.1 mg iron	7 mg vitamin C

Lime, Pickling: Calcium hydroxide. Its purpose is to make pickles crisp and it replaces alum, an aluminum salt that's no longer considered safe.

Limiting Amino Acids: Many plant foods contain a combination of amino acids, the building blocks of protein, but rarely all nine essential amino acids in amounts necessary for growth and maintenance of body tissues. When one of these essential amino acids is in short supply and that supply is exhausted, the body stops making protein and doesn't use the remaining amino acids for tissue building, but rather burns them for energy. The essential amino acid in shortest supply is thus called the limiting amino acid because it's the one that limits protein production.

Limonene (additive): A compound found in orange zest and oil of orange that has caused kidney tumors in male lab rats—not females, not mice of either sex, and the findings are probably not relevant to people. Limonene is a flavoring widely used by the food industry. GRAS when used within FDA guidelines.

Limonoids: Anticarcinogens in orange juice that have been shown to reduce the risk of mouth cancer. A biochemist studying limonoids at the Baylor College of Dentistry in Dallas predicts that limonoids may one day be added to toothpaste and mouthwash. Time will tell. See also PHYTOCHEMICALS.

Linaloe Oil, Lignaloe Oil, Bois de Rose Oil (additive): The scent is "wild rose," but this flavoring comes instead from several different tropical trees that grow in Mexico, Guyana and Brazil. As might be expected, linaloe oil is blended into soaps and perfumes. Food manufacturers use it, too, to boost the flavor of a huge variety of drinks (both hard and soft), candies, baked goods, sherbets and ice creams. Though considered safe, it's been known, on occasion, to cause allergic reactions.

Lingcod: An important market fish on the West Coast. Though lean and delicate, it is not a cod but a **greenling,** the biggest in fact of nine Pacific species and the only one of real commercial value. Lingcod sometimes tops the scale at 75 pounds. For approximate nutrient counts, see FISH, LEAN WHITE.

Lingonberries: Small, tart, bright red berries, the European cousins of our own cranberries. Lingonberries are especially popular in Scandinavia; the Swedes use them as a topper for omelets and pancakes. Until recently, no fresh lingonberries were available here, only preserves. Today, however, big-city boutique greengrocers are beginning to stock them. Like cranberries, lingonberries must be liberally sweetened before they can be eaten. **SEASON:** Late autumn.

NUTRIENT CONTENT OF 1 CUP COOKED SWEETENED LINGONBERRIES

(about 9¾ ounces; 272 grams)

433 calories	71 mg sodium
0 g protein	76 mg potassium
0 g fat, 0 saturated	4 g dietary fiber
0 mg cholesterol	5 RE vitamin A
106 g carbohydrate	0.05 mg thiamin
11 mg calcium	0.05 mg riboflavin
16 mg phosphorus	0.3 mg niacin
0.6 mg iron	6 mg vitamin C

Linguine: See PASTA.

Linoleic Acid: An essential, polyunsaturated fatty acid. **SOURCES:** Fish and vegetable oils (cottonseed, linseed, safflower, soybean), meat and milk (breast milk is four times as rich in linoleic acid as cow's milk). **DEFICIENCY SYMPTOMS:** Stunted growth, hair loss, scaly skin, slow-to-heal wounds.

Linolenic Acid: The alpha form is another essential fatty acid. Linolenic acid, researchers now know, can be converted by the body into the two most important omega-3 fatty acids: eicosapentaenic acid (EPA) and docosahexaenic acid (DHA), which are believed to fight heart disease. At present, scientists are studying linolenic acid on two fronts: the gamma form's usefulness as a treatment for certain types of cancer (breast, colorectal) and the alpha form's role in stroke prevention. Studies have so far shown that when middle-aged men considered to be prime candidates for heart disease have high blood serum levels of alpha-linolenic acid, their risk of stroke is substantially reduced. SOURCES: Fish oil is especially rich in linolenic acid, as are walnuts, soybeans, spinach, mustard greens and some vegetable oils (flaxseed, rapeseed [canola] and linseed). DEFICIENCY SYMPTOMS: Slow growth, weakened immune system.

Lipase: An enzyme that breaks down fats in the stomach and small intestine. Most of it is secreted by the pancreas.

Lipids: A fancy word for the fats found in plants and animals (and that includes our own bodies). Once isolated from plant or animal tissue, lipids consist largely of triglycerides (as much as 99 percent). The rest is a mix of monoglycerides, diglycerides, free fatty acids and phospholipids plus fragments that cannot be broken down. The lipid on everyone's mind these days is CHOLESTEROL. Another one that's zoomed into public awareness is LECITHIN, which self-styled nutritionists hustle as a sort of Roto-Rooter for cholesterol-clogged veins and arteries.

Lipoproteins: Lipids piggybacked aboard simple proteins, forming compound proteins. In the body, their job is to ferry lipids from the liver and intestinal tract to tissues where they're needed. Circulating in the blood at all times are five different lipoproteins, two of which have a familiar ring: **high-density lipoprotein** (HDL, or so-called "good" cholesterol) and **low-density lipoprotein** (LDL, or "bad" cholesterol). The others are **chylomicrons** (the largest but least dense lipoprotein), **very low-density lipoprotein** (VLDL, which ends up as cholesterol-laden LDL) and **intermediate-density lipoprotein** (IDL), which also metamorphoses into LDL. Age, health, diet and weight all determine the number and the mix of lipoproteins in the blood.

Liqueurs: See ALCOHOL, ALCOHOLIC BEVERAGES.

Liquid Diets: They produce rapid weight loss, yes. But they are not without risk. In the 1970s when the first of these high-protein diets burst upon us, they were "answered prayers" for the chronically or morbidly overweight. But they had a dark side. These early formulas lacked TRYPTOPHAN, an essential acid; they were not supplemented with vitamins, minerals and electrolytes; and worst of all, they were undertaken without medical supervision. As a result, sixty liquid-diet users died. Modern formulas (called **very low-calorie, high-protein** or **protein-sparing diets**) have corrected the nutritional balance and the strictest regimens (200 to 800 calories a day) are carefully supervised by physicians.

And what about the over-the-counter diet formulas recommended as substitutes for breakfast and lunch with a well-balanced but low-calorie dinner ending the day? Used as directed for a limited period of time, they are effective and harmless—for healthy people. But they should never replace solid food altogether. Nor should they be taken without your doctor's blessing. The trouble with all liquid diets is that once the pounds are shed, they pile back on unless good eating patterns are established together with a sensible program of exercise. Getting the weight off is one thing; keeping it off another.

Liquid Smoke: The brand name for a brush-on solution of condensed, filtered wood smoke used to suffuse home-grilled, -broiled or -roasted meats, poultry, seafood and vegetables with commercial "barbecue" flavor. The source of the smoke may be dampened sawdust, wood chips or charcoal; although most of the resins, tars and carcinogenic polycyclic aromatic hydrocarbons (see PAHs) have been filtered out, no studies have yet shown just how safe Liquid Smoke is. CONSENSUS: It's safer than charcoal grilling but may not be entirely risk free.

Liquor: See ALCOHOL, ALCOHOLIC BEVERAGES.

Listeria monocytogenes, Listeriosis: See BACTERIA.

Litchi Nuts: See LICHEE NUTS.

"Lite," "Light": Deceptive descriptions formerly used on packaged foods. The government's new nutritional labeling requirements, adopted in 1994, put a stop to false or misleading claims because these terms, once so cavalierly used, must now conform to rigid definitions. See also FOOD LABELING.

Littlenecks: See CLAMS.

Liver (as food):
Nutritionists have recently done a one-eighty on the merits of liver. In the old days, it was practically force-fed to anemic young women (well, not quite). There's no denying that liver is a powerhouse of iron, vitamins A and D, not to mention a good source of most of the B-complex. But it is also loaded with cholesterol and off-limits to anyone with high blood cholesterol or coronary heart disease. In addition, because of its role as a detoxer, liver contains many chemicals that may be hazardous to your health. The most delicate liver is **veal** or **calf's liver;** the two strongest, **beef** and **pork.** The richest in all creation? **Foie gras,** literally the "fat livers" of force-fed geese (or sometimes ducks); they are so full of fat they are almost white. Grilled or sautéed fresh foie gras has become the specialty of many young American chefs and it simply

NUTRIENT CONTENT OF 3 OUNCES (85 GRAMS) SAUTÉED CALF'S LIVER	
210 calories	113 mg sodium
26 g protein	375 mg potassium
10 g fat, 4 saturated	0 g dietary fiber
283 mg cholesterol	4,823 RE vitamin A
3 g carbohydrate	0.21 mg thiamin
10 mg calcium	2.88 mg riboflavin
376 mg phosphorus	14.5 mg niacin
4.5 mg iron	19 mg vitamin C

NUTRIENT CONTENT OF 3 OUNCES (85 GRAMS) SAUTÉED BEEF LIVER	
184 calories	90 mg sodium
23 g protein	309 mg potassium
7 g fat, 2 saturated	0 g dietary fiber
409 mg cholesterol	9,123 RE vitamin A
7 g carbohydrate	0.18 mg thiamin
9 mg calcium	3.52 mg riboflavin
391 mg phosphorus	12.3 mg niacin
5.3 mg iron	20 mg vitamin C

NUTRIENT CONTENT OF 3 OUNCES (85 GRAMS) BRAISED PORK LIVER	
140 calories	42 mg sodium
22 g protein	127 mg potassium
4 g fat, 1 saturated	0 g dietary fiber
301 mg cholesterol	4,590 RE vitamin A
3 g carbohydrate	0.22 mg thiamin
9 mg calcium	1.87 mg riboflavin
205 mg phosphorus	7.2 mg niacin
15.2 mg iron	20 mg vitamin C

oozes fat. "Squidgy" is the way someone once described its texture. Quite so. The tins of processed foie gras imported from France are no less sinful. The conventional wisdom today: Eat liver sparingly and, even then, only infrequently. See also CHICKEN LIVERS.

Liver (diet and):
The liver is the body's biggest organ and one of the most vital. Tucked underneath the diaphragm to the right of the stomach, the liver performs more major functions than any other single organ—and that includes the heart and lungs. It secretes bile, a sort of "atom smasher" of fat particles that's stored in the gallbladder, then released into the intestines when needed. It warehouses iron, all fat-soluble vitamins (A, D, E, K), all B vitamins. It also stores glycogen, then converts it to GLUCOSE (body fuel) whenever it's needed. There's more. The liver helps destroy bacteria and over-the-hill red blood cells, retrieving and storing any bits of iron they may contain. It detoxes a huge variety of harmful chemicals circulating in the blood—drugs, alcohol, medications. It manufactures part of the blood plasma proteins and is a major way station on the blood's journey through the body. Those with impaired liver function are usually put on a very low-protein diet, sometimes as low as 40 grams a day, because the metabolism of protein stresses the liver. Dietary fat may also be reduced; sometimes a doctor, working in concert with a registered dietitian, may recommend that it be replaced by medium-chain triglyceride oil (see MCT OIL). Finally, vitamin/mineral supplements may be prescribed.

Liverwurst:
A spicy, finely textured spread usually made of pork and pork liver although beef, even goose liver, may be used. Liverwurst is always cooked and packaged in links

large or small. **Braunschweiger,** a soft pink German liverwurst that came originally from the town of Braunschweig but is now widely made in the United States, is more delicate than regular pork liverwurst.

**NUTRIENT CONTENT OF 1 OUNCE (28 GRAMS)
BRAUNSCHWEIGER LIVERWURST**

103 calories	326 mg sodium
4 g protein	57 mg potassium
9 g fat, 3 saturated	0 g dietary fiber
45 mg cholesterol	1,023 RE vitamin A
1 g carbohydrate	0.07 mg thiamin
3 mg calcium	0.44 mg riboflavin
48 mg phosphorus	2.4 mg niacin
2.7 mg iron	3 mg vitamin C

**NUTRIENT CONTENT OF 1 OUNCE (28 GRAMS)
PORK LIVERWURST**

92 calories	244 mg sodium
4 g protein	48 mg potassium
8 g fat, 3 saturated	0 g dietary fiber
45 mg cholesterol	2,353 RE vitamin A
1 g carbohydrate	0.08 mg thiamin
7 mg calcium	0.29 mg riboflavin
65 mg phosphorus	1.2 mg niacin
1.8 mg iron	0 mg vitamin C

Lobelia: An herbal touted as a tranquilizer and an easy way to kick nicotine addition. The truth? It has caused runaway heartbeat, acute respiratory distress and coma. It has also killed.

Lobster: Given the stratospheric price of lobsters today, it's hard to believe the Pilgrims considered them poor man's meat. These, mind you, were not the inferior flat, spiny or rock lobsters but those great clawed beauties, American lobsters. Not quite three hundred years after the *Mayflower* landed, lobster had become "the king of shellfish," the darling of such fat cats as Diamond Jim Brady, whom New York restaurateur George Rector called "the best twenty-five customers I ever had" because he tackled "a deluge of lobsters, six or seven giants" along with the usual quota of oysters, clams and crabs, two entire canvasback ducks, steak and plenty of sweets.

The trouble with lobsters (in addition to being overfished) is that their life is such a series of crises that only 2 out of every 10,000 eggs laid ever reach maturity (the ripe old age of four). Despite all odds, some lobsters live long and happy lives, occasionally reaching awesome size. In the 1930s, a 42-pound leviathan was captured off the Virginia Capes and displayed in Boston's Museum of Science. Biologists believe it was at least one hundred years old.

Smaller lobsters—those in the 2-pound range—are what gourmets treasure. When perfectly prepared, they are, as historical novelist Kenneth Roberts described them in *Northwest Passage,* "not unlike hot curds, juicy and tender, and sweet as scorched honey from ocean depths."

Perfect Steamed Lobster

Makes 2 Servings

Don't buy any lobsters that aren't live and kicking.

1 quart water   **2 small live lobsters (about 2 pounds each)**

BRING WATER TO a vigorous boil in large heavy kettle with a rack in the bottom. Add lobsters; the minute the water boils vigorously again, cover kettle and steam 20 minutes—no more, no less. With tongs, place lobsters on their backs on a large cutting board covered with paper toweling. Split each lobster down the middle from head to tail with a sharp heavy knife. Serve at once with whatever accompaniments you fancy.

NUTRIENT CONTENT OF 3 OUNCES (85 GRAMS) BOILED/STEAMED LOBSTER

83 calories	323 mg sodium
17 g protein	299 mg potassium
1 g fat, o saturated	o g dietary fiber
61 mg cholesterol	22 RE vitamin A
1 g carbohydrate	0.06 mg thiamin
52 mg calcium	0.91 mg riboflavin
157 mg phosphorus	0.2 mg niacin
0.3 mg iron	o mg vitamin C

Locust Bean Gum: See CAROB-SEED GUM.

Loganberries: Often called a red blackberry, the logan-berry is actually a blackberry-raspberry cross developed in 1881 by J. H. Logan. Today loganberries are widely cultivated and available fresh, frozen and canned.

NUTRIENT CONTENT OF 1 CUP FROZEN, UNSWEETENED LOGANBERRIES
(about 5¼ ounces; 147 grams)

80 calories	1 mg sodium
2 g protein	213 mg potassium
1 g fat, o saturated	5 g dietary fiber
o mg cholesterol	5 RE vitamin A
19 g carbohydrate	0.07 mg thiamin
38 mg calcium	0.05 mg riboflavin
38 mg phosphorus	1.2 mg niacin
0.9 mg iron	23 mg vitamin C

Lollipops: Fruit-flavored hard candies on a stick. They are practically pure sugar (109 calories per ounce) and children who habitually suck them raise their chances of getting dental cavities.

London Broil: Flank steak. See BEEF.

Longans: Southeast Asian relatives of the lichee nut, gray fleshed rather than white and extremely flowery. In her benchmark book *Uncommon Fruits & Vegetables,* Elizabeth Schneider describes their flavor as "haunting, with hints of gardenia, spruce, and musk." Longans are now being grown in Florida and, according to Schneider, have "good commercial potential." Like lichees, they are delicious poached in syrup or sliced into fruit salads. Other than being a good

source of vitamin C, longans aren't very nutritious. The good news is that they're very low in calories and contain no fat or sodium. **SEASON:** Mid- to late summer.

NUTRIENT CONTENT OF 10 MEDIUM-SIZE RAW LONGANS
(about 1⅛ ounces; 32 grams)

19 calories	o mg sodium
o g protein	85 mg potassium
o g fat, o saturated	o g dietary fiber
o mg cholesterol	o RE vitamin A
5 g carbohydrate	0.01 mg thiamin
o mg calcium	0.04 mg riboflavin
7 mg phosphorus	0.1 mg niacin
o mg iron	27 mg vitamin C

Long Beans: See YARD-LONG BEANS under BEANS, FRESH.

Loquats: Golden egg-shaped fruits also called **Japanese plums** although they are native to China. Loquats now grow throughout much of the American southeast (Charleston gardens are full of them), but they're extremely fragile and don't ship well. So even though loquats are being grown commercially in Florida and California, they're more likely to appear at fancy greengrocers than in supermarkets. Their tart-sweet flesh is both soft and crisp, a rare combination. The Japanese relish loquats and harvest tons of them every year. They are no more difficult to prepare than apricots or peaches and can be substituted for them in almost any recipe. **SEASON:** Spring.

NUTRIENT CONTENT OF 10 MEDIUM-SIZE LOQUATS
(about 3½ ounces; 100 grams)

47 calories	1 mg sodium
o g protein	266 mg potassium
o g fat, o saturated	NA g dietary fiber
o mg cholesterol	153 RE vitamin A
12 g carbohydrate	0.02 mg thiamin
16 mg calcium	0.02 mg riboflavin
27 mg phosphorus	0.2 mg niacin
0.3 mg iron	1 mg vitamin C

Lotus Root: Fleshy fawn-skinned rhizome of a Southeast Asian aquatic plant that nature has linked like sausages. Each slice of lotus root looks like the star disk of a cookie press carved out of ivory. Lotus roots were precious to the ancient Egyptians and still are to millions of Thais, Japanese and Chinese. In the Chinatowns of New York, Los Angeles and San Francisco, fresh lotus roots can be bought. But the rest of America must be content with the canned or dried. They are extremely bland, rather like water chestnuts—or maybe artichokes. As for nutritive value, they are a good source of vitamin C and a first-rate one of potassium.

NUTRIENT CONTENT OF 10 SLICES BOILED LOTUS ROOT
(about 3 ounces; 89 grams)

59 calories	40 mg sodium
1 g protein	323 mg potassium
0 g fat, 0 saturated	1 g dietary fiber
0 mg cholesterol	0 RE vitamin A
14 g carbohydrate	0.11 mg thiamin
23 mg calcium	0.01 mg riboflavin
69 mg phosphorus	0.3 mg niacin
0.8 mg iron	24 mg vitamin C

Lotus Seeds: They look like black beans but are nutty-sweet (except for the bitter cores, which must be removed). The Chinese, who simmer lotus seeds in soups, grind them to paste for their beloved sweet buns, even roast them to eat out of hand, believe them powerful energizers. Chinese groceries sell lotus seeds both fresh and dried but connoisseurs prefer the dried. Like dried beans, they must be soaked. For all the Chinese claims of the tonic powers of lotus seeds, they are not particularly nutritious.

NUTRIENT CONTENT OF 1 OUNCE (28 GRAMS) RAW LOTUS SEEDS

29 calories	0 mg sodium
1 g protein	117 mg potassium
0 g fat, 0 saturated	NA g dietary fiber
0 mg cholesterol	0 RE vitamin A
6 g carbohydrate	0.05 mg thiamin
14 mg calcium	0.01 mg riboflavin
53 mg phosphorus	0.1 mg niacin
0.3 mg iron	0 mg vitamin C

"Low" (on labels): See FOOD LABELING.

Low-Acid Foods: Meats, poultry, fish and almost all vegetables. The acidity of food is a major concern for commercial processors and home canners. Because the heat-resistant spores of certain dangerous bacteria thrive in the airless, low-acid environments of canned meats, fish, fowl and vegetables, it's vital that all of them be destroyed. Hot-water baths won't do it. What's required is longer processing under 10, 15 or 20 pounds' pressure. **NOTE:** Modern tomatoes are lower in acid than those our grandmothers grew, so play it safe, and pressure-can these, too. See also BACTERIA.

Low-Methoxyl Pectin (additive): A pectin that gels in the absence of sugar, making it a perfect choice for diet jams, jellies and desserts. GRAS.

Lox: Smoked salmon. *Lox* is the Jewish word, *Lachs* the German. Smoked salmon is popular throughout Canada, the United States and Britain, northern Europe and also among Jews everywhere. They like tissue-thin slices of lox on bagels spread with cream cheese. Among the best known smoked salmons are Scottish, Norwegian and the unusually delicate, finely grained Nova Scotia. The curing and smoking of salmon vary from area to area and, in most places, the recipes and techniques are carefully guarded secrets. But all lox is high in sodium.

NUTRIENT CONTENT OF 3 OUNCES (85 GRAMS) LOX

99 calories	666 mg sodium
16 g protein	149 mg potassium
4 g fat, 1 saturated	0 g dietary fiber
20 mg cholesterol	22 RE vitamin A
0 g carbohydrate	0.21 mg thiamin
9 mg calcium	0.09 mg riboflavin
139 mg phosphorus	4.0 mg niacin
0.7 mg iron	0 mg vitamin C

Lunch: Although reams have been written about the virtues of breakfast, lunch has been largely overlooked. What is a good lunch? Not a lettuce salad and diet cola. Not a cheeseburger, milk shake and fries. Not a dab of cottage cheese and cup of coffee. Not a cup of fruit yogurt and glass of iced tea. A healthful lunch should provide about a third of the day's nutrients. The best way to touch all bases is to include something from each of the FOOD GUIDE PYRAMID's five major groups.

Luncheon Meats: A catchall term for a variety of ready-to-eat cold cuts. There are too many of them to detail, let alone to supply nutrient counts. As a rule, however, luncheon meats are high in fat, cholesterol, sodium, nitrates or nitrites, which the body can convert to cancer-causing NITROSAMINES. Look for those with lower percentages of fat, also of nitrates and nitrites (using antioxidants like vitamin E and preservatives like sodium erythorbate makes it possible).

Lycopene: A carotenoid pigment found in paprika, tomatoes, watermelons and pink grapefruit that some biomedical researchers believe reduces the risk of certain cancers.

Lye: Caustic soda. See SODIUM HYDROXIDE.

Lysine: One of the essential AMINO ACIDS. **GOOD SOURCES:** Cheese, fish and legumes. In addition to being necessary for the synthesis of protein, lysine is integral to the production of CARNITINE, which in turn is essential to the oxidation of fatty acids in the body. Finally, lysine is the limiting amino acid in wheat (see LIMITING AMINO ACIDS).

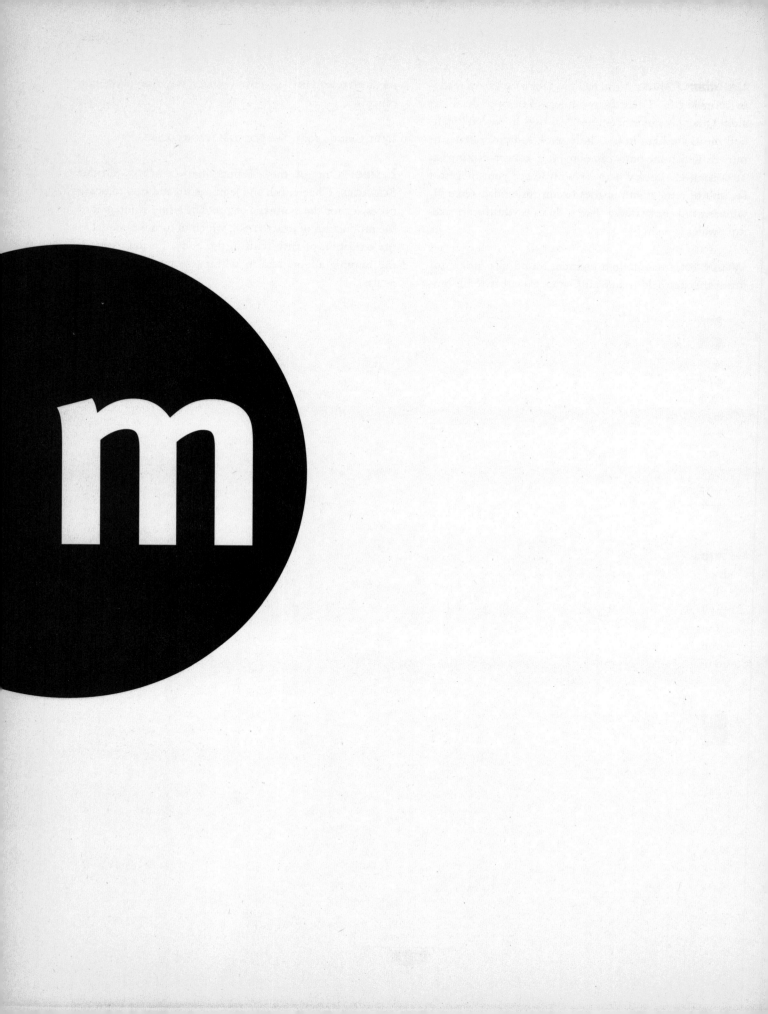

Macadamia Nuts: Crisp yet buttery round nuts native to the coastal wilds of Queensland, Australia. For centuries these Queensland nuts nourished the aborigines, a fact not lost on Dr. John MacAdam for whom the nuts were named. That was more than one hundred years ago. Today macadamias are grown commercially in parts of Africa and South America, but Hawaii is the major producer. Most macadamias come to market shelled, dehydrated (to bring their water content down to less than 2 percent), lightly roasted and vacuum packed. Macadamias are exceedingly rich and, alas, some of their fat is saturated. The good news is that they're high in monounsaturates.

NUTRIENT CONTENT OF 1 OUNCE (28 GRAMS) UNSALTED MACADAMIA NUTS

204 calories	2 mg sodium*
2 g protein	93 mg potassium
22 g fat, 3 saturated	2 g dietary fiber
0 mg cholesterol	0 RE vitamin A
4 g carbohydrate	0.06 mg thiamin
13 mg calcium	0.03 mg riboflavin
57 mg phosphorus	0.6 mg niacin
0.5 mg iron	0 mg vitamin C

*Salted macadamias contain 74 milligrams sodium per ounce.

Macaroni: An umbrella Italian word that includes all kinds of pasta. In the United States, however, it refers specifically to elbows big and little, made of durum flour and water. The American favorite, as every child knows, is macaroni and cheese, a sort of custard made with cooked macaroni, milk, eggs and coarsely grated Cheddar that's baked until crusty-brown. It's cheap and filling but unfortunately the fat, sodium and calorie counts all soar.

NUTRIENT CONTENT OF 1 CUP COOKED MACARONI (UNSEASONED)

(about 5 ounces; 140 grams)

197 calories	1 mg sodium
7 g protein	43 mg potassium
1 g fat, 0 saturated	2 g dietary fiber
0 mg cholesterol	0 RE vitamin A
40 g carbohydrate	0.29 mg thiamin
10 mg calcium	0.14 mg riboflavin
76 mg phosphorus	2.3 mg niacin
2 mg iron	0 mg vitamin C

NUTRIENT CONTENT OF ½ CUP HOMEMADE MACARONI AND CHEESE (MADE WITH MARGARINE)

(about 3½ ounces; 100 grams)

215 calories	543 mg sodium
8 g protein	120 mg potassium
11 g fat, 4 saturated	1 g dietary fiber
21 mg cholesterol	117 RE vitamin A
20 g carbohydrate	0.10 mg thiamin
181 mg calcium	0.20 mg riboflavin
161 mg phosphorus	0.9 mg niacin
0.9 mg iron	0 mg vitamin C

Mâche, Lamb's-quarter: See SALAD GREENS.

Mackerel: Not one fish but an immense family of Scombridae that even includes tuna (we discuss that fish separately). Mackerel are classified as "oily" fish, meaning their oils are distributed throughout their flesh instead of being concentrated in the liver, the case with cod. What makes them unique is that they contain both white meat and dark. The most important mackerel is the **Atlantic,** a cold-water fish that seldom swims farther south than Cape Hatteras, North Carolina. The South Atlantic and Caribbean are home to four other popular mackerels—**king, Spanish, cero** and **wahoo.** The biggest of these, giant king mackerel in particular, may carry ciguatoxins, responsible for a serious form of food poisoning (see CIGUATERA POISONING), and this applies to fresh, frozen, canned and salted mackerel alike. Those aware of the dangers of ciguatera eat only whole fish and ones small enough to fit on their dinner plate. The bigger the fish, the greater the concentration of ciguatoxins. Unfortunately, fillets can be cut from any size fish, even a 100-pound king mackerel.

NUTRIENT CONTENT OF 3 OUNCES (85 GRAMS) BAKED/BROILED MACKEREL

171 calories	94 mg sodium
22 g protein	443 mg potassium
9 g fat, 2 saturated	0 g dietary fiber
51 mg cholesterol	12 RE vitamin A
0 g carbohydrate	0.12 mg thiamin
25 mg calcium	0.46 mg riboflavin
136 mg phosphorus	9.1 mg niacin
1.3 mg iron	2 mg vitamin C

Macrobiotic Diet: A mostly vegetarian philosophy of nutrition and health loosely based on Japanese eating patterns. It decrees that whole grains comprise half of each meal and forbids meat, eggs and dairy products. Liberal macrobiotics do eat fish, but the more faithful subsist on whole grains, nuts, seeds, tofu and vegetables and limit their fluid intake. Although healthy people may be able to nourish themselves adequately on a macrobiotic diet, it is nothing to push as a cure for cancer. Despite the fact that no reputable scientific study has ever shown that a macrobiotic diet can send cancer into permanent remission, health faddists continue to hook the desperately ill, eager to cling to any hope, no matter how false. Many cancer patients have trouble eating and no high-fiber macrobiotic regimen can supply the nutrient-rich meals they need. Moreover, it can stress fragile gastrointestinal tracts because macrobiotic diets also restrict liquid intake.

Macrominerals: The seven minerals needed by the human body in relatively large amounts: CALCIUM, chlorine (see CHLORIDE), MAGNESIUM, PHOSPHORUS, POTASSIUM, SODIUM and SULFUR.

Madeira: Fortified wines, produced on the Portuguese island of Madeira, that range in sweetness from dry to syrupy. See WINES; also ALCOHOL, ALCOHOLIC BEVERAGES.

Madrilene: A tomato-blushed beef consommé that can be eaten hot or cold. It can also be mixed with gelatin and served like aspic. Delicate stomachs find it soothing.

NUTRIENT CONTENT OF 1 CUP MADRILENE

(8 fluid ounces; 244 grams)

90 calories	320 mg sodium
2 g protein	234 mg potassium
0 g fat, 0 saturated	1 g dietary fiber
0 mg cholesterol	32 RE vitamin A
21 g carbohydrate	0 mg thiamin
27 mg calcium	0.07 mg riboflavin
32 mg phosphorus	0.4 mg niacin
1.4 mg iron	2 mg vitamin C

Magnesium: A mineral essential for good health. Most of it goes into bones and teeth; the rest into muscles and soft tissues. Magnesium is vital to the metabolism of carbohydrates, proteins and fats and activates more than three hundred different body enzymes, particularly those that require three B vitamins (thiamin, riboflavin and pyridoxine), vitamins C and E. It also helps fight tooth decay by binding calcium to tooth enamel. **DEFICIENCY SYMPTOMS:** Muscular weakness, twitching, convulsions, nausea, vomiting and runaway heartbeat. With magnesium so widely distributed in plants and animals, deficiencies are rare except in alcoholics, in cases of kidney disease, in diuretic abuse, after severe vomiting and/or diarrhea or in those whose intestines aren't absorbing nutrients properly. **GOOD SOURCES:** Green vegetables, avocados, bananas, blackstrap molasses, chocolate, whole unprocessed grains, legumes, peanut butter, nuts and seeds. **PRECAUTIONS:** Too much magnesium can also cause trouble and, strangely, displays some of the deficiency symptoms—nausea and vomiting. But there may also be low blood pressure, sleepiness of almost drugged intensity and paralysis of the voluntary muscles.

RDA FOR MAGNESIUM

Babies:

Birth to 6 months	40 mg per day
6 months to 1 year	60 mg per day

Children:

1 to 3 years	80 mg per day
4 to 6 years	120 mg per day
7 to 10 years	170 mg per day

Men and Boys:

11 to 14 years	270 mg per day
15 to 18 years	400 mg per day
19 to 51+ years	350 mg per day

Women and Girls:

11 to 24 years	280 mg per day
15 to 18 years	300 mg per day
19 to 51+ years	280 mg per day

Pregnant Women:

	320 mg per day

Nursing Mothers:

First 6 months	355 mg per day
Second 6 months	340 mg per day

Magnesium Chloride (additive): Helps preserve the color and texture of canned peas. GRAS.

Magnesium Hydroxide (additive): An alkali that keeps canned peas green and processed cheeses smooth and bright. GRAS when used within FDA guidelines.

Magnesium Oxide (additive): An anticaking agent and stabilizer added to butter, cocoa, canned peas, sherbet, ice cream and frozen yogurt. GRAS when used within FDA guidelines.

Magnesium Sulfate (laxative; additive): The chemical name for **epsom salts.** When used as a laxative, epsom salts should be taken with juice on an empty stomach and, unless otherwise directed, followed by plenty of fluids. Apart from their bitter taste, epsom salts can cause nausea (see also LAXATIVES). To brewers, magnesium sulfate is a necessary additive, specifically, a flavor enhancer. GRAS when used within FDA guidelines.

Mahimahi: A game fish particularly popular in Hawaii. *Mahimahi* means ''dolphin,'' but this is not Flipper (a porpoise). These quicksilver fish, the dolphins of Greek myth, of Byron, swim all the world's warm waters and weigh anywhere from 2 to 85 pounds (the world record). They are firm fleshed, moist, sweet and moderately lean. Mahimahi are a superior source of phosphorus and potassium and a good one of niacin. Their roe is considered a particular delicacy.

NUTRIENT CONTENT OF 3 OUNCES (85 GRAMS) BROILED MAHIMAHI

100 calories	89 mg sodium
21 g protein	293 mg potassium
1 g fat, 0 saturated	0 g dietary fiber
58 mg cholesterol	9 RE vitamin A
0 g carbohydrate	0.07 mg thiamin
15 mg calcium	0.09 mg riboflavin
246 mg phosphorus	1.9 mg niacin
0.3 mg iron	0 mg vitamin C

Ma Huang: A Chinese botanical extracted from an evergreen that's sold as an energy booster and weight-loss aid (we know it as ephedrine). The truth? The FDA is investigating reports that it's caused high blood pressure, muscle injury, forgetfulness, psychosis, nerve damage, rapid heartbeat and stroke. In addition, the FDA warns that dietary supplements containing both *ma huang* and kola nut can be deadly. Not long ago there were more than one hundred reports of adverse reactions by people taking a *ma huang*-kola supplement. Some got hepatitis, some suffered heart attacks and some died. Scrutinize labels.

Maize: See CORN.

Malabsorption Syndrome: The body's inability to absorb one or more nutrients properly—carbohydrates, fats, proteins, vitamins and/or minerals. A number of different conditions cause malabsorption syndrome, among them celiac disease or sprue (see GLUTEN INTOLERANCE), cystic fibrosis, an intolerance to carbohydrates, impaired pancreatic function. Whatever the cause, the symptoms are not pleasant: painful bloating, fatty stools (stools with undigested fat) and/or diarrhea, anemia, anorexia, weight loss and wasted muscles. Treatment, quite obviously, depends on the underlying condition.

Malaga: A sweet, fortified Spanish wine. See WINES.

Malagueta. See HOT PEPPERS under PEPPERS, CAPSICUMS.

Malathion: A highly controversial, widely used pesticide that's periodically sprayed over huge swatches of California to control the Mediterranean fruit fly. The good news is that malathion disperses easily and doesn't become concentrated in food. The bad news is that it belongs to a toxic group of chemicals called organophosphates, which can cause everything from dermatitis, insomnia and depression to weakened immune systems to convulsions and death. Although tests by the National Cancer Institute suggest that malathion is one of the ''lesser'' organophosphates, that it does not cause cancer, some researchers think it may depower cancer fighters in the body. Further testing is due.

Malic Acid (additive): The major acid in apples, apricots, cherries and many other fruits. Food processors find its tartness a valuable flavor booster for candies, baked goods, jams and jellies, fruit drinks, ice creams and sherbets. Even wine makers use it. GRAS.

Malnutrition: Too little energy (calories) and too few of the right nutrients (**undernutrition**), or just the reverse, too many calories plus too many of the wrong nutrients (**overnutrition**). A simplistic definition, perhaps, but true. Nutritionists cite three major causes of malnutrition: (1) poverty and lack of food; (2) ignorance or indifference (i.e., junking out on snacks and soft drinks instead of eating well-balanced meals); (3) disease or substance abuse (alcohol, drugs, etc.). All three can be fatal unless corrected. The first step is a careful NUTRITION ASSESSMENT. See also the FOOD GUIDE PYRAMID.

Malt (additive): A protein- and carbohydrate-rich extract obtained from sprouted barley widely used by brewers. Malt's appearance in milk drinks began late in the last century in Racine, Wisconsin, when James and William Horlick concocted an easy-to-digest powdered baby formula. Called Diastoid at first, it was quickly—and fortunately—renamed Horlick's Malted Milk. Pretty soon Walgreen's soda jerks were buzzing up malted milks and shakes. The fad spread and the rest is history. GRAS.

NUTRIENT CONTENT OF 1 CUP MALTED MILK
(8 fluid ounces; 265 grams)

236 calories	215 mg sodium
11 g protein	529 mg potassium
10 g fat, 6 saturated	0 g dietary fiber
37 mg cholesterol	93 RE vitamin A
27 g carbohydrate	0.20 mg thiamin
347 mg calcium	0.54 mg riboflavin
307 mg phosphorus	1.3 mg niacin
0.3 mg iron	2 mg vitamin C

Maltodextrin (additive): A nonfermentable sugar obtained from cornstarch that's used as a texturizer/bulking agent in commercial candies, crackers and puddings. GRAS when used within FDA guidelines.

Maltol, Ethyl Maltol (additives): Flavor enhancers, both natural and synthetic, used to intensify the taste of chocolate, fruit and vanilla in a huge spectrum of processed foods. Although both compounds have been extensively tested for safety, they are wholly absorbed by the body and consumer watchdogs demand further proof that they are harmless.

Maltose: Malt sugar. It's more stable than table sugar (sucrose) but not as sweet. Maltose is used in everything from pancake syrups to commercial breads. See also CARBOHYDRATES.

Mammee Apples: See MANGOSTEENS.

Mandarins: See ORANGES.

Manganese: One of the metals the body needs in minute quantities for good health. Called a trace element or micromineral, manganese appears naturally in a variety of plants and animals. The human body uses it to activate enzymes that are integral to the metabolism of glucose and fatty acids; to build strong bones; to keep skin healthy; and to formulate urea. Although the body can't manufacture manganese, it is so readily available (in whole grains, legumes, nuts, fruits, leafy vegetables and tea) deficiencies are almost unheard of. On the other hand, those who persist in taking supercharged mineral supplements year after year or drink water contaminated with manganese do so at their own risk. Manganese overload produces dementia, psychiatric disorders that ape schizophrenia, and a debilitating neurological condition much like Parkinson's. Although there are no RDAs for manganese, the amount judged safe and adequate for adults is 2 to 5 milligrams per day. See also HEAVY-METAL TOXICITY.

Mangoes: In Southeast Asia where they originated, mangoes have been cultivated for more than six thousand years. Today, they feed more than a fifth of the world; indeed, they are more important in steamy climes than apples are farther north. Although mangoes are now grown in Florida and California, they are not as widely available as they might be. Too bad, for these butter-fleshed fruits taste of honey, of peaches, even faintly of pine. Their yellow-orange flesh suggests they're a powerhouse of beta-carotene. And so they are, but they are also rich in vitamin C and low in calories and sodium. Best of all, they contain zero fat and cholesterol. **SEASON:** Summer for the domestic crop (the choicest); late winter through fall for the imports.

NUTRIENT CONTENT OF 1 CUP THINLY SLICED MANGOES
(about 9½ fluid ounces; 265 grams)

107 calories	3 mg sodium
1 g protein	257 mg potassium
0 g fat, 0 saturated	3 g dietary fiber
0 mg cholesterol	642 RE vitamin A
28 g carbohydrate	0.10 mg thiamin
17 mg calcium	0.09 mg riboflavin
18 mg phosphorus	1.0 mg niacin
0.2 mg iron	46 mg vitamin C

Mangosteens: No relation to the mango, these giant deep purple berries also come from Southeast Asia. They often measure 3 inches across, yet their crimson-veined white flesh is so fragile it melts in your mouth. "Just like ice cream," aficionados say. They also claim that mangosteens contain the perfect balance of sugar and acid. Among their relatives are the huge **mammee apples** of tropical America. Once curiosities, mangosteens and mammee apples are both debuting at upscale big-city greengrocers. **SEASON:** Year-round.

NUTRIENT CONTENT OF 1 MEDIUM-SIZE MANGOSTEEN
(about 5 ounces; 140 grams)

80 calories	2 mg sodium
0 g protein	189 mg potassium
0 g fat, 0 saturated	7 g dietary fiber
0 mg cholesterol	0 RE vitamin A
21 g carbohydrate	0.05 mg thiamin
14 mg calcium	0.05 mg riboflavin
14 mg phosphorus	0.9 mg niacin
0.7 mg iron	6 mg vitamin C

NUTRIENT CONTENT OF 1 MEDIUM-SIZE MAMMEE APPLE
(about 1¾ pounds; 846 grams)

431 calories	126 mg sodium
4 g protein	397 mg potassium
4 g fat, NA saturated	25 g dietary fiber
0 mg cholesterol	195 RE vitamin A
105 g carbohydrate	0.17 mg thiamin
93 mg calcium	0.34 mg riboflavin
93 mg phosphorus	3.4 mg niacin
5.9 mg iron	118 mg vitamin C

Manioc: See CASSAVA.

Mannitol (sugar substitute): Extracted from seaweeds, this sweetener (actually a sugar alcohol) is only half as caloric as table sugar (sucrose) because it isn't wholly absorbed by the body. Mannitol is widely used in dietetic chewing gums and sweets. Presently considered GRAS, it can cause diarrhea and other digestive upsets and, if ingested in large quantities, can also burden the kidneys. Further tests are due before a final verdict is delivered on mannitol.

Maple Sugar: The sap of sugar maples boiled down until it crystallizes. It's about 95 percent sucrose, 2 percent fructose and the rest ash. It's available granulated, in blocks and as superbly creamy candies. You can substitute maple sugar for half the sugar in most recipes without coming to grief. But the maple flavor is usually too delicate to justify such extravagance.

NUTRIENT CONTENT OF 1 OUNCE (28 GRAMS) MAPLE SUGAR

100 calories	3 mg sodium
0 g protein	78 mg potassium
0 g fat, 0 saturated	0 g dietary fiber
0 mg cholesterol	1 RE vitamin A
26 g carbohydrate	0 mg thiamin
26 mg calcium	0 mg riboflavin
1 mg phosphorus	0 mg niacin
0.5 mg iron	0 mg vitamin C

Maple Syrup: The real thing—for there are dozens of imitations—is nothing more than the sap of sugar maple trees boiled down to syrup. It and maple sugar are the pride of Vermont, but other states produce both, too—New York and Michigan, to name two.

NUTRIENT CONTENT OF 1 TABLESPOON MAPLE SYRUP
(about ¾ ounce; 20 grams)

53 calories	2 mg sodium
0 g protein	41 mg potassium
0 g fat, 0 saturated	0 g dietary fiber
0 mg cholesterol	0 RE vitamin A
14 g carbohydrate	0 mg thiamin
14 mg calcium	0 mg riboflavin
0.5 mg phosphorus	0 mg niacin
0.3 mg iron	0 mg vitamin C

Maple Syrup Urine Disease: A rare metabolic defect, the inability to metabolize certain amino acids, that afflicts some newborns. Their urine smells sweet, malty. See ISOLEUCINE.

Maraschino Cherries: For hundreds of years, Italians have been marinating wild, bitter *marasca* cherries in maraschino, a liqueur made from the cherries. These are real maraschino cherries but they're virtually unknown in the United States. What we call maraschino cherries are Royal

Anns that have undergone a series of chemical assaults—brines, bleaches, artificial flavorings and colorings (these, contrary to popular belief, never included the cancer-causing Red Dye No. 2). No. 4, also now banned as a possible carcinogen, was used to redden maraschinos. But since the 1970s it's been Red No. 40, one of the most widely used of all food colorings.

Marasmus: An acute lack of calories and protein once known as **protein-calorie malnutrition.** Marasmus afflicts at least half the children in developing countries and its victims suffer extreme emaciation. There may also be diarrhea, anemia, skin disorders, enlarged livers and weakened immune systems. Treatment depends upon the degree of dehydration and electrolyte imbalance, specific vitamin deficiencies and presence of infection.

Marbling: The flakes of fat studding the lean of beef, lamb and other meats. Not so long ago, prime cuts of beef were chock-full of fat because, as everyone then believed, the greater the marbling, the juicier the steak or roast. Today cattle ranchers are following the lead of pork producers and turning out slimmed-down livestock. And to win back the beef eaters spooked by the amount of saturated fat and cholesterol in beef, they've mounted massive ad campaigns emphasizing the new *lean* beef.

Margarine: This butter substitute isn't an American invention. Nor is it very new. It was developed in the 1860s by a French chemist in response to a competition sponsored by Napoleon III, who was looking for an artificial butter. The first American margarine appeared in 1873, to the consternation of dairy farmers, who at one point insisted that all margarine be dyed purple to discourage people from buying it. Before World War II, butter was America's spread and shortening of choice. But by the late 1950s, margarine was outselling butter. Today many health-conscious Americans have banned butter in favor of vegetable-based margarines. But there's considerable confusion and misinformation. Margarines, for example, are not low calorie. In fact, stick margarine, like stick butter, weighs in at 100 calories per tablespoon (99 percent of these from fat). There is a difference, however. Butterfat is highly saturated and as such actually does more to raise blood levels of cholesterol than the cholesterol in food (real butter doesn't lack for that, either).

Margarines, on the other hand, are usually made from largely unsaturated vegetable oils—canola, corn, sunflower, safflower, etc.—then hydrogenated to give them the consistency of butter. Unfortunately, the hydrogenation does two things: It saturates some of the fat and it creates TRANS FATTY ACIDS, which may actually increase the risk of coronary heart disease by lowering the HDL, or "good" cholesterol, in the blood and increasing the LDL, or "bad." The point to remember is that the softer the margarine, the fewer saturated fats and trans fatty acids it contains. Here, then, is a quick rundown on the types of margarine now available (each is available both salted and unsalted):

Imitation Margarine, "Soft Diet" Margarine: It's about 40 percent fat (just half that of stick margarine) and anywhere from 38 to 57 percent water. Never substitute it for butter or stick margarine in baked goods. **CALORIES PER TABLESPOON:** 50.

Soft Margarine: Less hydrogenated than stick margarine, it contains fewer saturated fats and trans fatty acids. It's more spreadable, even straight out of the fridge, but should not be substituted for butter or even stick margarine in cakes, quick breads or pastries. **CALORIES PER TABLESPOON:** 100.

Squeeze Margarine: Margarine about the consistency of ketchup that's sold in plastic squeeze bottles. It does not contain less fat than stick margarine, merely less saturated fat. **CALORIES PER TABLESPOON:** 100.

Stick Margarine, Regular Margarine: A highly saturated, emulsified blend of refined vegetable oils, a minimal amount of preservatives, miilk, nonfat dry milk and/or water. It's hydrogenated to approximate the hardness of butter and often fortified with vitamins A and D. By law, stick margarines must be 80 percent fat and their labels must specify which fat they contain. **CALORIES PER TABLESPOON:** 100.

Whipped Margarine: Regular margarine pumped full of air. It's eminently spreadable and, measure for measure, contains about half the fat of stick margarine—6 to 7 grams per tablespoon versus 11. **CALORIES PER TABLESPOON:** 65.

There are also **fat spreads** containing about 60 percent fat, which cannot be called margarine. They may be a blend of vegetable oils or, in the case of **corn-oil spread,** compounded of a single oil. **CALORIES PER TABLESPOON:** 75.

Marigolds: See FLOWERS, EDIBLE.

Market-Basket Sample: Every three months FDA agents buy 234 "all-American foods" in cities across the United States, prepare them as they would at home, then analyze them for essential minerals, pesticides, industrial fallout (chemicals), toxic metals and radioactive contamination. They then compare the results with the acceptable daily intakes (ADIs) established by the UN's World Health Organization for eight different age-sex groups. Twenty-five years of market-basket samples have consistently shown pesticide residue levels well below the ADIs.

Marmalades: Citrus fruit preserves containing shreds of rind. They are mostly sugar. See also JAMS, JELLIES, MARMALADES, PRESERVES.

Marrons: See CHESTNUTS.

Marrow: Before people worried about fat and cholesterol, marrow (the soft connective tissue and fat in the hollows of animal leg bones) was the sort of delicacy trotted out to impress guests. Indeed, there were silver marrow spoons just for digging out the gorgeous quivery stuff. Today, few of us would forgo the marrow in osso buco; still, we are too health conscious to cook up a batch of "marrow bones" (veal or beef shanks).

Marsala: A sweet, fortified Sicilian wine. See WINES.

Marshmallows: In Victorian England, these airy sweets were made from the roots of mallow plants that grew in marshes. Leave it to American ingenuity to counterfeit them out of sugar, corn syrup and gelatin. Originally marshmallows were molded like chocolates. Today's high-tech puffs are extruded in great ropes and cut at precise intervals. Though every kid loves to toast marshmallows over a campfire, most of them show up in cups of cocoa, fruit salads and as toppings for candied sweet potatoes. Unfortunately, marshmallows are nutritional lightweights.

Marzipan, Almond Paste: Almonds ground to paste, then sweetened and flavored with almond extract. The difference between marzipan and almond paste is discernible only to chefs and connoisseurs. Marzipan is sweeter and finer; it is the "clay" confectioners tint and shape into fool-the-eye fruits, vegetables and animals. Almond paste is coarser, a precursor of marzipan. Marzipan may contain glycerin and egg whites as well as sugar and ground almonds, and may be **uncooked** (made with confectioners' sugar) or **cooked** (made with hot sugar syrup, the pastry chef's choice because of its malleability). Today many cooks shortcut the making of marzipan by beginning with almond paste, then adding sugar and smoothing the texture. Where did it all begin, this obsession with almond candies? Food historians point to the Middle East, to Persia in particular, where almonds were abundant and harem women had an insatiable sweet tooth. They further believe that Crusaders brought marzipan home to Europe, where the shaping of it was quickly elevated to fine art. The mas-

NUTRIENT CONTENT OF 1 OUNCE (28 GRAMS) MARZIPAN

133 calories	2 mg sodium
3 g protein	110 mg potassium
7 g fat, 1 saturated	1 g dietary fiber
0 mg cholesterol	0 RE vitamin A
16 g carbohydrate	0.03 mg thiamin
38 mg calcium	0.11 mg riboflavin
74 mg phosphorus	0.5 mg niacin
0.5 mg iron	1 mg vitamin C

NUTRIENT CONTENT OF 1 OUNCE (28 GRAMS) MARSHMALLOWS

90 calories	13 mg sodium
1 g protein	1 mg potassium
0 g fat, 0 saturated	0 g dietary fiber
0 mg cholesterol	0 RE vitamin A
23 g carbohydrate	0 mg thiamin
1 mg calcium	0 mg riboflavin
2 mg phosphorus	0 mg niacin
0.1 mg iron	0 mg vitamin C

NUTRIENT CONTENT OF 1 OUNCE (28 GRAMS) ALMOND PASTE

126 calories	3 mg sodium
3 g protein	183 mg potassium
8 g fat, 1 saturated	4 g dietary fiber
0 mg cholesterol	0 RE vitamin A
12 g carbohydrate	0.06 mg thiamin
65 mg calcium	0.21 mg riboflavin
126 mg phosphorus	0.8 mg niacin
1.8 mg iron	0 mg vitamin C

ters of marzipan today are the Sicilians, the Algarvian Portuguese and the Germans, but making marzipan remains a Christmas tradition all over Europe. Both marzipan and almond paste are sold in supermarkets, the most widely available being the plastic-wrapped, 7-ounce links imported from Denmark.

Masa Harina: A flour ground of corn kernels that have been puffed in a solution of wood ashes or lye, then parched. Also called simply **masa** or "tortilla flour," it is a Mexican staple. Because of our growing appetite for tacos and tortillas, *masa harina* is now being milled by giant U.S. food companies and stocked by supermarkets across the country. It's worth a try because it's an excellent source of iron, calcium, phosphorus and potassium as well as of the B vitamins thiamin, riboflavin and niacin.

NUTRIENT CONTENT OF 1 CUP UNSIFTED MASA HARINA
(about 4 ounces; 108 grams)

411 calories	9 mg sodium
11 g protein	360 mg potassium
5 g fat, 1 saturated	2 g dietary fiber
0 mg cholesterol	0 RE vitamin A
82 g carbohydrate	1.60 mg thiamin
231 mg calcium	0.87 mg riboflavin
258 mg phosphorus	10.5 mg niacin
8.8 mg iron	0 mg vitamin C

Mascarpone: A buttery, sweet Italian cheese the color and consistency of clotted cream. Mascarpone (also called **mascherpone**) comes originally from the countryside around Milan but is now widely produced elsewhere. It's made of cow's milk, specifically the top milk (a euphemism for heavy cream), and is more often used as a topping or recipe ingredient than as something to spoon up and eat. Mascarpone is 45 to 50 percent water; 45 to 55 percent fat. Before refrigeration, this fresh cheese was available only in winter. Today it comes to market year-round but is highly perishable. **NOTE:** Specific nutrient counts are unavailable for mascarpone, but there's no doubt that it's loaded with saturated fat and cholesterol.

Maté, Yerba, Paraguay Tea: A revitalizing bitter green tea drunk in South America almost since the beginning of time. It is brewed from the toasted leaves of a wild holly that carpets the mountains of Argentina, southern Brazil and Paraguay. Like coffee and tea, *maté* is a stimulant containing caffeine and tannin (like them, too, it is calorie, fat and cholesterol free when taken straight). Extracts of *maté* are also used as a flavoring by American soft-drink manufacturers. GRAS.

Matjes: See HERRING.

Matzo Balls: Passover dumplings made of matzo meal, eggs, shortening, salt and water. Now enjoyed right around the calendar, matzo balls may be poached in water or soup. They may also be enriched with chopped liver or nuts, marrow or parsley.

NUTRIENT CONTENT OF 3 OUNCES (85 GRAMS) MATZO BALLS

238 calories	398 mg sodium
6 g protein	66 mg potassium
15 g fat, 4 saturated	1 g dietary fiber
141 mg cholesterol	64 RE vitamin A
19 g carbohydrate	0.11 mg thiamin
20 mg calcium	0.24 mg riboflavin
79 mg phosphorus	0.9 mg niacin
1.2 mg iron	0 mg vitamin C

Matzo Crackers: Thin sheets of unleavened flour-and-water bread, the symbol of the Israelites' hasty flight from Egypt, that are integral to the Jewish celebration of Passover. Today Jews and Gentiles both enjoy matzo crackers year-round as a low-calorie, nonfat, low-sodium snack.

NUTRIENT CONTENT OF 1 OUNCE (28 GRAMS) MATZO CRACKERS

112 calories	1 mg sodium
3 g protein	32 mg potassium
0 g fat, 0 saturated	1 g dietary fiber
0 mg cholesterol	0 RE vitamin A
24 g carbohydrate	0.11 mg thiamin
4 mg calcium	0.08 mg riboflavin
25 mg phosphorus	1.1 mg niacin
0.9 mg iron	0 mg vitamin C

Matzo Meal: Matzo crackers ground fine or medium. Matzo meal is used to make matzo balls (*knaidlach*), *verenikes* (*latkes*) and other Jewish recipes. Ounce for ounce, the nutrient count of matzo meal is identical to that of matzo crackers.

Mayo Diet: A weight-reducing diet built around eggs, meats, grapefruit and a few vegetables that has no connection whatsoever to the respected Mayo Clinic. Hazardously high in fat and cholesterol, the Mayo Diet puts those with heart or kidney disease at severe risk. See also DIETS.

Mayonnaise: A fluffy emulsion of eggs (or yolks), oil, vinegar and seasonings used as both a salad dressing and sauce-and-sandwich-spread base. The real thing is loaded with fat and calories and the uncooked processor versions may be also contaminated with salmonella bacteria. Riding the fitness craze, manufacturers have developed new "light" mayonnaises, even fat-free ones.

NUTRIENT CONTENT OF 1 TABLESPOON MAYONNAISE	
(about ½ ounce; 14 grams)	
99 calories	78 mg sodium
0 g protein	5 mg potassium
11 g fat, 2 saturated	0 g dietary fiber
8 mg cholesterol	12 RE vitamin A
0 g carbohydrate	0 mg thiamin
2 mg calcium	0 mg riboflavin
4 mg phosphorus	0 mg niacin
0.1 mg iron	0 mg vitamin C

NUTRIENT CONTENT OF 1 TABLESPOON "LIGHT" MAYONNAISE	
(about ½ ounce; 14 grams)	
36 calories	78 mg sodium
0 g protein	2 mg potassium
3 g fat, 1 saturated	0 g dietary fiber
4 mg cholesterol	0 RE vitamin A
3 g carbohydrate	0 mg thiamin
0 mg calcium	0 mg riboflavin
0 mg phosphorus	0 mg niacin
0 mg iron	0 mg vitamin C

NUTRIENT CONTENT OF 1 TABLESPOON FAT-FREE MAYONNAISE	
(about ½ ounce; 14 grams)	
11 calories	169 mg sodium
0 g protein	13 mg potassium
0 g fat, 0 saturated	0 g dietary fiber
0 mg cholesterol	0 RE vitamin A
3 g carbohydrate	0 mg thiamin
NA mg calcium	0 mg riboflavin
NA mg phosphorus	0 mg niacin
NA mg iron	0 mg vitamin C

MCT Oil: *MCT* stands for "medium-chain triglycerides"; this fat-and-calorie supplement is especially synthesized for those who can't digest regular dietary fats properly.

Meals-on-Wheels: Community programs, now nationwide, developed to ensure housebound seniors and other shut-ins of nourishing food. Ideally, meals—usually a hot lunch and box supper—are prepared by volunteers and paid employees five days a week and delivered to those who request them. An individual's ability to pay determines the cost.

Meat: The edible flesh of livestock (see BEEF; HAM; LAMB; PORK; VEAL). Meat is a premium source of complete protein, but unfortunately doesn't lack calories, fat and cholesterol. The new FOOD GUIDE PYRAMID now lumps meat in with poultry, fish, dry beans, eggs and nuts and recommends that servings from this broad group be limited to two or three a day—and these, mind you, are 3-ounce portions.

Meatballs, Meat Loaves: You might call meatballs mini meat loaves because the mix is often the same— ground meat, onions, bread crumbs and seasonings plus just enough egg to hold everything together. Meatballs average 1 to 2 inches in diameter and are browned on the top of the stove instead of being pressed into loaves and baked. Meat loaf and meatball recipes vary hugely—from the meatballs that go into spaghetti sauce to the ketchup-glazed meat loaf to sweet-sour German Königsberger Klops. For most meatballs and loaves, beef is the meat of choice, yet any meat or combination of meats works well, provided there's enough fat or minced vegetables to keep them succulent. **NOTE:** Recipes vary too much for accurate nutrient counts, but you can be sure most meatballs and meat loaves run to fat, calories and cholesterol.

Meat Tenderizers: These consist mainly of crystallized PAPAIN, an enzyme extracted from papayas. In undeveloped parts of tropical America, women still tenderize meat by rubbing it with fresh papaya juice. It works.

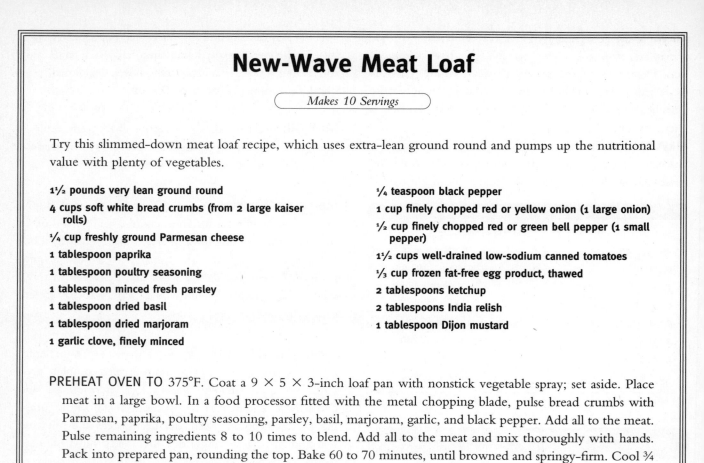

New-Wave Meat Loaf

Makes 10 Servings

Try this slimmed-down meat loaf recipe, which uses extra-lean ground round and pumps up the nutritional value with plenty of vegetables.

1½ pounds very lean ground round

4 cups soft white bread crumbs (from 2 large kaiser rolls)

¼ cup freshly ground Parmesan cheese

1 tablespoon paprika

1 tablespoon poultry seasoning

1 tablespoon minced fresh parsley

1 tablespoon dried basil

1 tablespoon dried marjoram

1 garlic clove, finely minced

¼ teaspoon black pepper

1 cup finely chopped red or yellow onion (1 large onion)

½ cup finely chopped red or green bell pepper (1 small pepper)

1½ cups well-drained low-sodium canned tomatoes

⅓ cup frozen fat-free egg product, thawed

2 tablespoons ketchup

2 tablespoons India relish

1 tablespoon Dijon mustard

PREHEAT OVEN TO 375°F. Coat a 9 × 5 × 3-inch loaf pan with nonstick vegetable spray; set aside. Place meat in a large bowl. In a food processor fitted with the metal chopping blade, pulse bread crumbs with Parmesan, paprika, poultry seasoning, parsley, basil, marjoram, garlic, and black pepper. Add all to the meat. Pulse remaining ingredients 8 to 10 times to blend. Add all to the meat and mix thoroughly with hands. Pack into prepared pan, rounding the top. Bake 60 to 70 minutes, until browned and springy-firm. Cool ¾ hour in the pan before slicing, then serve warm or cold.

APPROXIMATE NUTRIENT COUNTS PER SERVING

229 calories	16 g carbohydrate	3 mg iron	0.15 mg thiamin
19 g protein	2 g dietary fiber	273 mg sodium	0.27 mg riboflavin
10 g fat, 4 saturated	92 mg calcium	394 mg potassium	4.1 mg niacin
52 mg cholesterol	159 mg phosphorus	91 RE vitamin A	13 mg vitamin C

Mechanically Separated Meat (MSM): Is this robot meat? Not quite. Red meat or poultry carcasses are first hand trimmed and cut into large chunks. These are fed into high-pressure machines, which blend the soft tissue, bone powder and marrow. The process boosts the calcium and trace-mineral content, but also, alas, the fat and cholesterol. Because mechanically separated meats can cause problems for those with high blood levels of cholesterol or uric acid, the USDA only allows a fifth of any food product to contain mechanically separated meat. In addition, all processed red meat, chicken or turkey foods containing MSM must include that information in their ingredient lists.

Mediators: These chemicals, integral to the immune system, may cause allergic reactions in the hypersensitive. For example, IMMUNOGLOBULIN E (IgE) antibodies are major players in food allergies because they can trigger the release of such mediators as HISTAMINE, SEROTONIN and kinins, which can cause you to itch, twitch, sneeze and drip, vomit, even have trouble breathing.

Medications: If you take medicine or, worse, combinations of them regularly, you should know that drugs often interact with what you eat and drink. **Aspirin,** for example, may cause intestinal bleeding, thus depleting the body's supplies of iron; **antacids** (especially the aluminum- and magnesium-hydroxide-based ones) may accelerate bone loss by blocking the assimilation of phosphorus and fluoride; **anticoagulants,** if taken along with omega-3 fatty acids (fish-oil capsules), can cause bleeding; **anticonvulsants** may interfere with the absorption of folic acid, vitamin D (and thus of calcium); **diuretics** cause rapid potassium loss; **laxatives** may prevent the absorption of vitamin D and that in itself can exacerbate osteoporosis; **cholesterol-lowering drugs** also reduce the body's ability to process fat-soluble vitamins (A, D, E and K).

There's more. **Milk** blocks the body's ability to absorb tetracycline, **protein** kicks the body's medicine-processing center into fast forward and **antidepressants** (Darvon, Inderal, lithium, Valium, etc.) deliver greater punch when taken with meals. On the other hand, eating too many **high vitamin K foods** (liver, dark leafy greens) reduces the effectiveness of many anticoagulants. Finally, **alcohol** exaggerates or weakens the impact of more than a hundred different medications. Food/medication interaction is intimidatingly complex but all good physicians and pharmacists warn patients of potential problems. The lesson here: *Take as directed.*

Medicinal Plants: Our earliest ancestors knew that certain roots, leaves, barks and blossoms possessed healing powers. The traditional Chinese pharmacopoeia is largely herbal medicine and some of the West's "miracle drugs" are of plant origin: digitalis, quinine and taxol, to name three. The trouble is, many plants are potentially dangerous. Sipping lobelia or wormwood teas can be deadly and drinking infusions of comfrey or sassafras may increase your risk of liver cancer. Health hucksters are quick to push herbal preparations as cures for this and that, but buyer beware. See also HERBAL TEAS under TEA.

Mediterranean Diet: As defined at a 1993 international conference in Cambridge, Massachusetts, jointly sponsored by the Harvard School of Public Health and Oldways Preservation & Exchange Trust, and as set down by Nancy Harmon Jenkins in her valuable *Mediterranean Diet Cookbook,* the Mediterranean Diet consists of: "Plentiful fruits, vegetables, legumes and grains; olive oil as the principal fat; lean red meat consumed only a few times per month or somewhat more often in very small portions; low to moderate consumption of other foods from animal sources, such as dairy products (especially cheese and yogurt), fish, and poultry; and moderate consumption of wine (primarily at meals)." Out of this conference also came a Mediterranean Diet Pyramid, which parallels the USDA FOOD GUIDE PYRAMID in some respects but differs from it in others.

At its broad base is a bread/pasta/grain/potato group, which includes such Mediterranean staples as couscous, polenta and bulgur. Directly above are three food groups of equal height but varying width: vegetables (the largest), fruits (second) and a skinny category devoted to beans, other legumes and nuts. Just above, olive oil gets its own slot, a slim plank topped by an equally thin but shorter cheese and yogurt plank. Next, in ascending order (descending in importance as far as the daily Mediterranean Diet is concerned) come these separate categories: fish, poultry, eggs and sweets. Red meat is relegated to the very tip of the pyramid. People are advised to eat—daily and in moderation—from the food groups at the base of the pyramid through those three fourths of the way up; that is, through cheese and yogurt. It's also recommended that they drink wine in moderation each day and exercise regularly.

The food groups higher up on the Mediterranean Diet pyramid—fish, poultry, eggs and sweets—should be eaten a few times a week. And red meat only a few times a month. Some dietitians question the wisdom of recommending wine with meals. However, Dr. R. Curtis Ellison of the Boston University School of Public Health, after examining global population studies, concluded that one drink a day can reduce the risk of heart disease by as much as 30 percent. He is now weighing the particular merits, if any, of drinking wine with meals.

The Mediterranean Diet evolved, some nutritionists believe, from the 1960s research of Dr. Ancel Keys, who studied eating patterns in different parts of the world and tried to link them to disease (or the lack of it). Greeks, southern Italians and others in Mediterranean "olive country" who eat plenty of fresh fruits, vegetables and complex carbohydrates (rice, pasta, even pizza) and use olive oil as their primary fat are known to suffer fewer heart attacks and less cancer than red meat-loving Americans.

But there are many variables. How important is the way food is grown? Cooked? Packaged? Distributed? Is it the menu mix that's important? What role, if any, do single foods play? What role heredity? These are questions yet to be answered. Still, to quote Nancy Jenkins again, " . . . the Harvard conference revealed a developing consensus, based on the work of Keys and his many associates then and since, that the traditional diet of people in the Mediterranean is a major factor in their *generally* good health profiles, their *generally* long lives, their *general* lack of chronic and debilitating diseases."

Megaloblastic Anemia: A severe anemia caused by vitamin B_{12} and folic acid deficiency. Without these essential B vitamins, red blood cells never mature properly, lose their nuclei and die.

Megavitamin Therapy: Taking many times the RDA of one or more vitamins. When it comes to vitamins, many people believe "more is better." *Not true.* In fact, overdosing on such fat-soluble vitamins as A and D can be extremely toxic. Even prolonged megadosing on water-soluble Bs and C can prove troublesome. Never exceed any vitamin's RDA unless your doctor (or a dietitian he recommends) prescribes a particular therapy. For specific toxicities, see the individual vitamins, which are covered alphabetically elsewhere in this book.

Mellorine: Imitation ice cream made with vegetable oils. Although it contains no cholesterol, it is hardly fat free or low calorie.

NUTRIENT CONTENT OF 1 CUP VANILLA MELLORINE
(about 4³/₄ ounces; 133 grams)

265 calories	97 mg sodium
5 g protein	287 mg potassium
14 g fat, 12 saturated	0 g dietary fiber
0 mg cholesterol	0 RE vitamin A
32 g carbohydrate	0.05 mg thiamin
180 mg calcium	0.30 mg riboflavin
142 mg phosphorus	0.1 mg niacin
0.1 mg iron	1 mg vitamin C

Melons: Although close relatives of New World squashes, melons are decidely Old World. On his way to China, Marco Polo commented about those he saw in the markets of Afghanistan, "Here are found the best melons in the world and in very great quantity." Food historians put their place of origin in Persia, directly west, and believe that melons are one of the earliest foods grown (they are mentioned in the Old Testament). Melons were popular in ancient Egypt, Greece and Rome and were introduced to

Spain and Portugal by the Moors. By the end of the fifteenth century, melons were such a fad in France no meal was complete without them. Yet they were unknown in the New World until Europeans introduced them—the English brought them to the East Coast; the Spaniards to the West and Southwest.

The list of melons available today staggers; indeed, to keep bees from cross-pollinating them and creating even more varieties, gardeners must plant the different species

NUTRIENT CONTENT OF 1 CUP CUBED CANTALOUPE OR PERSIAN MELON
(about 5³/₄ ounces; 160 grams)

56 calories	14 mg sodium
1 g protein	494 mg potassium
0 g fat, 0 saturated	1 g dietary fiber
0 mg cholesterol	515 RE vitamin A
13 g carbohydrate	0.06 mg thiamin
18 mg calcium	0.03 mg riboflavin
27 mg phosphorus	0.9 mg niacin
0.3 mg iron	68 mg vitamin C

NUTRIENT CONTENT OF 1 CUP CUBED HONEYDEW MELON
(about 6 ounces; 170 grams)

60 calories	17 mg sodium
1 g protein	461 mg potassium
0 g fat, 0 saturated	1 g dietary fiber
0 mg cholesterol	7 RE vitamin A
16 g carbohydrate	0.13 mg thiamin
10 mg calcium	0.03 mg riboflavin
17 mg phosphorus	1.0 mg niacin
0.1 mg iron	42 mg vitamin C

NUTRIENT CONTENT OF 1 CUP CUBED CASABA OR CRENSHAW MELON
(about 6 ounces; 170 grams)

60 calories	17 mg sodium
1 g protein	461 mg potassium
0 g fat, 0 saturated	1 g dietary fiber
0 mg cholesterol	5 RE vitamin A
16 g carbohydrate	0.10 mg thiamin
10 mg calcium	0.03 mg riboflavin
17 mg phosphorus	1.0 mg niacin
0.1 mg iron	27 mg vitamin C

far apart. Perennial favorites: **cantaloupes, casabas** (introduced to California by Armenians emigrating from Kasaba, Turkey), the pale salmon-fleshed cultivars known as **Crenshaws,** the intensely orange **Persians** and honeyed little **Charentais** of France, the green-fleshed **honeydews, Galias** and **Christmas melons.** For all their sweetness, melons are low in calories. They are superior sources of vitamin C and, if orange fleshed, of beta-carotene as well. **SEASON:** Year-round; that is, one melon or another will be available right around the calendar. See also WATERMELONS.

NUTRIENT CONTENT OF 1 CUP FROZEN MIXED MELON BALLS
(about 6 ounces; 173 grams)

57 calories	54 mg sodium
1 g protein	484 mg potassium
0 g fat, 0 saturated	1 g dietary fiber
0 mg cholesterol	306 RE vitamin A
14 g carbohydrate	0.29 mg thiamin
17 mg calcium	0.04 mg riboflavin
21 mg phosphorus	1.1 mg niacin
0.5 mg iron	11 mg vitamin C

Melatonin: Is this hormone, produced by the tiny pineal gland in the middle of the brain, the fountain of youth? No reputable biomedical researcher will admit that it is. Still, years of tests both here and in Italy suggest that melatonin may actually boost the immune system, help prevent cataracts and protect body cells from scavenging free radicals (destructive by-products of metabolism that constantly circulate in the blood). Melatonin may reduce the risk of cancer and prolong life. Already this hormone, which helps regulate our biological clocks, has been used by flight crews to fight jet lag and by insomniacs to induce sleep. Without apparent side effects. In addition, a Virginia researcher, Dr. Michael Cohen, is exploring the contraceptive value of hefty (75 mg) doses of melatonin combined with progestin. In studies of a thousand European women, B-Oval, as he calls it, performed as well as conventional birth control pills. Cohen hopes to launch U.S. studies of B-Oval shortly and to show that his melatonin/progestin pill does double duty—prevents unwanted pregnancy *and* breast cancer all at the same time. Meanwhile, sales of melatonin capsules, tablets and lozenges, now available without prescription in many drugstores as well as in nearly every health-food store, are soaring. Much to the

chagrin of some scientists who caution that the effects of long-term melatonin use are wholly unknown. Proceed with caution. See also DHEA.

Memory (diet and): Does the food we eat—or don't eat—have anything to do with memory loss? Possibly. A University of New Mexico study of well-educated, well-heeled seniors between sixty and ninety-four found that the most poorly nourished scored lowest on memory tests. It also suggested that the nutrients most responsible for mental sharpness were protein, the B-complex vitamins and vitamin C.

Menadione: A synthetic form of vitamin K.

Menopause (diet and): Once women enter menopause, either naturally or posthysterectomy, bone loss trips into high gear and continues at an accelerated pace for about ten years; it then slows to the rate of men the same age. Estrogen therapy, often prescribed to brake bone loss, also helps control appetite and prevent the weight gain so common to menopausal women. Nutritionists still debate the effectiveness of calcium supplements in reversing, even slowing bone loss but do agree that certain things seem to help: exercising regularly, swearing off cigarettes and cutting down on alcohol. Unhappily, some medications—especially steroids and thyroid hormones—intensify bone loss.

Menstruation (diet and): During each menstrual period women lose about 15 milligrams of iron. Unfortunately, many women, especially young women, obsess about their weight and don't get the daily doses of iron they need. Result: anemia. To prevent it, the RDA for iron for women of child-bearing age is 15 milligrams a day. Bear in mind that there are two forms of iron—**heme** (from meats), which the body utilizes more efficiently than **nonheme** (from eggs, fruits, grains and vegetables).

Menthol (additive): A flavoring, both natural and synthetic, used in candies, soft drinks, ice creams, baked goods and chewing gums as well as in cough drops. GRAS.

Menu Claims: Chefs and restaurateurs in step with this Age of Fitness are filling their menus with "healthy" choices and "diet plates" despite the fact that few of them have had any training in nutrition. The trouble is, they've been free to say anything they like and much of their menu prose has been more fiction than fact. Enter the FDA. Through its new Nutrition Labeling and Education Act (the same ruling that requires nutritive contents to be listed on packaged foods), the FDA will also exercise some control over the phraseology of restaurant menus. For example, if a restaurant describes a dish as low fat or low cholesterol, it must support its claims with solid nutritional evidence. And if it chooses to key certain dishes or plates with hearts (meaning they're heart healthy), it must not only explain—on the menu—exactly what the heart symbol means but also be able to prove it. Those burger/cottage cheese/canned peaches diet plates so popular in fast-food restaurants will no longer pass FDA muster unless those burgers are made of lean meat and the cottage cheese is the low-fat variety.

Mercury: A highly toxic industrial metal that's polluting rivers and oceans and endangering anyone who eats fish taken from these waters. In the 1950s and 1960s, many Japanese died of a mysterious illness while others went blind, deaf or suffered general mental deterioration. The culprit: fish contaminated with a particularly insidious form of mercury called **methylmercury.** See also HEAVY-METAL TOXICITY.

Meringue: There are two types, the **soft,** which is swirled into turbulent seas atop cream pies and baked Alaskas, and the **hard,** which contains much more sugar and is baked long and slow until shattery-crisp. From a food-safety standpoint, hard meringues present no problems. But the soft definitely do. With so many eggs now contaminated with salmonella bacteria, the brief browning most soft meringues get may not provide enough heat to kill the bugs. **TWO SOLUTIONS:** Use an Italian meringue (made with boiling sugar syrup whipped into the whites) or, better yet, meringue powder made with dehydrated egg whites. Most bakery supply houses stock it. No meringue, by the way, supplies much more than calories and a dab of protein.

Mesclun: A salad mix originally grown in the South of France that consists of a variety of baby greens and often edible flowers, too. There may be nasturtiums, both the leaves and the blossoms; arugula; and assorted loose-leaf lettuces, each of them just out of the ground. Seed packets

of mesclun are now available here and all you need to grow it is a sunny windowsill. **NOTE:** Because mesclun mixes vary so, accurate nutrient counts are impossible. Still, it's safe to say they are good sources of vitamins A and C, not to mention a number of minerals.

Mesquite: A prickly, shrubby legume overrunning the American Southwest that trendy chefs use to fuel their grills. Its wood is soft and resinous and, according to one study, produces in regular ground beef burgers 8 times the cancer-causing polycyclic aromatic hydrocarbons (see PAHs) that charcoal briquettes do and 40 times the benzopyrene—the most dangerous PAH. Stick with charcoal or, better yet, use LIQUID SMOKE.

Metabolism: The chemical processes that go on in the body after food is absorbed from the digestive tract. Metabolism enables body cells to release the energy from food, to convert one substance into another (amino acids to protein, for example) and to prepare waste for excretion. See also BASAL METABOLISM.

Methane: Also known as **marsh gas** because it's produced as leaves and other organic matter decay in swampy areas, methane is one of the flatulents produced in the intestines. Certain foods—dried beans, for example—generate more of it than others.

Methanol: Methyl or wood alcohol—a deadly poison. Not to be confused with ETHANOL (ethyl or grain alcohol), the kind of alcohol in whiskeys and other spirits.

Methemoglobinemia: A rare but serious overload of nitrites sometimes seen in babies. When nitrites build up in the body, they displace the oxygen in hemoglobin and body tissues starve. Where do babies get so many nitrites? From the nitrates in well water, even from eating too much spinach or other high-nitrate vegetables. The digestive tracts of babies are nearly neutral instead of acidic, a situation in which nitrates are turned into toxic nitrites.

Methionine: One of the nine essential AMINO ACIDS. Its major role is to facilitate fat and protein metabolism; the body also uses it to manufacture cysteine, another amino acid. It is the LIMITING AMINO ACID in legumes and other vegetables. **GOOD SOURCES:** Grains, nuts and seeds.

Methylcellulose: The principal ingredient in many fiber pills (see DIET PILLS).

Methyl Cinnamate (additive): A synthetic, fruity flavoring used in everything from soft drinks, baked goods and gelatins to candies, ice creams and chewing gum. It is moderately toxic and the FDA strictly regulates its use.

Methyl Salicylate: Oil of wintergreen. Although the FDA allows food processors to use minute amounts of it to flavor candies, baked goods, ice creams, chewing gums, syrups, root beer and other soft drinks, oil of wintergreen *is* toxic. The lethal dose for children is so small (just 10 milliliters) the FDA wants all rubs and liniments containing more than 5 percent oil of wintergreen packaged in child-proof containers. Some drugstores sell oil of wintergreen, but never, ever use it to flavor food. Lock it away in the medicine cabinet.

Mettwurst: An extremely fatty German liverwurst.

Mexican Food, Tex-Mex Food: These are fast-food favorites, but nutrition analyses conducted by a Washington, D.C., consumer advocacy group, the Center for Science in the Public Interest, show that fast-food-chain tortillas, tacos, burritos and such are often riddled with fat. A chile rellenos platter was computed at 96 grams of fat (the same as a stick of butter), cheese nachos at 89 grams, beef chimichangas at 86 and taco salad at 71. Needless to add, the calories, cholesterol and sodium were sky high, too. Restaurateurs faulted the center's findings. And the center admits that one Tex-Mex dinner a month won't do you in. Still, its study does suggest that much of the Mex and Tex-Mex fast food, which many considered healthier than hamburgers, may be even more freighted with fat, calories, cholesterol and sodium. Healthier Tex-Mex choices? Grilled chicken and vegetables, any of half a dozen different bean dishes minus meat or cheese. Some fast-food chains now offer Tex-Mex "light."

Microminerals: Another term for **trace elements** or **trace minerals,** the twelve minerals we need in minute quantities for good health: ARSENIC, CHROMIUM, COPPER, FLUORINE, IODINE, IRON, MANGANESE, MOLYBDENUM, NICKEL, SELENIUM, SILICON and ZINC. Many nutritionists now believe that three others should be added to this list: BORON, TIN and VANADIUM.

Microorganisms: The miscroscopic organisms, some harmful, some beneficial, that exist all around us—in the air, in the soil, in the food we eat, in our own bodies. Each is discussed separately under BACTERIA; MOLDS; YEAST.

Microparticulation: The powerful industrial heating and shattering of egg whites and milk proteins into particles so small they feel creamy on the tongue. It's the process used to make Simplesse, the first fat substitute to receive FDA approval. So far it is used only by food manufacturers.

Microwave Cookery: Microwaves are short electromagnetic waves transmitted through the air at high frequency (2,450 million cycles per second). When absorbed by food—or even water—they set the molecules to vibrating, which generates enough heat to cook food—or boil water. This method of cooking is kinder to vitamins than most other forms of cooking. First, "nuked" vegetables require little or no liquid, so there's no danger of water-soluble B vitamins and C leaching out. Second, foods microwave so fast few heat-sensitive vitamins (again the Bs and C) are lost. Not everything microwaves well, but this speed demon does do fish, vegetables, rice and other grains to perfection.

Migraine Headaches (diet and): These brutal, paroxysmal headaches often occur only on one side of the head, and they're often accompanied by nausea and a heightened sensitivity to light. For years, no one knew what triggered migraine headaches, but nutritionists now know that they are frequently brought on by food allergies. The most common troublemakers? Milk, eggs, chocolate, oranges and wheat lead the list, with cheese, rye and tomatoes not far behind. And here's an irony: People—children, in particular—often crave the very foods that cause them so much pain.

Milk: If milk is not nature's perfect food, it is surely one of them. No mammal begins life without it and most of us drink milk from the cradle to the grave. Postmenopausal women drinking just a cup of it a day may negate—or at least minimize—the bone-thinning effects of decades of coffee drinking. So suggests a new four-year study of some thousand postmenopausal women conducted by the University of California.

Although everything from camel's milk to yak's milk is drunk in some part of the world, the only one of commercial value in the United States is cow's milk. As every farmer knows, however, not all cow's milk is created equal. Explaining the difference to a city slicker, a North Carolina dairyman said that if he put a silver dollar in a bucket and milked a Jersey cow into it, he'd get an inch of milk but wouldn't be able to see the coin. But if he milked a Holstein into the bucket, he'd be able to read the date on the dollar through ten inches of milk. His way of saying that Jerseys didn't give much milk but those few drops were "powerful rich" (about 5 percent fat) and that Holsteins were "milk machines," turning out gallons of watery stuff (actually, Holstein milk averages about 3 percent fat). What promises to turn all cows into "milk machines" is the fiercely controversial, genetically engineered bovine growth hormone, BOVINE SOMATOTROPIN (BST), which was recently approved by the FDA despite hot consumer opposition. The FDA made no snap judgments here; indeed, it moved cautiously before giving BST its blessing. With more than 120 studies conducted to determine BST's safety, it was, according to David A. Kessler, M.D., FDA commissioner at the time of its approval, "one of the most extensively studied animal drug products to be reviewed by the agency."

Before World War II there was fresh milk (both raw and pasteurized) and canned milk. Today the list of milks available is long and lengthening. And all of them sold across state lines, indeed by local creameries, are pasteurized or ultrapasteurized (heated to extremely high temperatures) to prolong shelf life. Raw (unpasteurized) milk is extremely risky. Here's a quick wrap-up of the types of milk now available:

Buttermilk: Originally a by-product of butter churning, buttermilk is now commercially soured with bacterial cultures. It's tart and thick even though most of it is made from either low-fat or skim milk. Because of its smooth

NUTRIENT CONTENT OF 1 CUP BUTTERMILK

(8 fluid ounces; 245 grams)

99 calories	257 mg sodium
8 g protein	370 mg potassium
2 g fat, 1 saturated	0 g dietary fiber
9 mg cholesterol	20 RE vitamin A
12 g carbohydrate	0.08 mg thiamin
284 mg calcium	0.38 mg riboflavin
218 mg phosphorus	0.1 mg niacin
0.1 mg iron	2 mg vitamin C

and creamy texture, buttermilk makes wonderful low-calorie sherbets and salad dressings (indeed, it can substitute partly or wholly for the oil). **NOTE:** There's also buttermilk powder, which can be reconstituted much like nonfat dry milk.

Evaporated Milk: Canned milk that's had 60 percent of its water removed. It's smooth, silky and, thanks to the high temperatures at which it's processed, tastes faintly of caramel. Three varieties are available: **whole milk, low fat** (2 percent) and **skim** (now often labeled "light" or "lite"). Evaporated milk—even the skim—makes stellar puddings, pie fillings, sherbets and ice creams. When using in cakes, cookies and breads, mix half and half with water.

NUTRIENT CONTENT OF ½ CUP EVAPORATED WHOLE MILK

(4 fluid ounces; 126 grams)

169 calories	134 mg sodium
9 g protein	382 mg potassium
10 g fat, 6 saturated	0 g dietary fiber
37 mg cholesterol	68 RE vitamin A
13 g carbohydrate	0.06 mg thiamin
329 mg calcium	0.40 mg riboflavin
256 mg phosphorus	0.2 mg niacin
0.2 mg iron	2 mg vitamin C

NUTRIENT CONTENT OF ½ CUP EVAPORATED SKIM MILK

(4 fluid ounces; 128 grams)

100 calories	147 mg sodium
10 g protein	422 mg potassium
0 g fat, 0 saturated	0 g dietary fiber
5 mg cholesterol	149 RE vitamin A
14 g carbohydrate	0.06 mg thiamin
369 mg calcium	0.39 mg riboflavin
249 mg phosphorus	0.2 mg niacin
0.4 mg iron	2 mg vitamin C

Homogenized (Whole) Milk: The standard, in which the fat and liquid have been processed into a smooth blend that does not separate on standing (see HOMOGENIZE). The composition of whole milk breaks down like this: 87 percent water, 3½ percent protein, 3¾ percent fat (the minimum allowed by the government's Grade A

Pasteurized Milk Ordinance is 3¼ percent), 5 percent carbohydrate and the rest ash. It's pasteurized and most of it fortified with vitamin D.

NUTRIENT CONTENT OF 1 CUP HOMOGENIZED (WHOLE) MILK
(8 fluid ounces; 244 grams)

149 calories	119 mg sodium
8 g protein	368 mg potassium
8 g fat, 5 saturated	0 g dietary fiber
33 mg cholesterol	76 RE vitamin A
11 g carbohydrate	0.09 mg thiamin
290 mg calcium	0.40 mg riboflavin
227 mg phosphorus	0.2 mg niacin
0.1 mg iron	2 mg vitamin C

Lactose-Reduced Milk: Milk (usually low fat or skim) that's been treated with lactase, the enzyme that breaks down lactose (milk sugar). It is designed for those with LACTOSE INTOLERANCE (the inability to digest lactose).

NUTRIENT CONTENT OF 1 CUP LACTOSE-REDUCED 1 PERCENT MILK*
(8 fluid ounces; 244 grams)

102 calories	123 mg sodium
8 g protein	381 mg potassium
3 g fat, 2 saturated	0 g dietary fiber
10 mg cholesterol	145 RE vitamin A
12 g carbohydrate	0.10 mg thiamin
300 mg calcium	0.41 mg riboflavin
235 mg phosphorus	0.2 mg niacin
0.1 mg iron	2 mg vitamin C

*Contains 70 percent less lactose than regular low-fat milk.

NUTRIENT CONTENT OF 1 CUP LOW-FAT (2 PERCENT) MILK
(8 fluid ounces; 244 grams)

121 calories	121 mg sodium
8 g protein	376 mg potassium
5 g fat, 3 saturated	0 g dietary fiber
18 mg cholesterol	139 RE vitamin A
12 g carbohydrate	0.10 mg thiamin
295 mg calcium	0.40 mg riboflavin
232 mg phosphorus	0.2 mg niacin
0.1 mg iron	2 mg vitamin C

Low-Fat Milk: Milk containing anywhere from ½ to 2 percent fat. The two most widely available low-fat milks are the 2 percent and 1 percent (often sold as "99 percent fat free"). All are pasteurized and may or may not be fortified with vitamins A and D, also with protein. Read the labels. **NOTE:** There is also low-fat chocolate milk.

NUTRIENT CONTENT OF 1 CUP PROTEIN-FORTIFIED LOW-FAT (2 PERCENT) MILK
(8 fluid ounces; 246 grams)

137 calories	145 mg sodium
10 g protein	447 mg potassium
5 g fat, 3 saturated	0 g dietary fiber
19 mg cholesterol	140 RE vitamin A
14 g carbohydrate	0.11 mg thiamin
352 mg calcium	0.48 mg riboflavin
276 mg phosphorus	0.3 mg niacin
0.1 mg iron	3 mg vitamin C

NUTRIENT CONTENT OF 1 CUP LOW-FAT (2 PERCENT) CHOCOLATE MILK
(8 fluid ounces; 250 grams)

178 calories	150 mg sodium
8 g protein	423 mg potassium
5 g fat, 3 saturated	4 g dietary fiber
17 mg cholesterol	143 RE vitamin A
26 g carbohydrate	0.09 mg thiamin
285 mg calcium	0.41 mg riboflavin
255 mg phosphorus	0.3 mg niacin
0.6 mg iron	2 mg vitamin C

NUTRIENT CONTENT OF 1 CUP LOW-FAT (1 PERCENT) MILK
(8 fluid ounces; 244 grams)

102 calories	123 mg sodium
8 g protein	381 mg potassium
3 g fat, 2 saturated	0 g dietary fiber
10 mg cholesterol	144 RE vitamin A
12 g carbohydrate	0.10 mg thiamin
300 mg calcium	0.41 mg riboflavin
235 mg phosphorus	0.2 mg niacin
0.1 mg iron	2 mg vitamin C

NUTRIENT CONTENT OF 1 CUP PROTEIN-FORTIFIED LOW-FAT (1 PERCENT) MILK

(8 fluid ounces; 245 grams)

119 calories	143 mg sodium
10 g protein	444 mg potassium
3 g fat, 2 saturated	0 g dietary fiber
10 mg cholesterol	145 RE vitamin A
14 g carbohydrate	0.11 mg thiamin
349 mg calcium	0.47 mg riboflavin
273 mg phosphorus	0.2 mg niacin
0.1 mg iron	2 mg vitamin C

Low-Sodium Milk: A special homogenized milk for those who must watch their sodium intake. Some 95 percent of its sodium has been removed, thus 8 ounces of low-sodium milk contain only 6 milligrams of sodium compared to 119 milligrams for whole milk. It's not widely available—just as well, maybe, because it tastes terrible.

NUTRIENT CONTENT OF 1 CUP LOW-SODIUM WHOLE MILK

(8 fluid ounces; 244 grams)

149 calories	6 mg sodium
8 g protein	617 mg potassium
8 g fat, 5 saturated	0 g dietary fiber
33 mg cholesterol	78 RE vitamin A
11 g carbohydrate	0.05 mg thiamin
246 mg calcium	0.10 mg riboflavin
209 mg phosphorus	0 mg niacin
NA mg iron	NA mg vitamin C

Nonfat Dry Milk: Dehydrated skim milk sold in powder form. It blends quickly and completely with water and, when properly reconstituted, tastes very much like fresh

NUTRIENT CONTENT OF 1 CUP SKIM MILK

(8 fluid ounces; 245 grams)

86 calories	126 mg sodium
8 g protein	404 mg potassium
0 g fat, 0 saturated	0 g dietary fiber
4 mg cholesterol	149 RE vitamin A
12 g carbohydrate	0.09 mg thiamin
301 mg calcium	0.34 mg riboflavin
247 mg phosphorus	0.2 mg niacin
0.1 mg iron	2 mg vitamin C

skim milk. Most of it is fortified with vitamins A and D to boost its content of these two nutrients to about that of fresh whole milk. See SKIM MILK for nutrient content.

Skim Milk: Milk stripped of most of its fat. By law it cannot contain more than ½ of 1 percent fat. Like other milks, it is pasteurized and may or may not have been fortified with vitamins A and D and protein.

NUTRIENT CONTENT OF 1 CUP PROTEIN-FORTIFIED SKIM MILK

(8 fluid ounces; 245 grams)

100 calories	144 mg sodium
10 g protein	445 mg potassium
1 g fat, 0 saturated	0 g dietary fiber
5 mg cholesterol	149 RE vitamin A
14 g carbohydrate	0.11 mg thiamin
350 mg calcium	0.48 mg riboflavin
274 mg phosphorus	0.2 mg niacin
0.1 mg iron	3 mg vitamin C

Sweet Acidophilus Milk: Unlike the tangy, thick buttermilklike acidophilus milk of old, this one's a dead ringer for homogenized milk—in looks, taste and texture. The difference is that it contains acidophilus bacteria, which go to work in the intestinal tract maintaining the proper balance of beneficial bugs. Its nutrient content approximates that of the milk from which it's made—usually 2 percent milk.

Sweetened Condensed Milk: Whole milk blended with sugar, relieved of more than half its water and canned. A key ingredient in Key lime pie, it's extremely rich and almost too thick to pour. Fortunately, there is now a low-fat sweetened condensed milk with 50 percent less

NUTRIENT CONTENT OF ½ CUP SWEETENED CONDENSED MILK

(4 fluid ounces; 153 grams)

491 calories	195 mg sodium
12 g protein	568 mg potassium
13 g fat, 8 saturated	0 g dietary fiber
52 mg cholesterol	124 RE vitamin A
83 g carbohydrate	0.14 mg thiamin
433 mg calcium	0.64 mg riboflavin
387 mg phosphorus	0.3 mg niacin
0.3 mg iron	4 mg vitamin C

fat. Its calorie count, alas, is nearly the same as that of regular sweetened condensed milk. Read the label carefully.

Milk Allergy: People who have difficulty digesting milk, cheese, ice cream and such aren't likely to have a true allergy. They are more apt to suffer from an intolerance (see LACTOSE INTOLERANCE). Still, some people are allergic to the protein in raw milk. Pasteurization denatures most of the protein—as does cooking—and lessens the possibility of an allergic reaction. If such still occurs, there are a variety of options: goat's or sheep's milk or fortified soy milk. These are usually less troublesome.

Milk Anemia: Although born with a reserve of iron, babies quickly lose it as they grow, and if milk is their sole source of this essential mineral, they may become anemic. By the time a baby's birth weight doubles, his store of iron is usually spent. At six months, babies need 10 milligrams of iron a day, which means they must be fed iron-enriched

formulas and/or cereals in addition to milk. Later (they're at greatest risk of developing "milk anemia" between six months and three years), they can begin eating meat and iron-rich legumes. Parents must also make sure their infants and toddlers get plenty of vitamin C (from fruits, vegetables and juices) because it maximizes the body's absorption of iron.

Milk Fat: The fat present in milk, cream, butter, cheese, ice cream; indeed, all dairy foods. It used to be called **butterfat.**

Milk of Magnesia: See LAXATIVES.

Milk Shake: Developed shortly before the turn of the last century, milk shakes (also called **frappés** and **frosteds**) might originally have been spiked with whiskey. Today they're nothing more than milk, chocolate (or vanilla or berry) syrup and a scoop or two of ice cream buzzed up to the consistency of soft ice cream. Sometimes malted-

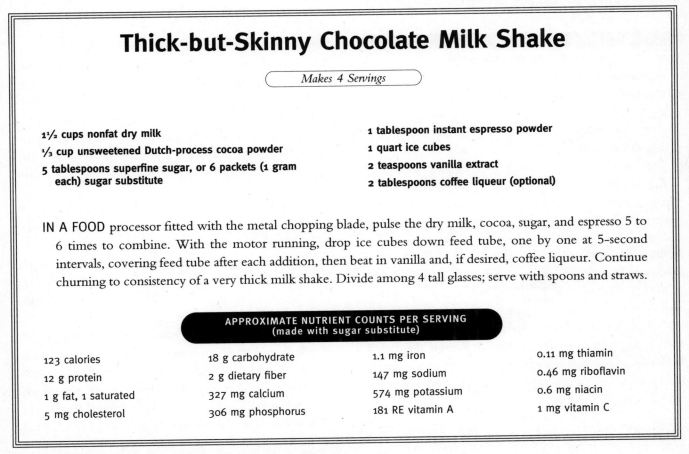

Thick-but-Skinny Chocolate Milk Shake

Makes 4 Servings

- 1½ cups nonfat dry milk
- ⅓ cup unsweetened Dutch-process cocoa powder
- 5 tablespoons superfine sugar, or 6 packets (1 gram each) sugar substitute
- 1 tablespoon instant espresso powder
- 1 quart ice cubes
- 2 teaspoons vanilla extract
- 2 tablespoons coffee liqueur (optional)

IN A FOOD processor fitted with the metal chopping blade, pulse the dry milk, cocoa, sugar, and espresso 5 to 6 times to combine. With the motor running, drop ice cubes down feed tube, one by one at 5-second intervals, covering feed tube after each addition, then beat in vanilla and, if desired, coffee liqueur. Continue churning to consistency of a very thick milk shake. Divide among 4 tall glasses; serve with spoons and straws.

APPROXIMATE NUTRIENT COUNTS PER SERVING
(made with sugar substitute)

123 calories	18 g carbohydrate	1.1 mg iron	0.11 mg thiamin
12 g protein	2 g dietary fiber	147 mg sodium	0.46 mg riboflavin
1 g fat, 1 saturated	327 mg calcium	574 mg potassium	0.6 mg niacin
5 mg cholesterol	306 mg phosphorus	181 RE vitamin A	1 mg vitamin C

Note: If made with sugar, add 54 calories and 16 grams carbohydrate.

milk powder is added, in which case the shake becomes a **malted-milk shake** or, simply, a **malted.** The best shakes, connoisseurs insist, are too thick to sip through the extra-wide straws that accompany them. Adolescents dote on milk shakes, defying (or at least turning a blind eye to) the saturated fats, calories and cholesterol they contain. They aren't nutritional ciphers, however, because milk shakes contain plenty of protein, carbohydrate, calcium and phosphorus.

Milk Sugar: See LACTOSE.

Millet:
These little golden pellets are better known as **birdseed.** But this Old Testament "gruel of endurance" isn't just for the birds. It brims with protein, B vitamins and such essential minerals as iron and phosphorus. Best of all, millet tastes a little like hot buttered popcorn—*if* it's toasted before it's boiled. That's easy: Place millet in a large, deep heavy saucepan (no more than 1 cup at a time), add no fat, set over moderately high heat and toast 5 minutes, shaking now and then to keep the grains moving.

NUTRIENT CONTENT OF 1 CUP BOILED MILLET	
(about 8½ ounces; 240 grams)	
284 calories	5 mg sodium
8 g protein	149 mg potassium
2 g fat, 0 saturated	3 g dietary fiber
0 mg cholesterol	0 RE vitamin A
57 g carbohydrate	0.25 mg thiamin
7 mg calcium	0.20 mg riboflavin
240 mg phosphorus	3.2 mg niacin
1.5 mg iron	0 mg vitamin C

Milling of Grains:
Milling and refining rob grains of many important nutrients, including iron and three important B vitamins—thiamin, riboflavin and niacin. In the early 1900s, when the poor subsisted largely upon breads made from highly refined flour and cornmeal, nutritional diseases like pellagra were common. As a result, the federal Enrichment Act was adopted in 1942 but is no longer mandatory. For details, see ENRICHED, ENRICHMENT PROGRAM.

Milo: See SORGHUM.

Mincemeat:
Was the pemmican of the Native Americans the original mincemeat? Some food historians think so. It was a mixture of dried fruits and meat (usually venison) compressed into cakes that could be eaten like candy bars or simmered into a kind of porridge. Today's mincemeat is apt to contain the mince of dried fruits but not the meat, not even suet, a popular ingredient before everyone began obsessing about fat and cholesterol. With bottled mincemeat available in every supermarket, few cooks bother to make it from scratch anymore. **NOTE:** Mincemeat recipes vary too much for a meaningful nutrient count but there's no denying that mincemeat is long on calories and carbohydrates. It won't lack for vitamins and minerals, either.

Mineral Oil: See LAXATIVES.

Minerals:
Inorganic (carbon-free) elements that turn to ash when burned. Of the more than three dozen known minerals, nineteen are necessary for good health. See MACROMINERALS; MICROMINERALS. See also the individual minerals—CALCIUM; COPPER; IRON; PHOSPHORUS; POTASSIUM; etc.

Mineral Water:
Two atoms of hydrogen, one of oxygen. Who would have dreamed that H_2O would become so trendy? Well, this is nothing new. Man's fascination with the magical powers of waters that come gushing out of middle earth is as old as man himself. But it was those great neurotics the Romans who glorified them by building spas and baths all over the face of Europe (two of the best preserved are in Germany at Baden-Baden and in England at—where else?—Bath).

Strangely, the more developed the country today, the greater the faith in "the cure." Germany abounds with spas, as do France, Italy, Japan and the United States. But you don't need to travel there to take the healing waters; you can buy them by the bottle at the supermarket. Some mineral waters sparkle, some are as flat as distilled water and most are mildly alkaline. But all of them are loaded with minerals—everything from calcium and magnesium to sodium and smelly hydrogen sulfide. Sodium's the one to watch out for, especially if you have high blood pressure, coronary heart disease or edema. Fortunately, the mineral content is detailed on every bottle of mineral water.

A MYTH THAT SHOULD BE SET STRAIGHT: Many people believe that bottled waters are pure, free of pollutants and harmful bacteria. Not necessarily true. Perrier, no less, was found to contain minute quantities of benzene, a powerful carcinogen, and although the problem has been corrected, Perrier is still scrambling to recover its image. Furthermore, routine samplings of some American spring waters have turned up *E. coli,* a sure sign of fecal contamination. **SUMMING UP:** You may be better off drinking from the tap than dropping a bundle on fancy spa waters.

Mirliton: See CHAYOTE.

Miso:
A heavily salted soybean paste fermented with barley, rice or other grain that's a Japanese kitchen staple. Miso may be white and sweet, yellow and nutty or red, an even saltier version, the farmer's favorite. Miso figures prominently in the MACROBIOTIC DIET.

NUTRIENT CONTENT OF 1 TABLESPOON MISO
(about 2/3 ounce; 17 grams)

36 calories	629 mg sodium
2 g protein	28 mg potassium
1 g fat, 0 saturated	1 g dietary fiber
0 mg cholesterol	2 RE vitamin A
5 g carbohydrate	0.02 mg thiamin
11 mg calcium	0.04 mg riboflavin
26 mg phosphorus	0.2 mg niacin
0.5 mg iron	0 mg vitamin C

Mixes: See CONVENIENCE FOODS.

Mizuna:
A deeply serrated, dandelionlike Japanese green that shows up regularly in tossed salads at cutting-edge restaurants and is now sold by many greenmarkets. Though *mizuna* has bite, it has a more delicate flavor than arugula, dandelion or watercress. **NOTE:** Nutrient counts are unavailable for *mizuna,* but for an approximation, see ARUGULA or DANDELION GREENS.

Modified Starch (additive):
Starch chemically treated to make it blend more easily, to fix its acidity and improve its texture. Food processors rely on modified starch to bind and thicken puddings, pie fillings, gravies, sauces and a huge array of instants and mixes. Baby-food manufacturers use modified starch to keep their products from weeping

(oozing liquid), as do frozen-food processors, who find that it keeps gravies and sauces creamy from freezer to oven to table. Some of the chemicals used to modify starch are aluminum sulfate (a key ingredient in many baking powders), propylene oxide, succinic anhydride and sodium hydroxide. Although modified starch is high on the FDA's must-reevaluate list, there is nothing new to report.

Molasses:
A by-product of sugar refining, specifically the dark brown ooze left after sugarcane sap has been reduced to syrup and the crystals have been filtered or centrifuged out. **First-strike molasses** is what remains after the first crystallization; **second-strike,** residue from the second; and **blackstrap,** bottom-of-the-barrel **third-strike** sludge (it does, as food faddists claim, contain more minerals than finer, earlier strikes—mainly iron, calcium and potassium—but nutritionists debate whether this extra iron is in a form the body can use). The cruder, darker molasses is often bleached by bubbling sulfur dioxide through it and, although almost all of the gas evaporates, this molasses is

NUTRIENT CONTENT OF 1 TABLESPOON UNSULFURED MOLASSES
(about 3/4 ounce; 21 grams)

55 calories	8 mg sodium
0 g protein	300 mg potassium
0 g fat, 0 saturated	0 g dietary fiber
0 mg cholesterol	0 RE vitamin A
14 g carbohydrate	0.01 mg thiamin
42 mg calcium	0 mg riboflavin
6 mg phosphorus	0.2 mg niacin
1.0 mg iron	0 mg vitamin C

NUTRIENT CONTENT OF 1 TABLESPOON BLACKSTRAP MOLASSES
(about 3/4 ounce; 21 grams)

48 calories	11 mg sodium
0 g protein	511 mg potassium
0 g fat, 0 saturated	0 g dietary fiber
0 mg cholesterol	0 RE vitamin A
12 g carbohydrate	0.01 mg thiamin
176 mg calcium	0 mg riboflavin
8 mg phosphorus	0.2 mg niacin
3.6 mg iron	0 mg vitamin C

labeled "sulfured." Today's top-quality molasses—all natural, fancy and unsulfured—is no longer a sugar-refining by-product. It is pure sugarcane juice boiled until syrupy, clarified, then blended for uniform color, consistency and sweetness. Molasses is the one sugar syrup with any food value.

Molds: Microscopic plants (fungi) that are both good and bad. The Japanese use mold to ferment rice water into *sake;* cheese makers turn curded creams into heavenly Gorgonzola, Roquefort and Stilton by injecting them with the mold *Penicillium roqueforti* or *Penicillium glaucum;* and wine makers rely on the mold *Botrytis cinerea* to induce the "noble rot" of grapes, which produces such ambrosial dessert wines as Sauternes and Beerenauslese. Needless to add, the healing powers of certain molds (penicillin, to name one) have revolutionized pharmacy and medicine.

But molds can be deadly, too. Although bacteriologists have long known that mycotoxins (mold-generated poisons) could cause people to sicken and die (the St. Anthony's fire of the Middle Ages was traced to moldy bins of rye), they had always considered molds less harmful than bacteria. *Until* the 1960s, when English turkeys began dying by the thousands. The culprit? Mycotoxins in imported peanut meal, among them the deadly AFLATOXIN. The trouble with toxins is that they are invisible, indestructible and proceed up the food chain: Animals eat contaminated feed; people eat contaminated plants and animals, often with dire results. Cooking doesn't destroy mycotoxins. As a result, scientists no longer consider moldy grains, legumes, nuts, breads, jams and fruits harmless. They may indicate the presence of harmful toxins that can work their way into food—often to depths of 1½ inches. So trimming off the mold is no longer good enough. The safest policy today: When in doubt, toss it out.

Mollusks: Bivalves (shellfish encased in hard, hinged shells). See CLAMS; MUSSELS; OYSTERS; SCALLOPS.

Molybdenum: A mineral the body needs in minuscule amounts as a component of several enzymes. With grains, leafy green vegetables, legumes, milk and liver all being good sources of molybdenum, deficiencies are unknown. On the other hand, too much molybdenum causes gout-like pain and swelling.

Monkfish, Goosefish, Anglerfish: Fierce of head but sweet of tail, this former "trash fish" has emerged as the chef's darling. Poor man's lobster, some call it, although monkfish is no longer cheap. It swims the North Atlantic, gobbling everything in sight: seabirds, sea bass, cod, herring, eels, lobsters, crabs, squid, even lobster pots. With their winglike pectoral fins, monkfish resemble skate and may weigh as much as 50 pounds although those coming to market are much smaller. Only the tail is edible. And what a treat it is—delicate but firm, moderately lean and as sweet as sea scallops.

NUTRIENT CONTENT OF 3 OUNCES (85 GRAMS) BAKED/BROILED MONKFISH	
83 calories	20 mg sodium
16 g protein	436 mg potassium
2 g fat, NA saturated	0 g dietary fiber
27 mg cholesterol	12 RE vitamin A
0 g carbohydrate	0.02 mg thiamin
9 mg calcium	0.06 mg riboflavin
218 mg phosphorus	2.2 mg niacin
0.4 mg iron	1 mg vitamin C

Monoamine Oxidase (MAO): An enzyme present in liver, lung and nerve tissues that speeds the breakdown of certain amines (nitrogen compounds), among them the tyramines present in wines and aged cheeses. Healthy people have enough MAO to handle TYRAMINES easily but those with a genetic lack of this crucial enzyme or those taking MAO inhibitors don't, and must watch what they eat to prevent potentially fatal food/drug interactions. Within hours, tyramines can build up to dangerous levels in the body, raising blood pressure, triggering excruciating headaches, irregular or rapid heartbeat, chest pain, tremors, dizziness, flushing and even, sometimes, death.

Monocalcium Phosphate: The active ingredient in phosphate baking powders. See LEAVENING AGENTS.

Monoglycerides (additives): A component of fats with which food processors stabilize sausages, lard, vegetable oils, margarines and shortenings. The most widely used of them is **monoglyceride citrate,** although the FDA imposes strict limits.

Monosaccharides: Simple (single) sugars. The three found in food are GALACTOSE, GLUCOSE and FRUCTOSE. See also CARBOHYDRATES.

Monosodium Glutamate (MSG) (additive; flavor enhancer): The sodium salt of glutamic acid, an amino acid that exists naturally in our bodies. What few people realize, however, is that MSG also exists naturally in plants—mushrooms and carrots are full of it. So are certain seaweeds from which the Japanese have been extracting MSG (now sold as AJI-NO-MOTO) for more than two thousand years, realizing that these odorless, almost tasteless white crystals intensify the flavor of sweets, sours and savories. The Chinese "pepper" everything with MSG, too, which explains why the headaches, burning and twitching it sometimes causes is called CHINESE RESTAURANT SYNDROME. For years the FDA has been testing MSG and continues to rate it GRAS (in 1995, scientific advisers to the FDA agreed that MSG was safe for almost everyone). However, as a concession to those few who are sensitive to it, the FDA requires that all food containing MSG be so labeled, even if the MSG is only a component of hydrolyzed vegetable or soy protein. (Some of these are 20 percent MSG.)

Monosodium Phosphate (additive): A stabilizer used in hams, bacon and other pork products to minimize the amount of liquid that cooks out. GRAS.

Monoterpenes: Anticarcinogenic antioxidants that exist naturally in basil, broccoli, cabbage, carrots, citrus fruits, cucumbers, eggplant, mint, parsley, peppers sweet and hot, squash, sweet potatoes and yams. They boost the body's immune system and also thwart the production of cholesterol. See PHYTOCHEMICALS.

Monounsaturated Fatty Acid: Fatty acids are molecules made up mostly of carbon and hydrogen. The more hydrogen they contain, the more saturated they are. And the stiffer. When one pair of hydrogen atoms is missing from a fatty acid—the case with oleic acid—it's said to be monounsaturated (*mono* simply means that one pair of hydrogen atoms is missing). When food processors turn vegetable oils into thick and fluffy shortenings, they do so by adding hydrogen. See HYDROGENATION; also FAT.

Monterey Jack: A pale, moderately mild, semihard Cheddar made from cow's milk. Though now produced all over the United States and Canada, Jack was first made in California, hence its name. The softer Jacks are aged three to six weeks; the hard, grating varieties at least six months. Soft Jacks average 20 to 21 percent fat; aged Jacks 23 to 30 percent.

NUTRIENT CONTENT OF 1 OUNCE (28 GRAMS) MONTEREY JACK	
106 calories	152 mg sodium
7 g protein	23 mg potassium
9 g fat, 5 saturated	0 g dietary fiber
25 mg cholesterol	72 RE vitamin A
0 g carbohydrate	0 mg thiamin
211 mg calcium	0.11 mg riboflavin
126 mg phosphorus	0 mg niacin
0.2 mg iron	0 mg vitamin C

Mood Fluctuations (diet and): For thousands of years people have attributed magical powers to food. Oysters, food lore tells us, are aphrodisiacal; so are chocolate and peanuts and olives. A glass of warm milk puts us to sleep at night; sugar sends children into rebellion. Even Dickens, in *A Christmas Carol,* had Scrooge justify his stinginess and foul temper on dyspepsia—"a fragment of underdone potato . . . an undigested bit of beef . . . a blot of mustard."

There's no denying that foods don't always "sit well" on the stomach. But most reputable nutritionists pooh-pooh their power to alter mood dramatically. Despite the recent jury-swaying, sugar-drove-him-to-it "Twinkies defense" of Dan White, the man who shot and killed San Francisco Mayor George Moscone, the truth is that sugar is more likely to calm than ruffle nerves. Studies show that an abrupt drop in blood sugar levels can make you depressed, sluggish and, yes, irritable—reason enough to eat regularly and sensibly. But these mood shifts are most likely to affect those with HYPOGLYCEMIA (chronically low blood sugar caused by an overproduction of insulin).

During the 1980s, hypoglycemia was the "new favorite disease" and neurotics blamed it for everything from headaches to dizziness to fatigue to sudden bursts of temper. In fact, true chronic hypoglycemia is rare.

In the mid-1970s, a California physician named Benjamin Feingold sent parents scurrying to buy his new book *Why Your Child Is Hyperactive*. His theory, now disproved, suggested that reversing hyperactivity was as easy as banning all food containing salicylates, either synthetic or natural, and the list of them was long: artificial food colors and flavors, almonds, apricots, peppermint and Worcestershire sauce, to name major culprits (see also FEINGOLD DIET).

Biomedical researchers studying the food/mood connection are now zeroing in on amino acids, the building blocks of protein. Several of them are needed (along with other nutrients) to synthesize neurotransmitters, which control all brain functions. Brain levels of the amino acid TRYPTOPHAN, for example, determine how much SEROTONIN is produced (it's the neurotransmitter that makes you sleepy and dulls your appetite and sensitivity to pain). And TYROSINE, another amino acid, seems to regulate the output of dopamine and norepinephrine, the neurotransmitters that determine, to some extent, how you handle stress. The subject is complex beyond belief, no simplistic conclusions can be drawn and studies continue.

Morels: See MUSHROOMS.

Morning Sickness (diet and):
Sometimes just opening the refrigerator door triggers them, the bouts of nausea that besiege about half the women who become pregnant. They can occur at any time of the day—not just the morning—but fortunately are usually confined to the first seventeen or eighteen weeks of pregnancy. No one knows what causes morning sickness. For years doctors (most of them men) considered the condition psychosomatic. Today, researchers are more inclined to hold a drop in blood sugar levels responsible. Or increased outputs of estrogen and progesterone, which heighten the sense of smell.

After treating hundreds of pregnant women at Brigham and Women's Hospital in Boston (a part of the Harvard Medical School), registered dietitian Miriam Erick, who wrote *No More Morning Sickness,* came to the conclusion that smells (stale coffee, cigarette smoke, cooking odors and so forth) are more likely to trigger morning sickness than food itself. She also considers the old white-and-tan list of easily tolerated foods obsolete. In fact, soda crackers, mashed potatoes, unsauced pasta and dry toast may not work at all. Erick's advice, based on years of experience: Eat whatever appeals—potato chips, if they will stop the vomiting. It's better to eat whatever you can keep down,

to consume calories, than to eat healthy only to have it all come up.

Ongoing morning sickness can cause weight loss and dehydration, both of which are bad for mother and child. Erick suggests that pregnant women keep a variety of foods on hand just to have something to nosh the instant hunger strikes. There should be sweets and sours, softs and crunchies, hots and colds, dries and wets, blands and spicies, earthies and fruities.

Erick's theories don't contradict standard nutritional advice: Eat several light meals during the day instead of three heavy ones, cut down on fat and drink liquids between meals, not *with* them. Some physicians prescribe vitamin B_6 supplements and in some cases they do seem to ease the nausea and vomiting. A few pregnant women (about 2 percent) suffer violent morning sickness the whole nine months, a potentially dangerous condition called HYPEREMESIS GRAVIDARUM that may require hospitalization and intravenous feeding.

Mortadella:
The original bologna, a giant pork sausage from Bologna, Italy, that's being widely (and poorly) counterfeited in this country. The best mortadellas are smooth and creamy, subtly seasoned and larded with strips of fat. They are boiled, ready to slice and slip into sandwiches or salads.

NUTRIENT CONTENT OF 1 OUNCE (28 GRAMS) MORTADELLA (BEEF AND PORK)	
88 calories	352 mg sodium
5 g protein	46 mg potassium
7 g fat, 3 saturated	0 g dietary fiber
16 mg cholesterol	0 RE vitamin A
1 g carbohydrate	0.03 mg thiamin
5 mg calcium	0.04 mg riboflavin
28 mg phosphorus	0.8 mg niacin
0.4 mg iron	7 mg vitamin C

Mouth Sores, Mouth Inflammation:
A smooth or slick tongue, a tongue splodged with patches of white, a fissured magenta tongue can all be symptoms of malnutrition. So are redness or cracks at the corner of the mouth. The deficiencies most apt to cause these conditions are of three B vitamins—B_2 (riboflavin), niacin and B_6 (pyridoxine). These important vitamins are discussed in detail under their own headings.

Mozzarella: A snowy and supple but compact Italian cheese that's gained fame as a pizza topper. Once exclusively a buffalo-milk cheese, mozzarella is now more often made with cow's milk, sometimes wholly or partly of skim milk (it averages 18 to 22 percent fat). Some mozzarella is smoked but more of it is simply curded, kneaded in near-boiling water until smooth and shiny, then given a quick brine dip. It's bland but has a subtle tang and faintly nutty flavor. Neapolitans like to slice mozzarella, fan it out with sliced tomatoes, drizzle all with a good, gutsy olive oil, add sprinklings of freshly minced basil and call it a meal. Delicious. Today mozzarella is available in part-skim milk and nonfat varieties, although the latter is unpleasantly rubbery.

NUTRIENT CONTENT OF 1 OUNCE (28 GRAMS) PART-SKIM MOZZARELLA

72 calories	132 mg sodium
7 g protein	24 mg potassium
5 g fat, 3 saturated	0 g dietary fiber
16 mg cholesterol	50 RE vitamin A
1 g carbohydrate	0.01 mg thiamin
183 mg calcium	0.09 mg riboflavin
131 mg phosphorus	0 mg niacin
0.1 mg iron	0 mg vitamin C

MREs: Nutrient- and energy-packed "meals-ready-to-eat," which the military now uses in place of the old K-rations of World War II. MREs are compact, portable, nonperishable thanks to such space age advances as freeze-drying and irradiation.

Mucous Membranes: They line the nose, mouth, digestive tract from start to finish as well as other inner body cavities. Their main functions are to protect against bacterial invasion, to provide a broad surface for secretion of enzymes and food absorption and to support blood vessels and lymph glands. If the mucosa are to remain vital and healthy, they need sufficient vitamin A or retinol (see A, VITAMIN).

Mucus: Secretions of the mucous membranes that not only serve as lubricants but also discourage viral and bacterial infection.

Muesli: A nut/whole-grain/dried-fruit mix developed in Switzerland as a healthful breakfast food; a European granola. Today most major American cereal manufacturers make their own versions of muesli. **NOTE:** Muesli recipes vary too much for a meaningful nutrient count. What can be said, however, is that most mueslis contain plenty of calories and fat as well as hefty doses of vitamins (especially the B group), minerals and dietary fiber.

Muffins: American muffins are getting bigger and sweeter, *much* sweeter. In fact, *muffin* has become a euphemism for *cupcake*. Good old-fashioned muffins rarely contained more than a tablespoon of sugar, not much fat and only a single egg. They were simply a wonderful way to put a hot bread on the table fast. Today's muffins, especially the "boutique"-baked sold in greenmarkets, delis and specialty food stores, drip with honey (or molasses) and are chock-full of nuts, seeds and dried fruits. Yet they're often passed off as health food. Read labels before you binge. See also ENGLISH MUFFINS.

NUTRIENT CONTENT OF 1 MEDIUM-SIZE PLAIN MUFFIN
(about 1²/₃ ounces; 45 grams)

135 calories	210 mg sodium
3 g protein	54 mg potassium
5 g fat, 1 saturated	1 g dietary fiber
19 mg cholesterol	13 RE vitamin A
19 g carbohydrate	0.13 mg thiamin
90 mg calcium	0.14 mg riboflavin
68 mg phosphorus	1.0 mg niacin
1.1 mg iron	0 mg vitamin C

Mulberries: Native to Persia, these dark purple berries of biblical antiquity gradually moved westward along the Mediterranean into northern Europe and on to North America when someone decided the colonies should get

NUTRIENT CONTENT OF 1 CUP FRESH MULBERRIES
(about 5 ounces; 140 grams)

60 calories	14 mg sodium
2 g protein	272 mg potassium
1 g fat, 0 saturated	2 g dietary fiber
0 mg cholesterol	4 RE vitamin A
14 g carbohydrate	0.04 mg thiamin
58 mg calcium	0.14 mg riboflavin
53 mg phosphorus	0.9 mg niacin
2.6 mg iron	51 mg vitamin C

into silk. Silkworms feed almost exclusively on mulberry leaves and although America's silk industry failed, the mulberries took to the southeastern wilds and thrive there to this day. Of the three types available—**black mulberries, red** and **white**—the best eating are the black. These rarely come to market and must be gathered wherever they grow. **SEASON:** Summer.

Mullet: A huge family of firm-fleshed fish, more than one hundred species strong, that swim the waters of the world. From a commercial standpoint, the most important are the **red mullet** of the Mediterranean (*rouget*) and the **striped** and **silver mullet** caught off the Carolinas and in the Gulf of Mexico. Though small (the best weigh only a pound or two), mullet contain both white meat (it's sweet and nutty) and a stronger, fatter dark meat. They are a superior source of protein and minerals, especially iodine.

NUTRIENT CONTENT OF 3 OUNCES (85 GRAMS) BAKED/BROILED MULLET	
127 calories	60 mg sodium
21 g protein	390 mg potassium
4 g fat, 1 saturated	0 g dietary fiber
54 mg cholesterol	36 RE vitamin A
0 g carbohydrate	0.12 mg thiamin
26 mg calcium	0.13 mg riboflavin
208 mg phosphorus	6.1 mg niacin
1.2 mg iron	8 mg vitamin C

Mung Beans: See BEANS, DRIED.

Mung-Bean Sprouts: See BEAN SPROUTS.

Munster, Münster: An ancient cheese first developed, it's said, by Irish or Italian Benedictine monks who came to the Munster Valley of eastern France more than one thousand years ago. Cow's milk is what they used to create this soft golden cheese. Today's Munster, still made from cow's milk, is easily identified by its rectangular shape, bright orange rind and sharp, salty flavor. The Germans have now adopted this French cheese as their own, and a well-aged German Munster packs considerable punch. Alas, American versions are bland and boring. True French Munster, protected by an *appellation d'origine contrôlée,* is bacterially fermented with lactobacillus and averages between 45 and 50 percent fat. It is buttery, biting, glorious.

NUTRIENT CONTENT OF 1 OUNCE (28 GRAMS) MUNSTER CHEESE	
104 calories	178 mg sodium
7 g protein	38 mg potassium
9 g fat, 5 saturated	0 g dietary fiber
27 mg cholesterol	90 RE vitamin A
0 g carbohydrate	0 mg thiamin
203 mg calcium	0.09 mg riboflavin
132 mg phosphorus	0 mg niacin
0.1 mg iron	0 mg vitamin C

Muscadines: See GRAPES.

Muscle Cramps: These may indicate a deficiency of calcium, sodium or two B vitamins—thiamin and pantothenic acid. Each nutrient is discussed in detail under its own heading.

Muscular Weakness: Many conditions cause muscular weakness, but ones not always identified are nutritional deficiencies, specifically of protein or vitamin C or D. A lack of any one of them might be to blame. Each nutrient is discussed fully under its own heading.

Mushrooms: "Either they are edible or they are poisonous. Either they grow among rusty nails or rotten rags or the holes of serpents or amongst trees bearing harmful fruits." Such mushrooms, advised the first-century Greek physician Dioscorides, were not to be eaten. The Romans, on the other hand, were cavalier about separating poisonous mushrooms from the nonpoisonous. Instead of taking time to learn which were edible, they devised an elaborate pharmacopoeia of antidotes, all of them useless.

We know better today. The surest way to sort the safe from the unsafe is to know your mushrooms even though you no longer need to forage for them. Snowy cultivated mushrooms (once called *champignons de Paris* because they were grown in limestone caves by Louis XIV's botanist) are the supermarket staple. And to think that not so long ago they were a "special order" in midsize American towns. Today wild woodland species show up with increasing frequency: Webbed brown **morels** . . . ruffled orange or black trumpets (**chanterelles**) . . . fleshy **porcini** (also called **cèpes, boletus** and **Steinpilzen**) . . . **shiitake** (brown Japanese "parasols" with woody stems) . . . silvery **pleurottes** or oyster mushrooms. **Cremini** (brown field mushrooms) are almost commonplace, as are big beefy **portobellos** and thumbtack-size **enoki.** With the exception of enoki (best tossed into salads), all mushrooms can be used interchangeably in recipes. Although the delicacy of cultivated mushrooms can't match the deep earthiness of wild mushrooms, they don't vary much nutritionally. **SEASON:** Year-round for cultivated mushrooms; spring and summer for the wild. **NOTE:** All raw mushrooms contain hydrazines, which have caused tumors in mice. Fortunately, cooking destroys a third of these carcinogens, as does a week in cold storage. Canning wipes them out altogether.

CAUTION: Never eat wild mushrooms you've gathered yourself or have been given unless you know your mushrooms and can tell the deadly from the edible. The differences between the two are often so subtle only an expert can detect them.

NUTRIENT CONTENT OF 1 CUP SLICED RAW MUSHROOMS
(about 2½ ounces; 70 grams)

18 calories	3 mg sodium
1 g protein	258 mg potassium
0 g fat, 0 saturated	1 g dietary fiber
0 mg cholesterol	0 RE vitamin A
3 g carbohydrate	0.07 mg thiamin
4 mg calcium	0.31 mg riboflavin
73 mg phosphorus	2.9 mg niacin
0.9 mg iron	3 mg vitamin C

NUTRIENT CONTENT OF 1 CUP CANNED MUSHROOM PIECES
(about 5⅔ ounces; 156 grams)

37 calories	662 mg sodium
3 g protein	200 mg potassium
0 g fat, 0 saturated	3 g dietary fiber
0 mg cholesterol	0 RE vitamin A
8 g carbohydrate	0.13 mg thiamin
17 mg calcium	0.03 mg riboflavin
103 mg phosphorus	2.5 mg niacin
1.2 mg iron	0 mg vitamin C

Muskellunge: Often called just **musky,** this lean-meated fish is a freshwater pike that swims the Great Lakes. Considered a delicacy among people of the upper Midwest, muskellunge is rarely available elsewhere. For approximate nutrient counts, see FISH, LEAN WHITE.

Muslim Diet Restrictions: See ISLAMIC DIETARY LAWS.

Mussels: Unlike oysters, scallops and clams, mussels have never been very popular in the United States despite the fact that because they're so fashionable abroad, they must be farmed. In the States, mussels are plentiful along both the Atlantic and Pacific coasts—from Alaska to San Francisco on the West Coast, from the Arctic to North Carolina's Outer Banks on the East Coast. They are cheaper than any other mollusk (i.e., clams, oysters, scallops) and can be substituted for them in any recipe. Although high in sodium, mussels are an impressive source of iron, phosphorus and potassium, even of niacin and vitamin C. **NOTE:** Because of the dangerous warm-weather red tide along the Pacific Coast, mussels (other mollusks, too) are available mostly between November and April. In recent years, alas, red or brown tides have begun to affect East Coast supplies of shellfish, too.

NUTRIENT CONTENT OF 3 OUNCES (85 GRAMS) STEAMED MUSSELS

146 calories	314 mg sodium
20 g protein	227 mg potassium
4 g fat, 1 saturated	0 g dietary fiber
48 mg cholesterol	77 RE vitamin A
6 g carbohydrate	0.26 mg thiamin
28 mg calcium	0.36 mg riboflavin
243 mg phosphorus	2.6 mg niacin
5.7 mg iron	12 mg vitamin C

Mustard: There are seeds, powders and, most important to the cook, a broad variety of prepared mustards: **yellow** (American) hot-dog mustard, spicy brown **Dijon,** fiery **Chinese** (a sinus-clearing dip popular with egg rolls), **German** (from the spicy Düsseldorf to the sweet Bavarian), the sharp and savory **English.** And oh, so many more—some smooth; some made with whole grains. One value of mustards is that they make it possible to cut down on butter, especially when dressing steaks, chops and vegetables. Prepared mustards are low in calories, averaging 10 to 12 calories per tablespoon. But they are extremely high in sodium (nearly 200 milligrams per tablespoon). Don't count on mustards to provide much in the way of minerals—they contain only smidgens of calcium, phosphorus, iron and potassium. When it comes to vitamins, they are nutritional ciphers.

NUTRIENT CONTENT OF 1 TABLESPOON PREPARED MUSTARD

(about ⅔ ounce; 16 grams)

12 calories	196 mg sodium
1 g protein	20 mg potassium
1 g fat, 0 saturated	0 g dietary fiber
0 mg cholesterol	0 RE vitamin A
1 g carbohydrate	0 mg thiamin
13 mg calcium	0 mg riboflavin
11 mg phosphorus	0 mg niacin
0.3 mg iron	0 mg vitamin C

Mustard Greens: The seeds are frequently mentioned in the Bible; the tops (greens) were relished by the Greeks and Romans. Today mustard is grown mostly for the seeds although the dark leafy tops, first cousins to kale and collards, brim with beta-carotene, vitamin C, calcium and potassium as well as sulfurous compounds believed to reduce the risk of cancer. Young mustard shoots are tender enough, delicate enough, to toss raw into salads. **SEASON:** Year-round, with supplies at their peak between December and April.

NUTRIENT CONTENT OF 1 CUP BOILED/STEAMED MUSTARD GREENS

(about 5 ounces; 140 grams)

21 calories	22 mg sodium
3 g protein	281 mg potassium
0 g fat, 0 saturated	2 g dietary fiber
0 mg cholesterol	424 RE vitamin A
3 g carbohydrate	0.06 mg thiamin
103 mg calcium	0.09 mg riboflavin
57 mg phosphorus	0.6 mg niacin
1 mg iron	35 mg vitamin C

Mutagens, Mutation: Mutagens are agents—chemical, physical, natural or synthetic—that can alter genetic material (DNA) and mutation is the genetic change itself. For years biochemists and molecular biologists have been studying mutagens in food, both the naturally occurring and the added, to learn their role in such diseases as cancer. A pioneer in the field, Dr. Bruce Ames of the University of California, Berkeley, says, "Of all the compounds that attack DNA, my guess is that 99 percent occur naturally, many of them in the common foods we eat. Every meal you eat is full of mutagens and carcinogens."

The mutagen/cancer connection is extremely complex, riddled with mysteries, contradictions, biochemical interactions and influences both internal and external. Scientists ponder why people in "rich" countries are prone to breast, colon, endometrial and prostate cancers while Third Worlders are to cervix, esophagus, liver and stomach cancers. Reasearchers suspect the fatter diets of the rich and the unsanitary conditions of underdeveloped nations may be factors but haven't proved it. They do know, however, that Mormons and Seventh-Day Adventists, neither of whom drink or smoke, suffer fewer breast, colon and lung cancers than drinking/smoking segments of society (tobacco smoke and alcoholic beverages both contain carcinogenic mutagens). Needless to add, studies are ongoing and intensive. Meanwhile, the safest plan is to eat wisely (see FOOD GUIDE PYRAMID), to drink moderately (no more than two beers *or* cocktails *or* glasses of wine a day) and to swear off tobacco.

Mutton: Fully grown sheep. Sinewy and tough, mutton is rarely eaten in the United States although the British still find room for it at their table.

Mycotoxins: Poisons produced by molds that can cause people and animals to sicken and die. More than a dozen different mycotoxins have been identified, among them AFLATOXIN, which contaminates seeds, legumes, grains and nuts. See also ERGOT; MOLDS.

Myoglobin: Muscle hemoglobin, or what makes meat red. When meat is first cut, it is dark purple, but as myoglobin absorbs oxygen from the air, it turns bright red.

Nachos: America's favorite new nibble, a Tex-Mex inspiration—tortilla chips scattered with grated Cheddar (or Monterey Jack) and minced green chiles, then broiled just until "melty." Nachos are high in fat, calories and sodium.

NUTRIENT CONTENT OF 1 OUNCE (28 GRAMS) NACHOS	
141 calories	201 mg sodium
2 g protein	61 mg potassium
7 g fat, 1 saturated	2 g dietary fiber
1 mg cholesterol	13 RE vitamin A
18 g carbohydrate	0.04 mg thiamin
42 mg calcium	0.05 mg riboflavin
69 mg phosphorus	0.4 mg niacin
0.4 mg iron	1 mg vitamin C

Napa Cabbage: See CHINESE CABBAGE.

Nasogastric (NG) Tube: A feeding tube threaded into the nose and down the esophagus to the stomach. It's a way of nourishing those who can't eat.

Nasturtiums: See FLOWERS, EDIBLE.

National Health and Nutrition Examination Survey (NHANES): This is an ongoing series of government studies designed to assess our nutritional health. The first study (NHANES I), conducted in the early 1970s, examined some twenty thousand Americans between one and seventy-four years of age, their diets, their general health and their body measurements. NHANES II (1976 to 1980), conducted like NHANES I, added a new focus—iron, zinc and copper, plus vitamin and mineral supplements. NHANES III is now under way. The results of NHANES surveys, reported in professional journals, are of particular interest to physicians, nutritionists and dietitians.

National Institutes of Health (NIH): The research arm of the Public Health Service, which is part of the U.S. Department of Health and Human Services. The NIH's jobs are to study diseases affecting public health and to support nutrition programs (via research and training) that treat and/or prevent disease. Their goal: better health for all Americans from the cradle to the grave.

National Research Council (NRC): To advise the federal government on matters scientific and technical, the National Academy of Sciences (NAS) established the National Research Council. That was in 1916. Today the NRC works with both the government and private sector. Its governing board, composed of members of the NAS, the National Academy of Engineering and the Institute of Medicine, recently approved the Food and Nutrition Board's overhaul of the RDA. Now in print as the *10th Edition of the RDA,* this is the most up-to-date table of recommended nutrient amounts now available.

National Science Foundation (NSF): A foundation established in 1950 to upgrade the quality of scientific education and research across America by offering grants to universities and nonprofit institutions.

"Natural Foods": Another term for ORGANIC FOODS. So far USDA guidelines apply only to meat and poultry, *natural* meaning they're free of synthetic colors, flavors, preservatives or other artificial additives. When it comes to fruits, vegetables and other foods, almost anything goes. The term is frequently applied to whole grains and cereals, the implication being that they're only minimally processed *without* additives. But the government has yet to crack down on the claims.

"Naturally Flavored": A misleading term. By law, a natural flavoring must be extracted from natural sources—from the rind, juice, leaves, roots or bark of fruits, herbs, spices or even animal tissues (as in "natural" beef extract). But don't count on a "naturally flavored" peach pie being chockablock with fresh peaches. It may in fact contain very few. See FLAVOR LABELING.

"Naturally Sweetened": A label description about which the FDA hasn't been too fussy. It means no artificial sweeteners but not necessarily no sugar. Sugar is, after all, natural. So is honey. But presumably *naturally sweetened* means no highly refined sweeteners. Scrutinize the ingredient list.

Natural Toxins: Some beans contain **hemagglutinins,** or blood clumpers; compounds in cabbage (and its many cousins) can thwart the body's ability to use iodine and lead to goiter (see GOITROGENS); the **pressor amines** in bananas, aged cheeses, chocolate, pineapple and wine can raise blood pressure; mushrooms are full of carcinogens (HYDRAZINES); spinach and rhubarb are rich in **oxalates,** causes of corrosive gastroenteritis, shock, even death; carrots, nutmeg and parsley harbor the hallucinogen **myristicin;** peach and apricot pits, cassava, and even certain types of beans contain deadly **hydrogen cyanide.** The point here: People are so spooked by additives they fail to realize that many *natural* compounds in food are toxic. These aren't likely to cause trouble, however, if you eat a wide variety of food and small amounts of each.

Natural Vitamins: Nutrients extracted from "real" food as opposed to the lab synthesized. Chemically, the two are identical and there is no nutritional advantage to natural vitamins despite all the health-food-store hype. Financial advantage is something else again. Natural vitamins usually fetch premium prices.

Nausea: Rough seas or air, twisty-turny highways, food poisoning, early pregnancy. All can bring on nausea, the queasiness that precedes vomiting. So can diseases of the central nervous system, gallbladder problems, even seeing something intensely upsetting. The first order of business is to remove the irritant and, if not possible (often the case with ocean crossings or cruise ships), to take "seasick pills." Old salts recommend munching dry toast and dry poached chicken breast and taking sips of tea. This usually works for all forms of motion sickness. Other bouts of nausea may require different treatment. Obviously, the underlying cause of the nausea determines the best medicine, the best diet. See also MORNING SICKNESS.

Navy Beans, Pea Beans: See BEANS, DRIED.

Nectarines: Honey-sweet, smooth-skinned first cousins of the peach. Nectarines (and there are more than a hundred varieties of them) are somewhat smaller than peaches and most of America's crop comes from California and

NUTRIENT CONTENT OF 1 MEDIUM-SIZE NECTARINE	
(about 5 ounces; 136 grams)	
67 calories	0 mg sodium
1 g protein	288 mg potassium
1 g fat, 0 saturated	3 g dietary fiber
0 mg cholesterol	101 RE vitamin A
16 g carbohydrate	0.02 mg thiamin
7 mg calcium	0.06 mg riboflavin
22 mg phosphorus	1 mg niacin
0.2 mg iron	7 mg vitamin C

Texas. Like peaches, nectarines can be freestone or cling. They are low in calories but high in beta-carotene and potassium and, make a note, contain zero sodium or cholesterol. SEASON: June to mid-September.

Negligible Risk Policy, De Minimis Rule: The FDA's reinterpretation of the Delaney Clause of 1958, which forbids the use of any carcinogenic food additives (pesticides included). The negligible risk policy, first used by the EPA to register and regulate pesticides used on food crops and later adopted by the FDA, empowered these agencies to determine pesticide and additive tolerances and set maximum allowable levels in food. What, exactly, constitutes "negligible risk"? The EPA and FDA define it as "one additional incidence of cancer per one million people over a 70-year life span." The negligible risk policy had scarcely gone into effect when a consumer advocacy group cried foul and challenged the FDA in court. Result: The U.S. Ninth Circuit Court of Appeals ruled the negligible risk policy in violation of the Delaney Clause of the Federal Food, Drug, and Cosmetic Act. That was in the summer of 1992. The U.S. Supreme Court has so far declined to review the case. See also DELANEY CLAUSE; FOOD ADDITIVES AMENDMENT.

Neufchâtel: One of France's best cheeses, fresh, soft and subtly flavored. The specialty of Normandy's Pays de Bray, it's uncooked, curded with lactic acid bacteria and its fat content varies according to whether it's made of whole cow's milk, or skim or enriched with cream. There are also low-fat domestic cream cheeses called Neufchâtel. See CREAM CHEESE.

NUTRIENT CONTENT OF 1 OUNCE (28 GRAMS) NEUFCHÂTEL CHEESE (FROM WHOLE MILK)	
74 calories	113 mg sodium
3 g protein	32 mg potassium
7 g fat, 4 saturated	0 g dietary fiber
22 mg cholesterol	75 RE vitamin A
1 g carbohydrate	0 mg thiamin
21 mg calcium	0.06 mg riboflavin
39 mg phosphorus	0 mg niacin
0.1 mg iron	0 mg vitamin C

Neural Tube Defects: Folic acid deficiencies in pregnant women can cause such horrific birth defects (a neural tube condition called **spina bifida** and **anencephaly,** a fatally malformed brain) that flours, breads, cereals and pastas, etc., will soon be fortified with this important B vitamin. See FOLACIN.

Neurotoxins: Poisons that attack nerve tissue causing paralysis and death. Neurotoxins are a problem with some pesticides and herbicides (chlordane, heptachlor and TCDD, among others) but they also exist naturally in food. For example, clams, mussels, oysters and bay scallops feeding upon the toxic plankton sporadically blighting mollusk beds from Alaska to California and Maine to Massachusetts contain SAXITOXINS, which cause paralytic shellfish poisoning. Its symptoms—incoherence, loss of coordination, rash, numbness, dry throat, tingling, paralysis—can appear within half an hour of eating. This is not the red tide that contaminates warmer coastal waters and produces equally deadly neurotoxins. As a preventive, the FDA's National Shellfish Sanitation Program monitors coastal waters and bans not only fishing in troubled waters but also the sale or distribution of fish taken from them. There's another neurotoxin to beware of and that's the one produced by *Clostridium botulinum,* a bacterium whose live spores germinate and grow in faultily canned low-acid foods—meats, fish, certain soups and vegetables (carrots, corn, beans, mushrooms, peas, potatoes, onions and so on). See also CLOSTRIDIUM BOTULINUM under BACTERIA.

New Zealand Spinach: Botanically not spinach but a tender, warm-weather green harvested while young. Like true spinach (*Spinacia oleracea*), New Zealand spinach (*Tegragona expansa*) is best steamed in the drops of rinse water that cling to its leaves. As its name suggests, it hails from New Zealand; although considered a minor herbage vegetable, it is a powerhouse of beta-carotene and also a good source of vitamin C and potassium. New Zealand spinach grows well in America, so look for it in greenmarkets and supermarkets. **SEASON:** Summer.

NHANES: See NATIONAL HEALTH AND NUTRITION EXAMINATION SURVEY.

Niacin, Nicotinic Acid (vitamin): Without this important member of the B-complex (sometimes called vitamin B₃), the body cannot utilize carbohydrates, fats and proteins to provide energy. Thus the amount of niacin the body needs depends on the number of calories consumed. But that's not niacin's only role. It also helps ensure the health and vitality of the skin, digestive tract and nerves. In the early 1900s, when impoverished Southerners subsisted on highly refined corn breads, asylums were full of patients whose dementia was traced to pellagra, a debilitating niacin-deficiency disease. Niacin supplements effected miracle cures and led, ultimately, to the enrichment of cornmeal down South much the way the federal Enrichment Act of 1942 required food processors to restore the iron, thiamin, riboflavin and niacin lost in the milling of wheat (see ENRICHED, ENRICHMENT PROGRAM).

In recent years, niacin has been used to treat those with high blood cholesterol and it can dramatically bring these levels down. But not without side effects, some of them serious. Researchers at two major medical colleges (Virginia and Pennsylvania) studied two dozen people for nine months, gradually upping their niacin dosage from 250 milligrams a day to 3,000 (for healthy adults, the RDA for niacin is 15 to 20 milligrams a day). They learned that although instant-release niacin tablets caused flushing, fatigue and/or skin discoloration, the time-release capsules led to upset stomachs, fatigue and impaired liver function (elsewhere there've been reports of jaundice and liver failure). Given niacin's potentially dangerous side effects, many physicians and nutritionists agree that this B vitamin should no longer be sold over the counter, especially in doses as high as 3,000 milligrams (10 to 20 milligrams are the usual strength). Taken indiscriminately, megadoses can be deadly. A less toxic form of niacin is **niacinamide** (also called **nicotinamide**) in which the oxygen-hydrogen (OH) or acid component is replaced by two molecules of hydrogen and one of nitrogen. Niacinamide does not cause the violent "hot flashes" that nicotinic acid does. And it doesn't lower blood cholesterol levels, either. **DEFICIENCY SYMPTOMS:** Digestive upsets, insomnia,

---

NUTRIENT CONTENT OF 1 CUP STEAMED CHOPPED NEW ZEALAND SPINACH

(about 6⅓ ounces; 180 grams)

22 calories	193 mg sodium
2 g protein	183 mg potassium
0 g fat, 0 saturated	1 g dietary fiber
0 mg cholesterol	652 RE vitamin A
4 g carbohydrate	0.05 mg thiamin
86 mg calcium	0.19 mg riboflavin
39 mg phosphorus	0.7 mg niacin
1.2 mg iron	29 mg vitamin C

headaches, irritability and, frequently, a sore, swollen, purple-red tongue. More desperate niacin shortfall leads to pellagra: skin and gastrointestinal lesions, inflamed mucous membranes, diarrhea, dementia and death. Now that most cereals, flours, pastas and cornmeals are enriched, full-blown pellagra is history. At least in the United States. **GOOD SOURCES:** Enriched cereals, meals and flours (plus anything made from them), whole grains, legumes, meat and organ meats, poultry, fish and peanut butter. Besides food sources, the body can obtain niacin by making it from TRYPTOPHAN, an essential amino acid. Nutritionists figure that 60 milligrams of tryptophan equal 1 milligram of niacin. Thus, to calculate the body's niacin requirements, both sources of niacin must be considered. The sum of the two is called the niacin equivalent (NE), and for RDAs today, it is the unit of measurement used. **PRECAUTIONS:** Being water soluble, niacin can leach out in cooking water and be lost unless that water is recycled. Fortunately, niacin isn't destroyed by heat or light like some of the other B vitamins.

RDA FOR NIACIN (VITAMIN B3)

Babies:

Birth to 6 months	5 NE* per day
6 months to 1 year	6 NE per day

Children:

1 to 3 years	9 NE per day
4 to 6 years	12 NE per day
7 to 10 years	13 NE per day

Men and Boys:

11 to 14 years	17 NE per day
15 to 18 years	20 NE per day
19 to 50 years	19 NE per day
51+ years	15 NE per day

Women and Girls:

11 to 50 years	15 NE per day
51+ years	13 NE per day

Pregnant Women:	17 NE per day
Nursing Mothers:	20 NE per day

*NE = niacin equivalent; 1 niacin equivalent = 1 milligram niacin or 60 milligrams of dietary tryptophan.

Niacinamide: An easily tolerated form of NIACIN available in various strengths as a supplement. It is also known as **nicotinamide.**

Nibbling: It's not necessarily bad, although mothers are forever telling their children, "Don't nibble! You'll spoil your appetite!" If the nibble is candy, cake, cookies or fat-laden chips, perhaps. But if it's an apple or orange, a carrot or celery stick, a handful of raisins or a couple of dried prunes or apricots, the snack is a good way to round out the day's nutritive requirements. Also, people with ulcers, hiatal hernias or other digestive problems are frequently told to graze—that is, to eat lightly throughout the day instead of settling for three heavier meals, which can tax the gastrointestinal tract.

Nickel: One of the minerals the body needs in minute quantities to produce some of the enzymes required for efficient metabolism. Nickel interacts with more than a dozen other minerals in the body and too little of it can stunt growth and curtail blood formation and upset the balance of iron, copper and zinc in the liver. Good sources of nickel are dried peas and beans, whole grains, nuts and—hooray!—chocolate. As with other heavy metals, nickel can be toxic (too much of it damages all vital organs—brain, heart, kidneys, liver and lungs). But nickel buildup is more apt to come from industrial fallout (chemical pollutants) than from eating. See HEAVY-METAL TOXICITY.

Nicotine: A toxic, addictive alkaloid found in tobacco. See CIGARETTE SMOKING.

Nicotinic Acid: A form of NIACIN that can cause problems when taken in large doses.

NIDDM: Non-insulin-dependent diabetes mellitus. For details, see DIABETES.

Night Blindness, Nyctalopia: The inability to see in the dark, especially when stepping abruptly from light to dark. A deficiency of vitamin A may be responsible; if so, more carrots—or other vitamin A-rich foods—may be all that's needed to reverse the condition. If the problem persists, see an ophthalmologist to determine if there's retinal disease. See also A, VITAMIN.

Nisin: A natural preservative now being tested by the USDA's Agricultural Research Service. Studies show that when mixed with citric and/or lactic acid, nisin inhibits growth of *Escherichia coli* and *Salmonella typhimurium,* the villains in several recent, serious outbreaks of food poisoning.

Nitrates, Nitrites: There's been much hue and hysteria about the use of sodium nitrite in bacon, ham, hot dogs and other cured meats; also the use of sodium nitrite and other nitrates, which the body converts to nitrites. These then bond with amines, an intermediary of protein digestion, forming NITROSAMINES, which are both toxic and carcinogenic. Since 1978, the USDA has been monitoring bacon for nitrosamine content and batches exceeding 10 parts per billion are pulled off the market. Reacting to consumer fears, food processors are using less sodium nitrite and fewer nitrates in curing meats and pumping up the ascorbate (an antioxidant and form of vitamin C), the vitamin E (another antioxidant) and the lecithin. So far, so good.

Despite all the controversy about nitrates and nitrites, the truth is that botulism (a deadly form of food poisoning) caused by improperly processed or preserved foods poses a greater health risk. In fact, cured meats are just one source of potential nitrosamines. Beets, cabbage, carrots, cauliflower, celery, lettuce, radishes and spinach also contribute their share of nitrates. Well water is another major source, as is human saliva. So in the process of digestion these, too, can end up as nitrosamines.

Still, cases of nitrate poisoning are rare. It's seen mostly in infants whose intestinal tracts don't yet contain the acid-producing bacteria necessary to thwart nitrite formation. The condition—METHEMOGLOBINEMIA—means newborns don't get enough oxygen and become "blue babies."

Tobacco smoke is a far greater source of nitrosamines than cured meats (just a pack of cigarettes a week adds 14 to 18 parts per million) and these, mind you, are *preformed* nitrosamines. So are those in beer, cheese, dried spices, dehydrated milk and fish, instant coffees and soups. Cosmetics also contain preformed nitrosamines, as do rubber baby-bottle nipples, pacifiers and the rubberized netting used to package hams. So cured meats aren't the "killers" they've been accused of being. They are part of the ongoing nitrosamine drama, true. And they should be minimized wherever possible. But compared to the major players, they're only extras.

Nitrogen: An element in the air and soil that is essential to all life. Plants can use the nitrogen in the air, but animals—and that includes us—must get their supply from food. They depend upon it to build and maintain protein tissue.

Nitrogen Balance: The equilibrium reached when the nitrogen consumed equals the amount excreted (via perspiration, urine and stools). If the intake is greater than the outgo, a person is said to be in **positive nitrogen balance** (this may occur during spurts of growth, pregnancy or nursing when extra protein—read nitrogen—is used for milk). In **negative nitrogen balance,** nitrogen outgo exceeds intake. Fasting trips the nitrogen balance into the negative column, as do high fever, surgery, burn or accident trauma.

Nitrosamines: Toxic, carcinogenic compounds that exist—preformed and full fledged—in tobacco smoke, beer, cheese and instant soups and coffees. The body also has the ability to manufacture nitrosamines. During digestion it converts nitrates (present in many vegetables and to a lesser degree in cured meats) to nitrites, which in turn bond with amines, forming nitrosamines. See also NITRATES, NITRITES.

Nitrous Oxide: This propellant/whipping agent used in squirt cans of nondairy whipped toppings is also known as **laughing gas.** GRAS.

NLEA (Nutrition Labeling and Education Act of 1990): This law finally went into effect in May 1994. It mandates far more detailed ingredient/nutrition labels for most foods sold in the United States. See also FOOD LABELING.

Nondairy Creamers: The chemical composition of these powders varies from brand to brand, but many contain highly saturated coconut oil. Alginates (seaweed ex-

NUTRIENT CONTENT OF 1 TEASPOON NONDAIRY CREAMER	
(about 1/14 ounce; 2 grams)	
11 calories	4 mg sodium
0 g protein	16 mg potassium
1 g fat, 1 saturated	0 g dietary fiber
0 mg cholesterol	0 RE vitamin A
1 g carbohydrate	0 mg thiamin
0 mg calcium	0 mg riboflavin
8 mg phosphorus	0 mg niacin
0 mg iron	0 mg vitamin C

tracts) are often added to make them creamy, sugar and natural or artificial flavorings to improve their taste, and synthetic colors to ape the appearance of the real thing. Nondairy creamers, despite their name, may also contain skim-milk solids. Read labels carefully and choose creamers containing unsaturated fats.

Nondairy Whipped Topping:
Like nondairy creamers, these are frequently formulated of highly saturated tropical oils—usually coconut and/or palm. They are pumped full of stabilizers and emulsifiers, artificial colors and flavors; in other words, they're an alphabet of additives. Some are whipped and frozen; others put into aerosol cans under pressure. Most provide very little other than calories and saturated fat. Scrutinize labels.

NUTRIENT CONTENT OF 1 TABLESPOON FROZEN NONDAIRY WHIPPED TOPPING

(about ¹/₇ ounce; 4 grams)

15 calories	1 mg sodium
0 g protein	1 mg potassium
1 g fat, 1 saturated	0 g dietary fiber
0 mg cholesterol	4 RE vitamin A
1 g carbohydrate	0 mg thiamin
0.5 mg calcium	0 mg riboflavin
0.5 mg phosphorus	0 mg niacin
0 mg iron	0 mg vitamin C

Nonessential Amino Acids:
They're called nonessential (also dispensable) because the body can synthesize as much of them as it needs. There are ten nonessential amino acids in all—alanine, ARGININE, asparagine, aspartic acid, GLUTAMIC ACID, GLUTAMINE, glycine, proline, serine and TAURINE. See also AMINO ACIDS.

Nonheme Iron:
The form of iron that occurs in plants. Nonheme iron is less easily and efficiently absorbed by the body than heme iron (that from animal sources), yet it supplies 85 percent of the iron in our diets. Some researchers believe that drinking tea with meals makes nonheme iron even less available to the body although between-meals cups or glasses of tea seem to have no effect.

Nonnutritive Sweeteners:
See ARTIFICIAL SWEETENERS.

Nonreactive Pans:
Recipes often call for cooking something—usually something acidic like tomatoes or pickles—in a nonreactive pan; in other words, one that won't react with the ingredients put into it and affect the color, flavor or texture of the finished dish. Such pans are made out of flameproof glass or one of the new inert space age materials, or they may be clad with porcelain.

Nonstick Pans:
Pans coated with heat-resistant compounds (often plastics like Teflon and Silverstone) that make it possible to use less cooking fat. An ongoing worry about such pans—despite repeated FDA assurances that nonstick coatings are inert and therefore safe—is that they may break down under intense heat and, over time, emit noxious (possibly carcinogenic) fumes that can migrate into food. Government scientists further claim that any flaking bits of nonstick coating, if accidentally eaten, are harmless because they pass through the body unchanged. Still, nervous Nellies choose to replace their blackened, scuffed, chipped nonstick pans with the new generation of nonsticks. Many of these are clad with something called Excalibur, a slick stainless-steel alloy that's fused to the pan. The toughest new nonsticks can take searing stove-top heat and oven temperatures as high as 425°F.

Nonstick Vegetable Cooking Sprays:
A dandy way to cut down on fat. To quote from the ingredient list of one popular brand, "All natural ingredients: canola oil, grain alcohol from corn (added for clarity), lecithin from soybeans (prevents sticking), and propellant." Some sprays are now butter flavored, some olive oil flavored, and all average about 2 calories, 0 cholesterol and negligible fat per average squirt. Nonstick cooking sprays can be used in skillets to reduce (even eliminate) fats for sautéing and stir-frying (for safety's sake, always apply to cold pans); they can be used to coat cake tins and cookie sheets; indeed, the flavored varieties can be sprayed directly on steamed vegetables or sliced bread.

Nonyl Alcohol (additive):
An artificial citrus flavoring used in candies, baked goods, ices, ice creams and soft drinks. Because it has caused nerve and liver damage in lab animals, further study is due.

Noodles:
See EGG NOODLES.

Nopales: See CACTUS PADS.

"No Preservatives": This may be a minus, not a plus. For example, preservatives thwart the growth of bacteria and molds that cause food poisoning. They also improve the quality and prolong the shelf life of a wide variety of food. "No preservatives," by the way, is not synonymous with "no additives." In fact, a "preservative-free food" may be riddled with synthetic colors, flavors, stabilizers and emulsifiers. Study a label's fine print.

Norepinephrine: A hormone produced in the brain that constricts blood vessels and raises blood pressure. Although related to EPINEPHRINE (adrenaline), norepinephrine doesn't speed up carbohydrate metabolism in the body.

Norwalk-Type Viruses: See VIRUSES.

"No Sugar Added," "No Added Sugar," "Without Added Sugar": Not only has no sugar been added at any point during processing or packaging but neither have any sugar-containing ingredients (fruit juices or sauces, dried fruits, etc.). Further, processing has not raised the sugar content of the food above the amounts normally present. Finally, the standard version of the same food (the food it replaces) usually has had sugar added. This revised definition, set forth by the new food-labeling laws, is far stricter than the old one, which merely meant that no refined sweeteners had been used.

"Nothing Artificial Added": Just what it says—the food so marked contains no synthetic colors, flavors, preservatives, stabilizers, emulsifiers, conditioners or other artificial additives. And that includes salt and sugar substitutes.

Nouvelle Cuisine: French for "new cooking." This movement, launched in the 1960s and 1970s by such French chefs as Paul Bocuse, the Troisgrois brothers and Roger Vergé, broke the strictures of classical haute cuisine. Specifically, it meant simpler recipes and menus, market-fresh food, rediscovery of regional specialties, an awareness of nutrition and a shunning, in general, of cream- and butter-laden sauces. *Nouvelle cuisine,* a phrase coined by French restaurant reviewers Henri Gault and Christian Millau, is not synonymous with *cuisine minceur,* the pared-down, low-fat, low-cal cooking of French chef Michel Guérard.

Nucleic Acids: The "mainframes" of DNA (deoxyribonucleic acid) and RNA (ribonucleic acid). Nucleic acids are highly complex, the core of nucleoproteins, the stuff of life, the holders and transmitters of genetic codes.

Nursing: See BREAST FEEDING.

Nursing Bottle Syndrome, Baby Bottle Syndrome (BBS): Buck teeth, misaligned jaw and extensive tooth decay caused by putting babies to bed with bottles of milk. The sucking action pushes the upper teeth out, the bottom teeth in, and misshapes the jaw. Moreover, milk sugars bathe the teeth, accelerating tooth decay. Doctors and dentists both urge mothers to put babies to bed without bottles and, if they can't fall asleep without them, at least to fill the bottles with water instead of milk or sugary fruit juice. They also recommend giving babies water after each feeding to rinse away residual sugars.

Nutmeg: The aromatic seed of tropical peachlike fruits that thrive in the East and West Indies (much of our supply comes from the island of Grenada). The reason for including nutmeg in a nutrition book is that it contains myristicin, a powerful hallucinogen. In the "turn-on, tune-out" 1960s, "nutmeg cocktails" (nothing more than nutmeg and water) were popular among teens who couldn't lay their hands on anything stronger. The amounts of nutmeg used in cooking are too small to send anyone to psychedelia.

Nutraceuticals: Foods or food components with the power to bolster health by preventing and/or helping to cure disease. Coined by Dr. Steven De Felice of the Foundation for Innovation in Medicine in Cranford, New Jersey, the term has been snapped up by nutritionists and writers and is finding its way into mainstream media. See also FUNCTIONAL FOODS; PHYTOCHEMICALS.

NutraSweet, Equal: Brand names for ASPARTAME, an artificial sweetener synthesized out of two amino acids—aspartic acid and phenylalanine. Like protein, aspartame weighs in at 4 calories per gram, but it is 200 times sweeter than sugar. Before it was granted FDA approval in 1981, aspartame underwent thirteen years of intensive testing. Still, it remains controversial. Some people insist that aspartame makes them dizzy or gives them headaches, and for those with PHENYLKETONURIA (PKU), it can be dangerous. Such people lack the enzyme needed to digest phenylalanine, so toxic levels of this amino acid can build up in the body, causing neurological damage. As a result, "contains phenylalanine" warnings must appear on all foods containing aspartame. Today aspartame is used in scores of processed foods and beverages, and most nutritionists and physicians agree that it poses no problems for healthy people who use it within moderation. Aspartame is also available in tablet form, in individual packets and more recently in crystals, which home cooks can measure out like sugar. Of course, aspartame can't be substituted for sugar in recipes, especially baked goods, because its physical and chemical properties are entirely different. Always use recipes developed specifically for aspartame.

Nutrient: A chemical or chemical compound, usually taken as food, that not only nourishes the body but also is essential to life. See also NUTRIENT CLASSIFICATION.

Nutrient Classification: To simplify and organize an unwieldy subject, nutritionists divide nutrients into the Basic Six—CARBOHYDRATES, FAT, MINERALS, PROTEIN, VITAMINS and WATER. Nutrients may be **inorganic** (minerals, water) or **organic** (everything else). Their functions vary. Carbohydrates, proteins and fats all provide energy; proteins, water, minerals and vitamins not only build and maintain body tissues but also regulate a variety of life processes (digestion, metabolism, respiration, etc.).

Nutrient Density: The ratio of essential nutrients (proteins, minerals, vitamins) in food to their energy value (calories). See INDEX OF NUTRIENT QUALITY.

Nutrition: The study of food and its role in nourishing the body and fostering good health. Too simplistic a definition, perhaps, because behavioral patterns, psychological states, even soil, climate and agricultural conditions all belong to the Big Picture. Nutrition is a highly specialized, constantly, rapidly, evolving science that requires years of training plus years of practical or clinical experience. See also NUTRITION ASSESSMENT; NUTRITIONIST; etc.

Nutritional Deficiency: The lack—either chronic or acute—of one or more essential nutrients in the body. Poverty may be the cause of it. But often nutritional deficiencies are the result of bad eating habits. Of junking out on chips and candy, for example, and of loading up on burgers, shakes and fries instead of following the FOOD GUIDE PYRAMID and eating a wide variety of food each day with the emphasis on whole grains, fruits and vegetables. Then, too, psychological disorders may underlie nutritional deficiencies (anorexia and bulimia, to name two). Or physical problems may be responsible—diabetes, over- or underactive thyroid, kidney or liver disease, alcoholism. Finally, MEDICATIONS often alter the way the body absorbs nutrients and, in some instances, blocks it altogether. Always ask your doctor about potential interactions. See also MALNUTRITION.

Nutritional Supplements, Supplemental Nutrition: We are not talking about vitamin pills here but about the nutrient-packed powder or liquid formulas now available as instant breakfasts or between-meals snacks (Ensure is one highly advertised, widely available brand). Originally formulated to supplement the diets of hospital patients unable to eat enough food to meet their daily nutritional requirements, these supplements—or more appetizing versions of them—have now landed on supermarket shelves. In a variety of flavors. Most nutritional supplements are milk- or skim-milk-based, high-protein formulas fortified with vitamins and minerals. Read labels carefully, paying particular attention to the fat and calorie contents, which vary from brand to brand.

Nutrition Assessment: Properly done, this is a four-step process conducted by a clinical nutritionist (often an M.D.) and/or a registered dietitian (R.D.). First, family diet and medical histories are taken; second, height, weight and circumferences of arms and legs are noted; third is a physical exam with special attention being paid to signs of malnutrition (hair loss, skin rashes, diarrhea, etc.); and fourth, blood and urine analyses are rated against the norm.

Nutritionist: A person with one or more degrees in nutrition (B.S., M.S., Ph.D.) from an accredited college or university. He or she will have spent many hours studying chemistry (inorganic, organic, biochemistry), microbiology, physiology, dietetics, nutrition, food technology and public health, together with such behavioral sciences as anthropology, psychology and sociology. In addition, the nutritionist may have studied anatomy, preventive medicine and pediatrics. Many nutritionists devote their lives to hard-core science, particularly research, to teaching, to communications and to developing more healthful food products. Unfortunately, there are many self-styled nutritionists who have bought degrees from diploma mills. These quacks are more likely to be found in health-food stores or companies manufacturing supplements of questionable value than in reputable universities, hospitals, government agencies or *Fortune* 500 corporations.

Nutrition Labeling and Education Act of 1990: See NLEA; also FOOD LABELING.

Nuts: The meaty, edible inner kernels of dried fruits, which are encased in woody or papery shells. With the exception of chestnuts, all nuts are high in fat, sometimes saturated fat. Let's clear up one misconception: Dry-roasted nuts are not significantly lower in fat than oil-roasted ones. For two reasons. First, oil-roasted nuts are whisked in and out of the oil so fast they absorb very little of it. Second, all the excess oil is drained away after the roasting. See entries for the most popular nuts—ALMONDS; CASHEWS; CHESTNUTS; HAZELNUTS; MACADAMIA NUTS; PECANS; PINE NUTS; PISTACHIO NUTS; WALNUTS. See also PEANUTS, although they are legumes, not nuts.

Nyctalopia: See NIGHT BLINDNESS.

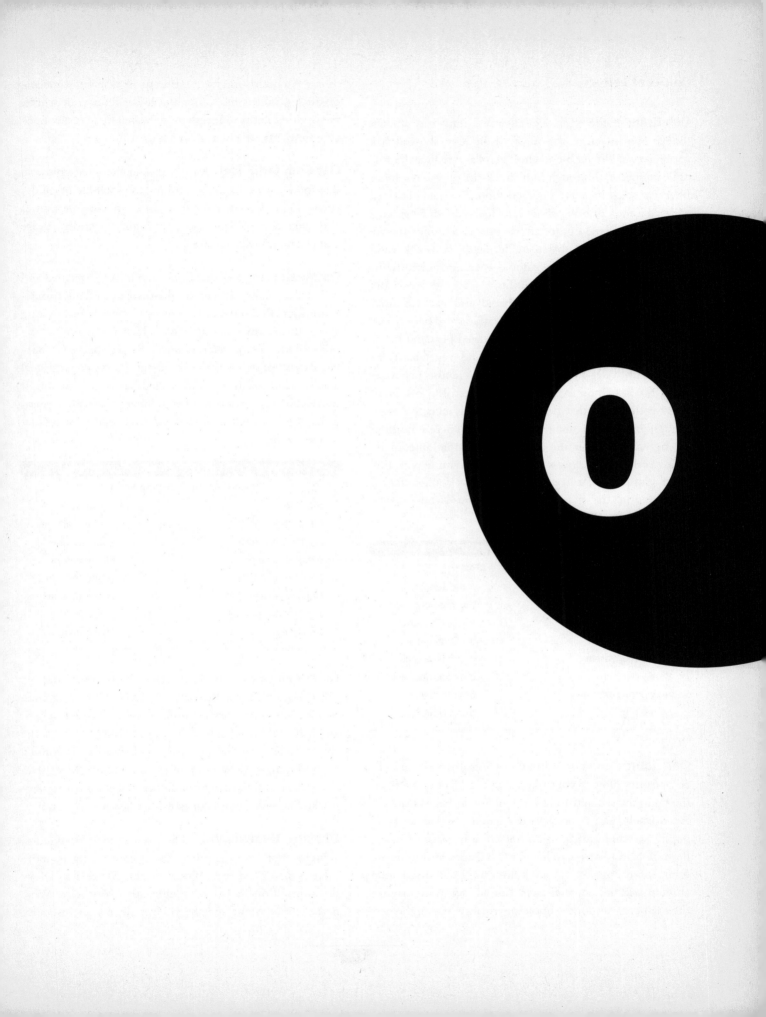

Oak Leaf Lettuce: See SALAD GREENS.

Oat Bran: A few years ago after two university studies (one at Northwestern, the other at Kentucky) showed that oat bran could lower blood cholesterol and reduce the risk of heart disease, this rough stuff chock-full of water-soluble fiber was being hailed as a miracle food. Two ounces a day were all it took to bring cholesterol levels down 5 percent, researchers pointed out (of course they also limited the fat and cholesterol their subjects ate during the six-week studies). Millers rushed to salvage floor sweepings, purify them, package them and ring up profits. And food processors began adding oat bran to cereals, breads and snacks to catch the wave of fanaticism. But the operative word here is *bran* (read dietary fiber), not *oat*. Apples, dried peas and beans (not to mention many other fruits and vegetables) are loaded with water-soluble fiber, which scientists believe is every bit as helpful in lowering cholesterol as oat bran. Now it turns out that rice bran is equally effective even though its fiber is not water soluble. There's nothing wrong with oat bran, mind you. It is a wholesome, high-fi, low-cal, low-fat, low-sodium food brimming with thiamin, phosphorus, iron and potassium. Just don't count on it to mop up the excess fat and cholesterol you eat. See also FIBER, DIETARY.

NUTRIENT CONTENT OF 1 CUP COOKED OAT BRAN	
(about 7³/₄ ounces; 219 grams)	
88 calories	2 mg sodium
7 g protein	201 mg potassium
2 g fat, 0 saturated	7 g dietary fiber
0 mg cholesterol	0 RE vitamin A
25 g carbohydrate	0.35 mg thiamin
22 mg calcium	0.07 mg riboflavin
261 mg phosphorus	0.3 mg niacin
1.9 mg iron	0 mg vitamin C

Oat Flour: Oats milled until fine and feathery; it varies in color from yellow to tan to faintly green. The more refined the flour, the less nutritious it is—unless it's been enriched. Read labels. Oat flour lacks the gluten needed to make good cakes and breads, so do not use it in place of wheat flour. In a bread recipe calling for 6 or 7 cups of all-purpose flour, substituting 1 cup of oat flour for 1 cup of the total amount will not court disaster. But adding more may tip the balance. Oat flour is not a supermarket staple; the best source is a health-food store. Because it contains some antioxidants, millers often mix a little oat flour with wheat, rye or other flours to lengthen their shelf life. **NOTE:** Specific nutrients are not available for oat flour.

Oat Gum (additive): An antioxidant extracted from oats that food processors use to prolong the shelf life of candy, cream and butter. Its thickening and stabilizing properties also make it valuable in the manufacture of cream cheese and cheese spreads. GRAS.

Oatmeal: Oat grains that have been husked, steamed and rolled flat. There are both **old-fashioned** and **quick-cooking rolled oats,** introduced, believe it or not, as long ago as 1921. **Instant oatmeal,** which needs only to be mixed with boiling water, is newer. **Scotch** and **Irish oatmeals** are not steamed and rolled but sliced thin with steel blades. They are firmer than rolled oats and taste almost nutty. The reason oatmeal keeps longer than other grains is that the heat used to process it destroys the enzymes that hasten staling.

NUTRIENT CONTENT OF 1 CUP COOKED OATMEAL	
(about 8¹/₂ ounces; 234 grams)	
145 calories	2 mg sodium
6 g protein	131 mg potassium
2 g fat, 0 saturated	5 g dietary fiber
0 mg cholesterol	5 RE vitamin A
25 g carbohydrate	0.26 mg thiamin
19 mg calcium	0.05 mg riboflavin
177 mg phosphorus	0.3 mg niacin
1.6 mg iron	0 mg vitamin C

Oats: One of the world's most nutritious grains and the one that grows better than any other in cold, wet climates. A third of the land farmed in Scotland is devoted to oats, and half of it in Ireland. Even so, the United States is the world's major producer of oats, with most of it coming from Illinois, Iowa, Wisconsin and Minnesota. More than 90 percent of the oats grown in the States are fed to livestock. The rest go into oat flour, oatmeal and oat gum.

Obesity, Overweight: The two are not synonymous, although both are caused by the body's taking in more calories than it expends. If overweight, you're a bit above the norm; if obese, you're significantly overweight. What *is* the norm? Some use the Metropolitan Life Insurance

Company height/weight tables as the standard for ideal body weight (IBW). But most professionals (nutritionists, dietitians and physicians) prefer the Quetelet Index, better known as the BODY MASS INDEX (BMI)—the body's weight (in kilos) divided by the square of its height (in meters). The ideal for men and women is a BMI of 20 to 25. A BMI between 25 and 30 is considered **overweight;** 30 to 34, **obese;** 35 to 44, **medically significantly obese;** 45 to 49, **morbidly obese;** and 50 or more, **super obese.** Again, these figures are for men *and* women.

What keeps one person forever thin, another forever fat? Researchers continue to puzzle it out. This much can be said: It isn't merely a matter of overeating; indeed, some "skinnies" scarf down gobs of food while "fatties" peck about like birds. Heredity, as studies with identical twins adopted by different families suggest, does predispose one to being fat or thin—67 percent of the time, according to one Danish study. Your genetic code may have programmed your neural and hormonal activity, determined the number and size of your fat cells, your general physique and, yes, your basal metabolic rate. Indeed, researchers at Rockefeller University recently discovered a "flawed" gene that upsets both the body's metabolism and its appetite control center. In other words, the brain doesn't get the message to tell the body to stop eating. But subsequent research at Jefferson Medical College in Philadelphia questions the "flawed" gene theory.

Some people nibble rich food while couching out in front of the TV. Diets can take unwanted pounds off, but keeping them off means eating a variety of low-fat foods with the emphasis on whole grains, fruits and vegetables, then backing up that regimen with a sensible one of exercise. There's another consideration, too. People tend to gravitate toward a given weight or SET POINT. According to Rockefeller University scientists, once you lose weight your body burns calories more slowly—sometimes 10 to 15 percent more slowly—so that you will return to your given weight. The reverse is true when you gain weight.

The rewards of desirable body weight are many and self-esteem is only one of them. Adults with a BMI below 30 are less likely to suffer from hypertension, coronary artery disease, certain types of cancer and non-insulin-dependent diabetes. See also LEPTIN.

Ob-Gene: The "fat" gene isolated at the end of 1994 by Dr. Jeffrey Friedman, a molecular geneticist at the Howard Hughes Medical Institute at Rockefeller University in New York City. Subsequent research by Friedman and his associates identified a hormone that the ob-gene produces. LEPTIN it's called, after *leptos,* the Greek word for *thin.* Leptin, the Rockefeller team suspects, may determine whether one is fat or thin or of normal weight. Although it isn't yet known exactly how this happens, a current theory is that the obese have a sluggish or inactive ob-gene. Result: The appetite centers (hypothalmus) in their brains never get the message to stop eating. See also LEPTIN.

Ocean Perch: Not a perch at all but a variety of redfish that swims the upper reaches of the North Atlantic. Small, white fleshed and lean, ocean perch is an important food fish both in America and abroad. In many parts of the United States, it is more available frozen than fresh. True perch, by the way, are primarily freshwater fish. For approximate nutrient counts, see FISH, LEAN WHITE.

Octopus: Never popular in the United States except in ethnic communities (Greek, Italian, Asian, Portuguese), the octopus, when properly prepared, is as delicate and tender as chicken. Although it sometimes grows to awesome size, the best-eating ones average 3 pounds apiece and have already been cleaned and dressed by the time they come to market. Like squid, the octopus is a cephalopod, a shellfish that carries its shell inside. You know it as cuttle, those slim white bones hung inside bird cages. As for food value, octopus is low in calories and fat but is a superior source of phosphorus, iron, potassium and niacin. Unfortunately, there are hefty shots of sodium and cholesterol, too.

NUTRIENT CONTENT OF 3 OUNCES (85 GRAMS) STEAMED/BOILED OCTOPUS	
139 calories	391 mg sodium
25 g protein	536 mg potassium
2 g fat, 0 saturated	0 g dietary fiber
82 mg cholesterol	69 RE vitamin A
4 g carbohydrate	0.05 mg thiamin
90 mg calcium	0.07 mg riboflavin
237 mg phosphorus	3.2 mg niacin
8.1 mg iron	7 mg vitamin C

Octyl Alcohol (additive): A component of a variety of artificial food flavors. Considered nontoxic.

Octyl Butyrate (additive): A versatile synthetic flavoring used to ape the taste of everything from butter to berries to lemons to melons. Food processors use it in baked goods, beverages, ice creams and candies. Considered nontoxic.

Octyl Formate, Octyl Heptanoate, Octyl Isobutyrate, Octyl Isovalerate, Octyl Octanoate, Octyl Phenylacetate, Octyl Propionate (additives): These octyls are all artificial fruit flavorings widely used by the food industry. All are considered nontoxic.

Offal: See VARIETY MEATS.

Oils: Liquid fats, usually of plant origin (a notable exception is cod-liver oil). Salad and cooking oils don't exist freely in nature and must be extracted from seeds, fruits and nuts. The reason they're liquid is that they are largely unsaturated; pumping hydrogen into oils to give them the consistency of butter or shortening not only saturates them but also produces unhealthy TRANS FATTY ACIDS. The **saturated** fats and oils (those containing hydrogen-rich myristic, palmitic and stearic acids) have been nailed as villains in coronary heart disease because they raise blood levels of cholesterol. In fact, most researchers now believe they do more harm than the cholesterol in food itself (vegetable fats and oils, make a note, never contain cholesterol).

So the race is on to find cooking oils full of **unsaturated fatty acids,** both the **polyunsaturated** (two of these—LINOLEIC ACID and LINOLENIC ACID—are so crucial to the body they're classified as essential fatty acids) and the **monounsaturated** (OLEIC ACID and palmitoleic acid being the most important). The emphasis today is on oils with the highest percentage of monounsaturates because these are thought to lower the amount of "bad" cholesterol (LDL) in the blood and raise the "good" (HDL). There is also some niggling concern that polyunsaturates may increase the risk of certain types of cancer although nothing has been proved.

Once limited to colorless blends (plus peanut and olive oil), cooks now face an arsenal of oils: CORN OIL, COTTONSEED OIL, OLIVE OIL, PEANUT OIL, RAPESEED OIL (CANOLA OIL), SAFFLOWER OIL, SOYBEAN OIL and SUNFLOWER-SEED OIL, not to mention such flavorful boutique oils as AVOCADO OIL, GRAPE-SEED OIL, HAZELNUT OIL, SESAME OIL both light and dark, WALNUT OIL and now even macadamia oil. Beware of tropical oils, especially CO-CONUT OIL and PALM OIL, the most saturated plant oils of all. Though not often sold by the bottle, they show up in hundreds of processed foods. And movie-theater popcorn drips with the stuff (one large bag, someone recently calculated, contains as much saturated fat as six Big Macs. And that's without the extra butter).

The dietary fat comparison charts the saturated/unsaturated fat ratios of the most widely used cooking oils, together with those of butter, lard, margarine and vegetable shortening. It also shows the cholesterol content of the animal fats. For additional information, see FAT; also the individual oils.

Oils, Flavored: If you're thinking about making basil oil, or chile oil, or lemon oil, or rosemary oil, better think twice. Herbs, dried chiles, peppercorns, garlic, shallots, indeed nearly every food, herb and spice may contain botulism spores, which can germinate in the airless environment of oils, producing toxins that can kill (see CLOSTRIDIUM BOTULINUM under BACTERIA). If you insist on making flavored oils, then play it safe. The *Gourmet* magazine test kitchen recently devised this method: Place ½ cup oil (plus garlic, herb or citrus zest) in a flameproof glass measuring cup, set in a shallow pan, insert a candy or deep-fat thermometer, and heat, uncovered, in a 300°F. oven until the oil reaches 250°F., then keep it at that temperature for 20 minutes. Strain the hot oil into a sterilized half-pint preserving jar, cover loosely with plastic food wrap, and store in the refrigerator. The flavored oil will keep for about a month—but it's unlikely it will last that long.

Okra: These mucilagenous, finger-shaped pods won't win any popularity contests. Yet the Africans who brought okra to the Deep South knew that this "glue" would thicken soups and also impart subtle flavor (it's part asparagus, part eggplant). Creoles and Cajuns, taking a tip from plantation slaves, loaded their gumbos with *ngombo,* the Angolan word for okra (and clearly the origin of the word *gumbo*). The youngest, tenderest pods can be sliced, dusted with cornmeal and bounced in and out of a hissing-hot skillet filmed with lard or bacon drippings—to this day a Southern favorite. Some people even like the sliminess of boiled or steamed okra. Over-the-hill okra is woody; indeed, its fibers are used to make paper. Once upon a time canned okra was available (not fit for much except gumbo). Today frozen okra (both whole and sliced) is stocked by many

COMPARISON OF DIETARY FATS

Legend:
- ■ Cholesterol mg/tbsp
- ■ Saturated Fat
- ■ Monounsaturated Fat
- ■ Polyunsaturated Fat
- □ Other Fats

Dietary Fat	Cholesterol mg/tbsp	Saturated Fat	Monounsaturated Fat	Polyunsaturated Fat	Other Fats
Canola oil (Puritan Oil)	0	6%	62%	31%	1%
Safflower oil	0	9%	12%	78%	1%
Sunflower oil	0	11%	20%	69%	
Corn oil	0	13%	25%	62%	
Peanut oil	0	13%	49%	33%	5%
Olive oil	0	14%	77%	9%	
Soybean oil	0	15%	24%	61%	
Margarine (fat)	0	18%	48%	29%	5%
Vegetable shortening (Crisco)	0	26%	43%	25%	6%
Cottonseed oil	0	27%	19%	54%	
Chicken fat	11	30%	47%	22%	1%
Lard	12	41%	47%	12%	
Animal fat shortening (Precreamed)	9	44%	48%	5%	3%
Beef fat	14	51%	44%	4%	1%
Palm oil	0	51%	39%	10%	
Butter (fat)	33	54%	30%	4%	12%
Coconut oil	0	77%	6%	2%	15%

The values shown for saturated and polyunsaturated fats are based on Federal Regulations, Title 21, Section 101.25 (c)(2)(ii)(a&b). These state that: (a) saturated fat is the sum of lauric, myristic, palmitic and stearic acids, and (b) polyunsaturated fat is cis, cis-methylene-interrupted polyunsaturated fatty acids. "Other Fats" include saturated and polyunsaturated fatty acids that are outside these definitions.

Provided as a Professional Service by Procter & Gamble ©1989 P&G

References:
Canola oil, animal fat (precreamed) shortening, vegetable shortening: data on file, Procter & Gamble.
Margarine: H.T. Slover et al. "Lipids in Margarines and Margarine-Like Foods," *Journal of the American Oil Chemists' Society,* vol. 62 (1985), 775–86.
All others: J.B. Reeves, and J.L. Weihrauch, *Composition of Food, Agriculture Handbook No. 84.* Washington, D.C.: United States Department of Agriculture, 1979.

supermarkets cross-country and by almost all of them down South. Still, fresh is best. As for food value, okra provides hefty doses of vitamin C and enough iron and calcium to matter. **SEASON:** Year-round, with supplies peaking in summer.

NUTRIENT CONTENT OF 1 CUP COOKED OKRA
(about 7³/₄ ounces; 219 grams)

68 calories	6 mg sodium
4 g protein	430 mg potassium
1 g fat, 0 saturated	5 g dietary fiber
0 mg cholesterol	94 RE vitamin A
15 g carbohydrate	0.18 mg thiamin
177 mg calcium	0.23 mg riboflavin
85 mg phosphorus	1.4 mg niacin
1.2 mg iron	22 mg vitamin C

Oleic Acid: A monounsaturated fatty acid present in canola, corn and, most of all, olive oil. High concentrations of it can lower blood levels of cholesterol. Oleic acid is also used by food processors to make synthetic butters and cheeses, and to flavor baked goods, candies, ice creams and soft drinks. GRAS.

Oleomargarine: See MARGARINE.

Oleoresin Turmeric (additive): A vivid yellow pigment extracted from turmeric root used primarily to color mustards, pickles and relishes. GRAS.

Olestra: A fat substitute created by Procter & Gamble, composed of sucrose (table sugar) and six to eight fatty acids. It's created a major buzz because it passes through the body unchanged, meaning *no calories*. Yet Olestra looks and cooks like real fat, tastes like it and has the same sensuous mouth feel. **OTHER PLUSES:** Tests show Olestra-fried potato chips produce significantly less heartburn (acid reflux) than deep-fat-fried chips. Olestra, moreover, blocks the absorption of dietary cholesterol as well as the reabsorption of that being recycled, so it is believed to lower blood cholesterol, too. The flip side is that Olestra also interferes with the absorption of vitamin E, a fat-soluble vitamin (although not, apparently, with A, D and K, also fat soluble). So far Olestra's tested "clean"—no evidence of its causing cancer or birth defects. Still, studies continue. If the FDA gives Olestra its blessing, the food industry will

use it for everything from french fries to high-calorie snacks to baked goods. However, Olestra will not replace 100 percent of the real fat in shortenings, etc. In those for home use, it will probably sub for about a third of the fat, and in those designed for the food industry for three fourths. Still, this will bring the per-gram calorie counts down to 6 and 2, respectively, as compared to 9 for the real thing. See also FAT SUBSTITUTES.

Oligosaccharides: Three to ten simple sugars (monosaccharides) bonded into a single molecule or complex sugar. The body can't digest the two oligosaccharides found in food—**raffinose** and **stachyose.** So intestinal bacteria go to work on them, producing lots of gas. Beans always get the rap for being "gassy" when in fact raw apples and onions and cooked cabbages win hands down. Even bananas up gas production by 50 percent, and apple juice and raisins double it. See also CARBOHYDRATES.

Olive Oil: Plato and Aristotle drizzled olive oil over their food. So did Christ and Julius Caesar. All lived in the Mediterranean basin and it's there, food historians believe, that olives originated. Some trace their beginnings to the Greek island of Crete because they were known there five thousand years ago. Small wonder olives, their leaves and twigs have worked their way into Greek myths and are so prominently mentioned in the Bible. It was an olive leaf a dove brought to Noah's Ark to announce the end of the Flood.

Today olive orchards tuft the slopes of Mediterranean Europe and the making of olive oil is big business in Greece, Italy, southern France, Spain and Portugal, although it's lapped by the Atlantic, not the Mediterranean. In most of those countries, the olives are cold pressed in stone mills although bigger operations have gone high-tech with hydraulic presses. The Portuguese, however, prefer gutsier oils ("rank" some call them). So they beat the olives out of the trees with sticks, then, instead of rushing them off to the crusher, leave them on the ground to ferment for a few days. Portuguese olives are also hot pressed, meaning the water used in the crushing is hot, and this, too, intensifies the flavor of the oil. A pitted ripe olive, by the way, is 20 to 30 percent oil—most of it monounsaturated (see OILS). The terms used to identify the different types of olive oil, codified by Italian law, generally apply to olive oils produced elsewhere. Here's a quick rundown:

Extra Virgin: The first pressing of top-quality ripe olives; the oil's acidity cannot exceed 1 percent.

Superfine Virgin: Top-quality, first-pressing oil with an acidity level between 1 and 1½ percent.

Fine Virgin: First-pressing oil with acidity up to 3 percent.

Simple Virgin: First-pressing oil with acidity between 3 and 4 percent.

Pure Olive Oil: Rougher oil or a blend of virgin and refined oils. **Refined** simply means that the oils have been filtered. It does not mean that they come from top-quality olives or a first pressing, either. They rarely do. Such olive oils are often called simply olive oil.

With the healthfulness of olive oils now so heavily hyped, some producers have developed **lights** and **extra-lights**—pale, bland oils with little olive taste. Ounce for ounce, these oils are no lower in fat or calories than thick, fruity oils. As a result, new FDA labeling rules ban the use of "light" and "extra light" on all oil labels lest shoppers think them less fattening. Some olive oil producers have already switched to **extra mild.** Their aim is to make extra-mild olive oils as much a kitchen staple as canola and corn oils. Connoisseurs prefer heavier, *fruitier* olive oils and rank those of Italy, especially Tuscany, at the very top. French olive oils are usually more delicate; those of Greece, Spain, Portugal, Tunisia and California, bolder. All are good multipurpose oils but should never be used for deep-frying; their smoke point is too low and their cost too high.

When it comes to nutritive value, olive oils offer nothing other than fat and calories: 1 tablespoon olive oil = 119 calories, 14 grams total fat (2 grams saturated). But make a note, olive oil contains no cholesterol and, because it's chock-full of monounsaturates, may actually lower blood cholesterol levels.

Olives: "Except the vine," wrote Pliny, "there is no plant which bears a fruit of as great importance as the olive." Its oil is the "butter" of millions throughout Mediterranean Africa, Asia and Europe, and the fruit itself is the key ingredient in thick spreads like *olivada* and *tapenade,* which have nourished peasants across the centuries, in olive breads, in *pissaladière* and *salade Niçoise.*

Which brings up the subject of olive varieties. The sharp, briny little black **Niçoise** olives, named for the Pro-vençal port of Nice where they're processed, are by most accounts the world's finest. Some prefer the cracked green **Provençal** (also French), some the fleshy yellow-green **Sicilian,** others the wrinkled jet-black oil-cured **Moroccan** and still others the purply **Greek Kalamatas** or firm, green **Spanish** giants. (With so many fine imports now available, we've graduated from the pimiento-stuffed that once garnished so many platters and tea sandwiches.)

The flavor differences in olives depend less on species than on climate, air, soil and cure. Thomas Jefferson, who did a hitch as America's minister to France, was so partial to Provençal olives he tried to grow them at Monticello, his Virginia country home. And when those slips died, he planted more in the Carolinas. These, too, failed. The Franciscans had better luck with Spanish varieties in California. To this day California is the only state where olives are grown on a large commercial scale. Many of them are cured in the town of Lindsay in huge vats through which air constantly bubbles (this oxygenation turns the olives as black as jet). Lindsay olives, as they're called, are sold by the can in nearly every deli, grocery and supermarket. For all their centuries of sustaining the poor, olives aren't very

NUTRIENT CONTENT OF 5 PITTED GREEN OLIVES
(about ¾ ounce; 20 grams)

23 calories	468 mg sodium
0 g protein	11 mg potassium
2 g fat, 0 saturated	0 g dietary fiber
0 mg cholesterol	6 RE vitamin A
0 g carbohydrate	0 mg thiamin
12 mg calcium	0 mg riboflavin
3 mg phosphorus	0 mg niacin
0.3 mg iron	0 mg vitamin C

NUTRIENT CONTENT OF 5 UNPITTED CANNED BLACK OLIVES
(about ⅞ ounce; 23 grams)

26 calories	146 mg sodium
0 g protein	2 mg potassium
2 g fat, 0 saturated	1 g dietary fiber
0 mg cholesterol	9 RE vitamin A
1 g carbohydrate	0 mg thiamin
20 mg calcium	0 mg riboflavin
1 mg phosphorus	0 mg niacin
0.7 mg iron	0 mg vitamin C

nutritious although they do supply some fat and smidgens of calcium, iron and potassium. Thanks to their brining, their major mineral, however, is sodium.

Omega-3 Fatty Acids: See FISH OILS.

Onion Flakes, Onion Powder, Onion Salt: These so-called instant onions are poor substitutes for the real thing because their ersatz flavor overpowers almost everything else. Onion salt, needless to add, is loaded with sodium.

Onions: What a big, beautiful family the onion family is. There are slim peppery **spring onions** and **scallions,** fawn-colored mild **Spanish** giants and delicate miniatures called **shallots,** sugary, big white-skinned **Bermudas,** pungent purple **Italian** onions, versatile **all-purpose yellows,** biting little **silverskins** that can be popped whole into stews, sharp **pearl** or **"martini" onions,** wispy green **chives,** and the sweetly succulent **Vidalias** and **Walla-Wallas** from Georgia and Washington, respectively. Finally, there are LEEKS and GARLIC, discussed individually.

All onions belong to the lily family, a species so ancient

NUTRIENT CONTENT OF ½ CUP CHOPPED RAW YELLOW ONIONS	
(about 3 ounces; 80 grams)	
30 calories	2 mg sodium
1 g protein	126 mg potassium
0 g fat, 0 saturated	1 g dietary fiber
0 mg cholesterol	0 RE vitamin A
7 g carbohydrate	0.03 mg thiamin
16 mg calcium	0.02 mg riboflavin
26 mg phosphorus	0.1 mg niacin
0.2 mg iron	5 mg vitamin C

NUTRIENT CONTENT OF 1 CUP BOILED SILVERSKIN ONIONS	
(about 7½ ounces; 210 grams)	
92 calories	6 mg sodium
3 g protein	348 mg potassium
0 g fat, 0 saturated	2 g dietary fiber
0 mg cholesterol	0 RE vitamin A
21 g carbohydrate	0.09 mg thiamin
46 mg calcium	0.05 mg riboflavin
74 mg phosphorus	0.3 mg niacin
0.5 mg iron	11 mg vitamin C

no one knows where it originated. Apparently man has always had onions; indeed, food historians believe that prehistoric clans were growing them in the Fertile Crescent long before the age of agriculture. Alexander the Great fed onions to his troops to increase their valor, and during the American Civil War, Ulysses S. Grant notified the War Department, "I will not move my army without onions." He got them.

This belief in the power of onions no doubt had to do with their intense sulfurous smell, their ability, as Benjamin Franklin once said, "to make even heirs and widows weep." We now know that onions supply a moderate amount of vitamin C (not to mention a surfeit of potassium). The good news is that they are low in sodium and calories, fat and cholesterol free but contain two compounds—ALLICIN and SULFORAPHANE—that are thought to lower the risk of certain cancers. **SEASON:** Year-round.

Open Dating: The dating of perishable foods that's supposed to be an indicator of freshness and safety. Some states require open dating but the federal government doesn't (*yet*). Unfortunately, four different types of dating are used, leaving shoppers more confused than informed:

"Packed On": The date a food was canned, frozen or packaged. Not much help unless you know that after several months of cold storage frozen foods dry out, losing color, taste and texture. Most canned goods begin to lose quality after a year. Even those within the pack date may, if improperly canned, bulge or leak. Get rid of them at once, placing where neither animals nor humans can get at them. See also FOOD PRESERVATION.

"Sell By": The final day a food should be sold. Also called the **pull date** because it tells grocers when to pull a perishable off the shelf, this date is stamped on egg, milk and yogurt cartons; packages of cheese and other dairy products; cold cuts, fresh pastas and pasta sauces; fresh fruit juice containers; and also on some baked goods. Most items are safe to eat a week beyond the sell-by date.

"Best If Used By": The last day food will be top quality, although it is still safe to eat. The "best if used by" term applies mostly to cheese.

Expiration Date (EXP): The toss-out date. It's stamped on packets of yeast, cans of baby formula and sometimes milk cartons, too. Foods older than the expiration date have lost their effectiveness and/or wholesomeness. Don't use.

Optifast Diet: A very low-calorie, vitamin- and mineral-fortified, high-protein, twelve-week liquid diet aimed at those who are at least 50 pounds overweight. Optifast is administered under medical supervision by hospitals and clinics but on an outpatient basis. It isn't cheap—in the thousands for the full twenty-six-week program (the twelve-week liquid fast is followed by a fourteen-week introduction to good eating/exercise habits). Unfortunately, the dropout rate is 50 percent. For most of those who hang in, however, the average weight loss is 40 pounds. Pretty impressive. Still, as talk show diva Oprah Winfrey so visibly proved, not everyone keeps the weight off. When pounds are shed in a hurry, nutritionists and physicians point out, it's three times tougher to keep them off than when they're lost slowly. They also object to the "one-formula-fits-all" philosophy of liquid fasts because everyone metabolizes them differently. Some people, for example, will lose more lean muscle than fat and that's dangerous. It can stress the heart and throw thyroid function out of whack. For that reason, many doctors and nutritionists believe that patients on liquid fasts should be monitored on a day-to-day basis. See also LIQUID DIETS.

Optivite: An over-the-counter vitamin/mineral supplement developed to relieve the symptoms of premenstrual syndrome (PMS). The theory is that PMS sufferers lack iron, magnesium and zinc as well as many vitamins (A, C, E and most of the B-complex, especially B_6). Anyone swallowing six Optivites a day as prescribed, however, will seriously exceed established nutritional recommendations. Such megadosing is not only expensive but also risky. Especially when no reputable research has proved that any amount of any of these nutrients cures PMS. In fact, the results of one study, printed in the *American Journal of Clinical Nutrition*, showed no link between PMS and deficiencies of vitamins A, B_1, B_6 or E, or of the mineral zinc.

Oral Contraceptives (diet and): Combination estrogen/progestin pills affect the metabolism of fats, carbohydrates and tryptophan (an essential amino acid). They can also lower blood levels of five important vitamins (riboflavin, folic acid, B_6, B_{12}, C) and two minerals (magnesium and zinc), thus some doctors recommend multipurpose vi-

tamin/mineral supplements. The newer, more widely used low-estrogen oral contraceptives interfere far less with bodily nutrition, and the only vitamin deficits of concern appear to be two of the B-complex—folic acid and B_6 (pyridoxine). The preferred course of action? Broadening the diet to include adequate amounts of these nutrients. Higher-estrogen pills (called estrogen-containing oral contraceptives) raise blood levels of vitamin A (at least in lab animals). This may sound beneficial; what it actually means is that the body's supply of vitamin A is being depleted and that over time there may be a deficiency (see A, VITAMIN). Once again, chronically malnourished women are the ones potentially at greatest risk.

Oral Hypoglycemic Agents (OHA): The medications most commonly given to those who have non-insulin-dependent DIABETES. Taken by mouth, OHAs (and there are several on the market) lower blood sugar levels either by jump-starting the pancreas into releasing insulin or by braking glucose production in the liver. **PERIOD OF EFFECTIVENESS:** From six to seventy-two hours. Physicians usually prescribe OHAs to patients who can't bring their blood sugar levels down through diet and exercise.

Orange Juice, Orangeade: From every standpoint—appearance, taste, vitamin and mineral content—freshly squeezed is best. And the less the juice is strained, the better (the pulp is where the fiber is). For most nutrients, frozen juice has the edge over canned. Certainly, there's no contest when it comes to flavor. But even canned orange juice is preferable to orangeade, which is both sweetened and watered down. Still, orangeade is healthier for between-meals sipping than colas or other soft drinks.

NUTRIENT CONTENT OF 1 CUP FRESHLY SQUEEZED ORANGE JUICE	
(8 fluid ounces; 249 grams)	
111 calories	2 mg sodium
2 g protein	496 mg potassium
0 g fat, 0 saturated	1 g dietary fiber
0 mg cholesterol	50 RE vitamin A
26 g carbohydrate	0.22 mg thiamin
27 mg calcium	0.07 mg riboflavin
42 mg phosphorus	1.0 mg niacin
0.5 mg iron	124 mg vitamin C

NUTRIENT CONTENT OF 1 CUP RECONSTITUTED FROZEN ORANGE JUICE

(8 fluid ounces; 249 grams)

112 calories	2 mg sodium
2 g protein	473 mg potassium
0 g fat, 0 saturated	1 g dietary fiber
0 mg cholesterol	20 RE vitamin A
27 g carbohydrate	0.20 mg thiamin
22 mg calcium	0.05 mg riboflavin
40 mg phosphorus	0.5 mg niacin
0.2 mg iron	97 mg vitamin C

NUTRIENT CONTENT OF 1 CUP CANNED ORANGE JUICE

(8 fluid ounces; 249 grams)

104 calories	5 mg sodium
1 g protein	436 mg potassium
0 g fat, 0 saturated	1 g dietary fiber
0 mg cholesterol	45 RE vitamin A
25 g carbohydrate	0.15 mg thiamin
20 mg calcium	0.07 mg riboflavin
35 mg phosphorus	0.8 mg niacin
1.1 mg iron	86 mg vitamin C

NUTRIENT CONTENT OF 1 CUP ORANGEADE

(8 fluid ounces; 249 grams)

127 calories	40 mg sodium
0 g protein	45 mg potassium
0 g fat, 0 saturated	0 g dietary fiber
0 mg cholesterol	5 RE vitamin A
32 g carbohydrate	0.02 mg thiamin
15 mg calcium	0.01 mg riboflavin
2 mg phosphorus	0.1 mg niacin
0.7 mg iron	85 mg vitamin C

Orange Oil, Oil of Orange (additive): Extracted from orange zest and used to flavor beverages, candies, gelatins, puddings, gum, condiments. GRAS.

Orange Roughy: A New Zealand saltwater fish, rough and orange of skin, that's frozen and exported all over the world. Orange roughy is lean, white, supremely sweet meated and versatile. Small wonder so many American chefs love it. For approximate nutrient counts, see FISH, LEAN WHITE.

Oranges: Paleobiologists believe that the orange is at least twenty million years old and that it originated in southern China. They further believe that oranges were cultivated there as early as 2400 B.C.—and certainly by 1500 B.C. because records of the time note that the emperor was urged to try "the bitter oranges of Chiang-p'u."

Arabs brought **bitter oranges** to Africa early on, then planted them in Spain and Portugal between the eighth and twelfth centuries A.D. (they came to be known as **bigarades** or **Sevilles**). Arabs are also thought to have carried **sweet oranges** westward although some food historians credit Genoese sailors. In any case, these were such a fad in France by the time of Louis XIV (1643–1715), elaborate orangeries (hothouses) were built for growing them. The one at Versailles held 1,200 trees, each bedded in a tub of silver, and it was there among the orange blossoms that Louis XIV liked to toss fancy-dress balls.

Columbus introduced oranges to Haiti on his second voyage, De Soto planted them in Florida fifty years later and a couple of centuries after that, the Franciscans set the first orange trees in California soil. Florida and California remain our major orange growers although south Texas contributes its share. These oranges are sweet—**Hamlins** and **Parson Browns** (two early-to-market Florida/Texas varieties), **Valencias** (America's top crop), **Temples** (a popular hybrid), **pineapples** (so honey-sweet they remain a best-seller despite all their abundance of seeds), **mandarins** (tangerinelike oranges with loose, leathery skin and pull-apart segments) and California's **navels** with their conspicuous belly buttons. Then there are such exotics as **blood oranges** (two varieties of this Mediterranean favorite—the **moro** and **ruby blood**—now grow here) and **clementines** (tiny, sugary mandarins).

NUTRIENT CONTENT OF 1 MEDIUM-SIZE NAVEL ORANGE

(about 5 ounces; 140 grams)

64 calories	1 mg sodium
1 g protein	249 mg potassium
0 g fat, 0 saturated	3 g dietary fiber
0 mg cholesterol	25 RE vitamin A
16 g carbohydrate	0.12 mg thiamin
56 mg calcium	0.06 mg riboflavin
27 mg phosphorus	0.4 mg niacin
0.2 mg iron	80 mg vitamin C

Bitter oranges are cultivated in the United States, too, although on a much smaller scale because they're used primarily for marmalade. Orange zest (the colored part of the rind) is intensely aromatic, a versatile seasoner for sweets and savories that makes it easy to cut down on salt. Oranges, as every child learns, are loaded with vitamin C. They are also a superior source of potassium. What's more, they contain FLAVONOIDS, which, some researchers believe, depower certain carcinogens in the body. **SEASON:** Year-round.

Orange Zest: See ORANGES.

Organic Foods: A chemist would define an organic food as anything containing carbon. But the popular definition is "a food untouched by synthetic fertilizers, pesticides, herbicides, artificial preservatives or other additives." Until the final implementation of the new Organic Foods Production Act (OFPA) passed as a part of the 1990 farm bill, no federal laws governed the production, processing, packaging and sale of organic foods. There were state laws, yes; indeed, many different ones, thus inconsistency and confusion reigned. For shoppers, there was no nationwide standard of certification; indeed, no guarantee that the "organic" foods for which they paid top dollar *actually were* organic, because "organic" had become as meaningless a sales pitch as "light" and "natural." Finally, foods marked "organic" will have to meet federal requirements (food processors who knowingly break the rules face not only decertification but also fines as high as ten thousand dollars). Among the major stipulations:

- No land can go organic until it has been free of federally prohibited fertilizers, insecticides, herbicides, etc., for three consecutive years.
- Farmers must keep accurate, detailed records of their food production and handling if their foods are to be verified as organic.
- Farmers wanting to sell their organic foods must register with the U.S. Department of Agriculture, then be certified by an agency it accredits.
- Livestock (and poultry) must be raised—without growth hormones or enhancers—on organic feed, free of plastic-pellet roughage and urea. No antibiotics or medications are allowed other than vaccinations. Dairy cows must follow this strict regimen for a full year before their milk can qualify as organic.

- Raw produce must be grown without toxic natural or synthetic materials (although synthetic insect pheromones are allowed as a pesticide).
- Organic food must meet all regulations for safety and quality (local, state and federal).

These are at the top of a long list being drawn up by the new National Organic Standards Board, whose members include environmentalists, scientists, certifying agents and consumer advocates as well as organic farmers, food processors and merchants. Working with the USDA, the board will determine which substances are permitted or prohibited, what residue tolerance levels are acceptable and how organic foods will be monitored for them.

The reach of the 1990 farm bill was long enough to include processed foods. For a processed food to qualify as organic, 95 percent of its ingredients (other than salt and water) must be organic. If the percentage drops but remains above 50 percent, the label may specify the organic ingredient—organically grown beans in a chili, for example, but only if they're more than half its weight.

In addition, no organic processed food may contain artificial ingredients, heavy metals, toxic residues, sulfites, nitrates or nitrites. Nor may it be packed in materials containing anything that might compromise its organic status (fumigants, fungicides, preservatives, etc.). Finally, any water used in processing must meet Safe Drinking Water Act standards.

Many people have the notion that organic foods are nutritionally superior. The truth is, many of them are extremely perishable. For example, bread made without mold inhibitors molds practically overnight. Organic grains and flours often crawl with insects and antioxidantless cooking oils quickly turn rancid. The biggest drawback of organic foods, however, is *price*. Many cost two or three times as much as their nonorganic counterparts.

Organ Meats: See VARIETY MEATS.

Origanum Oil (additive): A pungent rust brown oil extracted from oregano that's used to flavor everything from baked goods to sausage to root beer to vermouth. GRAS when used within FDA guidelines.

Orlistat, Tetrahydrolipstatin: A new, breakthrough "fat" pill (see DIET PILLS).

Ornish Diet (Life Choice Program): A low-fat (some say *very* low-fat), essentially vegetarian diet developed by Dean Ornish, M.D., president and director of the Preventive Medicine Research Institute in Sausalito, California, that became newsworthy in the nineties. Working with some thousand subjects, Ornish set out to reverse coronary heart disease by changing lifestyles. He reported his success in *Dr. Dean Ornish's Program for Reversing Heart Disease* (1990). Because participants in his study also lost weight (25 pounds, on average, over the first year), he followed up with *Eat More, Weigh Less*, which soared to the top of the best-seller lists in 1993, made Dean Ornish a household name and popularized his Life Choice Program as the Eat More, Weigh Less Diet.

Its daily dietary guidelines: 10 percent of the total calories from fat, 15 percent from protein and 75 percent from complex carbohydrate. The emphasis is on fruits, vegetables, grains and legumes. THE ONLY ANIMAL PROTEINS ALLOWED: Egg whites and such nonfat dairy foods as skim milk and yogurt. BANNED: Oils and oily foods; avocados, seeds, nuts, etc. ALLOWED: Up to 2 ounces of alcohol a day. ALSO ALLOWED: Unrestricted calories as long as they come from Ornish's list of recommended foods.

Ornish believes that most diet plans fail because they're based on deprivation (a recent government survey showed that 97 percent of them do fail over the long haul). His Eat More, Weigh Less plan is based on abundance. To make his recommended foods more palatable, Ornish has hired such culinary luminaries as Alice Waters and Wolfgang Puck (they're responsible for many of the low-fat recipes in his cookbooks). ConAgra is now manufacturing Ornish's ready-to-eat Life Choice meals and marketing them by mail.

Ornish also incorporates stress management and exercise into his Life Choice Program. To lower stress, he advocates changing either your environment or the way you react to it via an hour-a-day routine of meditating, breathing, stretching, relaxing. As for exercise, Ornish recommends a thirty-minute walk a day (or an hour-long walk three times a week). Consistency, he believes, counts more than feeling the burn.

SUMMING UP: Many doctors, dietitians and nutritionists believe Ornish's regimen too strict—and restricting—to work for most people. To which Ornish replies, "If you think it's important, you will do it." He also admits that his is not an "all-or-nothing program, that even small changes can be beneficial."

Orthomolecular Psychiatry: A dubious treatment for mental illness based on megavitamin therapy. It all began back in the 1950s when researchers thought massive doses of niacin (a B vitamin) would "ground" schizophrenics. Niacin, they said, kept epinephrine (a neurotransmitter) from being synthesized into a toxic hallucinogen. Although no studies showed niacin to be effective in stabilizing schizophrenics, this treatment remained popular in some quarters.

In 1968, Nobelist Linus Pauling announced that hefty doses of vitamin C would stave off the common cold, even, perhaps, certain cancers. He further claimed that while the government's RDAs may be adequate for normal, healthy persons, they weren't for those genetically predisposed to mental illness. The best preventive, he believed, was to create "the optimum molecular environment for the mind." He called this controversial new approach to psychiatry "orthomolecular."

Now convinced that schizophrenia was a deficiency disease, the niacin therapists grabbed the term. To this day no one has substantiated their claims. As a result, orthomolecular psychiatrists keep changing their treatment—adding some vitamins, dropping others, using hormones, medications, even electroshock. The one promising development of orthomolecular psychiatry is that megadoses of vitamin B_6 (pyridoxine) seem to bring a few autistic children into "the real world." Or so 1970s tests indicated. There've been no followup studies, however, so most reputable psychiatrists remain unconvinced.

Osteomalacia: Also called **adult rickets,** this deficiency disease is caused by a prolonged shortfall of dietary calcium and vitamin D (or too little sunlight). See D, VITAMIN.

Osteoporosis: The thinning and brittling of bones due to either a lack of the protein matrix that stores calcium or a shortage of dietary calcium (99 percent of the body's supply of this vital mineral is in the bones and teeth). More than twenty-five million Americans suffer from osteoporosis, which puts them at greater risk of hip and other bone fractures. Most are elderly women although men are not exempt. During their lives, men lose 20 to 30 percent of their peak bone mass—reached at age thirty—and women 30 to 40 percent. Between age thirty and menopause, the average woman loses about 1 percent of her bone mass every year, although some may lose three to five times that. After menopause, bone loss accelerates. What determines how fast bones thin, who gets osteoporosis? There are no hard-and-fast answers. But as a general rule, the women most likely to suffer osteoporosis are those who:

- Have a family history of osteoporosis.

- Are white or Asian (blacks have greater bone density).

- Are small boned and thin.

- Are poorly nourished, especially when it comes to calcium, phosphorus and vitamin D (this last not only enhances the absorption of calcium in the body but also regulates calcium and phosphorus metabolism). Sunlight, don't forget, is a major source of vitamin D. See D, VITAMIN.

Also women who have:

- Been anorexic during adolescence or childbearing years.

- Been on thyroid supplements (over time these accelerate bone loss).

- Taken such adrenal cortical steroids as prednisone, cortisone, hydrocortisone, etc.—all notorious leachers of calcium from bones.

- Exercised excessively and obsessively—premenopause. Marathoners are at risk, as are gymnasts and bodybuilders.

- Suffered from any of these diseases or disorders: hyperparathyroidism or hyperthyroidism (overactive parathyroid or thyroid glands); hyperprolactinemia (oversecretion of prolactin, a pituitary hormone that stimulates the production of breast milk); or multiple myeloma (a life-threatening, runaway synthesis in the bone marrow of plasma cells, which block the manufacture of red and white blood cells and lead, ultimately, to the destruction of bone tissue).

The men most apt to be afflicted with osteoporosis are alcoholics, heavy smokers, the bed or wheelchair bound, and those on medications known to deplete calcium reserves.

Is there any way to replace lost bone tissue (read calcium)? Probably not. The point is to stop further deterioration—or at least to retard it. Many doctors put menopausal women on artificial estrogen and though it does slow bone loss, its effects quickly ebb once the therapy is stopped. Estrogen may put women at greater risk of breast cancer, so it's risky for anyone with a family history of breast cancer.

The benefits of calcium supplements are questionable, even when coupled with vitamin D. The best preventive, most nutritionists agree, is eating plenty of calcium-rich foods—milk, yogurt, cheeses of all kinds, ice creams, sardines or salmon with bones. And the earlier you make it a daily habit, the better. Meaning in childhood. The conventional wisdom on the current RDAs for calcium and vitamin D for men and women over fifty is that they are too low. Several bone experts at the National Institutes of Health and Osteoporosis Foundation believe that the RDA for adults over the age of twenty-five should be upped from 800 milligrams a day to 1,000. The sad fact is that most adults get only half that. In addition, some nutritionists think the RDAs for vitamin D should be doubled from 5 micrograms per day to 10. They stress, too, the importance of regular exercise even if it's no more than walking half a mile a day.

Oven Frying: Just the ticket for trimming fat and calories. Instead of frying food in deep (or even shallow) fat, meats, fish, fowl and vegetables can be cooked in the oven with the lightest brushing of oil, melted butter or margarine. Sometimes all that's needed is a spritz of nonstick vegetable cooking spray, which sends the calories and grams of fat plummeting. Oven frying, to be honest, is really baking or roasting. No matter. It works.

Overeaters Anonymous: A support group that follows the lead of Alcoholics Anonymous. "It's very spiritual," says one member. "There are meetings several times a day and you can go as often as you like. We use the same creed as AA members except that our concern is food, not alcohol. We don't talk much about food at meetings, however. We just discuss problems in general; get rid of our anxieties. There are no set fees: A hat is passed at meetings and you drop in your contribution. In addition to regular meetings, we have special seminars with lecturers coming from all over the world. It's very helpful, but what means most is the support of the group and of your own personal sponsor."

Overnutrition: A form of MALNUTRITION.

Overweight: Being 10 to 20 percent above your normal (desirable) weight. See also OBESITY, OVERWEIGHT.

Ovovegetarians: Vegetarians who will eat eggs but no other animal food.

Spicy Oven-Fried Chicken

Makes 6 Servings

¾ cup buttermilk

¾ cup plain nonfat yogurt

2 garlic cloves, finely minced

½ teaspoon hot red pepper sauce

1 broiler-fryer (3 pounds), cut up for frying, skinned, and trimmed of fat

CRUMB MIXTURE:

2½ cups fine soft white bread crumbs

¼ cup freshly grated Parmesan cheese

2 tablespoons minced fresh parsley

2 teaspoons sweet paprika

2 teaspoons poultry seasoning

1 teaspoon dried marjoram

¼ teaspoon dried thyme

½ teaspoon salt

¼ teaspoon freshly ground black pepper

COMBINE THE BUTTERMILK, yogurt, garlic, and hot pepper sauce in a large shallow ceramic bowl. Add chicken pieces and turn until well coated. Cover and refrigerate overnight, turning chicken in marinade now and then.

WHEN READY TO cook chicken, preheat oven to 400°F. and position rack in lower third of oven. Also coat baking sheet with nonstick spray (preferably olive oil or butter flavor) and set aside. Combine crumb mixture in pie tin. One by one, lift chicken pieces from yogurt marinade, shaking off excess, and dredge evenly in crumb mixture, patting on chicken to make it stick. Arrange chicken pieces, not touching, on a baking sheet and spray lightly but evenly with nonstick spray. Bake, uncovered, 40 to 45 minutes or until chicken is crispy-brown and cooked through. Serve hot or cold.

APPROXIMATE NUTRIENT COUNTS PER SERVING

196 calories	9 g carbohydrate	1.8 mg iron	0.15 mg thiamin
27 g protein	1 g dietary fiber	346 mg sodium	0.27 mg riboflavin
5 g fat, 2 saturated	119 mg calcium	354 mg potassium	9.6 mg niacin
80 mg cholesterol	266 mg phosphorus	63 RE vitamin A	5 mg vitamin C

Oxalic Acid, Oxalates: Oxalic acid exists naturally in some foods—beet greens, chard, rhubarb and spinach, to name four—and binds with calcium in the body, forming useless calcium oxalate. For all the calcium in spinach, it's estimated that only 5 percent is absorbed by the body; the lion's share combines with oxalic acid, forming the insoluble oxalate. Cocoa contains oxalates, too, but not enough to block the absorption of the calcium in hot chocolate or chocolate milk.

Oxidation: It's what causes fats to go stale and the flesh of apples, avocados and peaches to brown after they're cut. In the body, oxidation plays a major role. Through an intricate series of steps it converts fats, carbohydrates and proteins to carbon dioxide (which we exhale), water and energy. Oxidation may mean the addition of oxygen atoms to a compound or the removal of hydrogen—the case when saturated fatty acids become unsaturated. Either way, oxidation is essential to life itself.

Oxtail: The muscular tail of beef, not oxen. It's rich of flavor, but tough and requires hours of slow, moist cooking to tenderize it. Oxtail stews are a particular favorite in England and France.

NUTRIENT CONTENT OF 3 OUNCES (85 GRAMS) SIMMERED OXTAIL	
205 calories	160 mg sodium
26 g protein	144 mg potassium
11 g fat, NA saturated	0 g dietary fiber
NA mg cholesterol	0 RE vitamin A
0 g carbohydrate	0.02 mg thiamin
12 mg calcium	0.02 mg riboflavin
120 mg phosphorus	2.8 mg niacin
3.2 mg iron	0 mg vitamin C

Oxygen: Chemically speaking, an element. Oxygen is in the air we breathe, the water we drink, the blood circulating in our veins. It is integral to every life process; indeed, without it, we'd die within minutes.

Oxymyoglobin: The red pigment in meat. See also MYOGLOBIN.

Oxytocin: A hormone produced by the hypothalamus gland that plays a major role in childbirth by causing powerful uterine contractions. It also stimulates lactation.

Oyster Mushrooms, Pleurottes: See MUSHROOMS.

Oyster Plant: See SALSIFY.

Oysters: Aficionados will forever argue the merits of one oyster over another: the subtle **bluepoints** of Long Island versus the briny **Wellfleets** of Cape Cod, the coppery **Chincoteagues** of Virginia versus the buttery West Coast **Olympias.** Then there's the ongoing debate about the superiority of the French **Belons** over every other. Heredity may affect the size, shape and color of a particular species of oyster, but habitat—particularly the salinity of the water—determines flavor.

Once blessed with an abundance of natural oyster beds off the shores of every surf-washed state, America's supply is now so depleted that we, like the Romans two thousand years before us, must grow our own if our appetites are to be satisfied. Judging from the middens of shells found along our coasts, Native Americans were almost as gluttonous in their consumption of oysters as the Romans. But America's first full-fledged oyster binge began early in the nineteenth century with the arrival of the "Oyster Express," lightweight wagons that raced from Baltimore to Pittsburgh, carrying fresh cargoes of oysters bedded in wet seaweed. Soon the craze spread farther west—to Cincinnati, where the places to be seen were the city's proliferating oyster parlors, and then farther still to Springfield, Illinois, where a young Mr. and Mrs. Abraham Lincoln threw parties at which they served nothing but oysters. Oyster madness abated only when the nation's supplies were imperiled late in the nineteenth century. And it is unlikely to resurface, given our conservationist turn of mind, to say nothing of the price of fine oysters.

There is something to the "R months" theory about the goodness of oysters. Not that May, June, July or August oysters will be hazardous to your health unless taken from waters infected with the dread red tide, an infestation of microscopic planktons that produce toxins. These build to dangerous levels in oysters, clams and other mollusks, and no amount of cooking will destroy them. But the main reason for avoiding non-R-month oysters is that they spawn during warm weather and most states forbid the taking of them. No matter; spawning oysters aren't very plump or tasty anyway. You can stretch the oyster season, of course, by resorting to canned or frozen oysters. But they are sorry substitutes.

Most fresh oysters are sold shucked nowadays although big-city markets (and oyster pounds at the source) also sell them in the shell and opened on the half shell. The best oysters will be plump, moist and ivory hued to pale tan. They will smell sweet but exude a distinct marine tang. Their liquor should be clear, never cloudy.

True oyster lovers prefer them raw, on the half shell. But eating raw oysters is increasingly dicey because of the prevalence of *Vibrio vulnificus,* a bacterium that grows naturally in warm seas, especially the Gulf of Mexico, between April and October. Oysters, clams and other mollusks, which feed by filtering seawater through their bodies, are apt to contain high concentrations of *V. vulnificus.* It can make you very sick; in fact, half of those with compromised immune systems or in generally weakened conditions die from *V. vulnificus* infections.

Then, too, there's the problem of seawater being pol-

NUTRIENT CONTENT OF 3 OUNCES (85 GRAMS) STEAMED ATLANTIC OYSTERS

116 calories	190 mg sodium
12 g protein	239 mg potassium
4 g fat, 1 saturated	0 g dietary fiber
89 mg cholesterol	46 RE vitamin A
6 g carbohydrate	0.16 mg thiamin
77 mg calcium	0.15 mg riboflavin
173 mg phosphorus	2.1 mg niacin
10.2 mg iron	5 mg vitamin C

NUTRIENT CONTENT OF 3 OUNCES (85 GRAMS) STEAMED PACIFIC OYSTERS

139 calories	180 mg sodium
16 g protein	257 mg potassium
4 g fat, 1 saturated	0 g dietary fiber
85 mg cholesterol	124 RE vitamin A
8 g carbohydrate	0.11 mg thiamin
14 mg calcium	0.38 mg riboflavin
207 mg phosphorus	3.1 mg niacin
7.8 mg iron	11 mg vitamin C

luted with other disease-causing bacteria (cholera and hepatitis, to name two of the more common). Cautious eaters reject all raw shellfish while others douse their raw oysters with fiery pepper sauce, believing it kills the harmful bugs. A controversial, unproved assumption. No one, however, denies that thorough cooking destroys dangerous bacteria. Or that it's best to play it safe by avoiding raw oysters—except, perhaps, those taken from cold waters in cold months, both of which discourage bacterial growth.

What about all the cholesterol in oysters? How harmful is it? Nutritionists and physicians now believe that the cholesterol present in food, particularly that in low-fat food, does less to damage arteries than saturated fats. Oysters are low in fat and saturated fat. And they don't contain that much cholesterol, either—at least compared to the amount in egg yolks or calf's liver. At the same time, oysters are a first-rate source of niacin, iron, phosphorus and potassium. Not a bad trade-off.

Oystershell: A powdered-oystershell calcium supplement widely sold by health-food stores. The truth is, the calcium present in oystershells is poorly absorbed by the body and even less so if fortified with magnesium. Save your money.

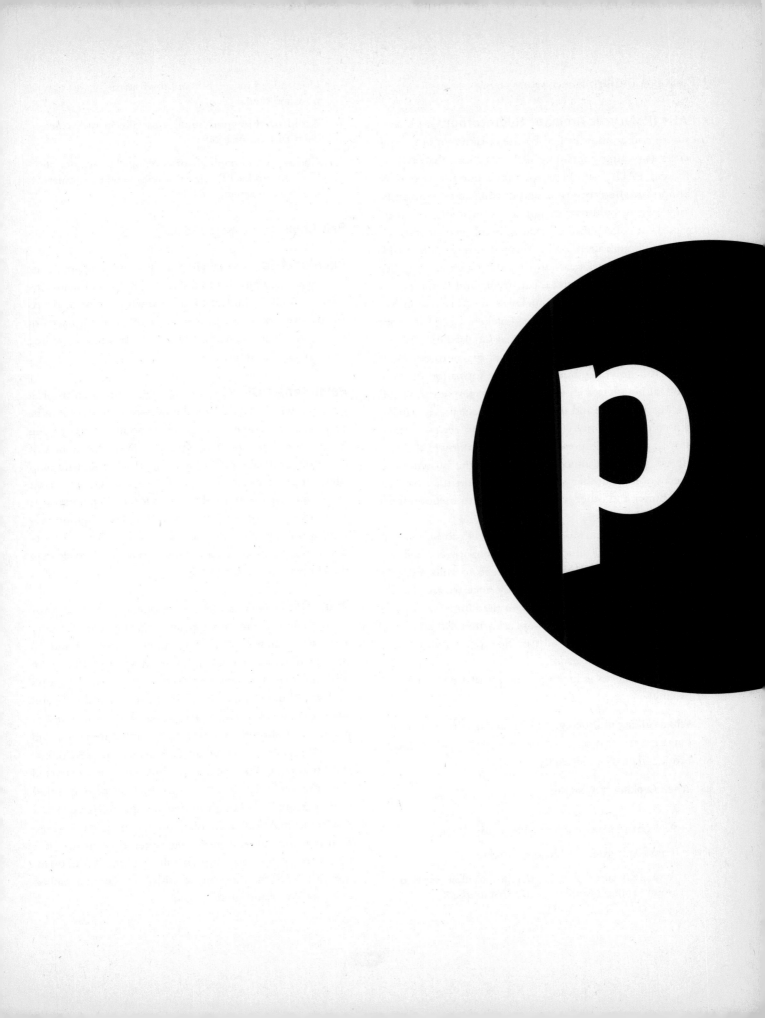

Package Dating: See OPEN DATING.

PAHs (Polycyclic Aromatic Hydrocarbons): Cancer-causing compounds formed by the breakdown of organic matter (anything containing carbon). More than twenty different PAHs have been identified but the two most common are **benzopyrene** and **quinoline compounds.** They exist in industrial air pollutants, in smoke given off by coal- or coke-burning furnaces, in tobacco tar and, yes, in food. Though attention has focused mostly on the PAHs formed when fatty meats are smoked or charcoal grilled (especially over MESQUITE), pan-frying and broiling produce plenty of them, too. High levels of PAHs have shown up in well-done bacon, burgers, chicken, eggs, fish, pork chops and sausage fried or broiled at intense heat.

But that's not all. The canning of high-protein foods (meat, fish, fowl, legumes) causes the formation of some PAHs, although to a lesser degree. So do fermentation and pickling (soy sauce and the Korean cabbage pickle, *kimchi,* both contain benzopyrene, a singularly powerful carcinogen). Even the cold pressing of peanut, safflower and sesame oils produces some PAHs, as does the browning of baked goods. Another source: the paraffin used to coat milk, butter and other food cartons, not to mention fresh fruits and vegetables.

A recent German study showed that 45 to 90 percent of the 250 to 1,000 micrograms of benzopyrene the average German ingested each year came from fruits and leafy vegetables. Pretty startling, especially since we are all now urged to eat more fresh produce. In the United States, the government controls PAH contamination by enforcing high purity standards for all paraffins used to wax fruits, vegetables and food cartons.

Is it possible to reduce the amount of PAHs in food? Absolutely.

When Grilling or Broiling: See dos and don'ts listed under CHARCOAL GRILLING. Most of these apply to foods broiled via gas or electricity.

When Cooking in General:

- Peel waxed fruits and vegetables before using.

- Trim all fat from food before cooking.

- Avoid fatty cuts of meat, opting, for example, for lean ground round instead of regular hamburger.

- Use smoked meats, fish and fowl sparingly and only now and then.

- Avoid overbrowning food, especially in the skillet, deep-fat fryer or broiler.

- Choose gentle methods of cooking that are not so likely to produce PAHs (steaming, stewing, simmering, microwaving).

Pak Choi: See CHINESE CABBAGE.

Palmitic Acid: A saturated fatty acid and a major component of solid fats. It's found in PALM OIL and many animal fats (milk or butterfat is 21 percent palmitic acid). As an additive, palmitic acid is used to enhance the flavor of butter and cheese spreads. But it must be used according to FDA specifications.

Palm-Kernel Oil: One of the highly saturated tropical plant oils widely used by food processors (85 percent of its fatty acids are saturated, 12 percent monounsaturated and 2 percent polyunsaturated). It comes from the kernels of the African oil palm rather than from the fibrous fruit pulp (the source of PALM OIL). Look for palm-kernel oil on labels and, whenever possible, avoid foods containing large amounts of it (candies and margarines). There's good reason for this. Biomedical researchers now believe that saturated fats do more to raise blood cholesterol levels than the cholesterol present in food.

Palm Oil: A beta-carotene-rich, orange-red oil so saturated it's sludgy at room temperature (51 percent of its fatty acids are saturated, 39 percent monounsaturated and 10 percent polyunsaturated). Like PALM-KERNEL OIL, palm oil comes from the African oil palm, which now also grows in Haiti, Honduras and Brazil. Brazilians call it **dendê** and use it to color and flavor such Bahian classics as *vatapá* (a porridge of shrimp or chicken, coconut, tomatoes and roasted peanuts) and *xin-xin* (a peppery chicken/dried-shrimp stew). Unlike palm-kernel oil, palm oil is extracted from the tree's fibrous fruit pulp, which averages from 30 to 70 percent fat. Though a kitchen staple in Brazil (and a motor fuel in Africa), palm oil is more often used elsewhere to make soap, tin and steel. Highly refined versions of it go into margarines and vegetable shortenings. Avoid them, opting instead for those made with less saturated canola, corn, safflower and sunflower oils.

Palm Sugar: See JAGGARY.

Panbroiling: Cooking food (usually steaks, chops, chicken or fish) in a skillet in a minimum of fat. You can even panbroil in a skillet coated with nonstick vegetable cooking oil spray. The advantage is obvious: less fat.

Pancakes: Flat breads, sometimes leavened, sometimes not, that are quickly browned in a skillet or on a griddle. Also called **griddle cakes** and **flapjacks,** these are the centerpiece of the hearty American breakfast. They may be made of white flour, whole-wheat, buckwheat, even mixtures of cornmeal and wheat. They may be plain, dressed with nothing more than pats of butter and drizzlings of maple syrup. Or they may be fancy—studded with blueberries, chopped apples or other fruit, with pecans, wild rice or bits of ham. They may be leavened with baking powder, yeast or sourdough starter—a California favorite. Nearly every nation makes pancakes of some sort. French **crêpes** have leaped the Atlantic (and tortillas the Rio Grande) to become as popular here as they are at home.

In the United States pancakes became a passion early on (Native Americans were making them by the time the colonists arrived). For generations they were as much a part of breakfast as steaming cups of coffee. Too much cooking, perhaps, for some at the start of the day. So two enterprising Missourians came up with self-rising pancake flour (combined with just the right amount of baking powder and salt) to make the job easy. It was introduced at the New Era Exposition in St. Joseph, Missouri, in 1889. Before long, the world knew it as Aunt Jemima pancake mix (the name, according to John Mariani in his endlessly fas-

cinating *Dictionary of American Food and Drink,* was taken from an old minstrel song).

Mariani goes on to say that the first of America's popular International House of Pancakes (IHOP) chain was opened in North Hollywood in 1958. It's going strong today. As are pancakes of every size, every flavor. For dedicated pancake eaters, however, any classic recipe is still the best.

Pancetta: Italian bacon. Unlike American bacon, *pancetta* is not smoked. Instead, it is lightly spiced and salted, rolled into a chunky link and cured. **NOTE:** No nutrient counts are available for *pancetta*, but it's safe to say they would approximate those of American bacon.

Pancreas: A vital organ, long and tapering, that lies just behind the stomach. By secreting pancreatic juice into the digestive tract, the pancreas aids in the digestion of carbohydrates, fats and protein. It also produces two vital hormones, INSULIN and glucagon, which work in concert to stabilize blood sugar (glucose) levels. To simplify, insulin lowers blood sugar in two ways—by directing it to body cells where it's used as fuel and by dispatching it to the liver to be stored. Glucagon, on the other hand, raises blood glucose levels by stimulating its release from the liver. This explains why diabetics, who secrete little or no insulin, have elevated blood sugar levels. See DIABETES.

Pancreatic Juice: An enzyme-loaded alkaline secretion of the pancreas that plays a major role in the digestion of carbohydrates, fats and proteins. It also helps neutralize the acidity of the stomach's gastric juice as food enters the small intestine.

Pancreatitis (diet and): Inflammation, either acute or chronic, of the pancreas. It can be triggered by gallbladder disease, alcoholism or abdominal injury, and symptoms range from mild stomach upset to searing pain, fever, nausea, vomiting, edema and shock. If untreated, pancreatitis can be fatal. The first job facing the physician is to give the pancreas a rest by restricting foods that stress it. In severe pancreatitis, no food and liquid are given by mouth. When the condition abates, they are gradually reintroduced—from clear liquids to semisoft foods with fat accounting for no more than 20 percent of the day's calories. Alcohol is banned and vitamin B_{12} supplements are sometimes prescribed.

NUTRIENT CONTENT OF 1 MEDIUM-SIZE HOMEMADE PANCAKE

(about 1 ounce; 27 grams)

61 calories	119 mg sodium
2 g protein	36 mg potassium
3 g fat, 1 saturated	0 g dietary fiber
16 mg cholesterol	15 RE vitamin A
8 g carbohydrate	0.05 mg thiamin
59 mg calcium	0.08 mg riboflavin
43 mg phosphorus	0.4 mg niacin
0.5 mg iron	0 mg vitamin C

Pan Drippings: The concentrated meat juices, melted fat and browned bits left in the bottom of the roasting pan after meat, fish or fowl has been roasted. Most cooks use pan drippings for gravy although some of them brim with saturated fat, especially if butter bastes have been used (often the case with turkey and pheasant). It's possible, of course, to skim off much of the fat. A good idea. It's also smart to use broth or water when making gravy instead of milk or cream.

Panfrying: Cooking food in fat in a skillet. It's also called **shallow frying** as opposed to deep-fat frying, although there may be half an inch of butter or oil in the pan. In France—and increasingly in the United States—panfrying is known as **sautéing.** The word sounds more elegant but the technique is the same. And it can present problems. If the temperature is too low, the fat soaks into the food, especially if that food is dredged or breaded or porous like eggplant and mushrooms. If the temperature is too high, the food browns before it cooks. The biggest disadvantage of panfrying, at least from a nutritional standpoint, is that it increases the fat content of food.

Pangamic Acid: Health-food stores hustle this as vitamin B_{15}, a panacea for, among other ailments, schizophrenia, hepatitis and heart disease. The truth? No reliable studies have proved pangamic acid of any therapeutic value. In fact, Canada has banned its sale.

Pangenic Acid: Not the same thing as PANGAMIC ACID, although health-food stores sometimes call it vitamin B_{15}. See DMG.

Pantothenic Acid (vitamin): Derived from the Greek word *pántothen,* meaning "from all quarters," this B vitamin is indeed a "do everything, be everywhere" nutrient. It is part of the chemical makeup of coenzyme A and thus key to the metabolism of carbohydrates, fats and proteins. Pantothenic acid is also involved in making fatty acids, cholesterol, acetylcholine (a form of choline, a vitaminlike substance), steroid hormones and nerve regulators. It occurs naturally in all plant and animal cells in concentrations ranging from impressive to infinitesimal. RDA: None so far. The Food and Nutrition Board of the National Research Council has set the Estimated Safe and Adequate Daily Dietary Intake for adults at between 4 to 7 milligrams of pantothenic acid a day. **DEFICIENCY SYMPTOMS:** None known for humans. However, in lab animals deprived of pantothenic acid, biomedical researchers have noted muscle cramps, weakened immune systems and impaired adrenal activity. **GOOD SOURCES:** Organ meats, most fish and whole-grain cereals contain the most pantothenic acid but all food groups contribute their share. **PRECAUTIONS:** Refined wheat flours and canned fruits and vegetables will have lost more than half their pantothenic acid, frozen ones anywhere from 7 to 47 percent. This B vitamin also breaks down when exposed to dry heat, acid or alkaline solutions.

Papain: An enzyme found in papayas, which Latin American women have been using for centuries to tenderize tough cuts of meat. They simply rubbed sinewy cuts of beef, goat, mutton or chicken with papaya juice and let it marinate several hours. Today papain is crystallized, bottled and sold in every supermarket as **meat tenderizer.** It is also used to treat stomach disorders, and many health-food stores sell it as a digestive.

Papaya Diet: A weight-loss diet popular among Hollywood glitterati some years ago that was supposed to keep you young, beautiful and in fighting trim. The truth? Papaya is a stellar source of vitamin C but no single-food diet is healthful—or even effective—over the long haul. The only way to lose weight, keep lost pounds off and feel vital is to combine a well-balanced diet with a sensible exercise program. See also FOOD GUIDE PYRAMID.

Papayas: Plump yellow to orange, these butter-fleshed tropical fruits brim with vitamin C and potassium. Once exotics that seldom showed up in heartland supermarkets, papayas are shipped in from Hawaii and now widely available. They are sweet but with an edge of tartness that

NUTRIENT CONTENT OF 1 CUP SLICED PAPAYA	
(about 5 ounces; 140 grams)	
54 calories	4 mg sodium
1 g protein	360 mg potassium
0 g fat, 0 saturated	4 g dietary fiber
0 mg cholesterol	39 RE vitamin A
14 g carbohydrate	0.04 mg thiamin
34 mg calcium	0.05 mg riboflavin
7 mg phosphorus	0.5 mg niacin
0.1 mg iron	86 mg vitamin C

Curried Crab and Papaya Salad

> *Makes 6 Servings*

A fresh-as-spring salad that's hearty enough for a main course.

2 ripe medium papayas (about 2¾ pounds each),
    peeled, halved, seeded, and cut into ½-inch cubes

1 pound lump crab meat, carefully picked over for bits of
    shell and cartilage

2 tablespoons minced fresh parsley

1 tablespoon minced fresh dill

2 tablespoons well-drained small capers

6 cup-shaped radicchio or bibb lettuce leaves

CURRY DRESSING:

1 small yellow onion, minced

4 teaspoons corn or peanut oil

2 teaspoons curry powder

Pinch of dried thyme

½ cup low-fat mayonnaise

⅓ cup light sour cream

1 teaspoon Dijon mustard

¼ teaspoon salt, or to taste

⅛ teaspoon freshly ground black pepper

PAT PAPAYA CUBES on several thicknesses of paper toweling to dry. Place in a mixing bowl along with crab, parsley, dill, and capers. Set, untossed, in refrigerator.

FOR DRESSING: IN a small heavy skillet, brown onion in oil for 5 minutes over moderate heat. Blend in curry powder and thyme, then turn heat to lowest point and heat 5 minutes. Pour into a blender or food processor fitted with the metal chopping blade, add remaining dressing ingredients, and churn 60 seconds to blend. Taste for salt and adjust as needed. Pour dressing over papaya mixture, toss lightly, cover, and chill several hours. Toss again and serve in radicchio cups.

APPROXIMATE NUTRIENT COUNTS PER SERVING

215 calories	16 g carbohydrate	1.1 mg iron	0.11 mg thiamin
17 g protein	3 g dietary fiber	465 mg sodium	0.13 mg riboflavin
10 g fat, 2 saturated	125 mg calcium	619 mg potassium	1.5 mg niacin
77 mg cholesterol	224 mg phosphorus	60 RE vitamin A	68 mg vitamin C

makes them as versatile as apples. Splendid in chutneys, fruit compotes, ice creams and sherbets, papayas are equally at home with curried fish or fowl. **SEASON:** Year-round with supplies peaking in spring and fall.

Paprika: It's more than a "blusher." Both the sweet paprika and the hot pack plenty of beta-carotene. And ounce for ounce, fresh paprika peppers contain more vitamin C than any citrus fruit. For discovering that fact, a twentieth-century Hungarian-American biochemist named Albert Szent-Györgi won the Nobel Prize. Although peppers (capsicums) are one of the foods the New World gave the Old, it was the Hungarians who learned to sun dry them and grind them into a powder called paprika that could be used to season, as well as to color, the stews they called *gulyás* (goulash). The choicest paprikas available today are imported from Hungary and they've become a staple at nearly every high-end grocery. The **sweet rose,** with its faintly musky, faintly lemony flavor, is the one to use for *paprikash,* goulash and all-purpose cooking. The **hot** requires a lighter hand; indeed, a pinch is all that's needed to spark the blandest dish.

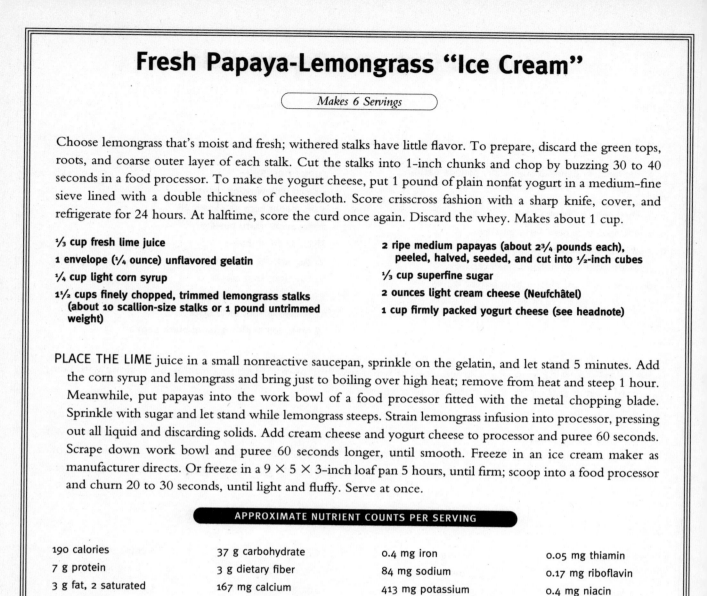

Fresh Papaya-Lemongrass "Ice Cream"

Makes 6 Servings

Choose lemongrass that's moist and fresh; withered stalks have little flavor. To prepare, discard the green tops, roots, and coarse outer layer of each stalk. Cut the stalks into 1-inch chunks and chop by buzzing 30 to 40 seconds in a food processor. To make the yogurt cheese, put 1 pound of plain nonfat yogurt in a medium-fine sieve lined with a double thickness of cheesecloth. Score crisscross fashion with a sharp knife, cover, and refrigerate for 24 hours. At halftime, score the curd once again. Discard the whey. Makes about 1 cup.

⅓ cup fresh lime juice

1 envelope (¼ ounce) unflavored gelatin

¼ cup light corn syrup

1½ cups finely chopped, trimmed lemongrass stalks (about 10 scallion-size stalks or 1 pound untrimmed weight)

2 ripe medium papayas (about 2¾ pounds each), peeled, halved, seeded, and cut into ½-inch cubes

⅓ cup superfine sugar

2 ounces light cream cheese (Neufchâtel)

1 cup firmly packed yogurt cheese (see headnote)

PLACE THE LIME juice in a small nonreactive saucepan, sprinkle on the gelatin, and let stand 5 minutes. Add the corn syrup and lemongrass and bring just to boiling over high heat; remove from heat and steep 1 hour. Meanwhile, put papayas into the work bowl of a food processor fitted with the metal chopping blade. Sprinkle with sugar and let stand while lemongrass steeps. Strain lemongrass infusion into processor, pressing out all liquid and discarding solids. Add cream cheese and yogurt cheese to processor and puree 60 seconds. Scrape down work bowl and puree 60 seconds longer, until smooth. Freeze in an ice cream maker as manufacturer directs. Or freeze in a 9 × 5 × 3-inch loaf pan 5 hours, until firm; scoop into a food processor and churn 20 to 30 seconds, until light and fluffy. Serve at once.

APPROXIMATE NUTRIENT COUNTS PER SERVING

190 calories	37 g carbohydrate	0.4 mg iron	0.05 mg thiamin
7 g protein	3 g dietary fiber	84 mg sodium	0.17 mg riboflavin
3 g fat, 2 saturated	167 mg calcium	413 mg potassium	0.4 mg niacin
9 mg cholesterol	119 mg phosphorus	61 RE vitamin A	67 mg vitamin C

Para-Aminobenzoic Acid (PABA): Though once considered a B vitamin, PABA is actually a component of folic acid, another of the B-complex. By itself it has no vitamin activity in humans and thus is no longer ranked as a vitamin.

Paraffin (additive): It's one of the compounds used to wax fresh fruits and vegetables, also to waterproof cartons used for milk, butter and other food. For that reason, paraffin is considered an additive and must be approved by the FDA. Further, it is sold by the block and remains popular among home cooks as a "sealer" for jams, jellies and preserves (a quarter of an inch of melted paraffin is all that's needed to shut out airborne microbes). **CAUTION:** As a petroleum derivative, paraffin is apt to contain cancer-causing PAHs. See also WAXING OF FRUITS AND VEGETABLES.

Paraguay Tea: See MATÉ.

Paralytic Shellfish Poisoning: It strikes without warning—usually within half an hour of your eating contaminated clams, mussels, oysters or scallops. And it can kill. The culprits? Microscopic dinoflagellates (algae) belonging to the *Gonyaulax* genus, which infect cold-water mollusk beds from Maine to Massachusetts and Alaska to California. *Gonyaulax* produce a powerful neurotoxin; the shellfish eat the algae, toxin and all, and it accumulates in them to levels that can make you deathly sick. **SYMPTOMS:** Numbness, tingling, drowsiness, lack of coordination, incoherence, dry throat and skin, paralysis and, in as many as 10 percent of the cases, death. No amount of cooking depowers this neurotoxin, you can't detect its presence in shellfish, but the FDA's National Shellfish Sanitation Program can. It constantly tests coastal waters and closes any where toxins in clam, mussel, oyster or scallop meat exceed 80 micrograms per 100 grams (about 3½ ounces).

This is not the RED TIDE that ravages warm inshore waters of Florida, the Gulf of Mexico and southern California. It, too, is caused by a dinoflagellate that produces dangerous neurotoxins (the government bans fishing in infected waters). Although red tide toxins produce symptoms similar to those of *Gonyaulax,* they are less deadly. See also CIGUATERA POISONING.

Parasites (in food or water): *Webster's* defines a parasite as "an organism living in or on another organism in parasitism." This means that it feeds on, draws strength from its host and, in the process, injures or even kills it. Unfortunately, parasites exist in food and drink and not just in the Third World. They are of four main types: **roundworms** (nematodes), **protozoa, tapeworms** (cestodes) and **flukes** (trematodes). Below we chart the various parasites, their sources, the diseases and symptoms they cause and the best preventives.

Parasitic Worms: Tapeworms are fairly common in this country. All it takes to get them is a bite of "infected" beef, pork or fish. Fortunately, tapeworms are big enough to see, so it's easy to avoid them. **Pinworms,** on the other hand, are so small a microscope is needed to identify them. Like **hookworms,** pinworms belong to the roundworm family. Even though thorough cooking kills parasitic worms, it's better to eat uninfected meat and fish. Toward that end, the federal government is tightening its inspection procedures and increasing their scope. See also PARASITES.

FOOD PARASITES

Type	Source	Disease and Symptoms	Preventives
ROUNDWORMS			
Trichinella spiralis★ (trichinae)	Raw or rare pork and wild game, especially bear, wild boar and cougar. When hogs were slopped or fed garbage, trichinosis was more common. Today about fifty new cases are reported each year in the United States although there are still occasional large outbreaks.	*Trichinosis.* These microorganisms burrow into muscles and intestinal walls, thwarting nutrient absorption, weakening muscles and causing much pain. If the trichinae riddle vital organs, serious illness and death may result.	Cooking to an internal temperature of 140°F., which kills trichinae. Most people prefer these meats well done (170°F.). Freezing also kills trichinae.
Ascaris lumbricoides	Raw or undercooked fish and shellfish. Also vegetables grown in contaminated soil or watered by sewage-polluted water.	*Roundworm Infection.* Larvae hatch in intestines, enter blood and may reach heart or lungs, causing considerable damage and frequent bouts of pneumonia.	Thorough cooking of all seafood and vegetables of questionable source.
Anisakidae★ (anisakid worms)	Raw or undercooked fish and shellfish. Recent major outbreaks in Seattle were traced to both raw and cold-smoked salmon, also to Pacific rockfish.	*Anisakiasis.* Larvae damage intestinal walls and impair absorption of food nutrients. There's fever, nausea, intense stomach and abdominal pain.	Cooking all seafood to well done, avoiding sushi, sashimi and cold-smoked salmon.

Type	Source	Disease and Symptoms	Preventives
PROTOZOA			
Cyclospora	Contaminated water; raw food taken from, washed or rinsed in that water; dirty hands; undisinfected cooking utensils.	Severe diarrhea and stomach cramps, nausea, debilitating fatigue, significant weight loss.	Drinking boiled or fizzy bottled water only; avoid ice, raw fruits and vegetables.
Giardia lamblia★	Contaminated water; raw food taken from, washed or rinsed in that water; improperly washed hands, cooking utensils.	*Giardiasis.* Diarrhea, abdominal cramps, gas, nausea, vomiting, flulike symptoms. New diagnostic tests are quick and reliable.	"Don't drink the water." Shun ice, salads, all raw food.
Entamoeba histolytica	Contaminated food or water; unsanitary kitchens and unclean food handlers. Travelers to Third World countries and those with weakened immune systems are most susceptible.	*Amoebic Dysentery.* Acute diarrhea with bloody stools; cirrhosis of the liver; and, unless treated, death.	Avoiding raw or partially cooked meat, fish, fowl and vegetables, all tap water and ice. Eat only thick-skinned fruits you have peeled.
Toxoplasma gondii★	Cat feces; partially or poorly cooked meat or poultry.	*Toxoplasmosis.* Those at greatest risk are pregnant women, who may suffer miscarriages, deliver stillborns or mentally retarded infants.	Being scrupulous about washing hands after fondling cats or disposing of cat litter. Also cooking all meat and poultry to well done.
TAPEWORMS★			
Taenia saginata, Taenia solium, Diphyllobothrium latum	Raw or rare beef. Underdone pork. Raw or underdone fish.	All these cling to intestinal walls and some may reach awesome length (30 feet). They interfere with digestion and cause abdominal cramps, appetite loss and weight loss. They're visible in stools as bits of ivory ribbon. Fortunately, they're easily killed.	Cooking all meat and fish to well done. Also reject any meat or fish with visible tapeworms.

FLUKES (trematodes)

These parasitic flatworms, prevalent in crowded areas of eastern Asia, are almost unheard of in the United States. Like tapeworms, they invade and destroy body tissue. At first there may be digestive problems and, unless treated, liver damage (some people carry flukes for twenty years or more). How do you get them? By eating raw or underdone fish taken from contaminated ponds or lakes. The cycle of infection works like this: Human feces contain fluke eggs, pollute water, snails eat the eggs, fish eat the snails and man eats the fish. The best preventive? Cooking all fish until well done, and that includes dried, salted and pickled fish, too.

★The most common food parasites in the United States.

Parasorbic Acid: A natural toxicant found in cranberries that has been shown to cause cancer in lab animals.

Parathormone: The hormone secreted by the parathyroid glands. It's crucial to the metabolism of calcium and phosphorus. Too much parathormone raises blood levels of calcium and, in addition, speeds its withdrawal from the bones whenever the diet lacks calcium. At the same time, excess parathormone lowers blood phosphorus by sending it off to the urine to be excreted.

Parathyroid Glands: Four small glands piggybacked on the thyroid that produce an essential metabolic hormone called PARATHORMONE.

Parboiled Rice, Converted Rice: See RICE.

Parboiling, Blanching: Both involve simmering or boiling food in water, but times vary. *Parboiling* means partially cooking something that will be finished by another method. It's particularly useful when short- and long-cooking foods are teamed in a single casserole. If the slower-to-cook foods are parboiled before they go into the casserole, they've a jump-start on the faster ones and both will be done at the same time.

Blanching, on the other hand, is little more than a quick dip in boiling water (beyond a few minutes, blanching becomes parboiling). Blanching serves many purposes. For example, before vegetables are frozen, they're blanched to set the color and deactivate any enzymes that might shorten freezer life. Bacons are often blanched to rid them of excess fat, smoky flavor and salt before they go into soups or stews. Meats likely to "throw a scum" (veal and sweetbreads, to name two) are given a fast simmer lest they muddy the recipes in which they star. Blanching precipitates the scum, most of which goes down the drain with the blanching water; the rest is simply rinsed off the meat. Certain raw fruits, vegetables and nuts are blanched to loosen their skins. Finally, the French way of cooking asparagus, green peas (especially the *mange-tout* or sugar snaps), *haricots verts* (snap beans) and other green vegetables is to blanch them briefly in boiling water, refresh (quick chill) in ice water, then come serving time, warm them briefly in sauce or butter. Vegetables never tasted better. And most of their vitamins—both the heat-labile and the water-soluble—remain intact.

Parenteral Feeding: The delivery of nutrients directly into the bloodstream by IV (intravenous feeding). It is administered to those who can't take food by mouth. The liquid is a high-energy mix of glucose and electrolytes. Sometimes parenteral and enteral (mouth tube) feeding are combined. If parenteral feeding is the only source of food, fat emulsions, amino-acid solutions, vitamins and minerals are also added to the formula or administered by additional IVs. See also ENTERAL NUTRITION.

Pareve, Parve: A Jewish food term meaning "milkless and meatless." Any food marked "pareve" will contain no milk or meat in any form and can thus be used with meat or dairy meals as dictated by Jewish dietary laws.

Parkinson's Disease (and diet): Although this disease, a degenerative nerve condition characterized by tremors, is incurable, a well-balanced diet does seem to boost the effectiveness of the medication used to treat it. Patients on levodopa who show little improvement may need to eat fewer protein foods, particularly at breakfast and lunch, and restrict pyridoxine (a B vitamin) to less than 5 milligrams a day. Drinking plenty of liquid should also help.

Parmesan: Although there are dozens of domestic Parmesan cheeses, they are salty, bitter, overbearing compared to **Parmigiano-Reggiano,** the Italian original from Parma and Reggio Emilia. This Parmesan is nut-sweet, the color of old ivory and superb eaten by the chunk or grated over everything from pasta to salad. It is even delicious as a dessert cheese. Parmesan is made of cow's milk, partially skimmed, then cooked, curded, compressed into chunky wheels and ripened. Mature at eighteen months, Parmesan is 31 percent protein and 25 percent fat. But a little of it goes a long way.

NUTRIENT CONTENT OF 1 OUNCE (28 GRAMS) PARMESAN	
111 calories	454 mg sodium
10 g protein	26 mg potassium
7 g fat, 5 saturated	0 g dietary fiber
19 mg cholesterol	42 RE vitamin A
1 g carbohydrate	0.01 mg thiamin
333 mg calcium	0.09 mg riboflavin
197 mg phosphorus	0 mg niacin
0 mg iron	0 mg vitamin C

NUTRIENT CONTENT OF 1 TABLESPOON GRATED PARMESAN

(about ¼ ounce; 7 grams)

28 calories	116 mg sodium
3 g protein	7 mg potassium
2 g fat, 1 saturated	0 g dietary fiber
5 mg cholesterol	11 RE vitamin A
0 g carbohydrate	0 mg thiamin
86 mg calcium	0.02 mg riboflavin
50 mg phosphorus	0 mg niacin
0 mg iron	0 mg vitamin C

Parsley: This first cousin to the carrot should be lavishly used instead of planted on plates as ruffs of green. **Flat-leaf Italian parsley** and the milder **curly parsley** are both flush with beta-carotene and vitamin C. The French had the right idea when they gelled gobs of parsley with bits of ham for that showy Easter classic *jambon persillé*. And Marylanders when they slashed their country hams and stuffed in fistfuls of finely minced parsley, spinach, watercress and scallions. **TIP:** To prolong the refrigerator life of parsley, trim off the stem ends with a sharp knife, cutting obliquely just as you would for long-stemmed roses. Stand the branches of parsley in a glass half filled with cold water, pop a plastic bag loosely on top and store in the refrigerator. Prepared this way, curly and flat-leaf parsley will keep fresh for a week to ten days.

**NUTRIENT CONTENT OF 2 SPRIGS PARSLEY
(1 TABLESPOON MINCED)**

(about ¹⁄₁₄ ounce; 2 grams)

1 calorie	1 mg sodium
0 g protein	11 mg potassium
0 g fat, 0 saturated	0 g dietary fiber
0 mg cholesterol	10 RE vitamin A
Trace carbohydrate	0 mg thiamin
3 mg calcium	0 mg riboflavin
1 mg phosphorus	0 mg niacin
0.1 mg iron	3 mg vitamin C

Parsley Root: Northern Europeans are partial to this ivory root, which looks like a dwarf parsnip. Parsley root is mellower, sweeter than leaf parsley and is usually added to soups and stews to add interest. But cooked and pureed, it perks up mashed potatoes no end (use about 1 part parsley root to 3 parts potatoes). It is becoming more available these days in American supermarkets. **SEASON:** Fall and winter. **NOTE:** Nutrient counts are unavailable for parsley roots, but they would approach those of turnips.

Parsnip: Looking like an anemic carrot, this pale but pungent root won't win any prizes for popularity. Yet it has its fans, New Englanders mostly, who find that the parsnip's carroty/turnipy flavor enlivens soups and stews. Some people like parsnips boiled and buttered, or mashed, or creamed. And very good these are. Parsnips may not contain the carrot's bounty of beta-carotene, but they are good sources of vitamin C, thiamin, phosphorus, fiber and potassium. Reason enough to put them on the menu. **SEASON:** October through January.

**NUTRIENT CONTENT OF 1 CUP BOILED/STEAMED
SLICED PARSNIPS**

(about 5½ ounces; 156 grams)

126 calories	16 mg sodium
2 g protein	573 mg potassium
0 g fat, 0 saturated	5 g dietary fiber
0 mg cholesterol	0 RE vitamin A
31 g carbohydrate	0.13 mg thiamin
58 mg calcium	0.08 mg riboflavin
107 mg phosphorus	1.1 mg niacin
0.9 mg iron	20 mg vitamin C

Partridge: The truth is, America has no true partridge although bobwhites and quails are sometimes called partridge. We do of course have GROUSE but not the partridge species of them.

Pasilla: See HOT PEPPERS under PEPPERS, CAPSICUMS.

Passion Fruit: This Brazilian native is not, as its name suggests, an aphrodisiac. As Elizabeth Schneider explains in her valuable book *Uncommon Fruits & Vegetables,* "passion" refers to the Passion of Christ, which someone early on thought its intricate purple-and-white flowers symbolized—cross, crown of thorns and all. Passion fruits—let's be honest—are ugly. The size and shape of limes, they are wizened when ripe and rusty purple (or ocher) depending on variety. Their shells are as stiff as parchment; their moist mustardy flesh is globular—like caviar. They're also riddled with crunchy black seeds no bigger than dust specks (small wonder the passion fruit is known in parts of the world as the **granadilla** or "little pomegranate"). But, oh, my, the flavor. Passion fruits are as perfumy as jasmine or gardenia, honeyed but with a welcome edge of tartness. Among America's trendy chefs, they are the fruit of the moment, nudging kiwis off the menu. Passion fruits also appear in upscale supermarkets but because most of them are imported from the ends of the earth (New Zealand, for example), they cost plenty. No matter; passion fruits are so intensely flavored it doesn't take much juice or puree to dominate a sauce, pudding, sherbet or ice cream. **SEASON:** Spring and early summer for the imports; late summer and fall for the Florida crop.

Pasta: Although it comes in dozens of shapes, classic golden Italian pasta contains two ingredients only—eggs and high-gluten durum flour, usually in the ratio of 3 to 2 (3 eggs to 2 or 2¼ cups flour). Not cheap. So big manufacturers often cut costs by adding fewer eggs to their pasta dough (sometimes none at all) and kneading in water until the consistency is perfect. Then there are the colored pastas: green (spinach), red (tomato), ocher (saffron), pink

NUTRIENT CONTENT OF 1 MEDIUM-SIZE PASSION FRUIT

(about ²⁄₃ ounce; 18 grams)

18 calories	5 mg sodium
0 g protein	63 mg potassium
0 g fat, 0 saturated	1 g dietary fiber
0 mg cholesterol	13 RE vitamin A
4 g carbohydrate	0 mg thiamin
2 g calcium	0.02 mg riboflavin
12 mg phosphorus	0 mg niacin
0.3 mg iron	5 mg vitamin C

Fusilli Primavera

Makes 4 Servings

1 tablespoon olive oil

4 scallions, including tops, minced

3 garlic cloves, minced

1 large carrot, peeled and diced

1 large red bell pepper, cored, seeded, and diced

2 cups broccoli florets

2 cups chopped ripe plum tomatoes (about 1 pound)

1 cup frozen peas, thawed

2 tablespoons chopped fresh basil, or 2 teaspoons dried basil plus 1 tablespoon minced fresh parsley

½ teaspoon salt

¼ teaspoon freshly ground black pepper

8 ounces fusilli, cooked according to package directions and drained

HEAT OIL FOR 1 minute in a large nonstick skillet over moderate heat. Add scallions and garlic, and cook, stirring occasionally, until softened, about 3 minutes. Mix in carrot and red pepper, and cook, stirring frequently, until softened, about 4 minutes. Add broccoli, stirring to coat, then stir in tomatoes and cook, uncovered, until sauce is lightly thickened and broccoli is tender, about 5 minutes. Stir in peas, basil, salt, and pepper and cook until peas are warmed through, about 2 minutes longer. Transfer to a large bowl and toss with the hot pasta. Serve with freshly grated Parmesan cheese, if you like.

APPROXIMATE NUTRIENT COUNTS PER SERVING

305 calories	55 g carbohydrate	3.7 mg iron	0.49 mg thiamin
11 g protein	7 g dietary fiber	341 mg sodium	0.29 mg riboflavin
5 g fat, 1 saturated	56 mg calcium	554 mg potassium	4.1 mg niacin
0 mg cholesterol	168 mg phosphorus	634 RE vitamin A	91 mg vitamin C

(beet), brown (mushroom) and black (squid ink). **NOTE:** Too little coloring is used to affect nutrient counts much. There is also a beige buckwheat pasta that's quite different (see PIZZOCCHERI).

When it comes to shape, the possibilities are as broad as the chef's imagination (some are now creating shadow prints by rolling whole herb leaves into lasagne and other broad pastas). Thirty years ago, the supermarket shopper had four or five types of pasta from which to choose: spaghetti and spaghettini (thin spaghetti), fettuccine and lasagne. Today the choices stretch the length of the aisle. There are **long, round pastas** of varying thickness (from angel hair to *bucatini,* the one with the hole in the middle that looks like a straw) and **long, flat ones** or **ribbons** (fettuccine, tagliatelle and pappardelle, to list from fine to broad). There are **tubes,** too (penne, *maccheroni* or macaroni, ziti and rigatoni). And no shortage of **fancy shapes** in a variety of sizes: farfalle (butterflies or bow ties), *conchiglie* (shells), *radiatori* (little radiators), fusilli (corkscrews), *gemelli* and *casareccia* (double-strand twists) and *ruote di carro* (little cartwheels). Then there's a huge assortment of **soup pastas:** alphabets; *quadrucci* (little squares); *semi, orzi* and *rizoni* (seed and rice shapes); *tubetti* and *ditali* (little tubes); *anelli* (rings of different sizes); *stelline* (little stars); *farfalline* (little bow ties); *funghetti* (little mushrooms) and *conchigliette* (little shells). And this is just for starters.

Finally, there are the **stuffed pastas,** many of which are freshly made and ready to cook: ravioli, tortellini, tortelloni and cappelletti (both little hats), lasagne, cannelloni and manicotti. The latest newcomer is an oven-ready lasagne that needs no boiling and no draining before it's layered into a casserole with cheese and tomato sauce and baked.

Why so many shapes? Italians know that shape determines sauce. For example, long pastas are best with olive oil and meatless tomato sauces. Ribbons and tubes team better with butter and cream sauces, fancy shapes with chunky meat or vegetable sauces because their hollows catch the chunks. Soup pastas—need it be said?—are for soup. Stuffed pastas may be floated in broth, tossed with melted butter and grated Parmesan or topped with smooth tomato sauces.

Pasteurization: A process of sterilization developed in France during the 1860s by Louis Pasteur. It was first used to keep wines and beers from spoiling. Around the turn of the century, U.S. food scientists began to pasteurize milk to reduce the incidence of undulant fever and tuberculosis. In the United States today all commercial milks and creams are pasteurized, meaning they are heated to 144°F., then held at that high temperature for half an hour. Or to save time, they may be heated to and held at 160°F. for 15 seconds (these milks and creams taste slightly caramelized or "cooked"). **Ultrapasteurization,** used primarily for heavy cream, subjects it to 280°F. for 1 second. It's a harsh process that changes the flavor of the cream and makes it much harder to whip. **TIP:** Ultrapasteurized cream will whip like a dream if you put it, the bowl and beater in the freezer for about 25 minutes.

Pastrami: A Jewish deli favorite that takes almost a month to make. First, beef plate or brisket is dry cured with salt and saltpeter (potassium nitrate) for three weeks, then smoked for up to twelve hours over hardwood chips or sawdust, then steamed several hours until tender. Pastrami is as red as corned beef and tastes something like it. Today there's even a **turkey pastrami,** which is lower in fat—but not sodium.

NUTRIENT CONTENT OF 3 OUNCES (85 GRAMS) BOILED EGG-FREE PASTA (WITHOUT SAUCE)	
105 calories	63 mg sodium
3 g protein	16 mg potassium
1 g fat, 0 saturated	1 g dietary fiber
0 mg cholesterol	0 RE vitamin A
21 g carbohydrate	0.15 mg thiamin
5 mg calcium	0.13 mg riboflavin
34 mg phosphorus	1 mg niacin
1.0 mg iron	0 mg vitamin C

NUTRIENT CONTENT OF 3 OUNCES (85 GRAMS) BEEF PASTRAMI	
297 calories	1,044 mg sodium
15 g protein	195 mg potassium
25 g fat, 9 saturated	0 g dietary fiber
78 mg cholesterol	0 RE vitamin A
3 g carbohydrate	0.09 mg thiamin
6 mg calcium	0.15 mg riboflavin
129 mg phosphorus	4.2 mg niacin
1.6 mg iron	3 mg vitamin C

NUTRIENT CONTENT OF 3 OUNCES (85 GRAMS) TURKEY PASTRAMI	
120 calories	888 mg sodium
16 g protein	221 mg potassium
5 g fat, 2 saturated	0 g dietary fiber
46 mg cholesterol	0 RE vitamin A
1 g carbohydrate	0.05 mg thiamin
8 mg calcium	0.21 mg riboflavin
170 mg phosphorus	3 mg niacin
1.4 mg iron	0 mg vitamin C

Pastry: There is butter-laden **puff pastry** (the classic ratio is 4½ pounds butter to 4 pounds flour), there is egg-rich **choux** or **cream-puff pastry** (1¼ pounds eggs and ½ pound butter to ¾ pound flour) and there is wispy-thin **phyllo pastry,** stacked up between slatherings of melted butter. But the one that concerns us here is old-fashioned **piecrust,** a more modest mix of flour, shortening and water. Hardly health food but not as ruinously rich as the first three. Basic one-crust recipes call for 1¼ cups flour, ⅓ cup shortening, ½ teaspoon salt and ¼ cup water; two-crust pies about twice that. Since both will be divided six or eight ways, the message is clear: Single-crust pies contain half the fat and calories and are obviously the better choice, especially when filled with fresh fruit.

NUTRIENT CONTENT OF ONE 9-INCH PIE SHELL (MADE WITH VEGETABLE SHORTENING)	
(about 6⅓ ounces; 180 grams)	
949 calories	976 mg sodium
12 g protein	121 mg potassium
62 g fat, 16 saturated	3 g dietary fiber
0 mg cholesterol	0 RE vitamin A
86 g carbohydrate	0.70 mg thiamin
18 mg calcium	0.50 mg riboflavin
121 mg phosphorus	6 mg niacin
5.2 mg iron	0 mg vitamin C

Note: These figures are for the entire pie shell. To determine per-serving counts, divide by 6 or 8—or however many times the pie is cut.

Pastry Flour: See FLOUR.

Pâté: Coarse or butter-smooth loaves made out of mixtures of liver (goose, duck, calf and/or pork), meat (usually pork) and assorted seasonings. They are served cold, thinly sliced, and most of them are as rich as all get out (saturated fat, cholesterol and calorie counts soar). Eat sparingly. There are also fish, vegetable and vegetarian pâtés that don't run to fat or cholesterol. **NOTE:** Recipes vary too much for meaningful nutrient counts. See also GOOSE LIVER.

Pathogen: A bacterium, virus, mold or other microorganism capable of causing disease.

Pattypan Squash: See SUMMER SQUASH.

Pawpaws: Some people call papayas pawpaws, but the two aren't remotely related. The pawpaw, which grows wild over much of the southeastern United States, is a member of the Annonaceae family, whose species number about six hundred. Most of them have edible fruits, among them the custard apples (cherimoyas), sweetsops, soursops and pawpaws. Pawpaws are ovoid, about 4 inches long and filled with flesh the color and consistency of custard. Their flavor melds cream, eggs, nutmeg and sugar, yet few people bother to eat pawpaws even though they're theirs for the picking. **SEASON:** Summer. **NOTE:** Nutrient counts are unavailable for pawpaws, but it's reasonable to say they'd approximate those of CHERIMOYA.

PBBs (Polybrominated Biphenyls): Chemical flame retardants that not only produce tumors in lab animals but also affect reproduction and liver function. In the early 1970s, thanks to a feed plant mishap, Michigan farmers unknowingly fed their livestock rations contaminated with PBBs. By the time the mistake was discovered, tainted meat, milk and eggs had reached the supermarket—and the consumer. What hadn't already been eaten was immediately destroyed—five million eggs, a million and a half chickens, thirty thousand cattle, fifteen thousand sheep and six thousand hogs. Ever since this costly mistake, the government has been tracking those affected to determine the impact on their health. To date no problems have surfaced, but the PBB watch continues.

PCBs (Polychlorinated Biphenyls): Nonbiodegradable industrial compounds used in the manufacture of everything from electronics to silo liners to recycled paper to food cartons. PCBs were synthesized early in this century and used right up until 1974, when their pollution of oceans, lakes and rivers and fish so alarmed the government they were banned. In the late 1960s, thousands of Japanese were poisoned by rice oil contaminated by PCBs that had oozed out of the machinery used to refine it. Some of the pregnant women who ate the PCBed oil delivered stillborns; others, babies with deformed fingernails, darkly pigmented skin, swollen eyelids.

Though no longer manufactured in the United States, PCBs still exist in older machinery and in major American waterways, among them the Great Lakes and the Mississippi and Hudson rivers, and they are virtually indestructible. (As someone said, "They have the half-life of infinity.") Scary thought. As long as PCBs pollute our waters, they contaminate our fish. The species most susceptible are "oily" fish whose fats are distributed throughout their flesh instead of being concentrated in their livers—the case with cod. These include Coho and Chinook salmon, lake trout, carp and other bottom feeders, and from inshore Atlantic waters, bluefish. Mother's milk also poses a risk because PCBs are stored in body fat, some of which goes into the production of breast milk.

Is there any way to reduce your exposure to PCBs? To some degree, yes. First, choose lean fish over fat (and only from the most reputable dealer). Second, cook the fish well because cooking destroys some of the PCBs. Third, broil or grill the fish so additional PCBs run off in the drippings. Finally, avoid eating fish skins and livers, where PCBs tend to concentrate.

P-Coumaric Acid: A natural compound recently isolated from tomatoes that seems to deactivate certain carcinogens in the body. See PHYTOCHEMICALS.

PEA (Phenylethylamine 192): A compound present in chocolate that arouses emotions. Or so some say because the body converts PEA into two neurotransmitters—epinephrine and norepinephrine, which do have the power to "turn you on." Maybe those old wives' tales about chocolate's being an aphrodisiac are right after all. On the other hand, maybe not. After stuffing themselves with chocolate, researchers at the National Institute of Mental Health found themselves headachy, *not* amorous.

Pea Beans: See BEANS, DRIED.

Peaches: Some say peaches came to Florida with the Spaniards; others to the Carolina colonies with the English. In either case, their arrival in America was roundabout. Indigenous to China, peaches have been grown there for thousands of years. Over time they made their way west to Persia and from there were carried farther west by the Romans. They, it's said, knew at least six kinds of peaches. Today there are thousands. Some are called **clingstones** (or clings) because their pits are hard to remove. Others are **freestones** with pits that pop right out. Peaches grow best in sandy soil at temperate climates, which explains why the bulk of our crop comes from California, Georgia, South Carolina and Washington State, although North Carolina and Michigan both grow plenty of them, too. Peaches are highly perishable and, once cut, quickly darken (a drizzling of lemon, lime or orange juice keeps them bright). Like apples, peaches are delicious eaten out of hand, sliced into compotes, cakes, puddings and pies. Un-

NUTRIENT CONTENT OF 1 MEDIUM-SIZE PEACH (PEELED)

(about 3 ounces; 87 grams)

37 calories	0 mg sodium
1 g protein	171 mg potassium
0 g fat, 0 saturated	2 g dietary fiber
0 mg cholesterol	47 RE vitamin A
10 g carbohydrate	0.02 mg thiamin
4 mg calcium	0.04 mg riboflavin
10 mg phosphorus	0.9 mg niacin
0.1 mg iron	6 mg vitamin C

NUTRIENT CONTENT OF 1 CUP SLICED CANNED PEACHES (IN HEAVY SYRUP)

(about 9 ounces; 256 grams)

189 calories	15 mg sodium
1 g protein	235 mg potassium
0 g fat, 0 saturated	3 g dietary fiber
0 mg cholesterol	85 RE vitamin A
51 g carbohydrate	0.03 mg thiamin
8 mg calcium	0.06 mg riboflavin
28 mg phosphorus	1.6 mg niacin
0.7 mg iron	7 mg vitamin C

like apples, they make splendid ice creams and sherbets. Peaches are low in calories but freighted with beta-carotene. **SEASON:** Late spring and summer.

NUTRIENT CONTENT OF 1 CUP SLICED CANNED PEACHES (IN JUICE)

(about 8¾ ounces; 248 grams)

109 calories	10 mg sodium
2 g protein	317 mg potassium
0 g fat, 0 saturated	2 g dietary fiber
0 mg cholesterol	94 RE vitamin A
29 g carbohydrate	0.02 mg thiamin
15 mg calcium	0.04 mg riboflavin
42 mg phosphorus	1.4 mg niacin
0.7 mg iron	9 mg vitamin C

Peanut Brittle: A crisp caramelized-sugar candy studded with peanuts. The molten syrup is poured onto marble slabs, then, when cold and hard, broken into manageable chunks. Peanut brittle, food historians believe, is an American invention that surfaced around the turn of the century. Its popularity has never waned.

NUTRIENT CONTENT OF 1 OUNCE (28 GRAMS) PEANUT BRITTLE

128 calories	128 mg sodium
2 g protein	59 mg potassium
5 g fat, 1 saturated	1 g dietary fiber
4 mg cholesterol	13 RE vitamin A
20 g carbohydrate	0.05 mg thiamin
9 mg calcium	0.02 mg riboflavin
31 mg phosphorus	1.0 mg niacin
0.4 mg iron	0 mg vitamin C

Peanut Butter: A St. Louis doctor first hit on the idea of churning peanuts to paste. A number of his patients had bad teeth, couldn't chew, and peanut butter was an easily swallowed, easily digested, high-protein food. That was in 1890. Fourteen years later peanut butter was being hustled as "health food" at the St. Louis Universal Exposition. And it was an immediate hit because people liked its mellow flavor and creamy texture. There was only one problem.

Peanut butter quickly separated into an ooze of oil and a grainy, not-very-spreadable "curd." Two decades later a California food packer learned to homogenize peanuts into a stable butter. Skippy Churned Peanut Butter, he called it. Today, most American homes have a jar of peanut butter at the ready—either the **creamy** or the **chunky** strewn with chopped roasted peanuts. According to recent figures, Americans scarf down more than three quarters of a billion pounds of peanut butter a year; that's nearly 3½ pounds per person. Most peanut butters contain salt, sweeteners and stabilizers, although modern labeling laws require that by weight they be 90 percent peanuts. Now peanut butter has gone light (or at least *lighter*). By subbing soy protein and corn syrup solids for some of the fat, two top brands have slashed overall fat content by 25 percent. So 1 tablespoon will contain 6 to 6.5 grams fat versus 8 or 8.5. **NOTE:** Ground-to-order "natural" peanut butters are more likely than the big name brands to contain aflatoxin, a powerful carcinogen produced by a mold that sometimes infects storage bins. See also AFLATOXIN.

NUTRIENT CONTENT OF 1 TABLESPOON PEANUT BUTTER

(about ½ ounce; 16 grams)

94 calories	76 mg sodium
4 g protein	115 mg potassium
8 g fat, 2 saturated	1 g dietary fiber
0 mg cholesterol	0 RE vitamin A
3 g carbohydrate	0.02 mg thiamin
6 mg calcium	0.02 mg riboflavin
52 mg phosphorus	2.1 mg niacin
0.3 mg iron	0 mg vitamin C

Peanut Oil: A pale golden oil extracted from peanuts. In Europe, Asia and America it is a popular cooking oil although some find its flavor too strong. Peanut oil is low in saturated fat, high in monounsaturates and polyunsaturates (for a specific profile, see OILS). Like other oils, peanut oil offers nothing more in the way of nutrients than fat and calories: 1 tablespoon peanut oil = 199 calories and 14 grams total fat (2 grams saturated).

Peanuts: They are legumes, not nuts (is this why they are called "pea" nuts?). Although slaves brought peanuts to Virginia plantations, these *gnuba* (or goober, from the

Angolan for "groundnut") had already made an earlier transatlantic voyage, this time eastward from Brazil to Africa in the holds of Portuguese ships. Fifteenth-century Portuguese navigators, still following the policies set forth by Prince Henry the Navigator half a century earlier, collected specimens of the plants they found on their travels. They carried peanuts not only to West Africa but also to their colonies in India, Indonesia and China. Although peanuts are difficult to grow (they die north of the thirty-sixth parallel, require sandy soil, abundant sun and moderate rain), Virginia, the Carolinas and Georgia provided the perfect habitat. Peanuts soon became popular throughout the South and were carried north by Yankee soldiers who'd acquired a taste for them during the Civil War.

But the man generally credited with spreading the "peanut gospel" is African-American George Washington Carver of Alabama's Tuskegee Institute. When the boll weevil killed "King Cotton" shortly after the Civil War, Carver urged farmers, big and small, black and white, to plant peanuts. Knowing that they were a healthful, high-energy food, he even developed dozens of recipes for using them—everything from soups to main dishes to desserts. Most people today, however, are happy just to munch roasted peanuts. They are a good source of protein, niacin, phosphorus and potassium, and although they're cholesterol free, they do run to fat (50 percent of it monounsaturated). There is good news, however. Plant breeders at the University of Florida in Gainesville have developed a new peanut—the Sunoleic 95R—with 80 percent monounsaturated fat, about the same as olives. These new "healthier" peanuts will be on the market soon. **A FINAL CAVEAT:** Beware of salted peanuts; they're loaded with sodium. Note, too, that dry-roasted peanuts are no lower in fat than the oil roasted.

NUTRIENT CONTENT OF 1 OUNCE (28 GRAMS) DRY-ROASTED PEANUTS (UNSALTED)	
166 calories	2 mg sodium
7 g protein	187 mg potassium
14 g fat, 2 saturated	2 g dietary fiber
0 mg cholesterol	0 RE vitamin A
6 g carbohydrate	0.12 mg thiamin
15 mg calcium	0.03 mg riboflavin
102 mg phosphorus	3.8 mg niacin
0.6 mg iron	0 mg vitamin C

NUTRIENT CONTENT OF 1 OUNCE (28 GRAMS) OIL-ROASTED PEANUTS (SALTED)	
165 calories	123 mg sodium
7 g protein	193 mg potassium
14 g fat, 2 saturated	3 g dietary fiber
0 mg cholesterol	0 RE vitamin A
5 g carbohydrate	0.07 mg thiamin
25 mg calcium	0.03 mg riboflavin
146 mg phosphorus	4 mg niacin
0.5 mg iron	0 mg vitamin C

Note: Unbelievable as it may seem, oil-roasted peanuts contain about the same amount of fat as dry roasted. They are roasted under pressure, which forces out 60 to 80 percent of their fat, offsetting the amount added during cooking.

Pearl Onions: See ONIONS.

Pears: **Anjou . . . Bartlett . . . Bosc . . . Comice . . . Seckel . . . Winter Nelis.** These are only six of the hundreds of varieties of pears. But they are the six best—and best known—in the United States. Pears are not a New World food. Food historians speculate whether they originated in central Eurasia. Or in China. There is no debate, however, about which country grows the finest pears. France. Or which country does them most proud. France again. French trappers introduced pears to the Iroquois, who took to them straight away. Spanish friars traveling the old mission trail north in California planted pears there. And the English brought them to Massachusetts (one planted there in 1630 was still standing 250 years later). Because eastern orchards were decimated by fire blight, America's finest pears grow on the West Coast and most of the orchards are given over to Bartletts, every artist's image of the perfect pear: long-necked but plump-bottomed, symmetrical, chartreuse of skin and pearly of flesh. When it comes to flavor, however, the Comice wins. Known as the Queen of Pears, it is, writes Waverley Root in *Food,* "sweetly and subtly perfumed . . . so soft it is best eaten with a spoon, a tenderness more appealing to gourmets than to those who have to pick, ship, handle and store it in constant fear of ruinous spoilage." By comparison, Bartletts are crisp and bland, Anjous sweet but firm, Boscs dryish and grainy, the Winter Nelis spicy and the Seckel gritty (not for nothing is it called "sand pear"). As for food value, pears are just a shade less nutritious than apples. Still, they contain more fiber than apples—and, alas, more calories, too. **SEASON:** Year-round, with different varieties coming to market at different times. Bartletts peak between July and November, Seckels from September through December, the Comice between October and April, the Anjou and Winter Nelis from October through May or June.

NUTRIENT CONTENT OF 1 MEDIUM-SIZE PEAR
(about 5¾ ounces; 166 grams)

98 calories	0 mg sodium
1 g protein	108 mg potassium
1 g fat, 0 saturated	5 g dietary fiber
0 mg cholesterol	3 RE vitamin A
25 g carbohydrate	0.03 mg thiamin
18 mg calcium	0.07 mg riboflavin
18 mg phosphorus	0.2 mg niacin
0.4 mg iron	7 mg vitamin C

NUTRIENT CONTENT OF 1 CUP SLICED CANNED PEARS (IN HEAVY SYRUP)
(about 9 ounces; 255 grams)

188 calories	13 mg sodium
1 g protein	165 mg potassium
0 g fat, 0 saturated	5 g dietary fiber
0 mg cholesterol	1 RE vitamin A
49 g carbohydrate	0.03 mg thiamin
13 mg calcium	0.06 mg riboflavin
18 mg phosphorus	0.6 mg niacin
0.6 mg iron	3 mg vitamin C

NUTRIENT CONTENT OF 1 CUP SLICED CANNED PEARS (IN JUICE)
(about 8¾ ounces; 248 grams)

124 calories	10 mg sodium
1 g protein	238 mg potassium
0 g fat, 0 saturated	5 g dietary fiber
0 mg cholesterol	2 RE vitamin A
32 g carbohydrate	0.03 mg thiamin
22 mg calcium	0.03 mg riboflavin
30 mg phosphorus	0.5 mg niacin
0.7 mg iron	4 mg vitamin C

Peas: Archaeologists have found peas on the Thai-Burmese border and carbon-dated them to 9750 B.C. They have found less prehistoric but still ancient peas at Troy

and in Swiss lake mud, which seems to trace their trek from Central Asia, where they are believed to have originated, into Europe. A twelfth-century A.D. inventory shows that among the provisions of the Barking Nunnery near London were "green peas for Lent." **English peas,** they came to be known, as well as **green peas** and **garden peas.** But there are other varieties of peas: **field peas,** which are dried both whole and split; **chickpeas** or **garbanzo beans** (see BEANS, DRIED); **snow peas** (those ex-

NUTRIENT CONTENT OF 1 CUP BOILED/STEAMED GREEN PEAS
(about 5¾ ounces; 160 grams)

134 calories	5 mg sodium
9 g protein	434 mg potassium
0 g fat, 0 saturated	8 g dietary fiber
0 mg cholesterol	96 RE vitamin A
25 g carbohydrate	0.41 mg thiamin
43 mg calcium	0.24 mg riboflavin
187 mg phosphorus	3.2 mg niacin
2.5 mg iron	23 mg vitamin C

NUTRIENT CONTENT OF 1 CUP BOILED/STEAMED SNOW PEAS OR SUGAR SNAPS
(about 5¾ ounces; 160 grams)

67 calories	6 mg sodium
5 g protein	384 mg potassium
0 g fat, 0 saturated	4 g dietary fiber
0 mg cholesterol	21 RE vitamin A
11 g carbohydrate	0.23 mg thiamin
67 mg calcium	0.14 mg riboflavin
88 mg phosphorus	3.0 mg niacin
3.2 mg iron	77 mg vitamin C

NUTRIENT CONTENT OF 1 CUP BOILED DRIED SPLIT GREEN PEAS
(about 7 ounces; 196 grams)

231 calories	4 mg sodium
16 g protein	710 mg potassium
1 g fat, 0 saturated	10 g dietary fiber
0 mg cholesterol	2 RE vitamin A
41 g carbohydrate	0.37 mg thiamin
27 mg calcium	0.11 mg riboflavin
194 mg phosphorus	1.7 mg niacin
2.5 mg iron	1 mg vitamin C

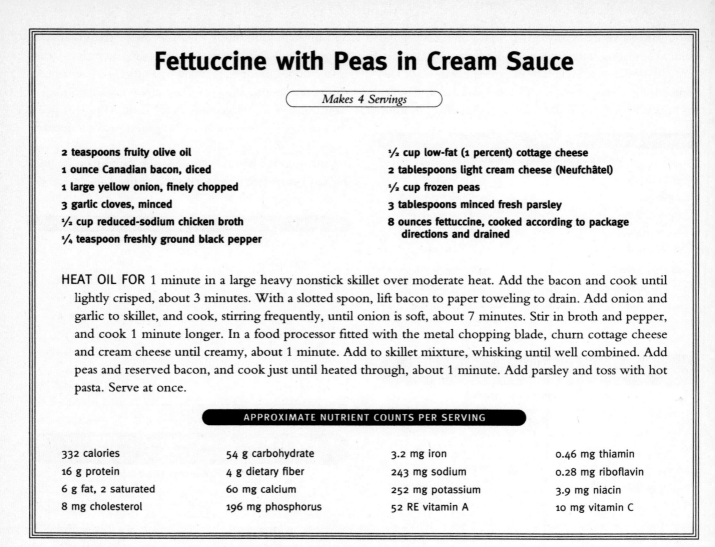

Fettuccine with Peas in Cream Sauce

Makes 4 Servings

2 teaspoons fruity olive oil

1 ounce Canadian bacon, diced

1 large yellow onion, finely chopped

3 garlic cloves, minced

½ cup reduced-sodium chicken broth

¼ teaspoon freshly ground black pepper

½ cup low-fat (1 percent) cottage cheese

2 tablespoons light cream cheese (Neufchâtel)

½ cup frozen peas

3 tablespoons minced fresh parsley

8 ounces fettuccine, cooked according to package directions and drained

HEAT OIL FOR 1 minute in a large heavy nonstick skillet over moderate heat. Add the bacon and cook until lightly crisped, about 3 minutes. With a slotted spoon, lift bacon to paper toweling to drain. Add onion and garlic to skillet, and cook, stirring frequently, until onion is soft, about 7 minutes. Stir in broth and pepper, and cook 1 minute longer. In a food processor fitted with the metal chopping blade, churn cottage cheese and cream cheese until creamy, about 1 minute. Add to skillet mixture, whisking until well combined. Add peas and reserved bacon, and cook just until heated through, about 1 minute. Add parsley and toss with hot pasta. Serve at once.

APPROXIMATE NUTRIENT COUNTS PER SERVING

332 calories	54 g carbohydrate	3.2 mg iron	0.46 mg thiamin
16 g protein	4 g dietary fiber	243 mg sodium	0.28 mg riboflavin
6 g fat, 2 saturated	60 mg calcium	252 mg potassium	3.9 mg niacin
8 mg cholesterol	196 mg phosphorus	52 RE vitamin A	10 mg vitamin C

quisitely sweet-crisp pods that take only minutes to cook); and **sugar snaps,** the newest entry, which resemble the French *mange-tout* and like them are eaten pod and all. They are sugary, crunchy—and almost as much a fad today as green peas were at the court of Louis XIV. "It is both a fashion and a madness," wrote Madame de Maintenon of the green-pea craze at the French court. As their sweetness suggests, green peas are a good source of carbohydrate. They also contain plenty of vitamins (A, C, thiamin, riboflavin and niacin) as well as impressive complements of phosphorus, iron and potassium. **SEASON:** March through July for green peas and sugar snaps, year-round for snow peas. Field peas are dried and available year-round.

Pecans: The pecan is an all-American nut; indeed, *pecan* is a Native American word. The pecan belongs to the hickory family. And like the hickory, it grows wild throughout the Southeast and as far west as Texas. Botanists believe the pecan may have originated in Texas, although Georgia tops it today in tons harvested. Strangely, pecans have never caught on in Europe, where hazelnuts and walnuts remain the nuts of choice. No matter. This means more

NUTRIENT CONTENT OF 1 OUNCE (28 GRAMS) PECAN HALVES

189 calories	0 mg sodium
2 g protein	111 mg potassium
19 g fat, 2 saturated	2 g dietary fiber
0 mg cholesterol	4 RE vitamin A
5 g carbohydrate	0.24 mg thiamin
10 mg calcium	0.04 mg riboflavin
82 mg phosphorus	0.3 mg niacin
0.6 mg iron	1 mg vitamin C

pecans for us home folks, more butter pecan ice cream, more pecan pralines, more pecan sandies, more pecan fudge and brownies. Pecans are so high in fat (about 70 percent) that their oil can be pressed right out. It's sweet and mellow, superb in green salads or drizzled over steamed asparagus, broccoli or cauliflower.

Pectin (additive): Complex carbohydrate extracted from apple pulp and citrus rinds that has the capacity to gel. Food processors use pectin to thicken and stabilize candies, syrups and frozen desserts as well as to set jellies, jams and preserves. Available to the home cook in liquid and powder form, pectin not only shortcuts jelly making but also means that nearly everything can be turned into quivery *gelées*—delicate herb or flower infusions as well as a nearly endless list of fruits and fruit juices. GRAS.

Pellagra: An acute niacin deficiency disease characterized by dermatitis, diarrhea and dementia. Once prevalent in the American South, especially among the poor who subsisted mostly upon highly refined cornmeal breads, it is very nearly a thing of the past. See also NIACIN.

Penicillin: A family of blue-green MOLDS. Some are powerful antibiotics; others are essential for the ripening of such cheeses as Camembert, Roquefort, Gorgonzola and Stilton.

Pepinos: Melon-pears with a curious cucumber/pear flavor. The Japanese love their delicacy, although they've won few fans here. They are now being imported from New Zealand and making occasional appearances at avant-garde greengrocers. If you should see them, give them a try. Eat out of hand like an apple, serve as you would honeydew with tissues of prosciutto or slip into a fruit compote. **SEASON:** Late winter through spring. **NOTE:** Specific nutrient counts are unavailable for pepinos, but their sunny gold flesh suggests that they're high in beta-carotene. And because they're neither buttery nor very sweet, it's safe to say that they are low in calories.

Pepitas: Pumpkin seeds. Once the province of health-food stores, hulled, roasted pepitas, both salted and unsalted, are now sold by the bag in many supermarkets. Go for the *unsalted* and look for them in the nut section. Pepitas taste somewhat like nuts, although they are less but-tery and have a musty aftertaste. They can be eaten out of hand, stirred into quick breads, tossed with dry cereals, even ground to paste and used, as Mexican women have done since pre-Columbian days, to thicken gravies and sauces.

NUTRIENT CONTENT OF 1 OUNCE (28 GRAMS) ROASTED PEPITAS (UNSALTED)

126 calories	5 mg sodium
5 g protein	260 mg potassium
5 g fat, 1 saturated	10 g dietary fiber
0 mg cholesterol	2 RE vitamin A
15 g carbohydrate	0.01 mg thiamin
16 mg calcium	0.02 mg riboflavin
26 mg phosphorus	0.1 mg niacin
0.9 mg iron	0 mg vitamin C

Pepper, Black and White: For this spice men scrambled to find the water route to its source, Columbus bumbling out into the Atlantic, convinced that the East Indies lay west of Europe, and the Portuguese Vasco da Gama, rounding the tip of South Africa, crossing the Indian Ocean, and bingo! For years the Portuguese ruled the pepper trade, then the Dutch wrested it from them, then the British snatched it from the Dutch. In medieval days, peppercorns fetched more than their weight in gold. They were the stuff of dowries, of bribes, of rents and taxes. All because they were rare—and made bland food exciting.

Black and white pepper both come from *Piper nigrum,* a vine native to Malaysia or India that produces catkins of fifty berries or more. Green when picked, the berries first turn red, then yellow, then brown, then black. And from smooth to wrinkled. White pepper, nothing more than black pepper stripped of its dark husk, is the milder of the two. In Europe, it is every cook's preference. Pepper owes its faintly lemony/cardamomy flavor to a volatile oil, its fire to an oleoresin.

But pepper does more than add flavor and fire. It increases the flow of saliva and gastric juices and actually cools the body (is this why incendiary dishes are so popular in steamy climates?). Because the amounts of pepper used in cooking rarely exceed a pinch or two, its nutritional content is of little consequence. Still, there is a nutritional plus: Clever use of pepper makes it possible to cut down on salt.

Peppercorns, Green: Unripe black peppercorns. Available dry or canned (wet), these have more flavor, less bite than mature pepper.

Peppercorns, Pink: These brittle peppercorns are wholly unrelated to true pepper. They are the dried berries of the Baies rose imported from Madagascar by way of France. When they first burst upon the culinary scene in the early 1980s, chefs used them every which way. Then word spread that they might be poisonous. After much controversy, the FDA has declared Baies rose peppercorns safe. **CAUTION:** A pink peppercorn grown in Florida, another species altogether, may trigger allergic reactions. Read the fine print.

Peppergrass: A delicate cress (also called **shepherd's purse** and **garden cress**), usually sold sprouted, by the box. Just a handful tossed into a green salad adds warmth and bite, not to mention a hefty dose of beta-carotene. **SEASON:** Spring and summer.

NUTRIENT CONTENT OF 1 CUP PEPPERGRASS	
(about 1¾ ounces; 50 grams)	
16 calories	7 mg sodium
1 g protein	302 mg potassium
0 g fat, 0 saturated	2 g dietary fiber
0 mg cholesterol	466 RE vitamin A
3 g carbohydrate	0.04 mg thiamin
41 mg calcium	0.13 mg riboflavin
38 mg phosphorus	0.5 mg niacin
0.7 mg iron	35 mg vitamin C

Peppermint Oil (additive): Extracted from dried mint leaves, oil of peppermint is used to flavor everything from candies to cordials to chewing gums to baked goods and beverages. Though it can trigger bouts of sneezing, skin rashes and even irregular heartbeat in those who are allergic to it, peppermint oil is rated GRAS when used within FDA guidelines.

Pepperoni: A highly spiced, air-cured, hard, dry Italian sausage sold in links a foot long or more. The mix is part beef, part pork. But there are flecks of fat, too, and no stinting on garlic or hot red pepper. Two popular ways to eat pepperoni: sliced on top of pizza or slipped into hero sandwiches. Both are good ways to run up the calories, saturated fat, cholesterol and salt.

NUTRIENT CONTENT OF 1 OUNCE (28 GRAMS) PEPPERONI	
140 calories	577 mg sodium
6 g protein	98 mg potassium
13 g fat, 5 saturated	0 g dietary fiber
22 mg cholesterol	0 RE vitamin A
1 g carbohydrate	0.09 mg thiamin
3 mg calcium	0.07 mg riboflavin
34 mg phosphorus	1.4 mg niacin
0.4 mg iron	0 mg vitamin C

Peppers, Capsicums: Columbus's great pepper hunt wasn't a total bust. He didn't find *Piper nigrum* in the New World, but he did find something equally valuable. As he wrote his Spanish sponsors, King Ferdinand and Queen Isabella, the natives weathered the chill of high island altitudes "with the aid of the meat they eat with very hot spices."

He called these "spices" pepper—as we do yet—although they are actually capsicums. Not even distant cousins of true pepper, these fleshy pods include hundreds of varieties ranging in temperature from cool to combustible. Not surprisingly, hot peppers were what impressed the Europeans.

Hot Peppers: Here, too, the varieties seem endless. And confusing. Which are explosive? Hot? Or merely tepid? Here's a tip. With few exceptions, the smaller the pepper

NUTRIENT CONTENT OF 1 MEDIUM-SIZE FRESH GREEN JALAPEÑO PEPPER	
(about 1⅔ ounces; 45 grams)	
18 calories	3 mg sodium
1 g protein	153 mg potassium
0 g fat, 0 saturated	1 g dietary fiber
0 mg cholesterol	35 RE vitamin A
4 g carbohydrate	0.04 mg thiamin
8 mg calcium	0.04 mg riboflavin
21 mg phosphorus	0.4 mg niacin
0.5 mg iron	108 mg vitamin C

NUTRIENT CONTENT OF 1 MEDIUM-SIZE FRESH RED JALAPEÑO PEPPER

(about 1²/₃ ounces; 45 grams)

18 calories	3 mg sodium
1 g protein	153 mg potassium
0 g fat, 0 saturated	1 g dietary fiber
0 mg cholesterol	484 RE vitamin A
4 g carbohydrate	0.04 mg thiamin
8 mg calcium	0.04 mg riboflavin
21 mg phosphorus	0.4 mg niacin
0.5 mg iron	109 mg vitamin C

or the more sharply pointed, the hotter it will be. There is also a 1 to 10 (cool to incendiary) scale for measuring the heat of peppers based on Scoville units developed in 1912 by a Parke-Davis pharmacologist named Wilbur L. Scoville. Today's test is high tech, a 1980 refining of the original method that can measure capsaicin (the hot stuff) to within 2 parts per million. **SEASON:** Year-round.

Sweet Peppers: These **bells** of all colors (green, gold, orange, red, purple), the sweet **pimientos** and pale yellow-green sweet **banana peppers** all rate zero on the heat scale, meaning they're as tepid as tomatoes. Most

MEASURING THE HEAT OF COMMON HOT PEPPERS

Fresh Peppers	Rating	Scoville Units
Sweet cherry peppers, Mexi-Bells, chile pimientos, sweet purple	1	100–500
NuMex Big Jim	2	500–1,000
Anaheim green or red peppers, Hungarian cherry peppers	2–3	500–1,500
Green or red poblanos, Española	3	1,000–1,500
Chawa, New Mexico red chile	3–4	1,000–2,500
New Mexico green chile	3–5	1,000–5,000
Sandia	4	1,500–2,500
Red or green de agua	4–5	1,500–5,000
Güero (Santa Fe Grande)	4.5–6.5	2,000–22,000
Red or green jalapeño	5	2,500–5,000
Red or green serrano, yellow wax hot, Dutch red chile, Fresno (red)	6	5,000–15,000
Fiesta, Fips	6–8	5,000–50,000
De Arbol, Korean	7	15,000–30,000
Aji, cayenne, pequin, rocoto, tabasco, tepín, Thai	8	30,000–50,000
Chiltepein, Jamaican hot, malagueta (piri-piri)	9	50,000–100,000
Scotch bonnet	9–10	50,000–200,000
Habanero	10	100,000–300,000

Dried Peppers	Rating	Scoville Units
NuMex eclipse, NuMex sunrise, NuMex sunset, New Mexico miniatures	2–3	500–1,500
New Mexico red chile	2–4	500–2,500
Ancho and mulato (dried poblanos), Hungarian cherry peppers	3	1,000–1,500
New Mexico green chile, pasilla	3–5	1,000–5,000
Pasado, pepperoncini	5	2,500–5,000
Chipotle (dried, smoked jalapeño)	5–6	2,500–15,000
Chiltepin	6	5,000–15,000
Serrano seco	7–8	15,000–50,000
Cayenne, pequin, tabasco, tepín	8	30,000–50,000
Malagueta (piri-piri)	9	50,000–100,000
Habanero	10	100,000–300,000

are fleshy and mellow and, weight for weight, can be used interchangeably in recipes. **SEASON:** Year-round.

When it comes to food value, a pepper's color is more of an indicator than its coolness or heat. The red and orange, for example, brim with beta-carotene, and though deep green peppers are a respectable source of it, too, they're no match for their redder, riper relatives. All peppers—except the dried—are good sources of vitamin C. And all, make a note, are fat and cholesterol free and extremely low in calories and sodium.

NUTRIENT CONTENT OF 1 MEDIUM-SIZE FRESH SWEET GREEN PEPPER	
(about 2⅔ ounces; 74 grams)	
20 calories	1 mg sodium
1 g protein	131 mg potassium
0 g fat, 0 saturated	1 g dietary fiber
0 mg cholesterol	47 RE vitamin A
5 g carbohydrate	0.05 mg thiamin
7 mg calcium	0.02 mg riboflavin
14 mg phosphorus	0.4 mg niacin
0.3 mg iron	66 mg vitamin C

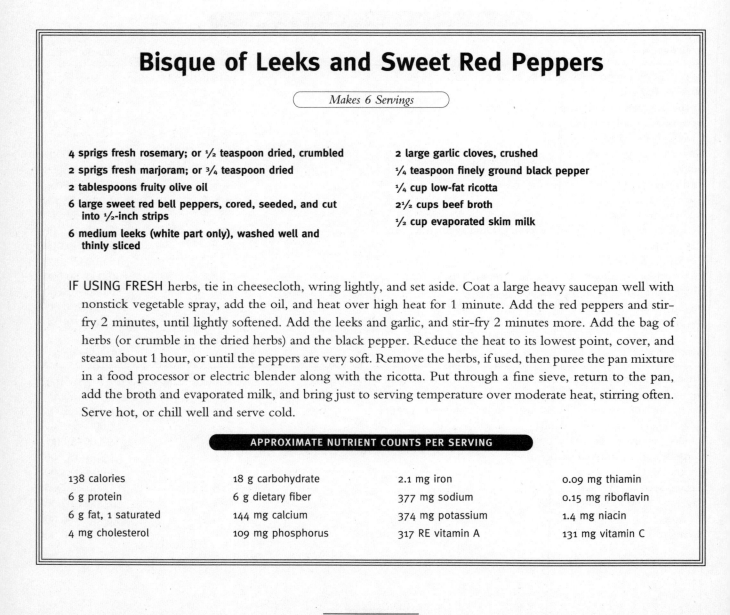

Bisque of Leeks and Sweet Red Peppers

Makes 6 Servings

4 sprigs fresh rosemary; or ½ teaspoon dried, crumbled

2 sprigs fresh marjoram; or ¾ teaspoon dried

2 tablespoons fruity olive oil

6 large sweet red bell peppers, cored, seeded, and cut into ½-inch strips

6 medium leeks (white part only), washed well and thinly sliced

2 large garlic cloves, crushed

¼ teaspoon finely ground black pepper

¼ cup low-fat ricotta

2½ cups beef broth

½ cup evaporated skim milk

IF USING FRESH herbs, tie in cheesecloth, wring lightly, and set aside. Coat a large heavy saucepan well with nonstick vegetable spray, add the oil, and heat over high heat for 1 minute. Add the red peppers and stir-fry 2 minutes, until lightly softened. Add the leeks and garlic, and stir-fry 2 minutes more. Add the bag of herbs (or crumble in the dried herbs) and the black pepper. Reduce the heat to its lowest point, cover, and steam about 1 hour, or until the peppers are very soft. Remove the herbs, if used, then puree the pan mixture in a food processor or electric blender along with the ricotta. Put through a fine sieve, return to the pan, add the broth and evaporated milk, and bring just to serving temperature over moderate heat, stirring often. Serve hot, or chill well and serve cold.

APPROXIMATE NUTRIENT COUNTS PER SERVING

138 calories	18 g carbohydrate	2.1 mg iron	0.09 mg thiamin
6 g protein	6 g dietary fiber	377 mg sodium	0.15 mg riboflavin
6 g fat, 1 saturated	144 mg calcium	374 mg potassium	1.4 mg niacin
4 mg cholesterol	109 mg phosphorus	317 RE vitamin A	131 mg vitamin C

NUTRIENT CONTENT OF 1 MEDIUM-SIZE FRESH SWEET RED PEPPER

(about 2²/₃ ounces; 74 grams)

20 calories	1 mg sodium
1 g protein	131 mg potassium
0 g fat, 0 saturated	1 g dietary fiber
0 mg cholesterol	422 RE vitamin A
5 g carbohydrate	0.05 mg thiamin
7 mg calcium	0.02 mg riboflavin
14 mg phosphorus	0.4 mg niacin
0.3 mg iron	141 mg vitamin C

NUTRIENT CONTENT OF ¼ CUP CANNED PIMIENTOS

(about 1³/₄ ounces; 48 grams)

11 calories	7 mg sodium
1 g protein	76 mg potassium
0 g fat, 0 saturated	1 g dietary fiber
0 mg cholesterol	128 RE vitamin A
2 g carbohydrate	0.01 mg thiamin
3 mg calcium	0.03 mg riboflavin
8 mg phosphorus	0.3 mg niacin
0.8 mg iron	41 mg vitamin C

Pepsin: An enzyme produced both by the pyloric and gastric glands that helps digest proteins in the acid environment of the stomach.

Peptic Ulcers (diet and): Painful lesions in the lining of the stomach (**gastric ulcers**) or of the duodenum or upper part of the small intestine (**duodenal ulcers**). Until recently no one knew what caused ulcers although stress was believed to play a greater role than diet. In any case, ulcers develop like this: First come weak spots in the lining of the stomach or duodenum, a baring of inner cells that have no mucous coating to protect them. These lesions are at the mercy of gastric juices (hydrochloric acid and pepsin), which eat at them, then burn into capillaries, causing the ulcers to bleed. Then, if unchecked, erode the wall of the stomach or duodenum, leading to perforated ulcers. Medical researchers once thought people might be genetically predisposed to ulcers. That they ran in families. Today there's a whole new theory about what causes peptic ulcers. Not that stress, poor diet, smoking and alcohol no

longer play roles. But the true culprit, medical researchers now believe, is a corkscrew-shaped bacterium (spirochete) called *Helicobacter pylori*. Physicians treating ulcers with a combination of antacids and antibacterials report a patient relapse rate of less than 20 percent. Compare that with the 50 percent rate of recurrence (after six months) and 95 percent (after two years) for those taking antacids only. Pretty convincing evidence against *H. pylori*. Now there's an even newer wrinkle. Recent studies at Washington University School of Medicine in St. Louis suggest that people with type O blood are more susceptible to *H. pylori* and thus to gastric ulcers and possibly to stomach cancer as well.

Where, then, does diet fit in? Instead of putting ulcer patients on a strict regimen of pap or bland soft foods (once standard treatment), most dietitians now recommend three to six regular meals a day. They also urge patients to avoid coffee (decaf as well as regular), alcohol and any foods that cause discomfort. These vary from person to person. Usually, trial and error will quickly identify problem foods.

Peptide, Peptide Linkage: Peptides are formed as the body breaks proteins down into simpler, more easily digested compounds. A **dipeptide** consists of two linked amino acids; a **polypeptide** of a larger number of them. The peptide linkage is the molecular "glue" that holds amino acids together.

Peptones (additives): By-products of protein digestion used to stabilize the foam in beer and to condition the doughs of baked goods. GRAS.

Perch: A market term for a group of lean freshwater fish with delicate but firm white flesh. These include the **yellow perch** (half-pounders that swim brackish lakes and ponds from Nova Scotia to the Carolinas) and the **white** (a small carnivorous drum or bass that also prefers temperate, brackish waters). Both fish are best when poached, sautéed or baked. For approximate nutrient counts, see FISH, LEAN WHITE.

Periodontal Disease: Gingivitis, pyorrhea or other gum disease that can lead to tooth loss. Vigilant brushing and flossing can help prevent it, as can swearing off sticky sweets that promote plaque buildup and tooth decay. See DENTAL HEALTH.

Peristalsis: The waves of stop/start muscular contractions that begin in the esophagus and spread, like rings radiating from a pebble dropped in a pond, the length of the digestive tract. Peristalsis is what moves food along during the process of digestion and, in the end, rids the body of waste.

Pernicious Anemia: A severe form of anemia caused by the body's inability to absorb vitamin B_{12}, which in turn frees folic acid (another B vitamin), which is essential to the manufacture of healthy red blood cells. At fault: a lack of INTRINSIC FACTOR. In healthy people, the stomach produces intrinsic factor. It piggybacks on B_{12}; the two pass into the small intestine, from which the B_{12} is absorbed and dispatched to do its appointed work. The standard treatment for pernicious anemia? B_{12} shots.

Peroxides (additives): **Benzoyl peroxide, calcium peroxide** and **hydrogen peroxide** are used, respectively, for bleaching cheese, flour and oil; for conditioning bread dough; and as an antioxidant and starch modifier. Hydrogen peroxide is also used as a preservative in milk and other dairy foods. Peroxides are strong stuff (they can harm the eyes and skin) and the FDA has put them on its "must review" list.

Persian Melons: See MELONS.

Persimmons: These are the small, wild persimmons of the American South, fruits no bigger than Ping-Pong balls that are superbly sweet when ripe. But woes be if you bite into a green one. It is so tannic it will turn your mouth inside out. More familiar, perhaps, are the big, orange, heart-shaped Japanese persimmons, a major California

NUTRIENT CONTENT OF 1 LARGE JAPANESE PERSIMMON	
(about 6 ounces; 168 grams)	
117 calories	2 mg sodium
1 g protein	270 mg potassium
0 g fat, 0 saturated	3 g dietary fiber
0 mg cholesterol	365 RE vitamin A
31 g carbohydrate	0.05 mg thiamin
13 mg calcium	0.03 mg riboflavin
29 mg phosphorus	0.2 mg niacin
0.3 mg iron	13 mg vitamin C

crop. Their flesh is soft, buttery and as sweet as honey. Whole, they can be sliced or diced and slipped into compotes, puddings and pies. Pureed, they can be substituted, measure for measure, for solid-pack pumpkin in any quick bread, cake, cookie or pie (so can the little wild persimmons). Given their vermilion color, Japanese persimmons are chockablock with beta-carotene. They are also good sources of potassium and vitamin C, yet they are low in calories and sodium. The nutritional profile of wild persimmons is less impressive, but they are yours for the picking and contain enough vitamin C to matter. **SEASON:** Late fall and winter for both persimmons. Gather the wild after the first hard frost.

NUTRIENT CONTENT OF 1 MEDIUM-SIZE WILD PERSIMMON	
(about 1 ounce; 25 grams)	
32 calories	0 mg sodium
0 g protein	78 mg potassium
0 g fat, 0 saturated	0 g dietary fiber
0 mg cholesterol	NA RE vitamin A
8 g carbohydrate	NA mg thiamin
7 mg calcium	NA mg riboflavin
7 mg phosphorus	NA mg niacin
0.6 mg iron	17 mg vitamin C

Pesticides: See HERBICIDES, PESTICIDES.

Pests: Ants, mice, rats, roaches and weevils plague the home cook as well as the restaurant chef, supermarket manager, food processor and farmer. At any stage down the line pests can destroy and/or contaminate food. One way to control them is by using pesticides (see HERBICIDES, PESTICIDES). But the homemaker has safer options. Ants, mice, roaches and weevils are crazy for sugars, starches, flours, cereals and other grains, even certain dried herbs and spices (for some reason, chile-pepper flakes and paprika are popular breeding grounds).

The first step is to avoid buying any foods that look infested—those with ripped bags, torn or unglued cartons. So far, so good. Once home, these foods require special attention before they go on kitchen or pantry shelf. Don't just stow the cartons. Instead, lock pests out—or, once in a great while, *in* (weevils sometimes lay eggs in grains and flours, and when these hatch, look out!). Half-gallon, quart, pint and half-pint screw-top preserving jars make marvelous minisilos because they not only keep "livestock" at bay but also showcase the food inside. If the jars are tightly sealed and kept in a cool, dark, dry spot, the sugars, starches, flours, cereals, grains, herbs and spices will keep for months—with nary a pest in sight. TIP: Always clip the how-to-cook label info and tuck inside the proper jar so you can grab it in a hurry.

Syrups, honeys and molasses also present problems. But a little tidy housekeeping keeps them pest free, too. Carefully rinse and dry the bottles after each use, paying particular attention to the lids and screwing threads. Regularly check shelves, too, and wipe away any dribbles.

Pewter: An alloy of tin and lead once commonly used for drinking mugs and tableware. Because lead is highly toxic and there's some danger of its leaching from container to food or drink, pewter is best used for show.

pH: It stands for "potential hydrogen." The pH scale is used in the chemistry lab to measure acidity—and in food and beverages, among other things. On this 1 to 14 scale, a pH of 7 is neutral—neither acidic nor basic (alkaline). The lower the number (pH), the more acidic something is; the higher the number, the more alkaline. When it comes to food, vinegars are acidic; so are most fruits and berries. Tomatoes used to be, but some modern varieties seem to have had the acid bred out of them. Meat, fish, fowl and most vegetables are low acid, neutral or even, sometimes, a shade alkaline—an important consideration when these foods are canned. The microorganisms of spoilage do not grow in acid mediums, which is why canned fruits, pickles and relishes require nothing more than a few minutes in a boiling water bath. Low-acid foods, on the other hand, provide a cozy environment for bacteria that thrive in the absence of air (anaerobes). If these are to be killed (along with their more heat-resistant spores), they must be processed under pressure (usually 10 or 15 pounds), which exposes the can contents to temperatures well above boiling (212°F.). See also CANNING under FOOD PRESERVATION.

Pheasant: A plump but lean white-meated game bird now being farm raised. Averaging 2 to 3 pounds apiece, pheasants are mostly breast and tricky to cook because they so easily toughen and dry. One solution is to bard them well (drape with thin slices of bacon or lard) before roast-

ing, but this ups the calorie, fat and cholesterol counts. Another is to poach or steam the boneless breasts (suprêmes), then sauce them. If you hold the butter and cream, using vegetable purees to thicken, the calories, fat and cholesterol shouldn't soar. Pheasant legs are sinewy and best tossed into the stockpot.

NUTRIENT CONTENT OF 3 OUNCES (85 GRAMS) ROASTED PHEASANT (WITHOUT SKIN)

181 calories	85 mg sodium
27 g protein	349 mg potassium
8 g fat, 3 saturated	0 g dietary fiber
75 mg cholesterol	45 RE vitamin A
0 g carbohydrate	0.03 mg thiamin
42 mg calcium	0.13 mg riboflavin
264 mg phosphorus	5.2 mg niacin
7.1 mg iron	2 mg vitamin C

Phenethyl Isothiocyanate (PEITC): A cancer-fighting compound that exists naturally in cabbage and turnips that has excited biomedical researchers. See PHYTOCHEMICALS.

Phenolic Compounds, Phenols, Phenolic Acids: Highly complex, deeply controversial compounds that exist in every plant. Some are known to be carcinogenic (the SAFROLE in sassafras, for example). Some, like the QUERCITIN in green beans and rhubarb, are thought to be mutagenic (capable of causing mutations in living cells). And some are clearly toxic (the COUMARIN in cabbage, radishes and spinach). Among the phenols are tannins (present in high doses in coffee, tea, red wine, beer, persimmons and other commonly eaten foods as well as in such herbal teas as bayberry, blackberry, comfrey and *maté*), which can bind protein and damage the liver. Other phenols include many plant pigments and natural antioxidants, some of which are known to reduce the risk of certain cancers.

The mixes, the ratios and concentrations of phenols vary from plant to plant. And their impact on health depends on how they interact not only with one another but also with the hundreds of other elements and compounds in food, in the body. All of which explains the ongoing dilemma in scientific circles. Which phenolic compounds are harmful? Which healthful? Or are they all Jekyll and Hydes, part good, part bad? Alas, there are no easy answers.

Two phenolic compounds, additives both, that have sounded the alarm among consumer advocates are butylated hydroxyanisole (see BHA) and butylated hydroxytoluene (BHT). Both are antioxidants used to extend the shelf life of cereals, dry soups, crackers, cold cuts, instant mashed potatoes and many other processed foods containing fat. The trouble with BHA and BHT is that in some tests with laboratory animals, they have been shown to impair liver function, to slow the production of DNA and RNA and thus slow cell growth. In other studies they've shown themselves to be carcinogenic, and in still others, just the opposite. For this reason—and because of a crusade on the part of consumer advocates—the FDA has targeted BHA and BHT for further tests. Meanwhile, both are being widely used. Scrutinize labels.

Phentermine: A mild stimulant/appetite suppressor prescribed in low doses to help dieters keep from regaining the weight they've lost. See DIET PILLS.

Phenylalanine: One of the essential AMINO ACIDS. The body uses phenylalanine to produce TYROSINE, a nonessential amino acid, and three important hormones (EPINEPHRINE, NOREPINEPHRINE and THYROXINE) as well as melanin, a brown skin pigment. **NOTE:** Phenylalanine is also one of the major components of the sugar substitute aspartame (see NUTRASWEET).

Phenylethylamine 192: See PEA.

Phenylketonuria (PKU): A buildup in the blood and body tissues of PHENYLALANINE or its derivatives. It's a genetic condition caused by a lack of the enzyme needed to convert phenylalanine to tyrosine, another amino acid. PKU can cause neurological disorders and, in infants, mental retardation. Though incurable, it can be controlled by restricting protein foods high in phenylalanine (meat, fish, fowl, eggs, milk and dairy products). As a rule, phenylalanine intake is limited to 15 to 25 milligrams per kilo (2.2 pounds) of body weight; age and phenylalanine tolerance will determine the exact amount. Babies must be fed special low-phenylalanine formulas, also fruits, vegetables and starches instead of meats, then phased on to a more normal diet gradually, cautiously, with frequent checks on blood phenylalanine levels. Anyone with PKU should avoid ASPARTAME, an articifial sweetener made with phenylalanine.

Phenylpropanolamine (PPA): An amphetaminelike appetite suppressant safe enough to be sold over the counter as a weight-loss aid (see DIET PILLS).

Phosphates: Phosphoric acid salts (primarily **monosodium phosphate** and **disodium phosphate**), which maintain the blood's acid/alkaline balance. Phosphates are also used as additives. **Ammonium phosphate** (GRAS) is used in baking and brewing as an acidifier, a buffer and a leavening. **Calcium phosphates** (GRAS) are used as anticaking agents (tribasic calcium phosphate), dough conditioners (dibasic) and firmer-uppers of canned vegetables and fruit jellies (monobasic). Brewers and wine makers add **potassium phosphate** (GRAS) to mash or must to feed the yeast and accelerate fermentation. And **sodium phosphate** (GRAS) is used as a buffer in evaporated milk.

Phospholipids: Fatty substances (two fatty acids + glycerol + a phosphate group) found in human cells. Able to absorb both fat- and water-soluble compounds, phospholipids act like emulsifiers during digestion. Because health-food stores are busy hustling it as a "cholesterol buster," LECITHIN is one phospholipid that's become a household word.

Phosphoric Acid (additive): It puts the fizz in many soft drinks and also acidifies and/or flavors a huge roster of baked goods, candies, frozen desserts and processed cheeses. GRAS. **NOTE:** Phosphoric acid, a form of phosphorus, is also found in every cell. Read on.

Phosphorus: A mineral as essential to the body as calcium or iron. Between 80 and 90 percent of the body's phosphorus is concentrated in the bones and teeth, usually in the form of calcium phosphate. More of it, as phosphoric acid, is present in DNA, in RNA, in all cells; indeed, cells can't form or grow without it. In addition, many enzymes and B vitamins need it to function, and it's key to the metabolism of carbohydrates, fats and proteins. Finally, phosphorus helps shuttle fats through the bloodstream and move nutrients in and out of cells. **DEFICIENCY SYMP-**

TOMS: Because phosphorus is so widely distributed in food, deficiencies are rare. However, by deliberately depriving experimental animals of phosphorus, researchers have been able to induce ricketslike symptoms, even full-blown rickets, a severe vitamin D deficiency characterized by calcium loss, soft bones and teeth (vitamin D regulates calcium and phosphorus metabolism in the body). **GOOD SOURCES:** All high-protein foods (cheese, egg, milk and other dairy products, meat, fish, fowl), legumes and whole grains such as oatmeal and brown rice. **PRECAUTIONS:** Nutritionists worry that those who drink too much soda pop or eat too much meat may be ODing on phosphorus. Not good. Excess phosphorus can not only interfere with the absorption of iron but can also upset the calcium/phosphorus ratio, which may lead to osteoporosis. On the other hand, phosphorus leaches into cooking water and, unless that water is recycled, is poured down the drain.

RDA FOR PHOSPHORUS	
Babies:	
Birth to 6 months	300 mg per day
6 months to 1 year	500 mg per day
Children:	
1 to 10 years	800 mg per day
Men and Boys:	
11 to 24 years	1,200 mg per day
25 to 51+ years	800 mg per day
Women and Girls:	
11 to 24 years	1,200 mg per day
25 to 51+ years	800 mg per day
Pregnant Women:	1,200 mg per day
Nursing Mothers:	1,200 mg per day

Phthalides: Compounds present in carrots, celery, parsley and other vegetables that reduce the risk of cancer. See PHYTOCHEMICALS.

Phytates, Phytic Acid: Compounds present in many foods, but especially whole wheat and rye, that bind calcium, iron, phosphorus and zinc, making them unavailable to the body. Other foods containing phytates include artichokes, blackberries, broccoli, carrots, figs, green beans and other legumes, nuts, potatoes, sweet potatoes and strawberries. In the Middle East, where quick-fermenting pita breads are a staple and diets lack variety,

zinc and iron deficiencies are common. The problem is that zinc- and iron-rich whole-wheat flours are used and the breads are made so fast there isn't time for the metal phytates to be reduced to a simpler, more assimilable form.

Phytochemicals: Neither vitamin nor mineral, these cancer fighters—also now called FUNCTIONAL FOODS—occur naturally in certain plants and they've piqued the interest of researchers. Can these compounds, they wonder, be extracted, concentrated and used to design "healing" or fountain-of-youth foods? Can they be formulated into a magic pill that goes vitamins two or three better? Or be used to boost the protective powers of existing foods? Phytochemicals are the New Nutritional Frontier, and already research has tripped into fast-forward. At a time when 80 percent of the most common cancers are diet related, the National Cancer Institute is so convinced of the potential of phytochemicals that it's loosed millions of dollars just for scientists to scrutinize them. Tens of thousands of phytochemicals exist in the foods we eat—nearly all of them in fruits and vegetables. And the race is on, in public and private sectors, to identify, isolate and learn how to use them to best advantage. These NUTRACEUTICALS, as they're sometimes called, may be the medications, minerals and vitamins of the twenty-first century. Time will tell. There isn't space to cover all of them. Or even the lion's share. On page 320 is a table of the most promising ones, what they do and where they're found.

The table lists just a few compounds from a long list of phytochemicals currently under scrutiny. And although the present focus is on the cancer fighters, the powers of phytochemicals don't stop there. Some are known to lower blood levels of cholesterol, others to reduce the risk of ulcers and still others to prevent tooth decay. With tens of thousands of phytochemicals in the nutritional gumbo, the twenty-first century may be one of major breakthroughs.

Phytoestrogens: Plant hormones similar to but weaker than human estrogens that are believed to reduce the risk of breast and prostate cancer; also to minimize the mood swings and hot flashes associated with menopause. Some medical researchers believe that phytoestrogens may one day supplant current estrogen-replacement therapy; unlike estrogen, their downside is nil. Phytoestrogens, now iden-

PHYTOCHEMICALS

Phytochemical	Source	Function
Allicin, allylic sulfides (including diallyl sulfide)	Onions, garlic and aged garlic extract	Detox cancer-causing chemicals and protect against stomach and digestive tract cancers.
Capsaicin	Chile peppers (the hot stuff)	Neutralizes carcinogenic benzopyrene, which not only occurs naturally in food but is also created or increased by processing and cooking.
Catechins	Green tea, strawberries, raspberries and other berries	Boost immune system and reduce risk of gastrointestinal cancers.
Chlorogenic acid	Tomatoes, green peppers, pineapple, strawberries	Blocks formation of carcinogenic nitrosamines during digestion.
Ellagic acid	Berries and other fruits, nuts, seeds, vegetables	Depowers a variety of cancer-causing compounds, notably AFLATOXIN and BENZOPYRENE.
Flavonoids, bioflavonoids	Abundant in fruits and vegetables, especially in skins and rinds; also beer, coffee, tea, wine	Keep estrogen and other possibly carcinogenic hormones moving in the body so they don't come to rest and cause trouble.
Genisteen	Soybeans	Seems to reduce risk of breast and prostate cancer.
Indoles (including indole-3-carbinol)	Cabbage, broccoli, brussels sprouts, cauliflower, collards, kale, mustard greens, turnips, rutabaga	Protect against breast, colon, esophageal, prostate and lung cancer. Indole-3-carbinol spurs enzymes to form a benign estrogen instead of one linked to breast cancer.
Isoflavones (e.g., genisteen, above)	Soybeans and soybean products	Reduce estrogen output in premenopausal women; may lower risk of breast cancer.
Limonoids	Citrus fruits, particularly their rinds	Increase production of protective enzymes.
Monoterpenes	Broccoli, cabbage, citrus fruits, cucumbers, eggplant, parsley, peppers, squash, tomatoes, yams	Antioxidants; boost immunity by stimulating activity of protective enzymes.
P-coumaric acid	Tomatoes, green peppers, pineapple, strawberries	Like chlorogenic acid, blocks production of cancer-causing nitrosamines during digestion.
Phenethyl isothiocyanate (PEITC)	Cabbage, broccoli, brussels sprouts, cauliflower, turnips, rutabaga	In lab rats and mice, has suppressed lung cancer induced by exposure to chemicals.
Phthalides	Carrots, celery, coriander, parsley, dill and other Umbelliferae	Moderate body's production of certain cancer-promoting substances.
Phytosterols	Soybeans and soybean products	Thwart or slow cholesterol absorption by body; may also be anticarcinogenic.
Sulforaphane	Broccoli, brussels sprouts, kale, turnips	In lab experiments, boosts production of cancer-fighting enzymes.
Triterpenoids	Licorice root extract, citrus fruits, tofu and other soy products	Suppress carcinogenic activity of estrogen.

tified in some three hundred plants, are grouped as **coumestans** (bean sprouts, red clover, sunflower seeds), **lignans** (rye, wheat, sesame seeds, linseed) and **isoflavones** (many fruits and vegetables, but most of all soybeans and soy products).

Phytosterols: Natural compounds abundant in soybeans that may reduce the risk of cardiovascular disease and cancer. See PHYTOCHEMICALS.

Pica: The eating of clay, dirt, cornstarch, plaster or other nonfood substances. *Pica* comes from the Latin word for magpie, a bird of indiscriminate taste. Also known as **geophagia,** pica afflicts some pregnant women, usually those in the tropics although it's also common in the American South and happens elsewhere in the United States, too. No one knows what triggers such bizarre behavior although there's no shortage of theories. It's been said, for example, that pica represents a craving for minerals present in soil; that it's a cheap way to stop hunger pangs and/or nausea; that it's a cry for a little TLC. Whatever the reason, pica can be hazardous to both mother and fetus. It can induce iron-deficiency anemia, deplete the body's supply of potassium, block the intestines, cause fetal lead poisoning (if the mother eats plaster) or parasitic infection (if the clay or soil is contaminated). Finally, it can kill.

Pickerel: A smallish, firm-fleshed, lean white fish related to the PIKE.

Pickles: Crisp, brined cucumbers or other vegetables. Though pickles contain a modicum of minerals and vitamins (in fact, dills are a modest source of beta-carotene), they are supersalty. Eat sparingly.

NUTRIENT CONTENT OF 1 MEDIUM-SIZE DILL PICKLE	
(about 2¹⁄₃ ounces; 65 grams)	
12 calories	833 mg sodium
0 g protein	75 mg potassium
0 g fat, 0 saturated	1 g dietary fiber
0 mg cholesterol	22 RE vitamin A
3 g carbohydrate	0.01 mg thiamin
6 mg calcium	0.02 mg riboflavin
14 mg phosphorus	0 mg niacin
0.3 mg iron	1 mg vitamin C

Pigeon Peas: Also known as **cajan peas** and **red gram,** these high-protein legumes nourish much of the tropical Third World. As forage, they rival alfalfa in importance and are especially palatable to poultry and livestock.

NUTRIENT CONTENT OF 1 CUP BOILED PIGEON PEAS	
(about 6 ounces; 168 grams)	
204 calories	8 mg sodium
11 g protein	646 mg potassium
1 g fat, 0 saturated	8 g dietary fiber
0 mg cholesterol	0 RE vitamin A
39 g carbohydrate	0.25 mg thiamin
72 mg calcium	0.10 mg riboflavin
198 mg phosphorus	1.3 mg niacin
1.9 mg iron	0 mg vitamin C

Pigments: The color of food is an indicator of nutritive value. For example, bright yellow or orange fruits and vegetables will be high in **carotenoids** (beta- and other carotenes), as will dark leafy greens. White to very pale yellow pigments (like those in onions) mean the presence of **flavones;** reds to purples (beets, red cabbage) signify **anthocyanins,** which, like flavones, are flavonoids (see PHYTOCHEMICALS). And green, of course, is **chlorophyll.** As a general rule, intensely colored fruits and vegetables will be richer in vitamin C than pallid produce.

PIH (Pregnancy-Induced Hypertension): A serious, sometimes fatal form of high blood pressure that occurs during pregnancy. See also ECLAMPSIA.

Pike: In his *Book of the Pike,* printed in England in 1865, H. Cholmondeley-Pennell writes that these freshwater fish were so precious in the days of Henry VIII that a "large one sold for double the price of a household lamb and a small one for more than a fat capon." Yet these sweet-meated fish have never been popular on this side of the Atlantic except among sportfishermen in the Great Lakes states and in Canada (whence the bulk of our commercial supply comes either fresh or frozen, whole, filleted or cut into steaks). The pike isn't a single fish but a small family of them that includes the **northern pike** (4 to 10 pounds), the feisty **muskellunge** (10 to 30 pounds) and the little **pickerel** (2 to 3 pounds). The **walleye** (often called **wall-eyed pike**) is actually a perch. All pike are bony but lean, white and firm of flesh. Although the French have made a classic of *quenelles de brochet* (poached pike dumplings), aficionados prefer them baked or poached whole. For approximate nutrient counts, see FISH, LEAN WHITE.

Pimientos: See SWEET PEPPERS under PEPPERS, CAPSICUMS.

Pineapples: No New World food went global more quickly or completely than pineapples. As far as anyone knows, the first Europeans to taste them were sailors on Columbus's second voyage. The place: Guadeloupe. The time: 1493. Pineapples are not native to Guadeloupe, however. Botanists point to Brazil as their place of origin, adding that they had spread north to the Indies long before Columbus. The Portuguese, and to a lesser degree the Spaniards, are responsible for carrying pineapples to the ends of the earth, for planting them in Africa, Asia, the East Indies and Polynesia.

People everywhere took to pineapples at first bite. Except for Louis XIV, who couldn't wait to have his peeled. With the royal lips lacerated, pineapples were banished from court. They faired better under the next Louis, who had hothouses built just so these tropical exotics could be grown near Paris. To Alexandre Dumas, pineapples tasted like Malmsey wine. George Washington was equally impressed. After trying them on a visit to Barbados in 1751, he noted that of all the local fruits he had tasted, "none pleases my taste as do's the pine." Still, pineapples reached mainstream America only at the turn of the twentieth century when they were grown—and canned—on a grand scale in Hawaii. To this day, Hawaii leads the world in the production of pineapples. Whether fresh, frozen or canned, pineapples are good sources of vitamin C and potassium. The fresh and frozen also contain BROMELIN, a natural digestive, which sometimes brings cooks to grief because it takes the "gel" out of gelatin. **SEASON:** Year-round.

NUTRIENT CONTENT OF 1 CUP FRESH PINEAPPLE CHUNKS

(about 5½ ounces; 155 grams)

76 calories	2 mg sodium
1 g protein	175 mg potassium
1 g fat, 0 saturated	2 g dietary fiber
0 mg cholesterol	3 RE vitamin A
19 g carbohydrate	0.14 mg thiamin
11 mg calcium	0.06 mg riboflavin
11 mg phosphorus	0.7 mg niacin
0.6 mg iron	24 mg vitamin C

NUTRIENT CONTENT OF 1 CUP CANNED PINEAPPLE CHUNKS (IN HEAVY SYRUP)

(about 9 ounces; 255 grams)

198 calories	3 mg sodium
1 g protein	265 mg potassium
0 g fat, 0 saturated	2 g dietary fiber
0 mg cholesterol	3 RE vitamin A
52 g carbohydrate	0.23 mg thiamin
36 mg calcium	0.06 mg riboflavin
18 mg phosphorus	0.7 mg niacin
1 mg iron	19 mg vitamin C

NUTRIENT CONTENT OF 1 CUP CANNED PINEAPPLE CHUNKS (IN JUICE)

(about 8¾ ounces; 250 grams)

150 calories	3 mg sodium
1 g protein	305 mg potassium
0 g fat, 0 saturated	2 g dietary fiber
0 mg cholesterol	10 RE vitamin A
39 g carbohydrate	0.24 mg thiamin
35 mg calcium	0.05 mg riboflavin
15 mg phosphorus	0.7 mg niacin
0.7 mg iron	24 mg vitamin C

NUTRIENT CONTENT OF 1 CUP PINEAPPLE JUICE (FROZEN, RECONSTITUTED)

(8 fluid ounces; 250 grams)

130 calories	3 mg sodium
1 g protein	340 mg potassium
0 g fat, 0 saturated	0 g dietary fiber
0 mg cholesterol	3 RE vitamin A
32 g carbohydrate	0.18 mg thiamin
28 mg calcium	0.05 mg riboflavin
20 mg phosphorus	0.5 mg niacin
0.8 mg iron	30 mg vitamin C

Pine Nuts, Pignoli, Piñons: Small, oily, slightly resinous nuts produced by several species of pine. They are indigenous to the Rocky Mountains and West Coast and for centuries have been a staple among the Native Americans living there. In the pueblos north and south of Santa

Fe, whole families go out after piñons, spreading blankets underneath the scrubby trees, then beating the nuts to the ground with sticks. In the Southwest, piñon nuts show up in everything from candies to breads to stews. Pine nuts are almost as popular in Italy, where they are called *pignoli*. They give pesto sauce a certain buttery smoothness and evergreen tang. Though pine nuts are very high in fat, most of it is unsaturated. They are also a good source of iron, thiamin, phosphorus and potassium. Yet they contain almost no sodium.

NUTRIENT CONTENT OF 1 OUNCE (28 GRAMS) PINE NUTS

146 calories	1 mg sodium
7 g protein	170 mg potassium
14 g fat, 2 saturated	1 g dietary fiber
0 mg cholesterol	1 RE vitamin A
4 g carbohydrate	0.23 mg thiamin
7 mg calcium	0.05 mg riboflavin
144 mg phosphorus	1.0 mg niacin
2.6 mg iron	1 mg vitamin C

Pinto Beans: See BEANS, DRIED.

Piri-Piri: See HOT PEPPERS under PEPPERS, CAPSICUMS.

Pistachio Nuts: Also known as **green almonds** (because of their grassy color and almondy flavor), these nuts of Old Testament antiquity grow throughout the Mediterranean basin. Probably they are native to Persia. But it is the Greeks who glorified them in dozens of honey-drenched pastries. Before pistachios are shipped abroad, many of them are brined in the shell. Some are also dyed

NUTRIENT CONTENT OF 1 OUNCE (28 GRAMS) SHELLED PISTACHIO NUTS

164 calories	2 mg sodium
6 g protein	309 mg potassium
14 g fat, 2 saturated	3 g dietary fiber
0 mg cholesterol	7 RE vitamin A
7 g carbohydrate	0.23 mg thiamin
38 mg calcium	0.05 mg riboflavin
142 mg phosphorus	0.3 mg niacin
1.9 mg iron	2 mg vitamin C

scarlet, but savvy shoppers, wary of the dangers of sodium and artificial colors, insist on unsalted nuts in their natural tan shells.

Pita Bread: Soft, flat Middle Eastern pocket bread that has become a supermarket staple in the United States. Available in both white and whole-wheat flour versions, it's the perfect container for lunch on the run. Fill it with shredded lettuce and chopped tomatoes, with chicken, tuna or other seafood salad. Or pop in a couple of chickpea fritters (FALAFEL) and a dollop of yogurt.

NUTRIENT CONTENT OF 1 WHITE PITA BREAD
(about 2 ounces; 60 grams)

165 calories	322 mg sodium
5 g protein	72 mg potassium
1 g fat, 0 saturated	1 g dietary fiber
0 mg cholesterol	0 RE vitamin A
33 g carbohydrate	0.36 mg thiamin
52 mg calcium	0.20 mg riboflavin
58 mg phosphorus	2.8 mg niacin
1.6 mg iron	0 mg vitamin C

NUTRIENT CONTENT OF 1 WHOLE-WHEAT PITA BREAD
(about 2 ounces; 60 grams)

160 calories	319 mg sodium
6 g protein	102 mg potassium
2 g fat, 0 saturated	5 g dietary fiber
0 mg cholesterol	0 RE vitamin A
33 g carbohydrate	0.20 mg thiamin
9 mg calcium	0.05 mg riboflavin
108 mg phosphorus	1.7 mg niacin
1.8 mg iron	0 mg vitamin C

Pizza: The Neapolitan cheese and tomato "pie" that America has made its own, spinning dozens of variations on the theme. Some of these, unfortunately, zoom the fat, calorie and cholesterol counts into the danger zone. The best pizzas, from a nutritional standpoint, are those made with a modicum of cheese and a garden of fresh vegetables—tomatoes, broccoli, onions and mushrooms, for example. The worst are cheese-laden pizzas freighted with pepperoni or other sausages. Even classic mozzarella and tomato pizza, if made with a heavy hand, can blow the day's quota for calories, fat and cholesterol. Choose carefully and try to settle for a wedge or two instead of a whole pie. This wedge, by the way, is also an excellent source of calcium, phosphorus, potassium, vitamin A, thiamin, riboflavin and niacin. So pizza isn't all bad.

NUTRIENT CONTENT OF 1 WEDGE CLASSIC MOZZARELLA/TOMATO PIZZA

(⅛ of a 15-inch pie; about 4¼ ounces; 120 grams)

268 calories	640 mg sodium
15 g protein	209 mg potassium
6 g fat, 3 saturated	2 g dietary fiber
18 mg cholesterol	140 RE vitamin A
39 g carbohydrate	0.35 mg thiamin
222 mg calcium	0.31 mg riboflavin
215 mg phosphorus	4.7 mg niacin
1.1 mg iron	2 mg vitamin C

Pizzoccheri: A speckled brown buckwheat fettuccine that's the specialty of Lombardy astride the Swiss border. *Pizzoccheri* is more strongly flavored than classic Italian pasta; indeed, there are hints of kasha. **NOTE:** Nutrient counts unavailable.

Placenta: A blood-vessel-webbed structure in the lining of the uterus that bonds mother to fetus. It is through the placenta that the developing baby obtains food and oxygen from its mother and rids itself of waste. The condition of the placenta determines the growth and health of the fetus.

Plaice: A popular European flat fish. See FLOUNDER.

Plantains: Also called **green bananas, hard bananas** and **vegetable bananas,** plantains are indeed first cousins of the banana. In flavor and taste, however, they are closer to potatoes. Like potatoes, plantains may be "chipped" and fried, baked whole in their skins, or peeled, sliced and boiled or steamed. Since the beginning of time, plantains have been a staple in the tropics and subtropics. They are never eaten raw and progress as they ripen from green to gold to black, mellowing each step of the way but never reaching the squishiness or perfumy sweetness of bananas. Only the ripest plantains should be refrigerated because cold stops the ripening process. Although the masses who subsist on plantains have no notion of their food value,

they could scarcely have chosen a better starch staple. Plantains are a stellar source of beta-carotene and potassium and a respectable one of dietary fiber and vitamin C. Yet they are fat free and very nearly sodium free, too. **SEASON:** Year-round.

NUTRIENT CONTENT OF 1 CUP BOILED/STEAMED SLICED PLANTAIN

(about 5½ ounces; 154 grams)

179 calories	8 mg sodium
1 g protein	716 mg potassium
0 g fat, 0 saturated	3 g dietary fiber
0 mg cholesterol	140 RE vitamin A
48 g carbohydrate	0.07 mg thiamin
3 mg calcium	0.08 mg riboflavin
43 mg phosphorus	1.2 mg niacin
0.9 mg iron	17 mg vitamin C

Plant Sterols: See PHENOLIC COMPOUNDS.

Plaque, Arterial: See CHOLESTEROL.

Plaque, Dental: See DENTAL HEALTH.

Plastic (food safety and): To reduce the risk of secondary additives (chemicals that may migrate from packaging into food), the government puts packagers and packages to the test. Do the materials used for packages, special finishes and coatings break down in any way and leach into food? If so, do the migrating chemicals pass FDA muster? As with primary additives, the FDA now requires that all new "indirect additives" used for packaging be carefully tested and proved safe before they go on sale.

Of particular concern are materials used for microwave food: popcorn, pizza and other brown- or crisp-and-serve bags, cartons and trays with built-in heat SUSCEPTORS; also plastic "dual ovenables" designed for conventional ovens as well as microwaves. Unfortunately, original FDA requirements failed to consider the intense microwave heat generated by heat-susceptor packages. The FDA's Center for Food Safety and Applied Nutrition recently tested microwave popcorn bags and discovered, in the susceptor portions, temperatures as high as 500°F. These susceptors are usually metalized plastic (polyethylene terephthalate, or

PET) laminated to cardboard. The PET film, designed to insulate the corn from the outer bag, not only failed at this intense heat but also sent secondary additives of its own into the popcorn. After three minutes of popping, nearly three fourths of the PET's chemical components (oligomers) landed in the corn. And after six minutes, 95 percent of them.

In conventional ovens, where thermostats are often off by 50°F. or more, there have been incidents of oligomer migration into food from dual-ovenable containers. These are designed for use at moderate oven temperatures, but at 400°F. or more there is some PET transfer to food. What isn't yet known is whether these migrating chemicals are harmful. And if so, *how harmful* they are. Microwave-age packages are overdue for further testing and review.

Meanwhile, you can play it safe by air popping corn the old-fashioned way and by transferring all frozen microwave side dishes and dinners to safe glass or ceramic ovenware. It's easy. Just pop the frozen blocks out and cover with a lid of heatproof glass. **A FEW ADDITIONAL CAUTIONS:** Never use margarine tubs, deli cartons or other plastic containers in the microwave (they may break down into chemicals that are hazardous to your health). And never "nuke" plastic foam (it will melt). Finally, use only plastic food wraps and bags that are microwave safe (read labels). Made of polyvinylidene, polyvinyl chloride or polyethylene, even these are best for brief heating (polyvinylidene softens at 250°F., polyvinyl chloride at 210°F. and polyethylene at 190°F., well below the boiling point of water; none should touch the food being microwaved). For longer microwaving, use ovenproof glass dome lids, which are sold by every five-and-dime.

Plastic Cutting Boards: For years "sanitarians" have been telling us to replace wooden cutting boards with sleek plastic models. They're easier to clean, the argument went; thus bacteria don't lodge in nicked, scratched surfaces the way they do in wood. Now, according to microbiologists at the University of Wisconsin, the most common bacterial contaminants (*Escherichia coli,* listeria and salmonella) like plastic better than wood. Tests show that none survives on wooden boards more than three minutes whereas they thrive on polyacrylic, polyethylene, polypropylene, polystyrene and hard rubber. The Wisconsin scientists can't explain why but insist that wood somehow checks bacterial

growth. And this holds true for all kinds of hardwood boards—ash, beech, birch, cherry, maple, oak. Other scientists, including those at the USDA, remain skeptical. Further tests are due. Meanwhile, whatever cutting board you choose, wash thoroughly in hot sudsy water after each use, rinse and air dry. Better yet, put them through the dishwasher where steam can seep into every nick and scratch. Finally, replace battered cutting boards.

Pleurottes: See MUSHROOMS.

Plums: Like their fellow drupes (stone fruits), plums are probably native to Asia. They now grow on four continents out of five (only Antarctica lacks them) and their varieties number in the thousands. The best plums, for both eating and commerce, are the **European** species (which include the **greengage** and small deep purple-blue **Italian**) and the **Japanese** (paler, plumper plums that range in color from gold to bloodred but are never blue). Then there are **damsons,** early European imports that now grow wild over much of the Deep South, and **beach plums,** which early colonists found Native Americans eating all up and down the East Coast. Neither of these is of commercial importance, but both are yours for the picking and make splendid jams and jellies. All plums are moderately good sources of fiber and vitamin C. Yet they are low in calories and contain zero fat, cholesterol and sodium. **SEASON:** May through October with supplies peaking between July and September.

NUTRIENT CONTENT OF 1 MEDIUM-SIZE PLUM	
(about 2⅓ ounces; 66 grams)	
36 calories	0 mg sodium
1 g protein	113 mg potassium
0 g fat, 0 saturated	1 g dietary fiber
0 mg cholesterol	21 RE vitamin A
9 g carbohydrate	0.03 mg thiamin
3 mg calcium	0.06 mg riboflavin
7 mg phosphorus	0.3 mg niacin
0.1 mg iron	6 mg vitamin C

PMS (Premenstrual Syndrome) (diet and): Ten days to two weeks before each period, some women become irritable, depressed, anxious and suffer such physical symptoms as bloating, weight gain, tender breasts, acne, constipation, headaches and fatigue. PMS it's called, and quack cures abound, most of them purveyed by health-food stores. Below are some of the more common.

Poaching: Cooking food at a gentle simmer in water or stock. Some of the fat and salt will leach out of the food and that's good. But so will water-soluble B and C vitamins. And that's bad. Poaching is more suited to fish and fowl than to meats and vegetables.

Poblanos: See HOT PEPPERS under PEPPERS, CAPSICUMS.

Poi: See DASHEENS.

Poisonous Plants: See FLOWERS AND PLANTS, POISONOUS.

Pole Beans: A variety of green bean (see BEANS, FRESH).

Polenta: A porridge of yellow cornmeal that's a staple throughout northern Italy. Classic cooks make it in a copper polenta pan, adding coarse-grained cornmeal to sim-mering water in a slow, steady stream. This is basic, everyday polenta. There are fancier versions, too, plumped up with cheese and butter, or sweet sausages, onions and tomatoes. Then there's fried polenta, nothing more than leftovers recycled much the way American cooks recycle cold cornmeal mush down South.

NUTRIENT CONTENT OF ½ CUP POLENTA (MADE WITH ENRICHED YELLOW CORNMEAL)	
(about 4 ounces; 119 grams)	
60 calories	0* mg sodium
1 g protein	17 mg potassium
0 g fat, 0 saturated	1 g dietary fiber
0 mg cholesterol	71 RE vitamin A
13 g carbohydrate	0.07 mg thiamin
1 mg calcium	0.05 mg riboflavin
17 mg phosphorus	0.6 mg niacin
0.5 mg iron	0 mg vitamin C

*No salt added when making polenta.

Pollack: A member of the cod family popular on both sides of the Atlantic that's also known as **coalfish.** Pollack are silver skinned, not brown speckled like cod. They are

COMMON PMS "CURES"		
"Cure"	**Claims**	**Facts**
Vitamin B₆ therapy (up to 2,000 mg per day)	Restores estrogen imbalance that causes depression and abrupt mood swings.	No reputable studies prove B₆ relieves PMS. Even fewer than 2,000 mg a day can damage nervous system.
Evening-primrose oil (efamol)	Reduces breast tenderness by supplying enzyme needed to correct prostaglandin E-1 deficiency.	Prostaglandin deficiency has never been shown to cause PMS. Taken on empty stomach, efamol irritates gastrointestinal tract.
Magnesium deficiency/calcium surplus	Too much calcium (via milk and cheese, etc.) deposes magnesium and causes PMS.	Apart from alcoholics and those with malabsorption disorders, women don't lack magnesium. Too much of it is laxative *and* toxic.
Megavitamin/mineral therapy	Shortfalls of vitamins A, C, E, B-complex (especially B₆), iron, magnesium and zinc cause PMS. Potent supplements like Optivite effect magic cures.	PMS is no deficiency disease. Continual vitamin/mineral megadosing is expensive, no PMS preventive or cure and possibly toxic enough to jeopardize health.

Note: Anyone with serious PMS should see her gynecologist. Others should eat a well-balanced diet every day and, in the two weeks before each period, cut down on alcohol, caffeine and salt.

smaller, too, topping out at about 35 pounds (market sizes average a more modest 4 to 5 pounds). Like cod, pollack are firm and lean of flesh. For approximate nutrient counts, see FISH, LEAN WHITE.

Pollen: See BEE POLLEN.

Polybrominated Biphenyls: See PBBs.

Polychlorinated Biphenyls: See PCBs.

Polycyclic Aromatic Hydrocarbons: See PAHs.

Polydextrose (additive): At 1 calorie per gram (versus 4 for sugar and 9 for fat), polydextrose is a multipurpose low-calorie bulking agent/partial fat substitute used in a huge array of commercial cakes, candies, dessert mixes, gelatins, frozen desserts, puddings and salad dressings. It is even used in chewing gum. Synthesized from dextrose (glucose), sorbitol and citric acid, polydextrose was given FDA approval only in 1981. Whenever levels of it exceed 15 grams, package labels must post this warning: "Sensitive individuals may experience a laxative effect from excessive consumption of this product."

Polyethylene Glycol (additive): A compound too complex for the body to metabolize that passes through the system unchanged. Polyethylene glycol is used mostly in diet sodas to reduce the thin flavor of artificial sweeteners and ape the richer "mouth feel" of sugar-sweetened soft drinks. GRAS.

Polyglycerols, Polyglyceryls (additives): Dispersants, emulsifiers, lubricants, plasticizers and gelling agents synthesized from saturated and unsaturated plant oils—coconut, corn, cottonseed, palm, peanut, safflower, sesame and soybean oils. Or from such saturated animal fats as lard and tallow. Not known to be toxic.

Polyneuropathy: A beriberilike nerve disease caused by a desperate lack of thiamin (B$_1$), pyridoxine (B$_6$) or pantothenic acid or possibly niacin or riboflavin. Polyneuropathy sometimes afflicts alcoholics, also those with stomach or liver disease. Usually thiamin or B-complex therapy relieves the symptoms—muscular weakness, leg pain, loss of

coordination and motor function, sometimes partial paralysis. Even so, recovery doesn't happen overnight. Some patients need a year before they can walk normally.

Polyphenols: See PHENOLIC COMPOUNDS.

Polypropylene Glycol (additive): A defoamer used in yeast and beet sugar. Not known to be toxic.

Polysaccharides: Complex sugars. See CARBOHYDRATES.

Polysorbates (additives): The numbers of these emulsifiers/stabilizers run from 1 through 85. Two of them, 60 and 80, have caused some concern because they have been linked with 1,4 dioxane, a contaminant that's caused malignancies in lab animals. Polysorbate 60, often used in coating chocolates to keep their fat from oozing out, also shows up in cakes and cake mixes, gelatin desserts, ice creams and sherbets, assorted dry instants and mixes, and egg yolk-less salad dressings. Polysorbate 80, less waxy and more liquid than 60, stabilizes coffee creamers and nondairy aerosol toppings. The other polysorbates are not known to be toxic.

Polyunsaturated Fats: Fats with a large percentage of fatty acids that lack more than one pair of hydrogen atoms. Most plants' OILS are high in polyunsaturated fats. So are fish, almonds, peanuts (and peanut butter), pecans, hazelnuts and walnuts. See also FAT.

Pomegranates: Symbol of fertility, stuff of legend, inspiration of artists, this ancient Middle Eastern fruit remains a curiosity. And small wonder. Inside its leathery shell is a cargo of "rubies"—seeds, or rather fleshy arils, that must be plucked out one by one, then eaten like nuts or scattered into recipes (they're best in salads and compotes). Pomegranates can be juiced but reaming them will spatter everything in sight. Elizabeth Schneider offers a neater method in her splendid book *Uncommon Fruits & Vegetables.* "Place the whole, unpeeled pomegranate on a hard surface," she writes, "press the palm of your hand against the fruit, then roll gently to break all the juice sacs inside. . . . Prick a hole and suck out the juice; or poke in a straw and do the same." Are pomegranates worth the trouble?

Maybe. They're sweet but tart, contain plenty of potassium and some vitamin C, yet are low in calories. **SEASON:** Fall and early winter.

NUTRIENT CONTENT OF 1 MEDIUM-SIZE POMEGRANATE
(about 5½ ounces; 154 grams)

104 calories	5 mg sodium
1 g protein	397 mg potassium
0 g fat, 0 saturated	3 g dietary fiber
0 mg cholesterol	0 RE vitamin A
26 g carbohydrate	0.05 mg thiamin
5 mg calcium	0.05 mg riboflavin
12 mg phosphorus	0.5 mg niacin
0.5 mg iron	9 mg vitamin C

Pomelos: See PUMMELOS.

Pompano: Is this America's finest saltwater fish? Many fish lovers swear so. Pompano is small (averaging 1½ to 2 pounds at the market), its flesh is as pale a parchment, yet firm and rich. As for flavor, some think pompano tastes a little like sea scallops; others liken its sweetness, its butteriness to nuts. Because of their size, pompano are best broiled or grilled whole. Or steamed *en papillote,* then sauced the New Orleans way with crab and shrimp. Although pompano swim the Atlantic as far north as New England and as far south as Brazil, fishermen know that they're most plentiful between the Carolinas and Florida and all along the Gulf Coast. For all their daintiness, pompano are powerful sources of thiamin, niacin, phosphorus and potassium. They aren't lean, but at least most of their fat is unsaturated.

NUTRIENT CONTENT OF 3 OUNCES (85 GRAMS) BROILED/BAKED POMPANO

180 calories	65 mg sodium
20 g protein	541 mg potassium
10 g fat, 4 saturated	0 g dietary fiber
54 mg cholesterol	31 RE vitamin A
0 g carbohydrate	0.58 mg thiamin
37 mg calcium	0.13 mg riboflavin
290 mg phosphorus	3.2 mg niacin
0.6 mg iron	0 mg vitamin C

Popcorn: The all-American snack. And, it turns out, the dieter's best friend *if* air popped and served without butter or salt because it's filling, full of dietary fiber, low in calories and free of saturated fat. Not so movie-theater popcorn, which recently loosed a torrent of media jabber because of its popping medium (coconut oil) and the staggering amount of saturated fat it contains. A medium-size bag of *unbuttered* movie popcorn averages as much saturated fat (28 grams) as two Big Macs and that's *with* fries. Drizzle the corn with "butter" (partially hydrogenated soybean oil plus fake color and flavor) and the saturated fat soars to 41 grams, 2 times what most nutritionists recommend as the daily max. (As a result of the media flak, some big-chain movie theaters have begun popping their corn in more nutritionally correct oils.) Popcorn may seem like a twentieth-century innovation. Actually, it's ancient. One of the foods Native Americans gave the world, one of the foods served at the Pilgrims' first Thanksgiving. The amount eaten today? About 65 quarts per person per year. Of

NUTRIENT CONTENT OF 1 CUP POPCORN (AIR POPPED, UNSALTED, UNBUTTERED)
(about ¼ ounce; 8 grams)

31 calories	0 mg sodium
1 g protein	24 mg potassium
0 g fat, 0 saturated	1 g dietary fiber
0 mg cholesterol	2 RE vitamin A
6 g carbohydrate	0.02 mg thiamin
1 mg calcium	0.02 mg riboflavin
24 mg phosphorus	0.2 mg niacin
0.2 mg iron	0 mg vitamin C

NUTRIENT CONTENT OF 1 CUP POPCORN (OIL POPPED, SALTED, UNBUTTERED)
(about ⅓ ounce; 11 grams)

55 calories	97 mg sodium
1 g protein	25 mg potassium
3 g fat, 1 saturated	1 g dietary fiber
0 mg cholesterol	2 RE vitamin A
6 g carbohydrate	0.02 mg thiamin
1 mg calcium	0.02 mg riboflavin
28 mg phosphorus	0.2 mg niacin
0.3 mg iron	0 mg vitamin C

course sales have exploded since the arrival of microwave popcorn. **CAUTION:** There are "secondary additives" in microwave popcorn—chemicals in the bag's heat susceptors that break down under the intense heat of popping and migrate into the corn. See PLASTIC. Presto's new PowerPop minimizes that risk and also makes it possible to pop corn in your microwave with or without oil. Best of all, nearly every kernel pops! No "grannies" to bust a cuspid!

Popovers: Egg-rich muffin-shaped quick breads baked at such intense heat they fairly explode. They are leavened by steam, not baking powder. Baked in a roasting pan, popovers become Yorkshire pudding.

NUTRIENT CONTENT OF 1 MEDIUM-SIZE POPOVER
(about 2 ounces; 54 grams)

122 calories	110 mg sodium
5 g protein	87 mg potassium
5 g fat, 1 saturated	0 g dietary fiber
64 mg cholesterol	39 RE vitamin A
15 g carbohydrate	0.13 mg thiamin
50 mg calcium	0.20 mg riboflavin
75 mg phosphorus	1.0 mg niacin
1 mg iron	0 mg vitamin C

Poppy Seeds: The tiny blue-black seeds of the opium poppy (*Papaver somniferum*) that are used to flavor breads and pastries. They are particularly popular in France, Germany and other northern European countries. **CAUTION:** Some people testing positive for drugs (heroin) were found to have done nothing more illegal than eat a poppy-seed Danish.

Porcine Somatotropin (PST): A hormone now widely used in research trials by hog growers to produce leaner animals (some PST hogs have 75 percent less fat than their non-PST cousins). PST also makes hogs grow faster. It's a natural hormone, but biotech labs can synthesize additional amounts for farmers to use. FDA approval is expected soon.

Porcini: See MUSHROOMS.

Porgies: A group of small (or mostly small) saltwater fish that rack up big sales along the Atlantic Coast. Also called **sea bream,** porgies are considered good catches by the sportsmen who go after them in deep-sea fishing boats off Long Island, New Jersey and other mid-Atlantic states. Though coarse of flesh, they are lean and white—just right for panbroiling or frying. In the New York area, the great favorite is the **sheepshead.** For approximate nutrient counts, see FISH, LEAN WHITE.

Pork: Exasperated by George Bernard Shaw during a theater rehearsal, Mrs. Patrick Campbell shrieked, "Shaw, someday you'll eat a pork chop, and then God help all women!"

The peppery playwright was a vegetarian and, unlike many people of Edwardian England, put no faith in the nutritive powers of meat. Pork, it turns out, has been nourishing mankind for nearly seven thousand years. Indeed, the first animal man is said to have domesticated (after the dog) was the pig.

NUTRIENT CONTENT OF 3 OUNCES (85 GRAMS) BROILED TRIMMED PORK LOIN CHOP

232 calories	64 mg sodium
28 g protein	356 mg potassium
12 g fat, 4 saturated	0 g dietary fiber
89 mg cholesterol	2 RE vitamin A
0 g carbohydrate	0.59 mg thiamin
9 mg calcium	0.30 mg riboflavin
203 mg phosphorus	5.9 mg niacin
1.2 mg iron	0 mg vitamin C

NUTRIENT CONTENT OF 3 OUNCES (85 GRAMS) ROASTED TRIMMED PORK LOIN/RIB

207 calories	39 mg sodium
24 g protein	360 mg potassium
12 g fat, 4 saturated	0 g dietary fiber
67 mg cholesterol	3 RE vitamin A
0 g carbohydrate	0.54 mg thiamin
9 mg calcium	0.27 mg riboflavin
217 mg phosphorus	4.6 mg niacin
0.9 mg iron	0 mg vitamin C

In ancient China pork was so esteemed it (and ham) accounted for two of the Eight Marvels of the Table. As recently as 1978 the CIA estimated that there were more than 280 million pigs in the People's Republic of China (as compared to 60 million in the United States).

The miracle of the hog is that it can subsist—fatten—on almost anything. In medieval Europe, for example, pigs were run through the streets to clean up table scraps. And in China today, hogs live largely upon cotton leaves, cornstalks, rice husks and water hyacinths.

The reason pork has remained such a world staple, despite the fact that two major religions—Judaism and Islam—forbid the eating of it, is that it's both economical and versatile. Nearly every part of a pig is edible ("everything but the squeal") and those few parts that cannot be eaten are turned into leather and bristles. Pliny, the first-century Roman scholar, claimed that he could discern fifty different flavors in pork. It may be so. Modern scientists have discerned something far more precious—abundant stores of thiamin (pork is a richer source of this important B vitamin than any other meat), niacin, phosphorus and potassium, even in today's leaner hogs (see PORCINE SOMATOTROPIN).

NUTRIENT CONTENT OF 3 OUNCES (85 GRAMS) ROASTED TRIMMED FRESH HAM (LEG)

249 calories	50 mg sodium
21 g protein	279 mg potassium
18 g fat, 6 saturated	0 g dietary fiber
79 mg cholesterol	3 RE vitamin A
0 g carbohydrate	0.54 mg thiamin
5 mg calcium	0.27 mg riboflavin
209 mg phosphorus	3.9 mg niacin
0.9 mg iron	0 mg vitamin C

NUTRIENT CONTENT OF 3 OUNCES (85 GRAMS) BRAISED SPARERIB MEAT

338 calories	79 mg sodium
25 g protein	272 mg potassium
26 g fat, 10 saturated	0 g dietary fiber
103 mg cholesterol	3 RE vitamin A
0 g carbohydrate	0.35 mg thiamin
40 mg calcium	0.33 mg riboflavin
217 mg phosphorus	4.7 mg niacin
1.6 mg iron	0 mg vitamin C

Port: A group of noble wines produced in Portugal's Douro Valley, then aged, bottled and shipped in Porto. The Portuguese call it **Porto** to distinguish it from other countries' imitations. See WINES; also ALCOHOL, ALCOHOLIC BEVERAGES.

Porterhouse: The biggest, choicest steak. It comes from the loin, contains a hefty chunk of tenderloin and in prime or choice grades is heavily marbled with fat (make that saturated fat). See BEEF.

Portobello: See MUSHROOMS.

Port-Salut: Originally called **Port-du-Salut,** this factory cheese was created by Trappist monks at the Abbey of Port-du-Salut shortly after the French Revolution. It is a cooked cow's-milk cheese of superior flavor (neither too harsh nor bland) and, when ripe, of spreadable consistency. There are now domestic Port-Saluts, but the imports are better.

NUTRIENT CONTENT OF 1 OUNCE (28 GRAMS) PORT-SALUT

100 calories	151 mg sodium
7 g protein	39 mg potassium
8 g fat, 5 saturated	0 g dietary fiber
35 mg cholesterol	105 RE vitamin A
0 g carbohydrate	0 mg thiamin
184 mg calcium	0.07 mg riboflavin
102 mg phosphorus	0 mg niacin
0.1 mg iron	0 mg vitamin C

Potassium: This mineral, working in concert with sodium, maintains the body's fluid balance—a vital function. Potassium is also believed to catalyze carbohydrate and protein metabolism. **DEFICIENCY SYMPTOMS:** Anxiousness, drowsiness, weakness, nausea, irrational behavior, irregular heartbeat. Spectators are used to watching marathon runners swig cups of fluid on the run to help them replace bodily fluids lost through sweating. Actually, far less potassium is lost through sweat than through prolonged vomiting, diarrhea or diuretics used to treat HYPERTENSION. **GOOD SOURCES:** Most fruits, vegetables, dairy products, fish, lean meats and poultry (bananas, cantaloupes, orange juice, baked potatoes and low-fat yogurt, in particular, are stellar sources). **NOTE:** The less fat food contains, the richer it's likely to be in potassium.

PRECAUTIONS: Potassium is sacrificed when grains are milled. It also leaches into cooking water if food is cut too fine and cooked too long, but recycling the "pot likker" salvages most of it. Because laxatives and diuretics both wash potassium from the body, they should be taken only as a physician directs. Some of the diuretics used to treat hypertension—hydrochlorothiazide and furosemide, to name two—deplete body potassium. Water is flushed out of the body along with potassium, thus blood volume is reduced as well as blood pressure. Anyone taking potassium-wasting diuretics must monitor his potassium intake carefully and make sure that the lost potassium is replaced. Drinking lots of orange juice, eating plenty of potatoes, bananas and other potassium-rich foods are good ways to go about it. **RDA FOR POTASSIUM:** Potassium is so widely distributed in food only general recommendations are given. For adults, 2,000 milligrams per day are the minimum. However, many nutritionists now recommend upping the daily quota to 3,500 milligrams to reduce the risk of high blood pressure.

Potassium Alginate: See ALGINATES.

Potassium Bicarbonate (additive): A slightly alkaline, tasteless white powder and multipurpose additive that's used in a variety of soft drinks and baked goods. GRAS.

Potassium Bromate (additive): A texturizer/dough conditioner used in commercial breads. Potassium bromate is also used to age flour and stabilize its baking properties. In the body, it's converted to POTASSIUM BROMIDE and excreted. There is, however, a report that potassium bromate may cause cells to mutate. And the FDA strictly limits amounts that can be used.

Potassium Bromide (additive): Many fruits and vegetables mass-produced today are given "preservative dips" in a mild solution of potassium bromide. The chemical can trigger nervous disorders, however, so the FDA imposes strict limits on its use.

Potassium Caseinate (additive): Milk protein used to smooth frozen custards, ice creams, sherbets. In sensitive individuals, potassium caseinate may trigger acne, depression, gastric disorders, headaches, muscular weakness. Still, the FDA continues to rate it GRAS.

Potassium Chloride (additive): A substitute for table salt (sodium chloride) that's often recommended to those with high blood pressure. Unfortunately, it is intensely bitter and does little to enhance food. GRAS.

Potassium Citrate (additive): A buffer widely used in jams, jellies, preserves and candies. GRAS.

Potassium Iodide (additive): The chemical most often used to iodize salt (two others, sodium iodide and cuprous iodide, are not so widely used). Iodized salt was introduced back in the 1930s as a way to combat goiter, which it did. Quite successfully. GRAS. See also GOITER; IODIZED SALT.

Potassium Nitrate (additive): Also known as **saltpeter,** this is one of the controversial nitrates used to cure meat. See NITRATES, NITRITES.

Potassium Phosphate (additive): Brewers and wine makers use all three forms (monobasic, dibasic and tribasic potassium phosphate) to speed the fermentation of yeast. GRAS.

Potassium Sorbate (additive): A widely used mold and yeast inhibitor that's added to everything from chocolates to baked goods to cheeses to jellies. Restaurant salad bars also count on potassium sorbate to keep slaws, salads and fruit cocktails "fresh." GRAS.

Potatoes: When Europe's fifteenth-century explorers went looking for the riches of the East, they found the West and a treasure that would ultimately prove more valuable—the potato. Today it is the world's single most important vegetable. But it took a long time to become so. When first carried to Europe by the Spaniards, potatoes failed to impress. Indeed, people whispered that they were poisonous. Potatoes, it's said, found scant room on world tables until the late eighteenth century when a Frenchman named Parmentier became their biggest booster. His first crop was so successful he presented a bouquet of potato blossoms to his king, Louis XVI, who stuck a single flower in his lapel and gave the rest to his queen, Marie Antoinette. An amusing tale that's probably apocryphal.

Not until the starving Irish peasants were driven to eat potatoes did the English discover how wholesome, versatile and delicious they could be.

It's said that the potato crossed the Atlantic seven times before it ever became popular in the United States. Certainly it wasn't established here until well along in the eighteenth century when a hearty Irish species took root in New Hampshire.

Today all white potatoes are known collectively as **Irish potatoes:** the round, all-purpose varieties called simply **Maine, eastern** or **boiling potatoes;** the nut-sweet little **news** or **redskins;** the **Finnish golds;** and the big fawn-skinned oval bakers sold as **Idahos.** All potatoes are superb sources of potassium and niacin and good ones of dietary fiber and vitamin C. Ounce for ounce, the different varieties do not vary much in food value. What about eating the skins? Rumors abound that they are full of poisonous chemicals. The only problem, say researchers, is a natural toxin called SOLANINE, which is present in green patches of skin and flesh (these develop when potatoes are exposed to bright light). Solanine can cause cramps, diarrhea, headache, even fever, but the preventive couldn't be simpler. Remove all green skin, taking with it any discolored patches underneath. There are advantages to eating potato skins—they're rich in fiber and iron.

NUTRIENT CONTENT OF 1 LARGE BAKED POTATO (WITH SKIN)

(about 7 ounces; 202 grams)

220 calories	16 mg sodium
5 g protein	844 mg potassium
0 g fat, 0 saturated	4 g dietary fiber
0 mg cholesterol	0 RE vitamin A
51 g carbohydrate	0.22 mg thiamin
20 mg calcium	0.07 mg riboflavin
115 mg phosphorus	3.3 mg niacin
2.8 mg iron	16 mg vitamin C

NUTRIENT CONTENT OF 1 MEDIUM-SIZE BOILED POTATO (WITHOUT SKIN)

(about 4³/₄ ounces; 136 grams)

118 calories	5 mg sodium
3 g protein	515 mg potassium
0 g fat, 0 saturated	2 g dietary fiber
0 mg cholesterol	0 RE vitamin A
27 g carbohydrate	0.14 mg thiamin
7 mg calcium	0.03 mg riboflavin
60 mg phosphorus	2.0 mg niacin
0.4 mg iron	18 mg vitamin C

NUTRIENT CONTENT OF 1 OUNCE (28 GRAMS) POTATO CHIPS

152 calories	169 mg sodium
2 g protein	361 mg potassium
10 g fat, 3 saturated	1 g dietary fiber
0 mg cholesterol	0 RE vitamin A
15 g carbohydrate	0.05 mg thiamin
7 mg calcium	0.06 mg riboflavin
47 mg phosphorus	1.1 mg niacin
0.5 mg iron	9 mg vitamin C

Potato Flour, Potato Starch (additive): Food processors capitalize on its ability to swell and gel when mixed with hot water. Potato starch is now being mixed into low-fat burgers to ape the juiciness and rich "mouth feel" of those that ooze fat. GRAS.

Potbelly (in children): A symptom of acute protein deficiency. See KWASHIORKOR.

Pot Cheese: See COTTAGE CHEESE.

Pot Liquor, Pot Likker: The cooking water, specifically that in which collards, kale, turnip salad and other greens are cooked. Down South pot likker is served either with the vegetables or separately (a good idea because it contains water-soluble vitamins and minerals). For sopping up every last drop, there is always plenty of fresh-baked corn bread.

Pot Roasting: The best way to cook big tough joints of meat (pot roasts) is to braise them; that is, to brown them nicely in butter or oil, then to cover and simmer slowly—either in the oven or on the stove top—in the company of vegetables or a little liquid. This gentle moist heat turns sinew to gelatin and produces meat of supreme succulence. The only drawback of pot roasting—the accumulation of fatty drippings—can be turned to an advantage. Skim off the fat and thicken the gravy with the pureed pot-roasted vegetables.

Poultry: Birds raised for the table. The individual fowl are discussed separately and in detail. See CHICKEN; DUCK; GOOSE; PHEASANT; TURKEY.

Powdered Sugar: Another—although not quite accurate way—of saying **confectioners' sugar.** See SUGARS.

PPB: A precise unit of measure meaning parts per billion. The federal government uses it—also PPM—to determine pesticide residue levels in food. For example, 1 ppb = 1 gram (0.035 ounce) of residue in 1 billion grams (1,102 tons of food). Or to translate these ratios to everyday terms, the weight of one dried apricot versus the tonnage of all of those produced in the United States in one year.

PPM: Parts per million. In practical terms, this would be the equivalent of the weight of one canned cherry in 10 tons of them.

Prawns: Although there are several families of prawns (most of them on the European side of the Atlantic), those sold almost everywhere in the United States as prawns are really giant SHRIMP.

Preeclampsia: A toxemia that occurs during pregnancy. It raises blood pressure to dangerous levels, causes the legs and feet to swell and, unless treated immediately, can be fatal. The condition is also known as **pregnancy-induced hypertension** (PIH). See also ECLAMPSIA

Pregelatinized Starch (additive): Starch that will swell in cold water, an essential ingredient in instant puddings, cake and soup mixes. It's nothing more than natural starch that's been cooked until thick, dehydrated and pulverized. GRAS.

Pregnancy (diet and): Since the government issued its last diet recommendations for pregnant women in 1970, the Food and Nutrition Board of the National Research Council has asked for an update. Small wonder, given the advances in nutrition and obstetrics. Already the updated report is in and, among other things, it does the following:

1. Establishes wider ranges for pregnancy weight gain (25 to 35 pounds for women of normal weight, 28 to 40 for the underweight and 15 to 25 for the overweight). *Rate of gain* is important, too. After the third month, women of normal weight should add 1 pound a week, underweight a few ounces more, overweight women 10 to 12 ounces.

2. Recommends iron supplements (30 milligrams a day for normal women, 60 milligrams for those with iron-deficiency anemia *plus* 15 daily milligrams of zinc and 2 of copper; the extra iron may interfere with the body's ability to absorb zinc and copper).

3. Further recommends the following daily doses for strict vegetarians: 400 IU vitamin D, 600 milligrams calcium (for women under twenty-five, not just vegetarians but also milk haters and others who get little dietary calcium) and 2 micrograms vitamin B_{12}.

4. Suggests that women who eat few fruits, vegetables and whole grains take 300 micrograms per day of folic acid.

5. Cautions all pregnant women to go easy on vitamin A during the first trimester because it may increase the risk of birth defects.

As for diet in general, most nutritionists urge women to follow the new FOOD GUIDE PYRAMID, keeping the day's calories in the 2,200 to 2,500 range. This means that each day they should get nine servings from the Bread Group, four from the Vegetable Group, three *each* from the Fruit and Milk groups and 6 ounces of meat or other protein food.

Pregnancy-Induced Hypertension: See PIH.

Premature Infants (diet and): Any infant born before the thirty-seventh week is considered premature. Because preemies lack fully developed digestive tracts, can't coordinate their sucking or swallowing and need huge amounts of water, protein, calories, vitamins, calcium and other minerals, feeding is generally supervised by hospital professionals—doctors, registered dietitians and nurses. They use high-tech equipment that can detect and correct any imbalances as soon as they occur.

Premenstrual Syndrome: See PMS.

Preservatives: Chemicals, natural or artificial, that prolong shelf life and improve the palatability of food. They fall into two broad categories: **antimicrobials** (which thwart the growth of the microorganisms of spoilage) and **antioxidants** (which prevent oxidation and thus any discoloration or rancidity due to it). Under food-labeling laws, all preservatives (with the exception of salt, sugar, vinegar and certain spices) must be listed not only by name but also by function. For example: calcium propionate (to retard mold). **NOTE:** The major food preservatives are discussed alphabetically elsewhere.

Pressure Canning: It's imperative for low-acid foods (vegetables, meat, fish and poultry) because only then can harmful microorganisms (and their heat-resistant spores) be killed. The problem bug is *Clostridium botulinum,* which produces a deadly toxin. If canned low-acid foods are to be safe, they must be processed for some minutes at 10 to 15 pounds pressure, which raises their temperature to 237°F. and 246°F., respectively. The downside of pressure canning is that it tends to make food squishy, dulls colors (especially those of green vegetables) but, more important, destroys heat-sensitive vitamins, mainly B$_1$ (thiamin) and C. See also CANNING under FOOD PRESERVATION.

Pressure Cooking: Indispensable to high-altitude cooks who could never boil hard vegetables *tender* without the higher temperatures pressure saucepans make possible. In the 7,000-foot altitude of Santa Fe, New Mexico, for example, water boils at around 198°F., meaning that it never gets hot enough to cook potatoes. Sea-level cooks find less use for pressure saucepans even though they do impressively shortcut cooking times. Pot roasts fare best in pressure saucepans; vegetables, the worst, because it's difficult to control cooking times. Too often vegetables are overcooked in pressure saucepans and lose more heat-sensitive vitamins (C and B$_1$) than those gently steamed on the stove top.

Pretzels: They come hard and soft, big and little, arrow straight or twisted into complicated curlicues. These aren't, as you might suspect, a twentieth-century invention. They date back to Roman times although a French monk is credited with twisting the pretzel into its now-classic shape (his idea of someone praying with arms folded). Thanks to the Dutch, pretzels reached America early on. Pretzel sticks, a safe munch for calorie counters, are low calorie and almost fat free. But do seek out the reduced salt or salt free.

NUTRIENT CONTENT OF 1 MEDIUM-SIZE SOFT PRETZEL	
(about 2 ounces; 55 grams)	
190 calories	772 mg sodium
5 g protein	48 mg potassium
2 g fat, 1 saturated	1 g dietary fiber
2 mg cholesterol	0 RE vitamin A
38 g carbohydrate	0.23 mg thiamin
13 mg calcium	0.16 mg riboflavin
44 mg phosphorus	2.4 mg niacin
2.2 mg iron	0 mg vitamin C

NUTRIENT CONTENT OF 1 OUNCE (28 GRAMS) PRETZEL STICKS	
108 calories	486 mg sodium
3 g protein	41 mg potassium
1 g fat, 0 saturated	1 g dietary fiber
0 mg cholesterol	0 RE vitamin A
23 g carbohydrate	0.13 mg thiamin
10 mg calcium	0.18 mg riboflavin
32 mg phosphorus	1.5 mg niacin
1.2 mg iron	0 mg vitamin C

Prickly Pears: Popular throughout the Mediterranean basin where they grow with abandon, these fleshy, egg-shaped fruits of the Opuntia cactus are little appreciated here. Except in the Southwest and Mexico. Too bad, for prickly pears are smooth and sweet as dead-ripe pears (the reason, no doubt, why they're also called **cactus pears**). Their flesh may be scarlet, papaya gold, even lavender; their spiked skin, avocado green or chartreuse or yellow. Prickly pears sometimes show up in supermarket bins, so by all means give them a try. Peel and dice them into fruit cocktail, puree and freeze into sherbet, or buzz into a high-vi shake. **SEASON:** Fall, winter and spring.

NUTRIENT CONTENT OF 1 MEDIUM-SIZE PRICKLY PEAR	
(about 3²/₃ ounces; 103 grams)	
42 calories	5 mg sodium
1 g protein	226 mg potassium
0 g fat, 0 saturated	2 g dietary fiber
0 mg cholesterol	5 RE vitamin A
10 g carbohydrate	0.01 mg thiamin
58 mg calcium	0.06 mg riboflavin
25 mg phosphorus	0.5 mg niacin
0.3 mg iron	14 mg vitamin C

Pritikin Diet: Two diets, one for those with cardiovascular disease and an even stricter regimen for those hoping to avoid it. Both were developed by Dr. Nathan Pritikin, now deceased. The diet most people associate with Pritikin is the stricter one, which limits dietary fat to 10 percent of the day's total calories, bans alcohol and caffeine as well as high-sugar foods. In addition to paring fat and calories, it pumps the heart rate to 70 or 80 percent of its potential via vigorous daily exercise. Though the Pritikin Diet has its fans, some nutritionists believe it's too dire to be practical over the long haul. At least for most people.

Prolactin: The hormone that stimulates milk production in new mothers.

Proline: One of the nonessential AMINO ACIDS.

Promoter: A substance that encourages the development of cancer although it does not initiate it.

Propionates (additives): Widely used since the 1930s as preservatives in baked goods and processed cheeses, **calcium propionate** and **sodium propionate** (salts of propionic acid) were recently reevaluated by the FDA. Although heavy doses of them did kill lab rats (by disordering their fat metabolism), these two propionates continue to be rated GRAS and to this day account, by weight, for 75 percent of all the chemical preservatives used by U.S. food processors. Germany has banned propionates.

Propionic Acid (additive): An acrid fatty acid that exists naturally in everything from apples to milk to wood pulp. For food processors it does double duty, flavoring butters, cheeses and baked goods and also inhibiting mold growth. GRAS.

Propylene Glycol (additive): A moisturizer (humectant) used to keep shredded coconut and ready-to-spread cake frostings from drying out. It's also a flavor carrier for candies and soft drinks. GRAS.

Propylene Glycol Alginate (additive): A seaweed extract used as a thickener/stabilizer in frozen desserts and salad dressings. GRAS.

Propylene Glycol Monostearate (additive): An emulsifier and dough conditioner used in a broad spectrum of baked goods. After tests showed that large doses of propylene glycol monostearate impaired kidney function in lab animals and depressed their central nervous systems, the FDA reviewed it, but continues to rate it GRAS.

Propyl Gallate (additive): A lab-synthesized antioxidant used in vegetable oils, processed meats, chicken soups and chewing gums. In studies, large doses of propyl gallate have damaged the kidneys and livers of experimental animals. Recently reevaluated by the FDA, it is now rated GRAS when used within strict government guidelines.

Prosciutto: The mahogany-hued, air-dried ham of Italy, known for its nut-sweet flavor. No specific nutrient counts are available but there's no denying that prosciutto is long on sodium, saturated fat and cholesterol.

Proteases (additives): Enzymes found in pineapples, figs and other fruits that are used as meat tenderizers, dough conditioners and beer clarifiers. Not known to be toxic.

Protein: We are protein. Our hair, our nails, our skin, our blood, our enzymes and hormones are protein; indeed, our bodies contain some ten thousand to fifty thousand kinds of protein. But these proteins are constantly being broken down into AMINO ACIDS, recycled and built anew, even oxidized to some extent to provide energy (1 gram of protein weighs in at 4 calories, the same as carbohydrate). In the typical American diet, about 20 percent of the day's total calories come from protein.

Just to sustain life, we need daily infusions of top-quality proteins because our bodies cannot store them (or their building blocks, the amino acids) the way they store fats. The proteins we eat may be **complete,** meaning they contain all the amino acids we need and in the portions necessary to good health. Or they may be **incomplete** (lacking one or more essential amino acids). They are further categorized as **simple proteins** (containing nothing more than amino acids) or **conjugated** (amino acids bonded with nonprotein molecules). Collagen, a form of connective tissue, is a good example of a simple protein; hemoglobin, of a conjugated one (it's composed of amino acids plus a heme [iron] group). It's important to know, too, that proteins can complement one another. That when a food lacking a specific essential amino acid is eaten with another food that supplies the missing amino acid, the result is a high-quality protein. Three examples of these **complementary proteins:** cooked dried beans eaten with rice, a peanut butter sandwich (i.e., bread plus peanut butter) and split pea soup accompanied by corn bread.

When a healthy adult (pregnant women excepted) receives and utilizes the amount of protein he or she needs, that person is said to be in **nitrogen equilibrium.** Pregnant women and growing children are in **positive nitrogen balance,** meaning their nitrogen intake exceeds that lost (they need it for growth, building of new tissue). On the other hand, those with illness or injury exhibit **negative nitrogen balance** because they excrete more nitrogen than they consume. As a general rule, the amount of good-quality protein needed to achieve nitrogen equilibrium is 0.8 grams per day per 2.2 pounds (1 kilogram) of body weight for adults. A dire shortfall of protein leads to MARASMUS, a severe form of PROTEIN-CALORIE MALNUTRITION common among children in developing countries. What determines the quality, the BIOLOGICAL VALUE OF PROTEIN? The amino-acid mix; specifically, the number, type and proportion. Egg whites, with a biological value of 100, contain the right amount of the right amino acids needed to meet the body's needs. Indeed, they are the standard against which other proteins are measured.

GOOD SOURCES OF COMPLETE PROTEIN: Eggs, meat, fish, poultry, milk and other dairy products. **GOOD SOURCES OF INCOMPLETE PROTEIN:** Legumes (especially peas, beans, soybeans and peanuts), grains (especially unrefined), potatoes. Vegetarians, in particular, must choose their proteins carefully if they are to receive each day all the essential amino acids they need because plant proteins, in general, have a lower biological value than animal proteins. An incomplete protein may keep you alive, but it won't promote growth.

Protein Allergies: See IMMUNOGLOBULIN E.

Protein-Calorie Malnutrition: Also called **protein-energy malnutrition (PEM)**, this dire shortfall of protein manifests itself in several ways, depending upon the foods eaten or not eaten. In MARASMUS, for example, protein and calories are both lacking. In KWASHIORKOR, protein foods are absent yet the day's calorie quota is usually met thanks to starchy (high-carb) diets. These protein deficiencies are common in developing countries, particularly among children. They mean drastic weight loss, bloated bellies, stunted growth and, unless reversed, death.

Protein-Sparing Modified Fast (PSMF): See LIQUID DIETS.

Protozoa: See PARASITES.

Provitamins: Vitamin precursors, or substances from which vitamins are made. Beta-carotene, for example, is a precursor of vitamin A.

Provolone: Everyone's image of an Italian cheese, provolone is shaped into balls, pears, pigs and sausages, trussed with string and suspended from the ceiling of every Italian deli. It is a hard cheese, pleasantly bland but salty, too,

RECOMMENDED DAILY PROTEIN INTAKE

Age	Weight	Calories Needed per Day	Protein Needed per Day
Children (boys and girls):			
1 to 3 years	29 lb (13 kg)	1,300	16 g
4 to 6 years	44 lb (20 kg)	1,800	24 g
7 to 10 years	62 lb (28 kg)	2,000	28 g
Men and Boys:			
11 to 14 years	99 lb (45 kg)	2,500	45 g
15 to 18 years	145 lb (66 kg)	3,000	59 g
19 to 24 years	160 lb (72 kg)	2,900	58 g
25 to 50 years	174 lb (79 kg)	2,900	63 g
51+ years	170 lb (77 kg)	2,300	63 g
Women and Girls:			
11 to 14 years	101 lb (46 kg)	2,200	46 g
15 to 18 years	120 lb (55 kg)	2,200	44 g
19 to 24 years	128 lb (58 kg)	2,200	46 g
25 to 50 years	138 lb (63 kg)	2,200	50 g
51+ years	143 lb (65 kg)	1,900	50 g
Pregnant Women:	—	an extra 300	60 g
Nursing Mothers:			
First six months	—	an extra 500	65 g
Second six months	—	an extra 500	62 g

thanks to its brine dip. Provolone is kneaded until compact and smooth, then cured with *Aspergillus* and *Penicillium* molds. Mature provolone is about 35 percent fat, 28 percent protein, 4 percent salt and the rest water. It's good as a snack, as dessert. When fully aged, provolone is hard enough to grate like Parmesan.

NUTRIENT CONTENT OF 1 OUNCE (28 GRAMS) PROVOLONE

99 calories	247 mg sodium
7 g protein	39 mg potassium
8 g fat, 5 saturated	0 g dietary fiber
20 mg cholesterol	75 RE vitamin A
1 g carbohydrate	0.01 mg thiamin
214 mg calcium	0.09 mg riboflavin
140 mg phosphorus	0 mg niacin
0.1 mg iron	0 mg vitamin C

Prudent Diet: A sane, well-balanced diet developed by the American Heart Association that limits dietary fat to 30 percent of the day's calories (with saturated, monounsaturated and polyunsaturated each accounting for 10 percent of the total). It also restricts cholesterol to 300 milligrams a day. Like the PRITIKIN DIET, the Prudent Diet is designed to prevent coronary heart disease. Unlike it, the Prudent Diet is much easier to follow.

Prunes: These fruits are not just dried plums but a sugary European fresh variety that can be dried, pit and all, without fermenting. They are firmer than other plums, more acidic but honey-sweet, too. Finally, prunes are freestone, like peaches, meaning their pits separate easily from their flesh—not true of other plums. Dried prunes, the most

NUTRIENT CONTENT OF 5 DRIED PRUNES (UNPITTED)
(about 1½ ounces; 42 grams)

100 calories	2 mg sodium
1 g protein	313 mg potassium
0 g fat, 0 saturated	3 g dietary fiber
0 mg cholesterol	84 RE vitamin A
26 g carbohydrate	0.03 mg thiamin
21 mg calcium	0.07 mg riboflavin
33 mg phosphorus	0.8 mg niacin
1 mg iron	1 mg vitamin C

familiar form, can be eaten out of hand like candy, pitted, chopped and stirred into a huge repertoire of breads, puddings and pies. They are quick sources of energy and contain hefty shots of iron, potassium and fiber.

NUTRIENT CONTENT OF 1 CUP STEWED PRUNES (UNPITTED)
(about 7½ ounces; 212 grams)

227 calories	4 mg sodium
2 g protein	708 mg potassium
0 g fat, 0 saturated	14 g dietary fiber
0 mg cholesterol	66 RE vitamin A
60 g carbohydrate	0.05 mg thiamin
49 mg calcium	0.21 mg riboflavin
74 mg phosphorus	1.5 mg niacin
2.4 mg iron	6 mg vitamin C

Prussic Acid, Hydrocyanic Acid: A deadly, fast-acting poison that exists naturally in many foods (cassava, bamboo shoots and dried beans) as well as in peach and apricot pits (from which flavorings are extracted). See also HYDROGEN CYANIDE.

PSMF (Protein-Sparing Modified Fast): See LIQUID DIETS.

Psoralens: Natural toxins present in celery, parsley and parsnips, small doses of which have been used for years to treat vitiligo, the pigment disorder that afflicts singer Michael Jackson. Psoralens promote tanning just as they accelerate the browning of celery and parsnips; indeed, the browner the vegetable, the greater its dose of psoralens. Today psoralens plus ultraviolet radiation (PUVA) are used to treat more than a dozen skin diseases, among them vitiligo, psoriasis and nonmelanoma skin cancers. It now appears that psoralens may actually protect against nonmelanoma skin cancers. But researchers continue to eye psoralens with caution because of their toxicity, their power to sensitize people to light and their potential to cause cellular mutations and perhaps cancer. Those handling a new pest-resistant celery developed phytophotodermatitis (skin disorders triggered by the interaction of psoralens and light). To date, no federal agency monitors or regulates natural toxins.

Psoriasis (diet and): This chronic, scaly-skin disorder may be triggered or eased by certain foods, but there's no proof positive. Some say that avoiding high-taurine foods (meat, organ meats and fish) may help; others that dosing on LECITHIN and vitamins does little good.

P:S Ratio: The proportion of polyunsaturated fats to saturated. Foods with a high P:S ratio (almonds, walnuts, corn, safflower and soybean oils, etc.) are considered beneficial in heart-healthy diets.

PST: See PORCINE SOMATOTROPIN.

Psychiatric Disorders (diet and): Does mood determine food? And vice versa? Certainly psychological problems underlie uncontrollable eating and bulimia, anorexia, alcoholism and drug abuse. To treat such addictions and eating disorders successfully, there must be a team effort with physicians, psychotherapists, registered dietitians and nurses all taking part. See also ORTHOMOLECULAR PSYCHIATRY.

Psyllium: A natural laxative full of soluble fiber extracted from the dried seeds of *Plantago psyllium*. Back in the 1980s there was considerable nutri-hype about psyllium's ability to flush "bad" cholesterol (LDL) out of the blood. Health-food stores began stocking the stuff, and two major food companies (General Mills and Kellogg) introduced cereals with psyllium. Not without flak (because of psyllium's laxative effect, the FDA considers it a drug). There were also plenty of consumer complaints because psyllium can produce serious side effects (intense allergic reactions, anorexia, abdominal cramps, gas). As a result, General Mills no longer makes Benefit cereal. And Kellogg now posts warnings on every package of Heartwise, explaining that those whose jobs expose them to psyllium dust (nurses, for example) may have become sensitive to psyllium.

Pteroylglutamic Acid (PGA): Chemical parlance for folic acid, a B vitamin.

Ptomaines, Ptomaine Poisoning: When meats and other high-protein foods decompose, ptomaines are formed. These, however, are not the culprits in food poisoning. That distinction belongs to certain microbes and the toxins they produce. So "ptomaine poisoning" doesn't exist. See BACTERIA.

Public Health Service (PHS): An important branch of the Department of Health and Human Services, the Public Health Service is subdivided into seven agencies, the better to safeguard our health: the Food and Drug Administration (FDA); the President's Council on Physical Fitness and Sports; the National Center for Health Statistics; the Alcohol, Drug Abuse and Mental Health Administration; the Centers for Disease Control (CDC); the Health Resources and Services Administration (which includes the Bureau of Health Care Delivery and Assistance, the Bureau of Health Maintenance Organizations and Resources Development, and the Indian Health Service); and, finally, the National Institutes of Health (NIH) and its six active arms: the National Cancer Institute; the National Heart, Lung and Blood Institute; the National Institute of Arthritis, Metabolism and Digestive Diseases; the National Institute of Dental Research; the National Institute on Aging; and the National Library of Medicine. See also HEALTH AND HUMAN SERVICES, U.S. DEPARTMENT OF.

PUFA: Short for polyunsaturated fatty acid.

Pufferfish Poisoning: Pufferfish, also called **blowfish** and **globefish,** gobble a species of dinoflagellates (plankton) that produce deadly tetrodotoxin. This poison concentrates in the pufferfish's internal organs (primarily the liver) and unless these organs are removed intact without nicks or tears, anyone eating the fish may sicken—even die—within twenty-four hours. In Japan, where pufferfish (*fugu*) is a delicacy of ritual proportion, chefs must be licensed to handle it.

Pulses: Another word for LEGUMES.

Pummelos, Pomelos: Also called **shaddocks** and **Chinese grapefruits,** these thick-skinned, pink- to yellow-fleshed citrus fruits are as popular in the Caribbean as in Indochina, where they're believed to have originated. Depending upon variety and ripeness, they can be honey-sweet or lemon-tart; use as you would grapefruit. Like other citrus fruits, pummelos are high in vitamin C and low in calories. **SEASON:** All too short: mid-January to mid-February.

NUTRIENT CONTENT OF 1 CUP PUMMELO SECTIONS
(about 6¾ ounces; 190 grams)

71 calories	2 mg sodium
1 g protein	411 mg potassium
0 g fat, 0 saturated	0 g dietary fiber
0 mg cholesterol	0 RE vitamin A
18 g carbohydrate	0.07 mg thiamin
7 mg calcium	0.05 mg riboflavin
32 mg phosphorus	0.4 mg niacin
0.2 mg iron	116 mg vitamin C

Pumpernickel: A family of dark, dense breads with a high percentage of rye flour. They owe their color, compactness and slightly caramel flavor to prolonged baking (sometimes a full twenty-four hours) in low-temperature steam ovens. Pumpernickel, often caraway scented, is popular throughout northern Europe but the Germans claim it as their own. In the industrial town of Osnabrück there's a Pumpernickel Tower, which, locals say, commemorates the first loaf baked there in the year 1400 during a famine. *Bonum paniculum* it was called. Does pumpernickel derive from *paniculum*? Maybe. Other Germans insist pumpernickel is named for Pumper Nickel, the miller who mixed and milled the grains. Then there's the Napoleon story. It seems that when he first tasted this leaden bread, he gagged and said, *"Pour Nicole!"* ("For Nicole!"—his horse).

NUTRIENT CONTENT OF 1 SLICE PUMPERNICKEL BREAD
(about 1 ounce; 32 grams)

80 calories	215 mg sodium
3 g protein	67 mg potassium
1 g fat, 0 saturated	2 g dietary fiber
0 mg cholesterol	0 RE vitamin A
15 g carbohydrate	0.11 mg thiamin
22 mg calcium	0.10 mg riboflavin
57 mg phosphorus	1.0 mg niacin
0.9 mg iron	0 mg vitamin C

Pumpkins: "A kind of melon or, rather, gourd" is the way one early European described pumpkins and winter squash. "Some of these are green, some yellow, some longish, others round like an apple, all of them pleasant food boiled and buttered and seasoned with spice. But the yellow . . . about the size of a pome . . . is the best kind." Of course pumpkins and squash all belong to the same big family, all of them native to the New World. Pumpkin pie is everyone's favorite, but pumpkins are equally delicious baked like butternut squash. They're even better when pureed and stirred into soup. All pumpkins are positively golden when it comes to beta-carotene and potassium and no slouch in the iron and riboflavin departments. Yet they are very low in calories and sodium, contain no fat or cholesterol.

NUTRIENT CONTENT OF 1 CUP CANNED SOLID-PACK PUMPKIN
(about 8⅔ ounces; 245 grams)

49 calories	2 mg sodium
2 g protein	564 mg potassium
0 g fat, 0 saturated	4 g dietary fiber
0 mg cholesterol	265 RE vitamin A
12 g carbohydrate	0.08 mg thiamin
37 mg calcium	0.19 mg riboflavin
74 mg phosphorus	1.0 mg niacin
1.4 mg iron	12 mg vitamin C

Pumpkin Seeds: See PEPITAS.

Pure Food and Drug Act: In 1906, the U.S. government, after defining "pure food" and "adulterated food," decreed that only "pure food" could be sold in the United States. Ten years later, a court ruled that caffeine could be added to soft drinks. Its reasoning: Although caffeine might be harmful in large or frequent doses, its use in soft drinks was harmless. To this day, caffeine is added to many colas. In 1938, the Food, Drug, and Cosmetic Act zeroed in on the toxic substances present in our food—mainly additives. The 1954 Miller Amendment broadened the act's reach to include pesticide residues and set strict limits on the amounts allowable. Then in 1958, the DELANEY CLAUSE was added, prohibiting the addition to food of any substance known to cause cancer in animals or human beings. At that time the GRAS list of additives was also established.

Purines: Nitrogen-rich compounds that break down into uric acid, a compound present in small amounts in urine. Once told to avoid meats or other protein foods high in purines, GOUT sufferers are now usually treated with medication.

Pyridoxine: See B₆, VITAMIN.

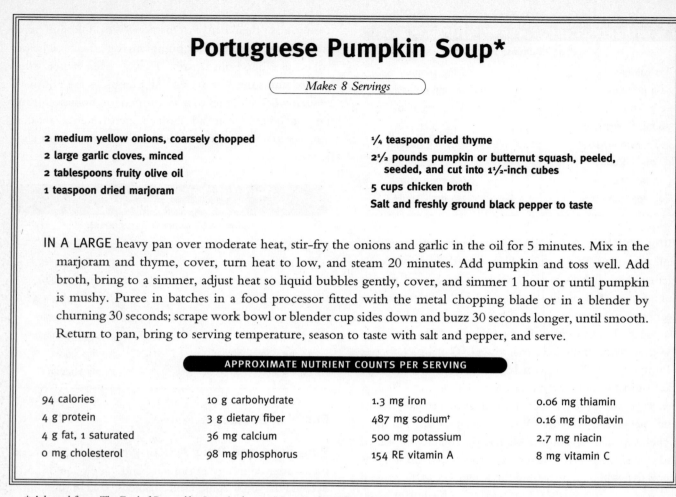

Portuguese Pumpkin Soup*

Makes 8 Servings

2 medium yellow onions, coarsely chopped

2 large garlic cloves, minced

2 tablespoons fruity olive oil

1 teaspoon dried marjoram

¼ teaspoon dried thyme

2½ pounds pumpkin or butternut squash, peeled, seeded, and cut into 1½-inch cubes

5 cups chicken broth

Salt and freshly ground black pepper to taste

IN A LARGE heavy pan over moderate heat, stir-fry the onions and garlic in the oil for 5 minutes. Mix in the marjoram and thyme, cover, turn heat to low, and steam 20 minutes. Add pumpkin and toss well. Add broth, bring to a simmer, adjust heat so liquid bubbles gently, cover, and simmer 1 hour or until pumpkin is mushy. Puree in batches in a food processor fitted with the metal chopping blade or in a blender by churning 30 seconds; scrape work bowl or blender cup sides down and buzz 30 seconds longer, until smooth. Return to pan, bring to serving temperature, season to taste with salt and pepper, and serve.

APPROXIMATE NUTRIENT COUNTS PER SERVING

94 calories	10 g carbohydrate	1.3 mg iron	0.06 mg thiamin
4 g protein	3 g dietary fiber	487 mg sodium†	0.16 mg riboflavin
4 g fat, 1 saturated	36 mg calcium	500 mg potassium	2.7 mg niacin
0 mg cholesterol	98 mg phosphorus	154 RE vitamin A	8 mg vitamin C

* Adapted from *The Food of Portugal* by Jean Anderson (New York: William Morrow, 1986).

† To reduce sodium, use a low-sodium chicken broth.

Pyridoxol Hydrochloride (additive): A form of vitamin B_6 added to baby formulas, evaporated milk, baked goods and other foods. GRAS.

Pyruvic Acid: An intermediate by-product of glucose metabolism, which strenuous exercise converts to lactic acid.

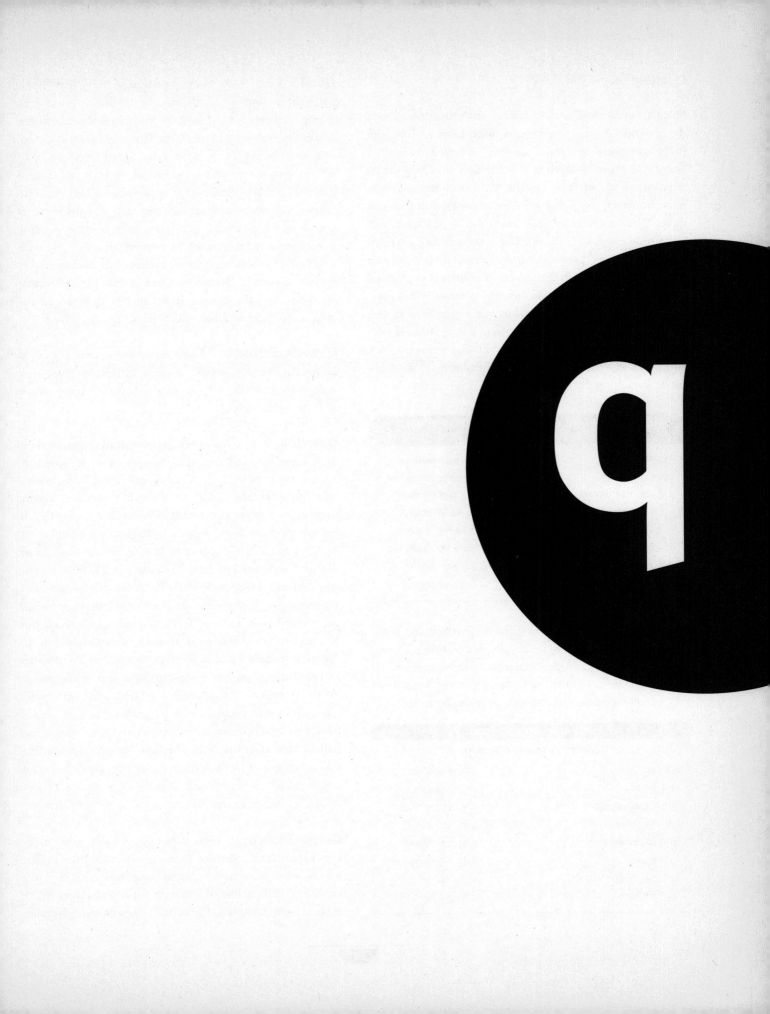

Quahog: See CLAMS.

Quail: Small, chunky chickenlike birds that forage about the ground for seeds, insects and fallen berries. Although there are several species of quail in the western United States, the eastern bobwhite is better known. Quail are so small one bird per person is the usual portion; trenchermen, however, can polish off a brace (two) with room to spare. Quail meat is dry and, unless the birds have found something tasty to eat, bland. But it is surprisingly rich in iron, phosphorus, potassium and niacin. The best way to cook quail is to brown them nicely in butter, bacon drippings or oil, then simmer in a covered casserole with a generous splash of sherry or dry white wine (they'll be tender in half an hour). In his classic but long out of print *Encyclopedia of Food,* Artemus Ward writes that the true quail "is a bird of the eastern hemisphere," then adds that "the Israelites, wandering through the desert, fed on quail."

NUTRIENT CONTENT OF 3 OUNCES (85 GRAMS) QUAIL (SKINNED, UNCOOKED)	
114 calories	44 mg sodium
19 g protein	202 mg potassium
4 g fat, 1 saturated	0 g dietary fiber
59 mg cholesterol	14 RE vitamin A
0 g carbohydrate	0.24 mg thiamin
11 mg calcium	0.24 mg riboflavin
261 mg phosphorus	7.0 mg niacin
3.8 mg iron	6 mg vitamin C

Quail Eggs: Not much bigger than hazelnuts, these brown-speckled tan eggs are all the rage just now among chefs, especially in Europe. Sometimes quail eggs are hard-cooked and served in the shell as an appetizer. Sometimes they're softly coddled and nestled in caviar or aspic.

NUTRIENT CONTENT OF 1 QUAIL EGG (about ⅓ ounce; 9 grams)	
14 calories	13 mg sodium
1 g protein	12 mg potassium
1 g fat, 0 saturated	0 g dietary fiber
76 mg cholesterol	8 RE vitamin A
0 g carbohydrate	0.01 mg thiamin
6 mg calcium	0.07 mg riboflavin
20 mg phosphorus	0 mg niacin
0.3 mg iron	0 mg vitamin C

Quark: A tart, fresh, spoon-up-thick, snow-white cheese made from skim or partly skim milk that is popular in Europe, especially Germany. Its texture is a cross between cream cheese and RICOTTA. Its flavor is ricottalike, too, only sharper. As for nutritive value, quark averages 70 to 80 percent water, 15 to 16 percent protein and 2 to 3 percent fat. Many health-food stores now sell quark, as do fancy-food stores and upscale big-city greenmarkets. If you're unable to find quark, you can fake it by blending pureed or sieved ricotta or fine-curded cottage cheese with a little crème fraîche, Devon cream, sour cream, cream cheese or yogurt. **NOTE:** Nutrient counts are unavailable for quark, but it's reasonable to say that they would approximate those of whole-milk ricotta cheese.

Quassia Extract: A bitter flavoring obtained from a South American tree used to make bitters, to flavor root beer and sarsaparilla, also to simulate vanilla, cherry, grape and other flavorings.

Quercitin: Red wines get their color from the grape skins on which they stand during the first stages of fermentation. At the same time, they pick up quercitin, a flavonoid, which may be the reason the French—who accompany their egg-, butter- and cream-rich meals with bottles of red wine—have fewer heart attacks than nationalities for which wine is less important. The death rate from heart disease among the French is 75 deaths per 100,000 as compared to more than twice that for Americans. Quercitin, University of Wisconsin researchers now believe, may not only raise blood levels of HDL ("good" cholesterol) but also act as a blood thinner. But there's a downside, too. In different studies, extracts of green beans, lettuce, paprika and rhubarb (all high in quercitin) have caused mutations, even cancer in lab rats. Onions, too, are loaded with quercitin, and cattle grazing fields overrun with wild onions have developed anemia; some have died. Other researchers believe that what's been dubbed the French paradox, the low incidence of heart disease among a people whose diet is notoriously high in fat and cholesterol, is due to a powerful antioxidant in red table wine called RESVERATROL.

Queso Blanco: A fresh skim- or low-fat cow's milk cheese popular throughout Mexico and Latin America that is now being made in the United States, too. It's soft, finely curded, slightly acidic, lightly salted, pressed and as white as snow, which explains the name "white cheese." Because of its low fat content, *queso blanco* has become a mainstay among those trying to trim fat, cholesterol and calories. A few years ago, *queso blanco* contaminated with *Listeria monocytogenes* made a number of people very sick in California and the Southwest (see BACTERIA). **Note**: Specific nutrient counts are unavailable for *queso blanco* but they would approximate those of low-fat cottage cheese.

Quetelet Index: Another term for BODY MASS INDEX.

Quiche: The French bacon-and-cheese tart that took America by storm and metamorphosed into a dozen flavor variations. The trouble is, all are supersaturated with fat, calories and cholesterol, averaging per serving some 500 calories, 40 grams fat (19 grams saturated) and 203 milli-

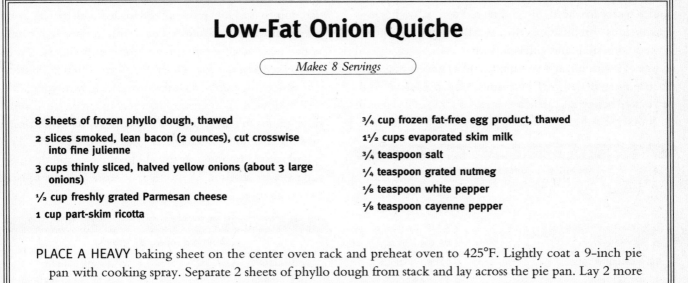

Low-Fat Onion Quiche

Makes 8 Servings

8 sheets of frozen phyllo dough, thawed

2 slices smoked, lean bacon (2 ounces), cut crosswise into fine julienne

3 cups thinly sliced, halved yellow onions (about 3 large onions)

½ cup freshly grated Parmesan cheese

1 cup part-skim ricotta

¾ cup frozen fat-free egg product, thawed

1½ cups evaporated skim milk

¾ teaspoon salt

¼ teaspoon grated nutmeg

⅛ teaspoon white pepper

⅛ teaspoon cayenne pepper

PLACE A HEAVY baking sheet on the center oven rack and preheat oven to 425°F. Lightly coat a 9-inch pie pan with cooking spray. Separate 2 sheets of phyllo dough from stack and lay across the pie pan. Lay 2 more sheets in the pan at right angles to the first set. Arrange 2 more sheets in pan on the diagonal to cover any gaps, and, finally, cover remaining gaps by adding 2 more sheets on another diagonal. Top with a double thickness of paper toweling wrung out in cold water, and gently press the phyllo into the contours of the pan. Carefully peel off the toweling and discard. Do not trim dough overhanging; instead, roll it loosely under on top of the rim, dampening as needed to prevent breaking and piecing.

BROWN THE BACON in a large heavy skillet over moderate heat for about 3 minutes; when crisp, lift browned bits to paper toweling to drain. Reduce heat to low, add onions to skillet, cover, and steam 15 minutes. Meanwhile, place all remaining ingredients in a blender or a food processor fitted with the metal chopping blade and churn 15 seconds. Scrape down work bowl sides and churn 15 to 20 seconds more until smooth. When onions have steamed 15 minutes, uncover, raise heat to moderate, and cook 1 minute to evaporate excess liquid. Arrange the onions in the crust, pour in the cheese mixture, and scatter reserved bacon bits evenly over top. Bake, uncovered, on baking sheet for 10 minutes. Reduce oven temperature to 350°F. and bake 18 to 20 minutes more, until quiche is set. Cool on a wire rack to room temperature before cutting.

APPROXIMATE NUTRIENT COUNTS PER SERVING

180 calories	15 g carbohydrate	0.8 mg iron	0.10 mg thiamin
12 g protein	1 g dietary fiber	490 mg sodium	0.29 mg riboflavin
8 g fat, 4 saturated	322 mg calcium	297 mg potassium	0.6 mg niacin
19 mg cholesterol	229 mg phosphorus	110 RE vitamin A	4 mg vitamin C

grams cholesterol. This "skinny" version slashes that unhealthy trilogy without compromising taste, texture or nutritional value.

Quince: An ancient fruit that still grows wild over much of the Middle East, its place of origin. Either round or pear shaped and as big as an apple, the ivory-fleshed quince, despite its flowery bouquet, is too hard, too sour to eat raw. Being naturally high in pectin, it's been used forever to make jams, marmalades and pastes (in Portugal, stiff quince pastes are sliced thin and served with salty cheese—a marvelous combination). In the Middle East, quince is stewed with lamb and chicken. Other than being a good source of potassium and vitamin C and a fair one of dietary fiber, quince is not very nutritious. And because it must be cooked before it's eaten, it even loses some of its vitamin C. **SEASON:** Fall.

NUTRIENT CONTENT OF 1 MEDIUM-SIZE QUINCE	
(about 3⅓ ounces; 92 grams)	
52 calories	4 mg sodium
0 g protein	181 mg potassium
0 g fat, 0 saturated	2 g dietary fiber
0 mg cholesterol	4 RE vitamin A
14 g carbohydrate	0.02 mg thiamin
10 mg calcium	0.03 mg riboflavin
16 mg phosphorus	0.2 mg niacin
0.6 mg iron	14 mg vitamin C

Quinine Extracts (additives): Quinine dihydrochloride and **quinine sulfate** are extracted from the bark of the South American chinchona tree. These intensely bitter white granules or needles are used to flavor carbonated beverages, primarily bitter lemon and tonic water. Quinine is also used in the manufacture of bitters and, of course, as a treatment for malaria. Because quinine is a toxic alkaloid, the FDA strictly limits the amounts of it that can be used.

Quinine Water, Tonic Water, Indian Tonic: A carbonated mixer containing quinine extract (usually quinine dihydrochloride or quinine sulfate), sugar and/or high-fructose corn syrup, citric acid and often the preservative sodium benzoate. The original Indian tonic also contained extracts of bitter orange, and many of those manufactured in Britain and continental Europe still do. They are mellower, richer than the made in the U.S.A. tonic waters. All mixers containing quinine have a bluish cast.

Quinoa: Pronounced *KEEN-wah*. This "new" supergrain is as old as the Incas. To them, these little sesamelike beads were the mother grain, a nutritional powerhouse that sustained them in hard times at high altitudes (we now know that quinoa is a high-protein food loaded with niacin, iron, phosphorus and potassium). For all this, quinoa is as bland as rice (except for a bitterish aftertaste) and, like rice, it is best served as a sop for gravies and stews. Quinoa's bitterness is due to saponin, a natural insecticide with which it's well endowed. To get the bitterness out, you need only rinse quinoa in a sieve under a cold tap. Purists don't rinse, insisting that quinoa's character goes down the drain. Try it both ways. In addition to whole quinoa, quinoa flour and pasta are available. A health-food store is the best place to buy all three.

NUTRIENT CONTENT OF ½ CUP DRY QUINOA	
(about 3 ounces; 85 grams)	
318 calories	18 mg sodium
11 g protein	629 mg potassium
5 g fat, 1 saturated	4 g dietary fiber
0 mg cholesterol	0 RE vitamin A
59 g carbohydrate	0.17 mg thiamin
51 mg calcium	0.34 mg riboflavin
349 mg phosphorus	2.5 mg niacin
7.9 mg iron	0 mg vitamin C

Quinolines: Cancer-causing chemicals that exist in food. See PAHs.

Quinones: A group of organic compounds that include vitamin K, both the naturally occurring (**phylloquinone** in plants, **menaquinone** in animals) and the lab-synthesized **menadione, Synkayvite** and **Hykinone** (originally called vitamins K_1, K_2 and K_3). Phylloquinone was isolated in 1939 from alfalfa meal, which remains a popular health food to this day. See also K, VITAMIN.

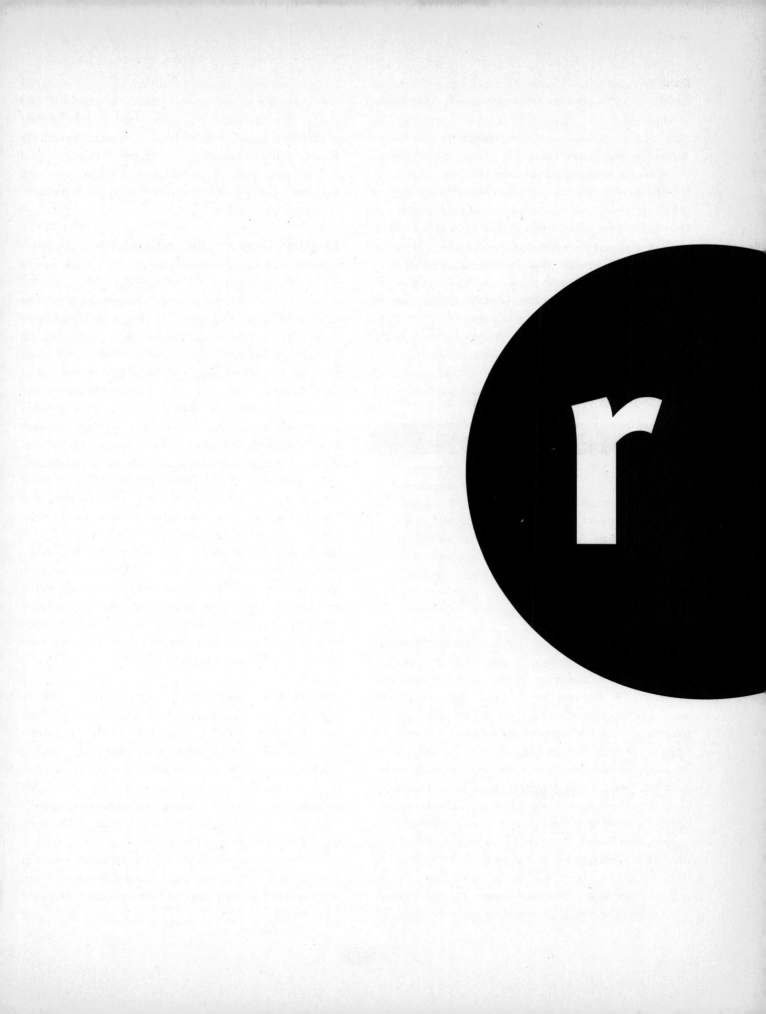

Rabbit: The Romans caught wild rabbits, caged them and fattened them for the table. Thomas Jefferson raised rabbits at Monticello. And although he imported certain species from France, rabbits were well known to the Native Americans long before Europeans arrived. Americans today don't eat much rabbit although the farm raised are as lean, as white, as delicate as chicken breast. Our images of the Easter bunny have turned most of us off rabbit although hunters are quick to bag (and eat) dark-meated jackrabbits. In truth, these are **hares,** dark-meated, bigger and gamier than rabbits. In France, food snobs consider rabbit blue-collar food and opt for hare every time. But when it comes to doing right by rabbits and hares, no people can top the Germans. They cook them in a jug, stew them and, if the animals are young and tender, roast or braise them. In the United States, oven-ready rabbits are available both fresh and frozen. They are low in saturated fat and calories yet high in iron, phosphorus, potassium and niacin.

**NUTRIENT CONTENT OF 3 OUNCES (85 GRAMS)
ROASTED RABBIT**

168 calories	40 mg sodium
25 g protein	326 mg potassium
7 g fat, 2 saturated	0 g dietary fiber
70 mg cholesterol	0 RE vitamin A
0 g carbohydrate	0.08 mg thiamin
16 mg calcium	0.18 mg riboflavin
224 mg phosphorus	7.2 mg niacin
1.9 mg iron	0 mg vitamin C

Radiation: Electromagnetic waves emitted by sunlight, dental and medical X rays, television sets, microwave ovens, etc. When microwave ovens debuted shortly after World War II, they cost the earth and were as big as telephone booths. Just as well because the average cook was terrified of them, considered them radioactive, a sure way to go sterile or get cancer. Even after the size and price of microwave ovens came down within reach of home cooks, Nervous Nellies across America refused to have anything to do with them. Only in the 1980s did microwave ovens become a must-have. And then only after decades of intensive consumer ed. To recap: Microwaves are not X rays; they are nonionizing rays and as such are not radioactive. Once cooking is done, there are no residual microwaves in the oven or in the food microwaved. To ensure microwave safety, the federal government approves all micro-

wave oven designs, requires that their doors be equipped with two independent interlocks that cut power the second they're opened. Further, the government sets the amount of nonionizing radiation that home microwave ovens may emit (1 milliwatt per square centimeter at a distance of 2 inches). As a result, the only microwave injuries to date have been the sorts of burns conventional ovens produce. See also IRRADIATION.

Radiation Therapy (diet and): Side effects vary in severity and frequency according to the dosage, the part of the body involved and the general health of the patient. As a rule, however, many people undergoing treatment suffer from nausea, vomiting, loss of appetite, heightened or diminished sense of taste and/or smell. If the head and neck are irradiated, there may also be mouth sores, tooth and gum destruction, lack of saliva and an inflamed esophagus. Abdominal radiation may mean diarrhea and faulty absorption of nutrients. And in most cases the immune system will be weakened. The dietitian's mission is to plan a well-balanced, strength-building, *appealing* eating program the patient can tolerate *before* he's lost weight, become malnourished and has no appetite. This may mean zipping up the seasonings for those who complain that "food has no taste," substituting other top-quality proteins for red meat when the sense of smell is heightened, recommending wet foods for those with dry mouth, modifying the lactose (milk sugar), fat and fiber for those with intestinal damage. If patients can no longer swallow, IVs or other tube feeding may be necessary. Because every case is individual, registered dietitians should join the medical team even before radiation therapy begins. Then fine-tune the patient's diet as treatment progresses.

Radicchio: A tightly headed, white-veined red chicory popular in Italy that's new to American salad bowls. Like other chicories, radicchio has a slightly bitter taste and a soft crunch. It pairs splendidly with salad greens, adding hot accents of color, and is best tossed with a good olive oil and balsamic vinegar. Never content to leave well enough alone, innovative American chefs have begun grilling radicchio or baking slivers of it atop pizza. Californians were the first to grow radicchio on a commercial scale in this country—but only in 1981. Today it is also grown in New Jersey and these two major sources manage to keep supermarket bins well supplied with radicchio. **SEASON:** Year-round.

NUTRIENT CONTENT OF ½ CUP SHREDDED RAW RADICCHIO

(about ¾ ounce; 20 grams)

5 calories	4 mg sodium
0 g protein	60 mg potassium
0 g fat, 0 saturated	NA g dietary fiber
0 mg cholesterol	1 RE vitamin A
1 g carbohydrate	0 mg thiamin
4 mg calcium	0.01 mg riboflavin
8 mg phosphorus	0.1 mg niacin
0.1 mg iron	2 mg vitamin C

Radionuclides: Radioactive substances that sometimes contaminate food. See MARKET BASKET SURVEY.

Radishes: For all their variety—peppery scarlet globes the size of marbles, snowy little icicles, pearly Asian giants (*daikon*) the shape of salami, "black turnips" (Spanish radishes) with all the fire of fresh horseradish—radishes belong to a single genus, *Raphanus*. They are ancient, probably Asian, although Egyptians were growing radishes early on because of the oil they could press from their seeds (this was before the arrival of the olive). Radishes belong to the family of CRUCIFEROUS VEGETABLES, which includes all the cabbages and turnips. Unlike cabbages and turnips, radishes are not very nutritious. As far as Pliny was concerned, the radish was "a vulgar article of the diet" because of its "remarkable power of causing flatulence and eructation." **SEASON:** Except for black radishes, year-round because many red radishes, white icicles and *daikon* are either hothouse grown or farmed in warm climates and shipped to the cold. The rarer black radishes are at their best in winter and early spring although in ethnic areas of great demand (New York City, for example, with its large Jewish population), they, too, are available year-round.

NUTRIENT CONTENT OF 5 SMALL RED RADISHES

(about ¾ ounce; 23 grams)

4 calories	5 mg sodium
0 g protein	52 mg potassium
0 g fat, 0 saturated	0 g dietary fiber
0 mg cholesterol	0 RE vitamin A
1 g carbohydrate	0 mg thiamin
5 mg calcium	0.01 mg riboflavin
4 mg phosphorus	0.1 mg niacin
0.1 mg iron	5 mg vitamin C

NUTRIENT CONTENT OF ½ CUP SLICED ASIAN RADISHES (DAIKONS)

(about 1½ ounces; 44 grams)

8 calories	9 mg sodium
0 g protein	100 mg potassium
0 g fat, 0 saturated	1 g dietary fiber
0 mg cholesterol	0 RE vitamin A
2 g carbohydrate	0.01 mg thiamin
12 mg calcium	0.01 mg riboflavin
10 mg phosphorus	0.1 mg niacin
0.2 mg iron	10 mg vitamin C

NUTRIENT CONTENT OF 1 MEDIUM-SIZE ICICLE RADISH

(about ½ ounce; 17 grams)

2 calories	3 mg sodium
0 g protein	48 mg potassium
0 g fat, 0 saturated	NA g dietary fiber
0 mg cholesterol	0 RE vitamin A
0 g carbohydrate	0.01 mg thiamin
5 mg calcium	0 mg riboflavin
5 mg phosphorus	0.1 mg niacin
0.1 mg iron	5 mg vitamin C

Radish Sprouts: The Japanese prize the peppery sprouts of the *daikon* (a big white Asian radish). They are now available in the United States, especially in big-city greenmarkets, and add welcome bite to salads and sandwiches. Season: Year-round.

NUTRIENT CONTENT OF 1 CUP RADISH SPROUTS

(about 1⅓ ounces; 38 grams)

16 calories	2 mg sodium
1 g protein	33 mg potassium
1 g fat, 0 saturated	1 g dietary fiber
0 mg cholesterol	15 RE vitamin A
1 g carbohydrate	0.04 mg thiamin
19 mg calcium	0.04 mg riboflavin
43 mg phosphorus	1.1 mg niacin
0.3 mg iron	11 mg vitamin C

Radon (in tap water): The EPA estimates that radon contaminates more well water and village water systems than lead, nitrates, bacteria, viruses, parasites and industrial wastes put together. This radioactive gas is particularly insidious because it's invisible, odorless and tasteless. Produced by uranium, radon exists in the earth's crust, seeps into houses and leaches into drinking water. The problem comes not from drinking the water, but from agitating it—washing dishes or clothes, showering—which frees radon gas. Unless it is vented outside, household levels of it build up to levels that can cause serious harm. The EPA estimates that inhaled radon is responsible for from 10,000 to 40,000 lung cancer deaths each year, 100 to 1,800 of these due to contaminated tap water. Known hot spots for radon-polluted water are Arizona, North Carolina, Maine, New Hampshire, Connecticut and, to a lesser degree, the other New England states. If you live in a high-radon area, test first for the amount of radon in your house, then, if those levels warrant it, for radon in your tap water. Some state agencies will do the testing for nominal fees; failing that, contact a private lab. What constitutes high radon levels for water? According to the EPA, 10,000 or more pico-curies per liter. Are there ways to get the radon out? Fortunately, yes. Carbon filter tanks (not small faucet attachments; these resemble water softener units) will remove about 90 percent of the radon. Home aerators are even more effective. Neither is cheap; in fact, cost plus installation may run into the thousands. Still, an ounce of prevention . . .

Raffinose: A compound sugar (galactose + glucose + fructose) present in legumes, molasses and sugar beets that's only partially digested. Bacteria in the colon feed upon it, producing lots of gas.

Raisins: The Egyptians, who have been growing grapes for more than six thousand years, were the first to appreciate raisins. They didn't dry grapes on purpose; merely noticed that those left unpicked shriveled under the down-pouring sun, growing more sugary and less perishable. Like

NUTRIENT CONTENT OF 1 OUNCE (28 GRAMS) DARK SEEDLESS RAISINS

85 calories	3 mg sodium
1 g protein	213 mg potassium
0 g fat, 0 saturated	2 g dietary fiber
0 mg cholesterol	0 RE vitamin A
22 g carbohydrate	0.04 mg thiamin
14 mg calcium	0.03 mg riboflavin
28 mg phosphorus	0.2 mg niacin
0.6 mg iron	1 mg vitamin C

Egypt, California discovered raisins (or, rather, their profitability) quite by accident. The year was 1873; the catalyst, a freaky hot spell that withered grapes on the vine. In a go-for-broke effort, one enterprising San Francisco grocer hyped these shriveled grapes as "Peruvian Delicacies." Today, California is the world's leading producer of raisins, turning the lush green Thompson seedless grapes into both dark raisins and golden (also sometimes called sultanas and often bleached with sulfur dioxide). Dried Zante currants are actually raisins, too, made from the tiny Black Corinth grapes. The other raisins of note are the big, meaty muscats. But California's dark seedless raisins account for 90 percent of all those produced.

NUTRIENT CONTENT OF 1 OUNCE (28 GRAMS) GOLDEN SEEDLESS RAISINS

86 calories	3 mg sodium
1 g protein	211 mg potassium
0 g fat, 0 saturated	2 g dietary fiber
0 mg cholesterol	1 RE vitamin A
23 g carbohydrate	0 mg thiamin
15 mg calcium	0.05 mg riboflavin
33 mg phosphorus	0.3 mg niacin
0.5 mg iron	1 mg vitamin C

Ramps, Rampions: Wild leeks that grow, untended, over much of the eastern United States. They resemble scallions but taste more like garlic. Ramps can be munched raw or substituted for scallions or leeks in recipes. **SEASON:** Spring. **NOTE:** No nutritional counts are available for ramps, but it's reasonable to say that they would approximate those of scallions.

Rancid, Rancidity: The staling of fats or fatty foods, resulting in a musty smell and acrid taste. The culprit is oxidation; that is, the breaking down of fatty acids into aldehydes and other chemical compounds. But that's not all. Some fat-soluble vitamins (mainly A and E) are also sacrificed.

Rape: A leafy green of the mustard family grown specifically for its seeds, which are pressed into oils low in saturated fats. Scandinavians have long used rapeseed oil for margarines and cooking oils. But only in this Age of Cholesterol Consciousness has the United States followed suit.

Rapeseed Oil: Best known as **canola,** nothing more than an acronym for the Canadian oil company that developed a new cultivar of rape and began growing it on a wide scale (see CANOLA OIL). In addition, rapeseed oil is used to stabilize peanut butter and the shortenings in cake mixes.

Rashes (diet and): These itchy/burning red skin blotches may be triggered by allergies or sensitivities to specific foods (common culprits are beans, chocolate, citrus fruits, corn, eggs, fish and shellfish, nuts, strawberries and tomatoes). Or nutrient deficiencies may be responsible. Shortfalls of certain B vitamins (niacin, riboflavin and B_6) can cause skin rashes. So can a lack of protein, linoleic acid and vitamin A. See also HIVES.

Raspberries: First cousins to blackberries, second cousins to roses, raspberries are believed to be native to Asia. Yet they grew wild over much of North America before the arrival of the Europeans. Did they, too, cross the land bridge joining Alaska and Asia? Perhaps, although no one knows for sure. What can be said is that raspberry seeds have been found in Stone Age sites in Denmark and Switzerland and in Iron Age ones in England. Raspberries always grew better in northern climes than in southern ones, which may explain why the Romans never bothered to cultivate them. Even today, raspberries are practically unheard of in Italy. Despite the fact that red and black raspberries grow wild across the northern tier of American states, the varieties we prize were developed from European varieties that had been cultivated for more than four hundred years. Red and black aren't the beginning and end of the raspberry palette. There are white raspberries, pearly ones, even golden ones. But these mutants are fairly rare. **SEASON:** Mid-April through November.

NUTRIENT CONTENT OF 1 CUP RED RASPBERRIES
(about 4⅓ ounces; 123 grams)

60 calories	0 mg sodium
1 g protein	186 mg potassium
1 g fat, 0 saturated	6 g dietary fiber
0 mg cholesterol	16 RE vitamin A
14 g carbohydrate	0.04 mg thiamin
27 mg calcium	0.11 mg riboflavin
15 mg phosphorus	1.1 mg niacin
0.7 mg iron	31 mg vitamin C

Ravioli: Little pasta pillows stuffed with ricotta cheese or forcemeat or, in the hands of a gifted chef, a puree of vegetables and/or herbs. Ravioli may be drizzled with melted butter and sprinkled with grated cheese, but more often they are smothered with a nippy tomato sauce. If stuffed with nonfat ricotta and sauced with a low-fat tomato sauce, ravioli are a filling but nourishing main course that's low on fat and cholesterol. **NOTE:** Recipes vary too much for a meaningful calorie count, although it's safe to say that classic ravioli are both high carb and high calorie. If made with whole-milk ricotta, they will contain a fair share of fat, too.

Raw Food (dangers of): Every traveler half expects to be waylaid by *turista,* and old hands know that the best way to avoid it is to follow the "boil it, cook it, peel it or forget it" rule of eating. But how many people realize that home cooking can also make them mighty sick? Precious few. Yet 33 percent of the cases of food poisoning can be traced to home kitchens, to sloppy food handling and dish washing. All raw foods contain disease-causing microorganisms, some (meats, poultry, seafood) more than others (fruits and vegetables). All require special handling if they're to remain safe to eat. Here are some tips:

Eggs: Store in their original cartons (not in the refrigerator egg bins; they'll last longer. Also cook eggs thoroughly (until the yolks are set) before eating (and this includes whole eggs, yolks or whites used for frostings, puddings, mousses, ice creams, sauces and salad dressings). Use eggs within a month.

Fish and Shellfish: Because of polluted waters, unsanitary conditions aboard ships and in fish markets (not to mention black marketers selling seafood taken from banned areas) and because, too, of proliferating sushi bars, the risk of getting sick from eating raw or improperly cooked seafood has soared to unacceptable levels. Illnesses range from viral intestinal infections to hepatitis to worms and parasites. Of the millions of seafood-borne illnesses diagnosed each year, 85 percent of them can be traced to eating raw shellfish (especially clams, mussels, oysters and scallops). **THE LESSON HERE:** Eat no seafood that hasn't been thoroughly cooked. Like meats and poultry, all seafood should be gotten home with dispatch, unwrapped, then placed on a clean plate and rewrapped—loosely—with plastic wrap. Cook or freeze fish and shellfish within twenty-four to thirty hours.

Fruits and Vegetables: Unbundle any bundled or banded vegetables (broccoli, asparagus, arugula, watercress, etc.), discard any soft or decaying pieces, then pop the rest into fresh plastic storage bags. Berries will also last longer if removed from their cartons and placed in a bowl (needless to add, moldy or rotting fruits should be tossed). All vegetables should be unwrapped, then transferred to pristine storage bags. Before serving or cooking, wash all fruits and vegetables carefully in several rinses of tepid water, then peel, if necessary.

Meats and Poultry: Rush them home from the store, unwrap at once, place on a clean plate, cover loosely with plastic food wrap and store in the coldest part of the refrigerator. Cook or freeze within two days. Ground meats are the most perishable of all; they've been handled more than other meats and thus contain more potentially harmful bugs. Before freezing, shape into patties, wrap snugly, date and place on the freezing surface of a 0°F. freezer. Before cooking, rinse poultry well under cool water (outside *and* in for whole birds). Blot red meats dry with paper toweling, then pitch the toweling into the trash at once. Cook all meat and poultry thoroughly before eating; for burgers and poultry, especially, this means no traces of pink in the middle. Beef, lamb, pork and veal should all be cooked to an internal temperature of 160°F.; whole turkeys, chickens, Cornish hens, ducks, geese, etc., to an internal temperature of 180°F.; and poultry breasts to 170°F. Lovers of rare meat will shriek, but if you aim to play it safe, these are the temperatures the USDA recommends.

Perhaps the greatest single challenge to the home cook is preventing **cross-contamination,** the transferral of microorganisms from infected food to uninfected ones. Here's where tidy housekeeping counts. This means washing hands thoroughly in hot soapy water after handling raw meat, poultry or seafood and before touching anything else (food or nonfood). It means meticulously washing all counters and cutting surfaces and all implements and utensils after every use, and getting rid of all materials used to package or wipe these foods. To play it safe, you can sanitize counters and cutting boards by swabbing with a weak chlorine solution (2 teaspoons chlorine bleach to 1 quart water). This helps kill salmonella and other microbes that lie dormant in dry nicks, cracks and crevices, then spring to life the next time these items are used. Even easier, run cutting boards through the dishwasher.

Home cooks also are too often careless about keeping cold foods cold and hot foods hot. About letting raw food (or even the cooked) languish at room temperature too long. **THE RULE HERE:** Never let food stand for more than two hours at temperatures between 40°F. and 140°F. You're flirting with food poisoning if you do. See also BACTERIA; PARASITES.

Raw Milk: For all the health faddists' claims of the superiority of raw milk, it has been known to cause undulant fever, tuberculosis and several forms of salmonella food poisoning. Even though **certified raw milk** must be produced and bottled under rigid standards of hygiene and meet bacterial limits even stricter than those set for pasteurized milk, it may still become contaminated somewhere down the line. During the 1980s, there were several outbreaks of *Salmonella dublin* food poisoning on the West Coast, the most serious of which sent 114 persons to the hospital and killed 2. All had drunk certified raw milk. Unfortunately, this and other bugs are not always destroyed in the cheese-making process, so even long-aged Cheddars made from raw milk may be cause for concern. **SUMMING UP:** Raw milk is not nutritionally superior to pasteurized milk, and from a bacterial standpoint it is definitely inferior. Indeed, it's so risky some areas ban its sale.

Raw Sugar: See SUGAR.

Ray: See SKATE.

R.D.: See DIETITIAN, REGISTERED.

RDAs (Recommended Dietary Allowances): Based on scientific consensus, these are the daily amounts of the different food nutrients deemed adequate for healthy individuals by the Food and Nutrition Board of the NATIONAL RESEARCH COUNCIL, an arm of the National Academy of Sciences. To build in a safety factor and account for the differences in people's ability to absorb proteins, assorted vitamins and minerals, etc., the RDAs are intentionally set somewhat higher than the body's actual physiological needs. To date, there are RDAs for protein, eleven vitamins (A, C, D, E, K, thiamin, riboflavin, niacin, B_6, folic acid and B_{12}) and seven minerals (calcium, iodine, iron, magnesium, phosphorus, selenium and zinc). The National Research Council periodically asks the Food and Nutrition Board to update the RDAs, usually every five to ten years. The latest update was in 1989.

The scope of the next RDA update may be broadened to include three sets of nutritional data. Or so the Food and Nutrition Board urges. It proposes the addition of two new categories—a deficiency level (at which healthy people would eventually show deficiency symptoms) and an upper safe level, beyond which nutrient intake might become toxic. The board further recommends renaming RDAs "Average Requirements," easier for nonprofessionals to understand. Will these proposals go through? And if so, when? First, no one knows. Second, don't hold your breath.

RDIs (Reference Daily Intakes): Formerly known as U.S. Recommended Daily Allowances (not to be confused with Recommended *Dietary* Allowances), RDIs are one of the standards used to determine the Daily Values (see DVs) now listed on new food labels. Also factored into the Daily Values are Daily Reference Values, which suggest, for the first time, healthful daily intakes for fat, carbohydrates, cholesterol, fiber, sodium and potassium. The reason for the name change to RDIs was to eliminate any confusion between U.S. Recommended Daily Allowances (set by the FDA) and Recommended Dietary Allowances (set by the National Research Council of the National Academy of Sciences).

RE (Retinol Equivalent): The new unit of measure for vitamin A and its precursor beta-carotene (the old measure was the international unit, or IU). Because many vitamin supplement labels still give vitamin A content in IU, we offer this quick conversion formula. To convert IU to RE: 1 RE = 3.3 IU if food source is an animal (retinol) and 10 IU if food source is a plant (beta-carotene).

Red Beans: See BEANS, DRIED.

Red Blood Cells, Red Blood Corpuscles, Erythrocytes: The most important cells in the blood. Their major component is iron-rich hemoglobin, which carries oxygen from the lungs to tissues throughout the body. Red blood cells also help maintain the pH (acid/alkaline) balance of the blood and ferry carbon dioxide back to the lungs to be exhaled. So essential to life are red blood cells that they account for 45 percent of the total volume of blood in a man, 40 percent of blood in a woman. An average blood cell lives about four months and the body constantly needs a healthy new supply. Red blood cells are synthesized in

the bone marrow, and if they are to be properly produced and maintained, they need three B vitamins—folic acid, pyridoxine (B_6) and B_{12}—plus iron, the carrier of oxygen. A lack of any one of them can lead to nutritional anemia. There are other anemias, too. Some are caused by iron and/or copper deficiencies. Others are genetic. In sickle-cell anemia, for example, the body is genetically programmed to produce deformed, short-lived red blood cells.

Red Cabbage: See CABBAGE, RED.

Red Dye Nos. 1, 2, 3, 4, etc.: See COLORINGS.

Redfish: Cajun chef Paul Prudhomme made this fish so famous supplies of it began to dwindle in the southern Atlantic and Gulf of Mexico. A temporary ban, now lifted, was imposed for a while. Home cooks want to coat redfish with spices and "blacken" them in white-hot skillets the way Chef Paul does. Also called **channel bass,** redfish are actually **red drums.** They can grow to awesome size (40 pounds or more) but the cook's choice are the 3- to 4-pounders ("puppy" drums). Redfish are lean, firm and white of flesh, marvelous stuffed and baked whole or chunked into chowders. For approximate nutrient counts, see FISH, LEAN WHITE.

Red Kidney Beans: See BEANS, DRIED.

Red Leaf Lettuce: See SALAD GREENS.

Red Mullet, Rouget, Salmonete: This popular little Mediterranean fish is not a mullet at all. It's a goatfish. Never mind. It is lean, white and supremely sweet and tender of flesh. To the Romans it was worth its weight in silver. And in Italy today it's not uncommon to see **triglia** (its Italian name) panned whole and served with a rosebud in its mouth. For approximate nutrient counts, see FISH, LEAN WHITE.

Red Peppers: See HOT PEPPERS and SWEET PEPPERS under PEPPERS, CAPSICUMS.

Red Snapper: There are many snappers but none tops the red snapper, which swims warm Atlantic waters from Cape Hatteras to Brazil. With its hot-pink color, a red snapper is dazzling to see. It's delicious to eat, too—lean, white and oh, so delicate. Although a snapper can weigh in at 30 pounds or more, those that come to market fresh are likelier to tip the scales at 4 or 5 pounds. **NOTE:** Red snapper is one of the fish apt to contain ciguatoxin, a poison not destroyed by cooking (see CIGUATERA POISONING). For approximate nutrient counts for red snapper, see FISH, LEAN WHITE.

Red Tide: An infestation of toxin-producing dinoflagellates (algae) that contaminate mollusks and may cause symptoms similar to those of PARALYTIC SHELLFISH POISONING in those who eat them. Not all red tides are poisonous, however. And not all toxic tides are red. Some are yellow, green, brown, even black. They are common at certain times of the year, primarily in the cold offshore waters of Maine, Massachusetts, New York and Pacific states including Alaska, and whenever, wherever they occur, fishing grounds are closed. Crustaceans (i.e., crabs, shrimps and lobsters), not being filter feeders, aren't affected by red tides. Nor are finfish.

"Reduced" (on food labels): According to the Nutrition Labeling and Education Act, passed in 1990 and implemented in the spring of 1994, the only foods that can be labeled "reduced" are those in which either the calories or a specific nutrient has been reduced by 25 percent. Those already low in calories or the specific nutrient don't qualify. See also FOOD LABELING.

Reducing (effects in cooking): So many recipes call for pan juices to be boiled down to a fourth or half of their original quantity, or sometimes until only a thick glaze remains on the bottom of the pan. How does this affect food value? Reducing will destroy such heat-sensitive vitamins as C, thiamin and folic acid. But it will also concentrate the nutrients not susceptible to heat—minerals, for example, and heat-stable vitamins (A, D, E, K and many of the B-complex).

Red Wines: See WINES; also ALCOHOL, ALCOHOLIC BEVERAGES. Finally, see QUERCITIN and RESVERATROL, which offer two theories for why the French, great eaters of fatty foods and great drinkers of red table wines, suffer fewer heart attacks than Americans, who are cutting down on fat and cholesterol. This is what's known as the FRENCH PARADOX.

Reference Daily Intakes: See RDIs.

Refining, Refined Foods: Refining is the removal of the coarse parts of food, most often of a grain, fruit or vegetable. White flour (the starchy wheat endosperm minus the bran and germ) is the refined food best known to one and all. Today white flours are routinely ENRICHED (had their lost thiamin, riboflavin, niacin and iron restored); still, they lack the fiber of whole grain, to say nothing of the zinc, copper and three important B-complexers (B_6, folic and pantothenic acids). Once highly refined, many cereals are now being FORTIFIED with bran, vitamins and minerals. White, or polished, rice, of course, has been stripped of its bran and so has cornmeal. Equally refined, though seldom thought of that way, are apple juices and ciders, which have lost nearly 100 percent of their fiber. Needless to say, all the instants lining supermarket shelves must also go into the refined category. Then there are the foods we ourselves refine by stripping them of their skins—apples, apricots, asparagus, carrots, cucumbers, peaches, pears, peppers, potatoes. And so on, and so on. Sometimes peeling is necessary because the skins have been waxed (see PARAFFIN). But often it is not, especially if the fruits and vegetables are homegrown.

Reflux Esophatitis, Acid Reflux: The backing up of stomach acids and partially digested food into the esophagus, where they inflame and burn. Overweight persons frequently suffer from acid reflux; also those with hiatal hernias. For more details, see ESOPHAGITIS.

Refreezing (dangers of): When frozen foods are thawed, then refrozen, they pass through the temperature danger zone three times—first on initial freezing, then on thawing, then again on refreezing. This zone—40°F. up to 140°F.—is where bacteria, molds and other disease-causing microorganisms multiply on fast forward. Only partially thawed frozen foods—those with ice crystals clearly discernible—should be refrozen. Thawed, refrozen foods are a particular problem at many supermarkets. It goes without saying that you should reject any that feel squishy, also those that seem misshapen, a pretty good indication that the contents have thawed, then refrozen. Although you may not get sick from eating refrozen food, it's best to err on the side of safety and avoid or discard them. Moreover, the quality (taste, texture, appearance) of refrozen foods is pretty punky. See also THAWING METHODS.

Refreshing: The French way to prepare many vegetables (asparagus, beans, broccoli, brussels sprouts, cabbage, cauliflower, green peas, summer squash and the like), which involves blanching them briefly in boiling water, quick chilling them in ice water, then, come serving time, warming them briefly in butter or sauce. There are nutritional advantages and disadvantages to refreshing. First, such heat-sensitive vitamins as C, thiamin and folic acid are more likely to be preserved than when the vegetables are boiled for longer periods of time. But, alas, if the vegetables are finely cut, the water-soluble vitamins (everything but A, D, E and K) plus many minerals are apt to leach into the blanching and/or chilling water and be lost.

Refrigeration: How cooks kept perishable foods cold before the arrival of mechanical refrigeration is a miracle. Of course, many of them didn't; food spoiled and people got sick. The point of keeping perishables cold, however, is not only to retard the growth of pathogens (disease-bearing microorganisms) but also to preserve as much freshness as possible. Today electric refrigerators are so common, so reliable we tend to take them for granted. We fail, for example, to check their temperatures from time to time to see that they're in the safe range (32°F. to 40°F. and the nearer 32°F. the better).

Temperatures constantly fluctuate inside a refrigerator, rising whenever the door is opened (never leave it open more than a few seconds), rising, too, whenever food, especially hot food, is added. Large batches of hot food should never be shoved straight into the fridge because they may raise temperatures to dangerous levels. Instead, spread large quantities of hot food in shallow containers and quick chill in ice baths before refrigerating.

Certain foods (bulky meats and poultry) chill more slowly than others; so do dense ones. The turkey refrigerated with its body cavity full of stuffing is sure to cause trouble. Always scoop out the stuffing and wrap it separately—in several packets, if necessary. And strip the turkey meat from the carcass, again portioning among several bundles to ensure quick chilling.

The most perishable foods—meats, poultry, fish—should always be stored in the coldest part of the refrigerator, meaning the bottom (hot air rises, cold air sinks). And they should be removed from their store wrappers, placed on clean plates and loosely covered with plastic food wrap so air can circulate around them, discouraging microbial growth. See also BACTERIA; MOLDS; RAW FOOD.

Regional Enteritis: Another name for CROHN'S DISEASE, a serious inflammatory disease of the small intestine.

Registered Dietitian: See DIETITIAN, REGISTERED.

Rehydration: The process by which athletes restore bodily fluids lost through perspiration (see HYDRATION). Also the soaking of dried or dehydrated foods to plump them to a facsimile of their original selves.

Rennet: See JUNKET.

Rennin: An enzyme excreted by the lining of a calf's stomach that can curdle ten million times its weight in milk. Rennin, especially the newly approved biotech form (chymosin), is widely used in the cheese industry. Rennin is also a component of rennet or JUNKET.

Residual Chemicals: See HERBICIDES, PESTICIDES.

Resins: Sticky liquid, semiliquid or semisolid substances, either natural or synthetic, many of which are used in plastic wraps and packages. Among the best known synthetic resins: polyvinyl, polyethylene and polystyrene. For details on these, their advantages and disadvantages, see PLASTIC.

Restaurant Nutrition Labeling: See MENU CLAIMS.

Restructured Meats: Meat trimmings (usually beef or veal) that are shredded or flaked, then shaped into minute steaks and cutlets. So that these bits of meat will hold their shape as steaks and cutlets, processors may bind them with gelatin or with egg, milk, soy or wheat protein. Among the advantages of restructured meats: They are boneless and of uniform size; they allow meat packers to adjust the proportion of fat to meat according to current demand and, finally, to upgrade odds and ends to the steak and cutlet category. Most restructured meats are frozen.

Resveratrol: One of the powerful antioxidants found in red wine and grape juice that is believed to lower blood levels of "bad" cholesterol (LDL) and thus reduce the risk of heart disease. There has been considerable media babble recently about the FRENCH PARADOX, the fact that the French, who don't stint on eggs, butter, cream or foie gras, have less cardiovascular disease and fewer heart attacks than Americans. The reason, some researchers suggest, is that the red wine the French drink with their meals contains resveratrol as well as another LDL-lowering compound called QUERCITIN.

Retina: The part of the eye that catches the light and focuses images. Essential to the proper function of the retina (specifically the visual purple or RHODOPSIN, a pigment lodged in the retina's rods) is vitamin A. One common symptom of vitamin A deficiency is night blindness. See also A, VITAMIN.

Retin-A, Tretinoin: The beauty industry is now touting this vitamin A derivative as a "youth cream" and "wrinkle and liver spot remover," but this is powerful stuff, available by prescription only. Its intended use: the treatment of ACNE. Retin-A tablets, prescribed for severe acne, should never be taken if you are pregnant (or expect to become pregnant) because they can harm the fetus.

Retinol: Another word for vitamin A, specifically the form found in animals (as opposed to beta-carotene, which exists in plants). See A, VITAMIN.

Rhodopsin: The medical term for **visual purple,** a pigment contained in the RETINA that helps the eye adjust to and see in dim light.

Rhubarb: For a plant that's been cultivated for nearly two thousand years, rhubarb was a long time reaching the kitchen. The Western kitchen, that is, for down the centuries this Asian plant was considered medicine (it was prescribed as a purgative). When people did begin to think of rhubarb as food, they invariably ate the wrong parts of the plant. The leaves, for example, are so full of oxalic acid they can be deadly. Ditto the fleshy rhizomes. Even the celerylike stalks, varying from scarlet to green depending on species, are too acid to eat raw. All that's needed to tame their tartness, however, is a little cooking and a lot

of sugar. Not for nothing has rhubarb been nicknamed **pie plant.** It does make splendid pies, cobblers and crisps, especially when teamed 50-50 with ripe strawberries. Rhubarb also makes lovely jams and preserves. **NOTE:** Despite rhubarb's impressive cargo of calcium, most of it combines with the plant's oxalic acid, forming calcium oxalate—useless, alas, to the body. **SEASON:** Spring and early summer.

NUTRIENT CONTENT OF 1 CUP DICED UNSWEETENED UNCOOKED RHUBARB

(about 4⅓ ounces; 122 grams)

26 calories	5 mg sodium
1 g protein	351 mg potassium
0 g fat, 0 saturated	3 g dietary fiber
0 mg cholesterol	12 RE vitamin A
6 g carbohydrate	0.02 mg thiamin
104 mg calcium	0.04 mg riboflavin
17 mg phosphorus	0.4 mg niacin
0.3 mg iron	10 mg vitamin C

NUTRIENT CONTENT OF 1 CUP DICED FROZEN RHUBARB (COOKED WITH SUGAR)

(about 8½ ounces; 240 grams)

278 calories	2 mg sodium
1 g protein	230 mg potassium
0 g fat, 0 saturated	5 g dietary fiber
0 mg cholesterol	17 RE vitamin A
75 g carbohydrate	0.04 mg thiamin
348 mg calcium	0.06 mg riboflavin
19 mg phosphorus	0.5 mg niacin
0.5 mg iron	8 mg vitamin C

Riboflavin: Another name for vitamin B_2. See B_2, VITAMIN.

Rice: For half the world's people, rice is the staff of life. It is a grain so ancient no one knows where it originated. China, some say. India, others insist. Now comes word of archaeological digs in Thailand where rice grains have been carbon-dated at 3500 B.C. Wherever rice first sprang to life, one thing is sure: It was in a monsoonal land, a land of puddling torrents followed by hot dry spells that provided the perfect habitat for *Oryza sativa.* How rice made its trek westward into the Mediterranean basin isn't known either, although food historians believe that the Moors introduced it to Portugal and Spain, whence it spread eastward to Italy. The rest of Europe never was—and isn't yet—keen on rice. Wheat and rye are the staples there.

Americans, on the other hand, do dote on rice. And have done since colonial days. In 1647, William Berkeley sowed half a bushel of rice on his James River plantation—and reaped thirtyfold! Still, the first colony to become a major rice grower was South Carolina. From the late seventeenth century onward, "Carolina gold" was exported far and wide. Then came the Civil War and the decimation of the crop. Today, most of America's rice comes from Arkansas, California, Louisiana, Mississippi, Missouri and Texas. Their combined harvests make the United States the world's twelfth largest producer of rice (and the second biggest exporter—after Thailand).

Rice these days isn't just a matter of **short** or **long grain, converted** (parboiled) or **instant** (precooked or dehydrated)—or even **brown** (the whole grain with its bran intact) or **white** (polished). There are dozens of varieties, both domestic and imported. Here's the short list: **aromatic rices** (Jasmine, Popcorn, Texmati, Wild Pecan, etc.), **basmati** (a slender, long-grain Indian rice of superior flavor), **glutinous** (a sweet, sticky "dessert" rice popular in China and the rest of East Asia), **Italian** (of these, the chunky, medium-grain risotto rice called **arborio** is the best known) and **wehani** (a rust brown California cousin of basmati). See also WILD RICE, which is not a rice at all but a wild aquatic grass native to North America.

All rices are high-carbohydrate, low-fat, low-sodium foods with good supplies of iron and many of the B vita-

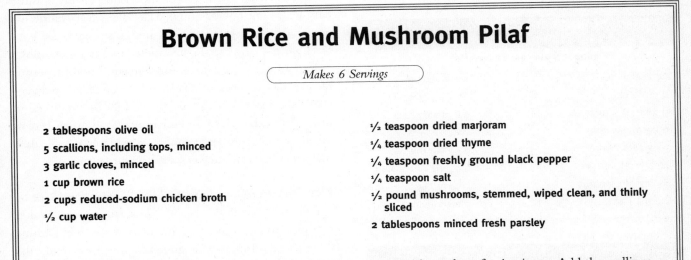

Brown Rice and Mushroom Pilaf

Makes 6 Servings

2 tablespoons olive oil

5 scallions, including tops, minced

3 garlic cloves, minced

1 cup brown rice

2 cups reduced-sodium chicken broth

½ cup water

½ teaspoon dried marjoram

¼ teaspoon dried thyme

¼ teaspoon freshly ground black pepper

¼ teaspoon salt

½ pound mushrooms, stemmed, wiped clean, and thinly sliced

2 tablespoons minced fresh parsley

HEAT 2 TEASPOONS of the oil in a large heavy saucepan over moderate heat for 1 minute. Add the scallions and garlic, and cook, stirring occasionally, until softened, about 3 minutes. Add the rice, stirring to coat. Stir in the broth, water, marjoram, thyme, pepper, and salt, and bring to a boil. Adjust heat so mixture bubbles gently, cover, and simmer 45 minutes or until all the liquid is absorbed.

MEANWHILE, IN A large heavy skillet over moderate heat, heat the remaining 4 teaspoons oil. Add the mushrooms and sauté until lightly browned and mushrooms have given up their juices, 3 to 5 minutes. Stir mushrooms and any juices into the simmering rice during the final 10 minutes of cooking. Mix in parsley and serve in place of potatoes.

APPROXIMATE NUTRIENT COUNTS PER SERVING

183 calories	28 g carbohydrate	1.6 mg iron	0.13 mg thiamin
5 g protein	3 g dietary fiber	122 mg sodium	0.15 mg riboflavin
6 g fat, 1 saturated	35 mg calcium	275 mg potassium	4.0 mg niacin
0 mg cholesterol	144 mg phosphorus	14 RE vitamin A	7 mg vitamin C

mins—and this applies to both brown rice and white (because most of it is now enriched with iron, thiamin and niacin). Where brown rice has the edge is fiber.

NUTRIENT CONTENT OF 1 CUP COOKED LONG-GRAIN WHITE RICE

(about 7¼ ounces; 205 grams)

267 calories	2 mg sodium
6 g protein	72 mg potassium
1 g fat, 0 saturated	1 g dietary fiber
0 mg cholesterol	0 RE vitamin A
58 g carbohydrate	0.33 mg thiamin
21 mg calcium	0.03 mg riboflavin
88 mg phosphorus	3.0 mg niacin
2.5 mg iron	0 mg vitamin C

NUTRIENT CONTENT OF 1 CUP COOKED CONVERTED WHITE RICE

(about 6 ounces; 175 grams)

200 calories	5 mg sodium
4 g protein	65 mg potassium
0 g fat, 0 saturated	1 g dietary fiber
0 mg cholesterol	0 RE vitamin A
43 g carbohydrate	0.43 mg thiamin
33 mg calcium	0.03 mg riboflavin
74 mg phosphorus	2.5 mg niacin
2.0 mg iron	0 mg vitamin C

NUTRIENT CONTENT OF 1 CUP COOKED LONG-GRAIN BROWN RICE

(about 6⅞ ounces; 195 grams)

216 calories	10 mg sodium
5 g protein	84 mg potassium
2 g fat, 0 saturated	3 g dietary fiber
0 mg cholesterol	0 RE vitamin A
45 g carbohydrate	0.19 mg thiamin
20 mg calcium	0.05 mg riboflavin
161 mg phosphorus	3.0 mg niacin
0.8 mg iron	0 mg vitamin C

Rice Bran: With oat bran, you get the husk. With rice bran, you get the husk *and* the germ, both of which are removed during the polishing process. The husk contains not only vitamins and minerals but also plenty of insoluble fiber, which has gained a reputation as a cholesterol fighter.

But the germ oil lowers blood cholesterol, too, making rice bran even more effective than heavily hyped oat bran. A sawdusty but delicately sweet brown powder that was for years the province of health-food stores, rice bran has gone mainstream and is being mixed into everything from English muffins to rice cakes to breakfast foods. One major American cereal maker recently introduced **Kenmei,** exotic-sounding rice-bran flakes available either plain or teamed, muesli-style, with almonds and raisins. Plain rice bran is highly perishable and should be stored in tightly covered containers in the refrigerator.

Rice-Bran Oil: Extracted from the germ, rice-bran oil is rich in beta-sitosterol and is believed to reduce blood levels of "bad" cholesterol, or LDL (but neither raises nor lowers amounts of the "good" HDL). Consisting mainly of three fatty acids—the polyunsaturated LINOLEIC ACID, monounsaturated OLEIC ACID and small amounts of saturated PALMITIC ACID—this mostly unsaturated oil has a high smoke point and is a good choice for sautéing. Food processors blend it into all-purpose salad/cooking oil blends and vegetable shortenings. It can also be bought by the bottle in many Asian groceries and some health-food stores. Buy in small amounts and store snugly capped on a cool, dark shelf; rice-bran oil quickly stales and turns rancid.

Rice Diet: A low-sodium diet developed in the 1940s by a Durham, North Carolina, physician named Walter Kempner to treat those with high blood pressure. Because those on Dr. Kempner's regimen shed many pounds, the Rice Diet soon became better known as a surefire way to lose weight. The original Rice Diet consisted of boiled rice, fruit and fruit juice—nothing more. Later, vitamin pills and sugar were added. People still go down to Durham to try the Rice Diet. And some of them lose impressive amounts of weight. Whether they keep the lost pounds off depends upon whether they adopt sound eating habits and sensible programs of exercise once they've completed the Rice Diet.

Rice Flour: A gluten-free powder milled from broken kernels of long-, medium- or short-grain rice that's used in many commercial baby foods, cereals, processed meats and breaded foods. Although rice flour is too tender for breads, cakes, pastries and cookies, Scottish cooks count on it to give shortbread that dissolve-on-the-tongue texture.

NUTRIENT CONTENT OF 1 CUP RICE FLOUR
(about 5½ ounces; 158 grams)

578 calories	0 mg sodium
9 g protein	120 mg potassium
2 g fat, 1 saturated	4 g dietary fiber
0 mg cholesterol	0 RE vitamin A
127 g carbohydrate	0.22 mg thiamin
16 mg calcium	0.03 mg riboflavin
155 mg phosphorus	4.1 mg niacin
0.6 mg iron	0 mg vitamin C

Rice Noodles: See CELLOPHANE NOODLES.

Rickets: A debilitating, deforming deficiency disease caused by a lack of vitamin D. See also D, VITAMIN.

Ricotta: A soft, bland, white, cooked Italian cheese of fine curd made from the whey of ewe's or cow's milk. To give ricotta its creamy texture, cheese makers routinely blend in whole milk or cream and stabilize the mix with egg protein, citric or tartaric acid. Standard ricotta is 50 to 60

NUTRIENT CONTENT OF ½ CUP WHOLE-MILK RICOTTA
(about 4⅓ ounces; 123 grams)

214 calories	103 mg sodium
14 g protein	128 mg potassium
16 g fat, 10 saturated	0 g dietary fiber
62 mg cholesterol	165 RE vitamin A
4 g carbohydrate	0.02 mg thiamin
255 mg calcium	0.24 mg riboflavin
195 mg phosphorus	0.1 mg niacin
0.5 mg iron	0 mg vitamin C

NUTRIENT CONTENT OF ½ CUP PART-SKIM RICOTTA
(about 4⅓ ounces; 123 grams)

170 calories	153 mg sodium
14 g protein	154 mg potassium
10 g fat, 6 saturated	0 g dietary fiber
38 mg cholesterol	139 RE vitamin A
6 g carbohydrate	0.03 mg thiamin
335 mg calcium	0.23 mg riboflavin
225 mg phosphorus	0.1 mg niacin
0.5 mg iron	0 mg vitamin C

percent water, 23 to 26 percent protein, 15 percent fat and 3 percent lactose (milk sugar). Fortunately, there are now part-skim and nonfat ricottas although they lack the rich "mouth feel" of the real thing. Ricotta is the cheese Italians use for making lasagne, for stuffing ravioli and other pasta and for producing cheesecakes of supreme delicacy. It is very good, too, served with fresh berries, sliced peaches, pears or apricots. Although ricotta can be substituted for cottage cheese, its texture and flavor are both unique and superior.

Roasting: Cooking, uncovered, in the oven with little or no liquid and a wonderful way to cut down on fat. Properly roasted, meats and birds are elevated on racks so that their fatty drippings drain away from them and into the bottom of the pan. Most vegetables roast splendidly, too. Try roasting breaded eggplant slices instead of frying them, for example. The fat and calories both plummet. Another advantage to roasting is that it caramelizes some of the starches in food, intensifying and enriching the flavor so that little butter, margarine or oil is needed for seasoning.

Rock Cornish Hens: Although they are often called **game hens,** there is nothing wild about these little birds, which every supermarket sells both fresh and frozen. These bantamweights are especially bred and fed chickens averaging 1½ pounds or less. Rock Cornish hens are almost all breast, meaning their meat is white and dry (but frequent basting will keep them moist). Being moderately low in fat (especially saturated fat) and calories, yet a good source of phosphorus, potassium and niacin, Rock Cornish hens are an acceptable choice for dieters. Allow ½ bird per person.

NUTRIENT CONTENT OF 3 OUNCES (85 GRAMS) ROASTED ROCK CORNISH HEN

202 calories	56 mg sodium
23 g protein	188 mg potassium
12 g fat, 3 saturated	0 g dietary fiber
75 mg cholesterol	40 RE vitamin A
0 g carbohydrate	0.05 mg thiamin
13 mg calcium	0.14 mg riboflavin
154 mg phosphorus	7.2 mg niacin
1.1 mg iron	0 mg vitamin C

Rocket: The British name for ARUGULA.

Rockfish: A huge family of lean, white-meated saltwater fish that includes **Pacific Ocean perch, yellowtail** and **red rockfish,** often palmed off as red snapper but another fish entirely. Rockfish are particular favorites in California Chinatowns and lend themselves to a variety of sweet-sour recipes. The best of them are small enough to bake, steam, even deep-fry whole. For approximate nutrient counts, see FISH, LEAN WHITE.

Roe: See FISH ROE.

Rolled Oats: See OATMEAL.

Romaine: See SALAD GREENS.

Romano: The full name for this hard, sharp, Italian grating cheese is **pecorino Romano.** The original is a firm, fine-textured cooked ewe's-milk cheese, although most domestic varieties are made of cow's milk. True pecorino Romano, which dates at least as far back as the first century, is believed to be Italy's oldest cheese. It is still made the age-old way during the fall, winter and spring on farms outside Rome or in Sardinia. When drums of it emerge from their eight-month dry-salt cure, they are as pale as Parmesan, but saltier, sharper. Italian pecorino Romano averages about 30 percent water, 33 percent fat, 26 to 28 percent protein and 4 to 5 percent salt. Domestic cow's–milk Romanos are slightly moister (32 percent water), higher in protein (32 to 33 percent) and lower in fat (25 to 27 percent).

NUTRIENT CONTENT OF 1 OUNCE (28 GRAMS) ROMANO CHEESE (DOMESTIC)

109 calories	339 mg sodium
9 g protein	25 mg potassium
8 g fat, 5 saturated	0 g dietary fiber
30 mg cholesterol	40 RE vitamin A
1 g carbohydrate	0.01 mg thiamin
300 mg calcium	0.01 mg riboflavin
215 mg phosphorus	0 mg niacin
0.2 mg iron	0 mg vitamin C

Root Beer: A bubbly soft drink originally but no longer flavored with sassafras bark because the safrole it contains has caused cancer in laboratory animals. Today's root beer, whether sweetened with sugar or one of the low-cal sub-stitutes, is artificially flavored. Unlike Grandma's home-made root beer, which was often made with yeast and left to ferment and bubble, modern versions are mechanically carbonated. In *The Dictionary of American Food and Drink,* John Mariani writes that root beer, at first called herb tea, was developed by Philadelphia druggist Charles E. Hires in 1875 as the "National Temperance Drink." It was served for the first time at the 1876 Philadelphia Centennial Exposition.

NUTRIENT CONTENT OF 8 FLUID OUNCES (247 GRAMS) ROOT BEER (NATURALLY SWEETENED)

101 calories	32 mg sodium
0 g protein	2 mg potassium
0 g fat, 0 saturated	0 g dietary fiber
0 mg cholesterol	0 RE vitamin A
26 g carbohydrate	0 mg thiamin
12 mg calcium	0 mg riboflavin
0 mg phosphorus	0 mg niacin
0.1 mg iron	0 mg vitamin C

NUTRIENT CONTENT OF 8 FLUID OUNCES (240 GRAMS) ROOT BEER (DIET)

2 calories	46 mg sodium
0 g protein	70 mg potassium
0 g fat, 0 saturated	0 g dietary fiber
0 mg cholesterol	0 RE vitamin A
0 g carbohydrate	0 mg thiamin
6 mg calcium	0 mg riboflavin
6 mg phosphorus	0 mg niacin
0.9 mg iron	0 mg vitamin C

Roquefort: "The Queen of the Blues," this superbly creamy, tart yet nutty French cheese of ancient lineage is made exclusively from ewe's milk. Shaped into cylinders weighing about 5 pounds apiece, it comes from the commune of Roquefort northeast of Toulouse very near the town of Millau. Roquefort is aged for three months in natural caves and owes its blue veins and piquancy to *Penicillium roqueforti,* a mold. Only cheeses made in this area in this way can bear the *appellation d'origine contrôlée* and be called Roquefort. Well-aged Roquefort averages 36 to 38 percent water, 32 to 36 percent fat and 22 to 24 percent protein. It's plenty salty, too.

NUTRIENT CONTENT OF 1 OUNCE (28 GRAMS) ROQUEFORT CHEESE	
104 calories	511 mg sodium
6 g protein	26 mg potassium
9 g fat, 5 saturated	0 g dietary fiber
26 mg cholesterol	85 RE vitamin A
1 g carbohydrate	0.01 mg thiamin
187 mg calcium	0.17 mg riboflavin
111 mg phosphorus	0.2 mg niacin
0.2 mg iron	0 mg vitamin C

Rosacea (diet and): Chronic acnelike bumps accompanied by flushing. Alcoholic beverages seem to exacerbate rosacea, as do highly spiced foods.

Rose Hips: The fleshy fruits of roses in general and wild roses in particular. Health faddists have for years been touting the nutritional bonanza to be found in rose hips, especially the huge amounts of vitamin C. Many "natural" vitamin C supplements claim to be made with rose hips. What they're careful *not* to say is exactly how much vitamin C is obtained from rose hips, how much from elsewhere. Once rose hips have been dried, pulverized and stored, the amount of vitamin C they contain is both variable and questionable. What they are high in is pectin, a fiber-rich carbohydrate that acts like a mild laxative and/or diuretic.

Rosemary: Although herbs are not a main concern here, we mention this resinous, richly aromatic plant because it makes it possible to cut down on salt. Carrots, green peas, sweet corn, summer and winter squash are all improved if cooked with a sprig of fresh rosemary or a pinch of the dried. So are lamb, most fowl and such strongly flavored fish as tuna, salmon and swordfish. Season with a light touch, however. Rosemary is strong stuff.

Rosé Wines: See WINES; also ALCOHOL, ALCOHOLIC BEVERAGES.

Roughage: See FIBER, DIETARY.

Royal Jelly: A waxy substance worker bees manufacture to feed to their queen. Because queen bees are three or four times the size of the workers, some practitioners of alternative medicine attribute magical powers to royal jelly.

One health-food store bills it as a synergistic performance booster, adding that for brute strength all you need are six 50-milligram tablets a day. Another claims that royal jelly is "known to aid bronchial asthma, liver disease, pancreatitis, insomnia, stomach ulcers, kidney disease, bone fractures and skin disorders" and that it is also a "potentiator of the immune system." There is no reputable scientific proof for any of these claims.

Rum: See ALCOHOL, ALCOHOLIC BEVERAGES.

Runner's Anemia: See SPORTS ANEMIA.

Rutabagas: In the strictest botanical sense, rutabagas, often called **yellow turnips,** are not turnips but turnip-cabbage hybrids, members of the mustard family, first cousins to broccoli, brussels sprouts, cauliflower, kale and kohlrabi. But their flavor and texture, if not their whopping size, so closely resemble true turnips that they can be prepared and cooked the same way. Because of their yellow-orange flesh, rutabagas are stellar sources of beta-carotene. They also contain more than middling amounts of vitamin C, calcium, phosphorus, potassium and thiamin. Yet they are low in calories, fat and sodium and contain zero cholesterol. **SEASON:** Year-round, with supplies peaking in October and November.

NUTRIENT CONTENT OF 1 CUP MASHED COOKED RUTABAGA (about 8½ ounces; 240 grams)	
94 calories	48 mg sodium
3 g protein	782 mg potassium
1 g fat, 0 saturated	4 g dietary fiber
0 mg cholesterol	134 RE vitamin A
21 g carbohydrate	0.20 mg thiamin
115 mg calcium	0.10 mg riboflavin
134 mg phosphorus	1.7 mg niacin
1.3 mg iron	45 mg vitamin C

Rutin: A bioflavonoid now being sold by health-food stores. To quote one catalog, rutin "enhances the absorption of vitamin C, helps relieve pain, bumps and bruises, has an antibacterial effect, promotes circulation, stimulates bile production, helps lower blood cholesterol, and prevents cataracts." There's more. Rutin also helps relieve symptoms of oral herpes. The truth? No one has ever proved that rutin, or any other bioflavonoid for that matter, is necessary for health, growth or life. Researchers are studying rutin, it's true. But not for its nutritional value or any of the cure-all claims made for it. They see it as an alternative sweetener.

Rye: Although it has been cultivated for more than two thousand years, rye is new as grains grow. It appeared first as a weed, probably in northeastern Europe (but perhaps in Afghanistan, Caspian Sea or Black Sea lands), over-running fields of wheat. To this day, 90 percent of the world's rye comes from northern Europe. In medieval France, embattled farmers let the two grains coexist, ground them into a mixed flour and baked it into sturdy tan loaves (*maslin* bread is still popular, although today the rye and wheat are grown separately). The wonder of rye is its ability to grow on poor soil in harsh climates, often at startlingly high altitudes. For that reason, it was called the grain of poverty. For centuries, rye sustained the poor of Germany, Poland, Russia and Scandinavia. Unfortunately, it also killed millions. Time and again during the Middle Ages, bins of rye fell prey to *Claviceps purpurea,* a mold that produces a toxin, which in turn causes a deadly disease known as St. Anthony's fire (see ERGOT).

Rye Bread: Russians and Germans, in particular, like the leaden loaves that rye flour produces. Some of these—PUMPERNICKEL, to name one—are baked in steam ovens for days so that their starches caramelize, making the bread as dark as chocolate. More likely to determine the color and texture of a loaf of rye, however, are the grind of the flour, the seasonings and other ingredients used. As for shape—long, round, oval—it's a matter of regional preference. Regardless of where and how rye breads are made, the majority of them are sour (even those strewn with caraway seeds), compact and dense (some are unleavened or barely leavened, with yeasty starters doing the job). Rye breads are moist, excellent keepers. They also contain some B vitamins and minerals.

NUTRIENT CONTENT OF 1 SLICE RYE BREAD	
(about ⅞ ounce; 25 grams)	
65 calories	165 mg sodium
2 g protein	42 mg potassium
1 g fat, 0 saturated	2 g dietary fiber
0 mg cholesterol	0 RE vitamin A
12 g carbohydrate	0.11 mg thiamin
18 mg calcium	0.08 mg riboflavin
31 mg phosphorus	1.0 mg niacin
0.7 mg iron	0 mg vitamin C

Rye Flour: See FLOUR.

Rye Whiskey: See ALCOHOL, ALCOHOLIC BEVERAGES.

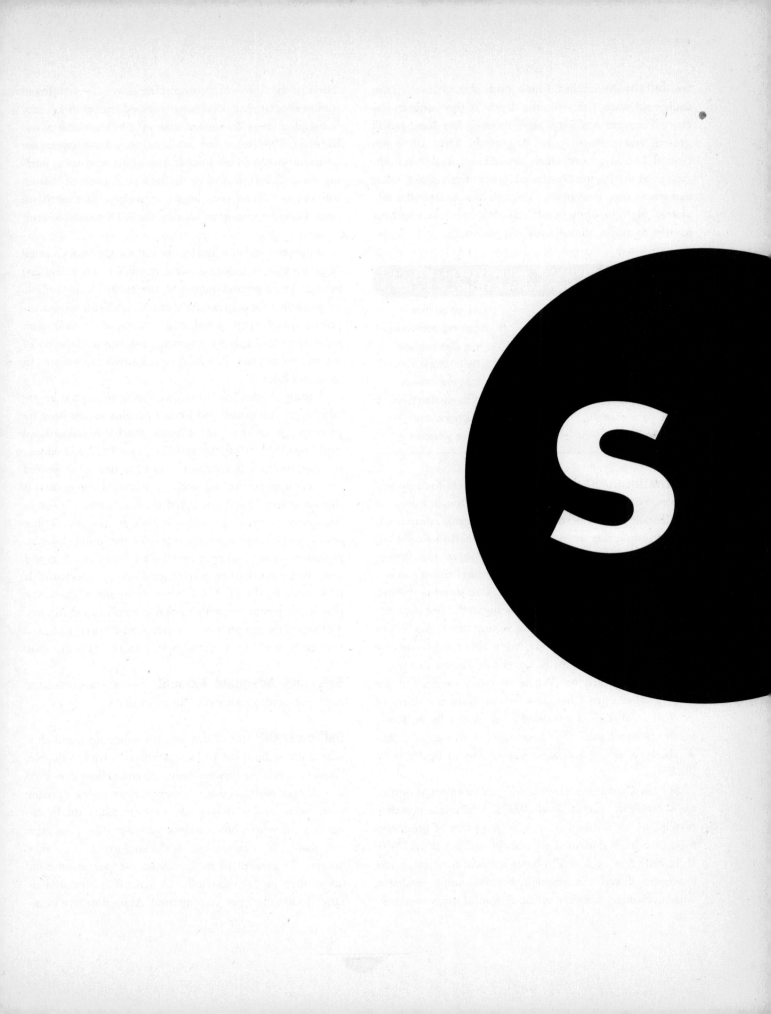

Sablefish: Also called **black cod,** though not a cod, these cold-water fish swim the depths of the northern Pacific. They are not very big—about 3 feet long at full growth and perhaps 35 to 40 pounds. They are white fleshed, but oily, more widely available smoked than fresh. Except in the Pacific Northwest, where fresh steaks, fillets and whole fish are available. Though high in fat and moderately high in cholesterol, sablefish are also excellent sources of niacin, phosphorus and potassium.

NUTRIENT CONTENT OF 3 OUNCES (85 GRAMS) BAKED/BROILED SABLEFISH	
213 calories	61 mg sodium
15 g protein	390 mg potassium
17 g fat, 4 saturated	0 g dietary fiber
54 mg cholesterol	86 RE vitamin A
0 g carbohydrate	0.10 mg thiamin
38 mg calcium	0.10 mg riboflavin
183 mg phosphorus	4.4 mg niacin
1.4 mg iron	0 mg vitamin C

Saccharin: In 1879, while developing new food preservatives, a young Johns Hopkins chemistry research assistant accidentally discovered that one of the organic compounds he was testing was intensely sweet. Saccharin he called it, after *sakcharon,* the Greek word for *sugar.* He further learned that it passed through the body unchanged and was thus a safe sweetener for diabetics. The weight-obsessed soon learned that saccharin, unlike sugar, did not pack the pounds on. And food processors, noting that it was 500 to 700 times sweeter than sugar, were able to cut costs by using it. Even Theodore Roosevelt, a diabetic, championed saccharin early on. When, in 1907, the chief of the USDA's Bureau of Chemistry fretted about the safety of saccharin and wanted it banned from canned foods, Roosevelt was bombastic. "My doctor gives it to me every day. Anybody who says saccharin is injurious to health is an idiot!"

Still, saccharin was banned, only to be restored during the sugar-short years of World War I. Available as powders or pills, to say nothing of in a huge variety of processed foods, saccharin remained popular throughout World War II. Its only drawback was its bitter metallic aftertaste. Food processors licked that problem by combining saccharin with cyclamate, another artificial noncaloric sweetener.

Then in the 1960s came disturbing news. Two different studies suggested that cyclamate caused cancer in lab rats. Subsequent tests concurred and in 1969 cyclamate was banned. With no other artificial noncaloric sweetener available, saccharin use soared. Americans were soon scarfing down 2,500 tons of saccharin a year, most of it from soft drinks. When tests began to suggest that saccharin caused bladder tumors in lab rats, the FDA moved to limit its use.

If the protests launched by the Calorie Control Council (a group that includes saccharin manufacturers and users) weren't heard around the world, they were clearly audible in the halls of Congress. As a result, saccharin won a reprieve in order that testing might continue, even though some suspected that its continued use was a violation of the DELANEY CLAUSE, which bans known carcinogens in food and drink.

Already Britain has banned saccharin (except as an at-table sugar substitute) and France permits its use only by prescription. In the United States, saccharin was deleted from the FDA's GRAS list in 1972. Since 1977, hazardous-to-your-health warnings not only have had to be posted on every item containing saccharin but must also point out that saccharin "has been determined to cause cancer in laboratory animals" (specifically bladder cancers). Those believed to be at greatest risk in general are young children, pregnant women, white men who are heavy smokers and nonwhite women. The current legal status of saccharin? It is classified by the FDA as a weak cocarcinogen, meaning that it may promote (though not necessarily cause) tumors. The saccharin product most widely available in the United States is Sweet'n Low. See also ARTIFICIAL SWEETENERS.

Safe and Adequate Amount: See ESTIMATED SAFE AND ADEQUATE DAILY DIETARY INTAKE.

Safflower Oil: In India, where it's indigenous, and elsewhere throughout the tropics, safflower is triply valuable. From its thistlelike flowers come red and yellow dyes used to color cosmetics, foods and fabrics; from its leaves come salad greens; and from its seeds comes an edible oil. In this age of cholesterol consciousness, safflower oil—pale, clear and bland—has become one of the cooking oils of choice because 78 percent of its fatty acids are polyunsaturated (more than in any other oil), 12 percent are monounsaturated and only 9 percent saturated. As for nutritive value, safflower oil offers nothing other than fat and calories: 1 tablespoon = 120 calories, 14 grams total fat (1.2 grams saturated). Being a vegetable oil, safflower oil contains zero cholesterol. To compare the composition of safflower oil with that of canola, corn, olive and other cooking oils, see OILS.

Safflower Seeds: They look a little like corn kernels. Or perhaps small pine nuts. And like pine nuts they are extremely oily. The oil pressed from safflower seeds is classified as a drying oil, meaning that it air dries into a thin elastic film. Such oils are used in the manufacture of paints, soaps and varnishes. But SAFFLOWER OIL is also edible.

Safrole: A phenolic compound that accounts for 80 percent of the aromatic oils extracted from sassafras bark and roots and once used to impart a licorice flavor to root beer and other soft drinks. Safrole was banned by the FDA in 1960 after it was found to be carcinogenic. It is also present to some extent in nutmeg and star anise.

Sage: The reason for including this herb here is that its lemony/salty/musky flavor makes it possible to cut down on salt. Sage pumps up the flavor of such bland foods as chicken, turkey and veal. It's very good, too, in all manner of stuffings, and just a sprig (or pinch) added to a pot of potatoes, corn, polenta or rice does wonders.

Salad Bars (dangers of): "The greening of America," you might call this proliferation of salad bars. Heartland restaurants are full of them; so are chain supermarkets plus hundreds of delis that have recently sprung up in major metro areas. People like the convenience of salad bars, the creative options they offer and the sociability. Salad bars look innocent enough, nutritious even, but the truth is often not so pretty. Because of the dangerous allergic reactions sulfites can trigger, the FDA now bans their use on raw fruits and vegetables (their purpose was to keep food looking fresh). But the small government policing corps can't begin to watchdog America's millions of salad bars. Sloppily tended salad bars, moreover, are breeding grounds for BACTERIA and VIRUSES, some of which have caused serious outbreaks of food poisoning. The more finely cut a food is, the more often it's handled (exposed to less than pristine knives, cutting boards and counters), the greater its chance of contamination. Then there are all those people sidling down the salad bar, helping themselves to this and that—often with their hands instead of the serving implements, people sneezing into salad bars, coughing, wheezing, laughing and talking. Add to this the fact that not all salad bars are kept properly cold, that flies sometimes buzz about—well, you get the picture.

Salad Dressings: Simple vinaigrettes (olive oil, herbs and vinegar or lemon juice) are best. Yet supermarket shelves bulge with so many instants and mixes one wonders if mass America ever makes dressings from scratch (hardly a culinary tour de force). Ranch (buttermilk) dressing? It's there on the shelf. Russian, French, Italian, Thousand Island, Green Goddess, blue cheese. Name your flavor and you can get it—in low-fat or nonfat versions as well as regular. There are mayonnaises to fit every health concern, too (low or no cholesterol, reduced fat or fat free, reduced or low calorie). Unfortunately, the majority of these prepared dressings are "chemical gumbos" freighted with preservatives, emulsifiers, stabilizers, texturizers, artificial colors and flavors. Most are also too sweet, too salty, too expensive. Scrutinize labels. Better yet, try making your own salad dressing. It's a snap. See also MAYONNAISE.

Salad Greens: Not so long ago the list of supermarket salad greens could be listed on one hand—**iceberg, Bibb** and **Boston lettuce; romaine;** and **Belgian endive.** And in deepest America, it was iceberg or nothing. Today an entire alphabet of salad greens is showing up in small-town farmer's markets as well as in big-city greenmarkets. Among the top tossers: ARUGULA, a biting, dark green also called rocket; **butterhead lettuce** (soft medium green leaves); **chicory** (curly endive, especially the frilly curly chicory called *frisée* by the French); DANDELION GREENS (yes, the blight of lawns adds zest to the salad bowl); **escarole** (a green of medium pungency); **lamb's-quarter** or **mâche** (delicate little rosettes beloved by the French); **mizuna** (a spiky Japanese green that resembles dandelion but lacks its bite); **oak leaf lettuce** (gorgeous bronzy "greens" as deeply convoluted as oak leaves); RADICCHIO (tightly headed crimson endive popular in Italy); **red leaf lettuce** (bright and crinkly leaves). And there are even more exotics on the way (one to look for is a bright mix of newly sprouted greens, sometimes with nasturtium blossoms tumbled in, called MESCLUN). How nutritious are the various lettuces? Pale, bland iceberg, as you might suspect,

Low-Calorie, Nonfat Yogurt-Dill Dressing

Makes 1⅓ Cups

1 cup plain low-fat yogurt

2 tablespoons buttermilk or skim milk

2 tablespoons balsamic vinegar or red wine vinegar

2 tablespoons honey

1 tablespoon snipped fresh dill, or ½ teaspoon dried

½ teaspoon salt

⅛ teaspoon hot red pepper sauce

COMBINE ALL THE ingredients in a tightly capped shaker jar; shake to blend, and thin, if needed, with a little additional skim milk. Store in the refrigerator. Shake well and use to dress mixed green salads.

APPROXIMATE NUTRIENT COUNTS PER TABLESPOON

14 calories	3 g carbohydrate	0 mg iron	0.01 mg thiamin
1 g protein	0 g dietary fiber	61 mg sodium	0.03 mg riboflavin
0 g fat, 0 saturated	23 mg calcium	32 mg potassium	0 mg niacin
1 mg cholesterol	18 mg phosphorus	2 RE vitamin A	0 mg vitamin C

is no nutritional powerhouse. As a general rule, the more colorful the "green," the more vitamins and minerals it will contain. Dark leafy greens, for example, will invariably contribute some beta-carotene, calcium and iron. Nearly all lettuces are fair to good sources of vitamin C, and all are exceedingly low in calories. See also WATERCRESS.

SEASON: Year-round for the majority of lettuces because most of them are hothouse grown; those grown out of doors come to market in late spring and continue in good supply throughout the summer.

NUTRIENT CONTENT OF 1 CUP CHOPPED CHICORY LEAVES
(about 6⅓ ounces; 180 grams)

42 calories	81 mg sodium
3 g protein	756 mg potassium
1 g fat, 0 saturated	2 g dietary fiber
0 mg cholesterol	720 RE vitamin A
8 g carbohydrate	0.11 mg thiamin
180 mg calcium	0.18 mg riboflavin
85 mg phosphorus	0.9 mg niacin
1.6 mg iron	43 mg vitamin C

NUTRIENT CONTENT OF 1 CUP BROKEN BUTTERHEAD LETTUCE LEAVES
(about 2 ounces; 56 grams)

7 calories	3 mg sodium
1 g protein	143 mg potassium
0 g fat, 0 saturated	1 g dietary fiber
0 mg cholesterol	54 RE vitamin A
1 g carbohydrate	0.03 mg thiamin
18 mg calcium	0.03 mg riboflavin
13 mg phosphorus	0.2 mg niacin
0.2 mg iron	4 mg vitamin C

NUTRIENT CONTENT OF 1 CUP BROKEN ICEBERG LETTUCE LEAVES
(about 2 ounces; 56 grams)

7 calories	5 mg sodium
1 g protein	88 mg potassium
0 g fat, 0 saturated	1 g dietary fiber
0 mg cholesterol	19 RE vitamin A
1 g carbohydrate	0.03 mg thiamin
11 mg calcium	0.02 mg riboflavin
11 mg phosphorus	0.1 mg niacin
0.3 mg iron	2 mg vitamin C

NUTRIENT CONTENT OF 1 CUP BROKEN ROMAINE LETTUCE LEAVES

(about 2 ounces; 56 grams)

9 calories	4 mg sodium
1 g protein	162 mg potassium
0 g fat, 0 saturated	1 g dietary fiber
0 mg cholesterol	146 RE vitamin A
1 g carbohydrate	0.06 mg thiamin
20 mg calcium	0.06 mg riboflavin
25 mg phosphorus	0.3 mg niacin
0.6 mg iron	13 mg vitamin C

Salami: A family of hard, dry, rough-textured pork (or pork-and-beef) sausages of Italian origin (but domestic manufacture). Salamis were developed centuries ago when the only ways of preserving meats were salting, smoking and drying. There are dozens of different salamis, most named for the communities where they were first made (by most accounts, **Genoa salami** is the choicest). Salamis are usually garlicky, many are flecked with peppercorns and bits of fat, more of them have been air cured than smoked and most owe their longevity (not to mention their bright rosy hue) to nitrates. Salamis can be bought whole or sliced into cold cuts.

NUTRIENT CONTENT OF 1 OUNCE (28 GRAMS) SALAMI (PORK AND BEEF)

71 calories	302 mg sodium
4 g protein	56 mg potassium
6 g fat, 2 saturated	0 g dietary fiber
19 mg cholesterol	0 RE vitamin A
1 g carbohydrate	0.07 mg thiamin
4 mg calcium	0.11 mg riboflavin
33 mg phosphorus	1.0 mg niacin
0.8 mg iron	3 mg vitamin C

Salatrim: The trademarked name of a new fat, developed by Nabisco chemists, that contains only 5 calories per gram, as opposed to 9 for conventional fats. How did they do it? By combining stearic acid (a long-chain fatty acid, which the body can't fully absorb) with a number of short-chain fatty acids that release fewer available calories during digestion. Nabisco intends to use Salatrim—both its solid and liquid forms—in new lines of snacks, cookies and dairy products.

Salicylates: Compounds that exist naturally in certain foods (almonds, apples, apricots, bananas, blueberries, licorice, green peas, peaches, peppermint, potatoes) and also in aspirin that may exacerbate hives, an allergenic skin condition. Back in the early 1970s, Dr. Benjamin Feingold also reported that 50 percent of the hyperactive children he put on a diet devoid of artificial colors, flavors and natural salicylates showed dramatic improvement. Subsequent tests by the National Institutes of Health refuted Feingold's claims. See also FEINGOLD DIET; HIVES.

Saliva: Digestion begins in the mouth when saliva attacks and partially breaks down carbohydrates. But that's not its only role. Rich in calcium and phosphorus, saliva neutralizes plaque acids and helps fight tooth decay. It helps flush food particles from the gums and teeth and also destroys many potentially harmful bacteria in the mouth.

Salmon: If Americans were asked to name their favorite fish, salmon would surely make the top five. Apparently, it was always thus for Columbia River digs have turned up salmon bones carbon-dated at 11,000 B.C. Europeans have been feasting on salmon even longer, judging from the vertebrae found in Stone Age middens. Only a handful of important salmon species now find their way to U.S. markets: **Atlantic salmon** (most of it imported from Canada or Europe because U.S. eastern rivers are too polluted to support spawning) and five from the Pacific. These are the **chinook** or **king salmon;** the **sockeye** or **red salmon** (its flesh is the darkest of all); the mostly farm-raised **coho;** the orange-meated **chum;** then last (and also least), the **pink salmon,** most of which goes into cans. All salmon species are firm of flesh and "oily," meaning that the natural oils are evenly distributed throughout the meat instead of being concentrated in the liver (the case with

NUTRIENT CONTENT OF 3 OUNCES (85 GRAMS) BAKED/GRILLED SOCKEYE SALMON

184 calories	56 mg sodium
23 g protein	319 mg potassium
9 g fat, 2 saturated	0 g dietary fiber
74 mg cholesterol	54 RE vitamin A
0 g carbohydrate	0.18 mg thiamin
6 mg calcium	0.15 mg riboflavin
235 mg phosphorus	5.7 mg niacin
0.5 mg iron	0 mg vitamin C

cod and halibut). The tastiest whole salmon weighs 5 pounds or less and bakes, poaches and grills superbly (as do steaks and fillets). Fresh salmon is a good source of niacin, phosphorus and potassium, and the canned, because of the soft, edible bones it contains, is a potent source of calcium. Salmon is a fairly fatty fish, it's true, but the fat is mostly unsaturated. Smoked salmon is extremely salty and off-limits for those on low-sodium diets. So is brined salmon (what the Hawaiians call *lomi-lomi*). See also LOX.

NUTRIENT CONTENT OF 3 OUNCES (85 GRAMS) BAKED/GRILLED ATLANTIC SALMON FILLET

155 calories	48 mg sodium
22 g protein	534 mg potassium
7 g fat, 1 saturated	0 g dietary fiber
60 mg cholesterol	11 RE vitamin A
0 g carbohydrate	0.23 mg thiamin
13 mg calcium	0.41 mg riboflavin
218 mg phosphorus	8.6 mg niacin
0.9 mg iron	0 mg vitamin C

NUTRIENT CONTENT OF 3 OUNCES (85 GRAMS) POACHED/STEAMED COHO SALMON FILLET

156 calories	45 mg sodium
23 g protein	387 mg potassium
6 g fat, 1 saturated	0 g dietary fiber
49 mg cholesterol	27 RE vitamin A
0 g carbohydrate	0.10 mg thiamin
39 mg calcium	0.14 mg riboflavin
254 mg phosphorus	6.6 mg niacin
0.6 mg iron	1 mg vitamin C

NUTRIENT CONTENT OF 3 OUNCES (85 GRAMS) CANNED CHUM SALMON (DRAINED)

120 calories	414 mg sodium
18 g protein	255 mg potassium
5 g fat, 1 saturated	0 g dietary fiber
33 mg cholesterol	15 RE vitamin A
0 g carbohydrate	0.02 mg thiamin
212 mg calcium	0.14 mg riboflavin
301 mg phosphorus	6.0 mg niacin
0.6 mg iron	0 mg vitamin C

NUTRIENT CONTENT OF 3 OUNCES (85 GRAMS) CANNED PINK SALMON (NO SALT ADDED, DRAINED)

118 calories	64 mg sodium
17 g protein	277 mg potassium
5 g fat, 1 saturated	0 g dietary fiber
47 mg cholesterol	15 RE vitamin A
0 g carbohydrate	0.02 mg thiamin
181 mg calcium	0.16 mg riboflavin
280 mg phosphorus	5.6 mg niacin
0.7 mg iron	0 mg vitamin C

NUTRIENT CONTENT OF 3 OUNCES (85 GRAMS) CANNED SOCKEYE SALMON (NO SALT ADDED, DRAINED)

130 calories	64 mg sodium
17 g protein	321 mg potassium
6 g fat, 1 saturated	0 g dietary fiber
37 mg cholesterol	45 RE vitamin A
0 g carbohydrate	0.01 mg thiamin
203 mg calcium	0.16 mg riboflavin
277 mg phosphorus	4.7 mg niacin
0.9 mg iron	0 mg vitamin C

Salmonella: See BACTERIA.

Salmon Trout: These are not salmon; they are trout—in fact, three close relatives, **brown trout, lake trout** and **sea trout,** all of which are more popular in Britain and continental Europe than they are in the United States. Salmon trout are smallish (the best freshwater catches average 1 pound or 2 apiece; the sea-runs, somewhat more), their flesh is firm and, depending on their diet, can range from pale pink to bright orange (for crayfish eaters).

NUTRIENT CONTENT OF 3 OUNCES (85 GRAMS) BAKED/GRILLED SALMON TROUT (SEA TROUT)

113 calories	63 mg sodium
18 g protein	372 mg potassium
4 g fat, 1 saturated	0 g dietary fiber
90 mg cholesterol	30 RE vitamin A
0 g carbohydrate	0.06 mg thiamin
19 mg calcium	0.18 mg riboflavin
273 mg phosphorus	2.5 mg niacin
0.3 mg iron	0 mg vitamin C

NUTRIENT CONTENT OF 3 OUNCES (85 GRAMS)
POACHED/STEAMED SALMON TROUT (SEA TROUT)

128 calories	60 mg sodium
21 g protein	390 mg potassium
4 g fat, 1 saturated	0 g dietary fiber
90 mg cholesterol	34 RE vitamin A
0 g carbohydrate	0.09 mg thiamin
26 mg calcium	0.09 mg riboflavin
208 mg phosphorus	5.4 mg niacin
1.2 mg iron	0 mg vitamin C

Salsa: The Spanish word for "sauce," but in culinary terms it means a Mexican sauce that's a confetti-bright mix of chopped fresh tomatoes, onions, parsley and peppers sweet and hot. Salsa's equally popular north of the border and is especially good on grilled or sautéed fish, fowl, meat or vegetables. Salsa is now so "hot" it comes in bottles. Just like pasta sauce. The fresh, needless to say, is more nutritious and usually less salty than the processed versions; recipes vary from cook to cook. Salsa's big plus is that it's fat and cholesterol free, extremely low in calories, yet exploding with flavor. It also contains a modicum of vitamins and minerals.

NUTRIENT CONTENT OF 1 TABLESPOON HOMEMADE SALSA
(about ½ ounce; 15 grams)

3 calories	58 mg sodium
0 g protein	24 mg potassium
0 g fat, 0 saturated	0 g dietary fiber
0 mg cholesterol	25 RE vitamin A
1 g carbohydrate	0 mg thiamin
2 mg calcium	0 mg riboflavin
3 mg phosphorus	0.1 mg niacin
0 mg iron	6 mg vitamin C

Salsify: There are two salsifies, one **black** (actually black skinned), one **white,** both alternatively known as **oyster plant** because they taste faintly of oysters, especially when creamed or bubbled into chowder. Although members of the huge Compositae family, the two salsifies are of different genera and different species. Both are fleshy, carrot-shaped roots with flat, coarse grassy tops. Both are ivory fleshed but turn rust brown the minute they're peeled (a quick dip in acidulated water—1 tablespoon vinegar or

lemon juice per pint of cool water—will keep them bright). Their brown juices will stain your hands, may even cause a rash, so wear rubber gloves when handling salsify. Salsify is believed to be native to southern Europe, perhaps Spain (black salsify's botanical name, *Scorzonera hispanica,* certainly suggests Iberian roots). Thomas Jefferson was partial to salsify, had it grown at Monticello, which may explain why it has long been popular down South. Salsify is an excellent source of riboflavin and potassium and a moderate one of vitamin C and fiber. It's low in sodium and contains zero fat and cholesterol. **SEASON:** Fall, winter, early spring.

NUTRIENT CONTENT OF 1 CUP BOILED/STEAMED SALSIFY
(about 4¾ ounces; 135 grams)

92 calories	22 mg sodium
4 g protein	382 mg potassium
0 g fat, 0 saturated	3 g dietary fiber
0 mg cholesterol	0 RE vitamin A
21 g carbohydrate	0.08 mg thiamin
64 mg calcium	0.23 mg riboflavin
76 mg phosphorus	0.5 mg niacin
0.7 mg iron	6 mg vitamin C

Salt: Sodium chloride. But that's just the beginning of a story that dates back to the Stone Age and includes whole chapters when salt was more precious than gold. Recently salt's gotten a bad rap as an elevator of blood pressure. Too much salt is bad, it's true. But too little is equally bad. Our body fluids all contain salt, in about the same proportion as seawater, and without salt we would die (see SODIUM). Our focus here, however, is on salt as seasoner. Which of the many types now available is best? It depends on use.

Flavored Salts: Most cooks worth their salt would never dream of using these ersatz seasonings, although **celery salt, garlic salt, onion salt** and other flavored salts do have their fans, especially among grill enthusiasts who use them as dry rubs and Cajuns who like their flavors intense.

Iodized Salt: Table salt to which sodium or potassium iodide has been added (about 1 part per 5,000). Iodized salt was developed early in the twentieth century as a way to eliminate GOITER (see also the main entry for IODIZED SALT). Iodine gives salt a slightly medicinal taste, so this salt shouldn't be used in canning, pickling and preserving. It may also alter the color of the food somewhat, graying the greens, for example.

Kosher Salt: Also called **cheese, dairy** or **flake salt,** kosher salt was originally produced under rabbinical supervision, but today *kosher salt* is an umbrella term that includes all coarse-grained, additive-free natural salts. It's the pro's choice because as Julia Child says, it's so easy to pick up by the pinch, so easy to scatter evenly.

Pickling Salt: An additive-free salt of exceptional purity that dissolves quickly and completely, leaving no cloudy traces.

Rock Salt: Salt mined from deep in the earth where ancient evaporated seas left extensive deposits. Also called **ice cream salt** or **melting salt,** rock salt is coarse grained and gray because of the impurities it contains. Most of these are harmless, but some rock salt may contain arsenic. Those safe to eat are marked "edible."

Sea Salt: According to Elizabeth David, Britain's late poet laureate of food writers, "Food cooked with sea salt tastes so much better than that cooked with powdered rock salt that people who are accustomed to it notice a startling difference when deprived of it." Seawater, of course, contains minerals other than sodium and it's the mix that gives sea salt its clear, pure taste. "Sea" salt is something of a misnomer because most of it is produced by evaporating lagoon or marsh water into crystals large or small. Of all the sea salts, the English **Malden** is considered the very best because of its delicate flavor.

Table Salt: Pan-evaporated, vacuum-purified solutions of rock salt that have been pulverized until uniformly fine. To keep table salt free-running, carbonates (usually magnesium), bicarbonates or starch may be added. For this reason, table is a poor choice for pickling and preserving. Its additives cloud the brine.

Salt Cod: Because the Portuguese (who were the first to dry it at sea) eat more dried salt cod than any other people on earth, we cover it under its Portuguese name, BACALHAU.

"Salt-Free," "No Salt Added," "Reduced Salt," "Low Sodium," "Very Low Sodium": Labels are full of such terms, but since the Nutrition Labeling and Edu-

cation Act went into effect in the spring of 1994, food must meet strict government requirements to qualify for any of these designations. For example:

"Salt-Free": No more than 5 milligrams sodium per serving.

"No Salt Added": Exactly what it says. No salt has been added and this includes additives that may have built-in salt.

"Reduced Salt": The salt content has been reduced by 25 percent. **NOTE:** If the food is already low in salt, "reduced" cannot be used.

"Low Sodium": No more than 140 milligrams sodium per serving; and for servings of 2 tablespoons (30 grams) or less, no more than 140 milligrams sodium per 50 grams of the food.

"Very Low Sodium": No more than 35 milligrams of sodium per serving; and for servings of 2 tablespoons (30 grams) or less, no more than 35 milligrams sodium per 50 grams of the food.

Saltines: A type of cracker. See SODA CRACKERS.

Saltpeter: See POTASSIUM NITRATE.

Salt Pork: Brined pork fat often streaked with a little lean. Called **streaky** down South, it is frequently added to a pot of greens or beans for flavor. It is so very salty, many recipes calling for salt pork need no additional salt.

NUTRIENT CONTENT OF 1 OUNCE (28 GRAMS) SALT PORK (COOKED)	
193 calories	344 mg sodium
3 g protein	12 mg potassium
20 g fat, 7 saturated	0 g dietary fiber
21 mg cholesterol	0 RE vitamin A
0 g carbohydrate	0.08 mg thiamin
2 mg calcium	0.03 mg riboflavin
34 mg phosphorus	0.6 mg niacin
0.5 mg iron	0 mg vitamin C

Salt Substitutes: Seasonings containing either no sodium or a reduced amount. **Potassium chloride** is the oldest and best known, but it can cause irregular heartbeat in those with kidney trouble or those on potassium-retaining diuretics. Too much potassium chloride, moreover, can throw the body's fluid balance out of whack because potassium and sodium work together in maintaining this extremely delicate ratio. Other problems: Potassium chloride has a bitter aftertaste and it's so much blander than salt that people tend to shake it on with a heavy hand. Fortunately, other salt substitutes are now available—**calcium chloride** or **ammonium chloride,** plus assorted dehydrated vegetable/herb/spice blends and some of them quite specific (for chicken, for fish, for vegetables, etc.). A number of these contain considerable sodium, however, so scrutinize package labels. Then there's **sour salt** (powdered citric acid), pinches of which add a certain salinity to soups, sauces and stews (simmering these with a strip of orange or lemon zest builds flavor without adding salt, too). Finally, drizzlings of **lemon juice** or **balsamic vinegar** can sub for salt on grilled fish, fowl and vegetables. And certain **herbs**—dill, sage, rosemary—have a lemony/salty savor that adds zest to veal, fish and fowl as well as to asparagus, broccoli, cabbage, carrots, corn, green beans and peas. With a little improv, you'll learn which herbs work best with which foods.

Sandwiches:

The original fast food, created, it's said, so the earl of Sandwich could eat at the gaming table. The trouble with these meals-in-one is that often they're loaded with fat, cholesterol and salt. Think of pastrami on rye, for example. Bologna and cheese with no hold on the mayo. Even BLTs stint on important nutrients but don't lack for saturated fat, cholesterol and sodium. The most healthful sandwiches begin with whole-grain breads, use mustard or fat-free salad dressings as spreads and lean slices of turkey or chicken breast as fillers, along with red-ripe tomatoes, shredded carrots, slaw or roasted sweet peppers. Peanut butter makes a nutritionally acceptable sandwich, especially if the bread isn't slathered with butter, mayonnaise or jelly. Tuna, turkey or chicken salads plumped up with minced carrots or sweet peppers and onions and bound with fat-free mayos are good, too, if served on whole-grain bread topped with cress or bright green lettuce.

Sapotes:

These sweet, perfumy plum-shaped fruits are Caribbean and Central American staples. The choicest sapote is the white variety, a fruit about the size of a small grapefruit, blessed with exceptionally fine and juicy flesh the color of country cream. White sapotes are now being grown on a limited scale in Florida and California. They are best when pureed and stirred into puddings, ice creams and sherbets. Sapotes are good sources of vitamin C and niacin, also of fiber, iron and potassium, yet they are very low in sodium. **SEASON:** Fall.

NUTRIENT CONTENT OF 1 MEDIUM-SIZE SAPOTE	
(about 6 ounces; 170 grams)	
228 calories	17 mg sodium
3 g protein	585 mg potassium
1 g fat, 0 saturated	4 g dietary fiber
0 mg cholesterol	70 RE vitamin A
58 g carbohydrate	0.02 mg thiamin
66 mg calcium	0.03 mg riboflavin
48 mg phosphorus	3.1 mg niacin
1.7 mg iron	34 mg vitamin C

Sapsago:

A hard-enough-to-grate Swiss cheese made from the milk of cows that graze blue melilot clover, which explains its green color and musty/grassy flavor. Shaped into squatty cones, sapsago is an acquired taste but many like it grated over pasta, even pizza. It averages about 41 percent protein, 37 percent moisture and the rest fat. **NOTE:** Specific nutrients are unavailable for sapsago.

Sardines:

What few people realize is that sardine is not a species of fish but a generic term applied to a variety of small herrings—**Atlantic** and **Pacific herrings, bluebacks, pilchards, sprats** (or **brislings**). On the streets of Lisbon during the spring and summer sardine season, plump fresh sardines are grilled on little terra-cotta braziers, popped into chewy rolls and eaten for lunch. Wonderful! Most of the rest of the world must settle for canned sar-

NUTRIENT CONTENT OF 2 OUNCES (57 GRAMS) CANNED SARDINES (OIL PACKED, DRAINED)	
146 calories	286 mg sodium
14 g protein	226 mg potassium
10 g fat, 2 saturated	0 g dietary fiber
80 mg cholesterol	38 RE vitamin A
0 g carbohydrate	0.05 mg thiamin
216 mg calcium	0.13 mg riboflavin
278 mg phosphorus	3.0 mg niacin
1.7 mg iron	0 mg vitamin C

dines, a poor second when it comes to taste and texture. Sardines may be packed in oil (usually olive or soybean). Or they may be packed in water. Note the calcium content of sardines (below). They're one of the best nondairy sources available for this precious mineral.

NUTRIENT CONTENT OF 2 OUNCES (57 GRAMS) CANNED SKINLESS SARDINES (WATER PACKED, DRAINED)

110 calories	520 mg sodium
14 g protein	253 mg potassium
6 g fat, 2 saturated	0 g dietary fiber
47 mg cholesterol	22 RE vitamin A
0 g carbohydrate	0.07 mg thiamin
48 mg calcium	0.18 mg riboflavin
184 mg phosphorus	2.5 mg niacin
0.9 mg iron	1 mg vitamin C

Sashimi, Sushi: The Japanese dote on sliced raw fish (sashimi) and sushi (vinegared rice topped with strips of raw fish or rolled up in dried seaweed sheets with strips of vegetable or raw fish). So do American habitués of sushi bars. In the best of times, raw fish are perfectly wholesome. Today, however, with many fish riddled with parasites and/or contaminated with such bacteria as *Vibrio vulnificus,* it's eat at your own risk. See also BACTERIA; PARASITES.

Sassafras: An aromatic tree native to the American South. The Native Americans of the eastern woodlands prized the licorice flavor of sassafras roots and bark and brewed them into tea. They also discovered that when dried and pulverized, sassafras leaves had the power to thicken soups and stews (Creoles call this powder *gumbo filé*). Alas, SAFROLE, the very essence of sassafras, the flavoring used for years in root beer and other soft drinks, is now known to cause cancer. The FDA banned it as an additive in 1960.

Satiety Value: The ability of a food to make you feel full, satisfied. High-fat and high-protein foods have greater satiety value than carbohydrates, especially simple sugars.

Saturated Fat: See FAT.

Sauces: Say "sauce" and butter and cream come to mind. Not all sauces are chockablock with fat, calories and cholesterol, however. On the contrary. In this age of fitness, more and more cooks—both pros and amateurs—are concentrating on freshly made SALSAS; on reduced, skimmed pan juices; and on vegetable purees, creamed, perhaps, with a little low-fat yogurt or ricotta or evaporated skim milk. Good thinking. Such sauces are not only lower in the no-nos but also higher in important vitamins and minerals.

Sauerkraut: Although everyone associates this brined, shredded cabbage with Germany, it originated in China. Quite by accident. In the third century B.C., laborers building the Great Wall discovered that their rations of cabbage were spoiling. In an effort to preserve what was left, they chopped the cabbage, mixed it with rice wine and barreled it. Before long the cabbage began to fizz and foam and presto! Sauerkraut. Genghis Khan's armies later traveled with brined sauerkraut, carrying it as far west as the Middle East, from which it was a relatively short leap to Western Europe, including Germany. The fresh sauerkraut of Germany is crunchy, delicately salted and far superior to any canned American varieties. Fortunately, upscale supermarkets now stock 1-pound plastic bags of fresh sauerkraut. It is an impressive source of vitamin C, a good source, too, of iron, potassium and fiber and is extremely low in calories. Unfortunately, it's on sodium overload, but thorough rinsing will bring these counts down.

NUTRIENT CONTENT OF 1 CUP CANNED SAUERKRAUT (UNDRAINED)

(about 8½ ounces; 236 grams)

45 calories	1,559 mg sodium
2 g protein	401 mg potassium
0 g fat, 0 saturated	6 g dietary fiber
0 mg cholesterol	5 RE vitamin A
10 g carbohydrate	0.05 mg thiamin
71 mg calcium	0.05 mg riboflavin
47 mg phosphorus	0.3 mg niacin
3.5 mg iron	35 mg vitamin C

Note: Although figures are unavailable, fresh sauerkraut would be significantly higher in vitamin C than canned; other food values would remain about the same.

Sausage: There are thousands of sausages; indeed, Germany alone produces hundreds of different wursts. But these are not our concern here. This is about fresh pork sausage, the meat sold in bulk, links and patties in nearly every supermarket. A particular favorite down South, pork sausage was a by-product, originally, of hog killing, the odds and ends of the annual butchering ground up together with plenty of salt, pepper and sage. Many sausage recipes remain closely guarded family secrets. The same can be said for fresh Italian sausages, both sweet and hot, which have made their way into mainstream America. Unfortunately, sausage is surfeited with the very things that bring some people to grief—fat, saturated fat, cholesterol, calories, sodium and often nitrates, too. To downsize some of these culprits, meat packers are now making turkey sausage. It's

somewhat leaner and significantly less salty than pork sausage although cholesterol counts remain just the same (the figures in the following food value charts are for 1 ounce and, sad to say, few people would limit themselves to portions that small). For coverage of other classic sausages, see BLOOD SAUSAGE; BOLOGNA; BRATWURST; FRANKFURTERS; KIELBASA; KNACKWURST; LIVERWURST; PEPPERONI; SALAMI; THURINGER; VIENNA SAUSAGE; WEISSWURST.

Sautéing: The French word for FRYING.

Sauternes: A group of sweet or semisweet white wines produced in the Bordeaux region of France. See WINES; also ALCOHOL, ALCOHOLIC BEVERAGES.

Savoy Cabbage: See CABBAGE, SAVOY.

Saxitoxins: Powerful neurotoxins that cause PARALYTIC SHELLFISH POISONING. They show up in clams, oysters, mussels and bay scallops living in beds contaminated with toxic marine plankton (a dinoflagellate called gonyaulax, to be specific). And woes be to anyone who eats these mollusks. See also NEUROTOXINS; RED TIDE.

Scallions: See ONIONS.

Scallops: "The caviar of mollusks" scallops have been called. Not a bad description if the scallops in question are the tiny nut-sweet **bay scallops** taken from the waters off eastern Long Island, New York. They are as fine as lobsters or blue crabs, infinitely more enjoyable than clams, mussels and oysters. Or so scallop fanciers insist. Now plentiful, **sea scallops** were once so rare dishonest fishmongers faked them by punching disks out of cod and skate wings.

NUTRIENT CONTENT OF 1 OUNCE (28 GRAMS) COOKED PORK SAUSAGE LINKS

96 calories	336 mg sodium
6 g protein	94 mg potassium
8 g fat, 2 saturated	0 g dietary fiber
22 mg cholesterol	0 RE vitamin A
0 g carbohydrate	0.20 mg thiamin
8 mg calcium	0.06 mg riboflavin
48 mg phosphorus	1.2 mg niacin
0.4 mg iron	0 mg vitamin C

NUTRIENT CONTENT OF 1 OUNCE (28 GRAMS) COOKED PORK SAUSAGE PATTY

100 calories	349 mg sodium
5 g protein	98 mg potassium
8 g fat, 3 saturated	0 g dietary fiber
22 mg cholesterol	0 RE vitamin A
0 g carbohydrate	0.20 mg thiamin
9 mg calcium	0.07 mg riboflavin
50 mg phosphorus	1.2 mg niacin
0.3 mg iron	0 mg vitamin C

NUTRIENT CONTENT OF 1 OUNCE (28 GRAMS) COOKED TURKEY BREAKFAST SAUSAGE

65 calories	191 mg sodium
6 g protein	76 mg potassium
5 g fat, 2 saturated	0 g dietary fiber
23 mg cholesterol	0 RE vitamin A
0 g carbohydrate	0.03 mg thiamin
5 mg calcium	0.08 mg riboflavin
52 mg phosphorus	1.4 mg niacin
0.5 mg iron	0 mg vitamin C

NUTRIENT CONTENT OF 3 OUNCES (85 GRAMS) POACHED/STEAMED SCALLOPS

91 calories	157 mg sodium
14 g protein	239 mg potassium
3 g fat, 0 saturated	0 g dietary fiber
27 mg cholesterol	39 RE vitamin A
2 g carbohydrate	0.01 mg thiamin
21 mg calcium	0.05 mg riboflavin
135 mg phosphorus	0.9 mg niacin
0.2 mg iron	2 mg vitamin C

But the discovery in the mid-1930s of vast scallop beds off the New England shore ensured a good supply of the real thing. Sea scallops are bigger, firmer and less delicate than bay scallops. But they're often safer, too, because the waters from which they come are less likely to be polluted or afflicted with the dread RED TIDE. Scallops are invariably sold shucked and, because they are highly perishable, should be served within twenty-four hours of purchase.

NUTRIENT CONTENT OF 3 OUNCES (85 GRAMS) BAKED/BROILED SCALLOPS

113 calories	435 mg sodium
17 g protein	332 mg potassium
3 g fat, 1 saturated	0 g dietary fiber
34 mg cholesterol	49 RE vitamin A
2 g carbohydrate	0.01 mg thiamin
26 mg calcium	0.07 mg riboflavin
225 mg phosphorus	1.1 mg niacin
0.3 mg iron	2 mg vitamin C

Scampi: The Italian word for prawns. See SHRIMP.

Scarsdale Diet: A high-protein, low-carbohydrate, limited-fat, two-week weight-loss diet devised by the late Dr. Herman Tarnower of Westchester County, New York. It skimps on fruits, vegetables and breads and short-shrifts vitamin A, calcium and riboflavin (B_2). See also DIETS.

Schizophrenia (niacin and): Back in the 1970s, a number of scientists began hyping the healing powers of vitamin megadoses, specifically of niacin, which they believed would relieve the agonies of schizophrenia. Dubbed ORTHOMOLECULAR PSYCHIATRY by Nobelist Linus Pauling, megavitamin therapy caused such a media stir that the American Psychiatric Association commissioned a special task force to study its effect on the mentally ill, schizophrenics included. They found nothing to support the claims of the orthomolecular "psychiatrists" and damned them for their headline-grabbing, false-hope theories.

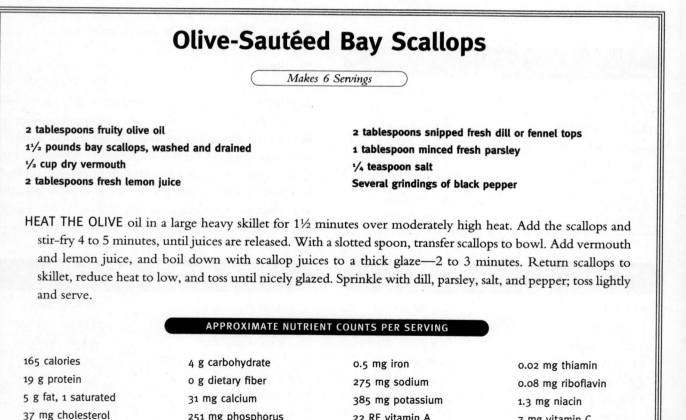

Olive-Sautéed Bay Scallops

Makes 6 Servings

2 tablespoons fruity olive oil
1½ pounds bay scallops, washed and drained
½ cup dry vermouth
2 tablespoons fresh lemon juice

2 tablespoons snipped fresh dill or fennel tops
1 tablespoon minced fresh parsley
¼ teaspoon salt
Several grindings of black pepper

HEAT THE OLIVE oil in a large heavy skillet for 1½ minutes over moderately high heat. Add the scallops and stir-fry 4 to 5 minutes, until juices are released. With a slotted spoon, transfer scallops to bowl. Add vermouth and lemon juice, and boil down with scallop juices to a thick glaze—2 to 3 minutes. Return scallops to skillet, reduce heat to low, and toss until nicely glazed. Sprinkle with dill, parsley, salt, and pepper; toss lightly and serve.

APPROXIMATE NUTRIENT COUNTS PER SERVING

165 calories	4 g carbohydrate	0.5 mg iron	0.02 mg thiamin
19 g protein	0 g dietary fiber	275 mg sodium	0.08 mg riboflavin
5 g fat, 1 saturated	31 mg calcium	385 mg potassium	1.3 mg niacin
37 mg cholesterol	251 mg phosphorus	22 RE vitamin A	7 mg vitamin C

Schmaltz: Rendered chicken fat, which many traditional Jewish cooks prefer to other cooking fats and oils. Like other fats, schmaltz contains 120 calories per tablespoon. But as an animal fat, it also contains cholesterol and a higher percentage of saturated fatty acids than most vegetable oils.

School Breakfast Program: One of the five federal assistance programs administered by the Food and Nutrition Service of the U.S. Department of Agriculture. Its purpose is to provide schoolchildren with a free or bargain-priced breakfast that is nutritionally adequate: 1 cup milk, ½ cup fruit or fruit or vegetable juice plus two servings bread and/or cereal is the bare minimum.

School Lunch Program: Another of the USDA's Food and Nutrition Service programs designed to see that American schoolchildren receive healthful lunches at prices they can afford (the lunches are sometimes free or reduced in price—family income determines). The aid consists of cash reimbursements or donated food. To qualify for the School Lunch Program, schools must serve lunches that meet the requirements set by the secretary of agriculture. This originally meant 1 cup milk, 2 ounces meat or meat substitute, ¾ cup each of 2 or more fruits or vegetables, 1 slice enriched or whole-grain bread (or ½ cup pasta, rice or other grain). But the rules have changed. Junior and senior high school students must be offered this menu but they have the option of settling for only three or four of the foods offered. See also FRESH START, a program implemented late in 1993 to improve the nutritive value of school lunches.

Scombroid Poisoning: Severe allergylike reactions triggered by eating fish with extremely high levels of histamine, specifically bonito, mackerel, sardines, tuna (all scombroids) and such oily-fleshed nonscombroids as amberjack (yellowtail) and mahimahi. Symptoms, which can occur anywhere from ten minutes to an hour and a half after eating, range from rashes to violent headaches to dizziness, breathlessness, diarrhea, vomiting and shock. Because heat doesn't destroy the harmful histamines, canned, salted and smoked fish are just as dangerous as the fresh or frozen. Fortunately, the histamines are sometimes detectable—the fish tastes sharp, peppery. Still, the best medicine, no question, is prevention. And that's as easy as quick chilling these fish the minute they're caught. In any left at room temperature three to four hours, histamine levels can zoom to 400 times the normal level.

Scorzonera: Another word for black salsify. For details, see SALSIFY.

Scotch: See ALCOHOL, ALCOHOLIC BEVERAGES.

Scoville Units: The scale used to measure the heat of chile peppers. See HOT PEPPERS under PEPPERS, CAPSICUM.

Scrapple: Also called **pawnhaus** by the Pennsylvania Dutch, this breakfast staple is a pork-and-cornmeal mush that's cooled, sliced, then browned in butter. Laden with calories, fat, cholesterol and sodium, it's hardly "the breakfast of champions."

Scrod: Young COD.

Scup: Another name for porgy (see PORGIES).

Scuppernongs: See GRAPES.

Scurvy: A severe, often fatal disease caused by a prolonged deficiency of vitamin C. In centuries past, it was the scourge of sailors, who lacked fresh fruits and vegetables at sea. See C, VITAMIN.

Sea Bass: **Black sea bass,** to give these small (1½- to 5-pound) fish their full name, swim the Atlantic from New England to Florida but are most abundant between New York and North Carolina. George Washington used to fish for them off New Jersey's Sandy Hook. Sea bass are lean and white of flesh but so full of needle-sharp bones they must be eaten with care. Sea bass are a particular favorite among the Chinese, who steam and deep-fry them whole. For approximate nutrient counts, see FISH, LEAN WHITE.

Seafood Safety: In the early 1990s, after investigative reporters attacked the seafood industry for its lax standards and the U.S. Congress for failing to pass seafood-safety laws, the Food and Drug Administration announced tough new rules that lie within its jurisdiction to ensure the wholesomeness of our fish and shellfish. In addition to ongoing government inspections, all shellfish must now be identified as to where it was taken and these identifying tags must be kept by all companies handling fish (five thousand at last count) for ninety days. This way, any outbreaks of sickness are easier to trace. Eventually, if Congress gets around to legislating it, all seafood will be subject to Hazard Analysis and Critical Control Points (see HACCP), a highly accurate method of testing the purity of food at a series of checkpoints that was originally developed for NASA. Until HACCP is implemented, the FDA's only course of action is to require all seafood processors, vendors and handlers to police themselves. Meanwhile, the surest way to avoid getting sick from contaminated seafood is to make sure it's well cooked. See also RAW FOOD.

Searing: The purpose is to brown food, particularly meat or seafood, quickly, forming a crust that seals in juices. But searing may also seal in some of the fat. And if there is surface fat, the searing may produce ACROLEIN, a noxious aldehyde that can harm mucous membranes.

Sea Salt: See SALT.

Sea Urchins: The porcupines of the sea. These spiny creatures may be as small as an orange or as big as a basketball, but their innards—specifically their creamy pink-orange roes—are considered a great delicacy. Only in high-end metropolitan fish markets can sea urchins be bought by the home cook, however. And only in fancy big-city restaurants can they be sampled. Sea urchins have an intense marine flavor, a texture sometimes described as "squidgy" and clearly are an acquired taste. For most Americans they will remain more a swimmer's hazard than something to savor. **NOTE:** Nutrient counts are unavailable for sea urchins.

Seawater: In the not so long ago, people insisted that lobsters should never be cooked in anything but seawater; that it was best, too, for poaching salmon and certain other fish. But that was before industrial runoffs flowed downstream into the Atlantic and Pacific, raising ocean levels of mercury and other heavy metals, before other contaminants, both bacterial and chemical, began showing up in test samples. As for the health faddists' claims that bottled seawater is "the fountain of youth," forget it.

Seaweed: To the Japanese, seaweeds are kitchen staples, nutritious gifts from the sea to be treated with artistry and respect. Among their favorites are **kombu** (a giant olive brown kelp that is dried into sheets, then simmered into *dashi* or stock), **nori** (dried tissues of seaweed, forest green or purple, which are the classic sushi wrappers) and **wakame** (curly green or brown seaweeds, also dried, then bubbled into soups and stews). All have a delicate deep-sea flavor. In the United States, food companies have for years used gelatinous seaweed extracts to smooth puddings, fillings, frostings and ice creams. And health-food stores have long touted KELP and SPIRULINA as vitamin and mineral powerhouses, cures for almost everything that ails you. "Reported to be beneficial to sensory nerves, membranes surrounding the brain, the spinal cord and brain tissue" begins one pitch for kelp. Then it goes on to extol the virtues of kelp as a cure for hair loss, goiter, ulcers and obesity, even as a "protector from effects of radiation." Seaweeds are rich in minerals, mainly iodine, but they are not miracle workers. See also AGAR; CARRAGEENAN.

Seitan: A meat analogue made of wheat gluten. See also ANALOGUE.

Selenium: A trace mineral that functions in concert with vitamin E and is essential to good health. It helps detox cell-scavenging free radicals as well as heavy metals like arsenic, cadmium, mercury and silver. Some researchers also now believe that selenium reduces the risk of certain cancers (although a new Harvard study questions whether this is true). Selenium may even slow the progress of AIDS. Although selenium deficiencies crop up in remote corners of the world (notably the Keshan Province of China, where young boys and pregnant women were felled by heart-muscle disorders), they are rare in the United States. Overdoses of selenium are more likely because health-food stores push selenium supplements (some of them nearly five times the RDA for women) as the key to sturdier immune systems, stronger hearts, healthier pancreatic function, greater skin and muscle tone. In fact, high doses of selenium (1 milligram or more a day) are extremely toxic, causing hair and nail loss, nerve damage, skin lesions, irritability, fatigue, diarrhea, nausea and abdominal cramps. **GOOD SOURCES:** Brazil nuts, eggs, lean meats, seafood, legumes and whole grains. **NOTE:** Many cattle and poultry feeds are fortified with selenium because the soil in some areas (and thus the grains and grass grown on them) lack this important mineral.

RDA FOR SELENIUM

Babies:

Birth to 6 months	10 mcg per day
6 months to 1 year	15 mcg per day

Children:

1 to 6 years	20 mcg per day
7 to 10 years	30 mcg per day

Men and Boys:

11 to 14 years	40 mcg per day
15 to 18 years	50 mcg per day
19 to 51+ years	70 mcg per day

Women and Girls:

11 to 14 years	45 mcg per day
15 to 18 years	50 mcg per day
19 to 51+ years	55 mcg per day

Pregnant Women: 65 mcg per day

Nursing Mothers: 75 mcg per day

Seltzer, Soda Water: Carbonated water, either natural or man-made. The first bubbly waters to be called seltzer were the mineral waters of Nieder Selters, Germany. In the mid-1800s, soda fountains sprang up across America, their original purpose being to dispense seltzer as a digestive. Before long, flavors were added and, presto, the age of soda pop. Unlike soda water (club soda), seltzers usually contain little or no salt. Of course many soda waters sold today are available in low- or no-sodium versions. See also MINERAL WATER.

Semivegetarians: Vegetarians who shun red meat but may occasionally eat fish and fowl. They are also known as **white vegetarians** (because the meats they do eat are white) and **quasi-** or **partial vegetarians.**

Semolina: The golden heart of durum wheat, an exceptionally hard, high-protein wheat. Semolina grains, sometimes called **Moroccan pasta,** boil up nice and fluffy and make a welcome change of pace from rice or potatoes. Good Italian cooks lighten their gnocchi by mixing in some semolina; they even make a marvelous semolina flour cake. See also COUSCOUS.

NUTRIENT CONTENT OF ½ CUP SEMOLINA FLOUR
(about 3 ounces; 84 grams)

301 calories	1 mg sodium
11 g protein	156 mg potassium
1 g fat, 0 saturated	2 g dietary fiber
0 mg cholesterol	0 RE vitamin A
61 g carbohydrate	0.68 mg thiamin
14 mg calcium	0.48 mg riboflavin
114 mg phosphorus	5.0 mg niacin
3.6 mg iron	0 mg vitamin C

Senior Citizens: See ELDERLY PERSONS; also AGING.

Serine: One of the nonessential AMINO ACIDS.

Serotonin: A neurotransmitter (chemical messenger) manufactured by brain nerve cells that makes you sleepy, lessens pain and decreases appetite. Its production, like so many body processes, involves a delicate chain reaction. Eating carbohydrates stimulates insulin secretion, which causes amino acids circulating in the blood to be deposited in muscle tissue. All amino acids, that is, except TRYPTOPHAN. This one amino acid is ferried to the brain, where it triggers the manufacture of serotonin. Of particular interest to biochemical researchers is the role serotonin may play in eating disorders, particularly bulimia. Two recent studies (one at the University of Pittsburgh School of Medicine; one at Massachusetts General Hospital in Boston) suggest that low levels of serotonin trigger eating binges. Research continues.

Serranos: See HOT PEPPERS under PEPPERS, CAPSICUMS.

Serving Size: In our athletic, pioneering past, men, women and children ate as if there were no tomorrow. Often there wasn't. But the reason they scarfed down such huge quantities of food was that they needed energy to clear land, build houses, do the daily chores, many of which amounted to hard labor. With machines taking the drudge out of drudgery, our lives have become softer, more sedentary, and there's no reason to chow down as our ancestors did. Most nutritionists now agree that the following constitute adequate portion sizes for healthy persons: 2 to 3 ounces meat, fish or poultry; ½ cup fruits and vegetables; 8 ounces milk; 1 slice bread or 1 ounce cereal. The *number* of portions will depend on age, sex and lifestyle—whether you're a jock or a couch potato. Thus a healthful meal will consist of a variety of portions or servings that meet the daily requirements for protein, fat, carbohydrate, essential vitamins and minerals. See also FOOD GUIDE PYRAMID.

Sesame Oil: Sesame seeds are about 50 percent oil, a fact not lost on the Chinese and East Indians who have been cooking with sesame oil for centuries. Top-quality sesame oil is cold pressed, as pale as straw and very nearly tasteless. Asians favor oil made from pressed **roasted** or **toasted** sesame seeds because of its warm brown hue and rich, nutty flavor. Often it is too strong and its smoke point too low to use solo, so Asian cooks team it with a blander, more heat-stable vegetable oil. Then there's **chile** or **red pepper oil,** a fiery red sesame oil in which chile peppers have been steeped (proceed at your own risk). Like other oils, sesame oil is all fat (in this case, 40 percent each mono- and polyunsaturated fatty acids, 18 percent saturated and 2 percent other); 1 tablespoon sesame oil equals 120 calories.

Sesame Paste: See TAHINI.

Sesame Seeds: The small, flat, pearly seeds of an annual herb native to Asia but now an important crop in tropical regions of Africa, Mexico and Latin America. For a time, sesame seeds were also grown in the South Carolina/Georgia low country, first by the slaves who brought them from Africa and called them **benne** and later by their masters. To this day, benne wafers, cookies and candies are low country specialties. Elsewhere, sesame seeds are more likely to be sprinkled onto rolls, flat breads and bread sticks. Or

NUTRIENT CONTENT OF 1 OUNCE (28 GRAMS) SESAME SEEDS	
167 calories	11 mg sodium
7 g protein	115 mg potassium
16 g fat, 2 saturated	2 g dietary fiber
0 mg cholesterol	2 RE vitamin A
3 g carbohydrate	0.20 mg thiamin
37 mg calcium	0.02 mg riboflavin
220 mg phosphorus	1.3 mg niacin
2.2 mg iron	0 mg vitamin C

to be ground to paste or pressed into oil. **NOTE:** Raw sesame seeds have a slightly bitter green-peanut taste. To bring out their nutlike mellowness, spread in a pie pan and toast 5 to 10 minutes in a 350°F. oven—or just until pale tan. Overbrowning will make sesame seeds bitter. See also SESAME OIL; TAHINI.

Set Point: A controversial theory that maintains that people are genetically programmed to be a certain weight in adulthood. Studies with prisoners show that when those of normal weight were put on high-calorie diets to induce obesity, they returned to their original weights—their set points—once the tests were over. For much the same reason, researchers believe, "fatties" who lose significant amounts of weight usually regain the lost pounds when they abandon their diets. A new study conducted by Rockefeller University researchers seems to corroborate the set-point theory. Their subjects gravitated toward given weights, weights that they seemed genetically (or otherwise) programmed to maintain. Subjects who lost weight were found to have slowed metabolisms, encouraging them to regain the lost pounds. And those who gained weight exhibited revved-up metabolisms, the better to trim the excess baggage and return to their set points. Can set points be changed? Researchers say yes, that regular exercise can lower them. They believe, too, that set points rise as you grow older and/or heavier. But that around the age of sixty-five or seventy they may lower, explaining why some older people begin to lose weight. See also OBESITY, OVERWEIGHT; OB-GENE; and LEPTIN.

Seviche: Chunks of raw fish or shellfish that are said to be "cooked" by the lime juice or vinegar in which they marinate. Both lime juice and vinegar are acidic and they will firm the fish and turn it opaque. But in no way do they *cook* fish or shellfish. For that you need heat. Thus the risks of eating seviche are the same as for eating any raw fish: the chance of being infected by PARASITES and/or BACTERIA.

Sevruga: See CAVIAR.

Shad: Although shad do exist in Europe, they're no match for the American shad. It is plump, firm of flesh and as rich as herring, the family to which it belongs. Like salmon, shad ascend great rivers in spring to spawn; only the shad streams all lie along the Atlantic. There's a saying along the James in Tidewater Virginia that "shad run when the shadbush blooms." That's early spring. But there are December runs in the St. Johns River of north Florida, usually right around Christmas. It's possible to clock spring's northward march by following the shad runs—from Georgia's Ogeechee to Virginia's James to New York's Hudson to Canada's St. Lawrence. Although Native Americans have always prized shad, grilling or baking it on slabs of bark before open fires, the New England colonists thought little of it. Perhaps because of its frightening number of needle-sharp bones (people joke that only a surgeon can bone a shad). No one has yet improved on the Native American method of cooking shad although hickory planks have replaced slabs of bark. The best planking size for shad: 3 to 5 pounds.

NUTRIENT CONTENT OF 3 OUNCES (85 GRAMS) BAKED/GRILLED SHAD (BONED, SKINNED)	
214 calories	55 mg sodium
18 g protein	418 mg potassium
15 g fat, 4 saturated	0 g dietary fiber
82 mg cholesterol	31 RE vitamin A
0 g carbohydrate	0.16 mg thiamin
51 mg calcium	0.26 mg riboflavin
297 mg phosphorus	9.2 mg niacin
1.1 mg iron	0 mg vitamin C

Shaddocks: See PUMMELOS.

Shad Roe: See FISH ROE.

Shallots: See ONIONS.

Shark Cartilage: The buzz is that sharks don't get cancer and that taking shark cartilage supplements will keep you cancer free, too (in addition to easing the pain and stiffness of injury or inflamed joints). The truth? Sharks do get cancer. Even cancer of the cartilage. Indeed, there's no reliable evidence that shark cartilage performs any of the miracles attributed to it.

Sheepshead: A type of porgy. See PORGIES.

Shellfish: They fall into two categories: **crustaceans** or legged creatures (CRABS, CRAYFISH, LOBSTER, SHRIMP) and **mollusks** (CLAMS, MUSSELS, OYSTERS, SCALLOPS, plus OCTOPUS and SQUID). All are lean or moderately lean and mineral rich.

Sherbet: Milk-based frozen-fruit desserts of exceptionally fine grain. Commercial sherbets usually contain stabilizers of some sort to keep them creamy, and for calorie counters, many of them are artificially sweetened. Although the sherbets most familiar to us are fruit flavored, some of America's innovative young chefs are now serving savory sherbets as between-courses palate clearers—tomato, Champagne, fresh basil or rosemary. Some chefs are also dreaming up new ice creamlike flavors—caramel, cappuccino, espresso, even chocolate. See also ICE MILK.

NUTRIENT CONTENT OF 1 CUP ORANGE SHERBET (about 6¾ ounces; 192 grams)	
264 calories	88 mg sodium
2 g protein	184 mg potassium
4 g fat, 2 saturated	0 g dietary fiber
10 mg cholesterol	39 RE vitamin A
58 g carbohydrate	0.05 mg thiamin
104 mg calcium	0.13 mg riboflavin
77 mg phosphorus	0.2 mg niacin
0.3 mg iron	4 mg vitamin C

Sherry: A fortified wine produced in and around Jerez, Spain. See WINES; also ALCOHOL, ALCOHOLIC BEVERAGES.

Shigella, Shigellosis: See BACTERIA.

Shiitake: See MUSHROOMS.

Shortening: See VEGETABLE SHORTENING.

Shrimp: Of all the species of shellfish, shrimp are the best known, best loved, most available and most versatile. They abound in coastal waters surrounding much of the United States, but the bulk of them—not to mention the finest—come from the warm waters of the Gulf of Mexico. The choicest are the **Gulf white;** second best, the **pink;** third, the **brown,** which tend to taste of iodine. In addition to these three domestics, there are three imports that often find their way into American fish markets: **black tigers,** farmed in Asia; another farm-raised Asian shrimp called **Chinese white;** and, most abundant of all, the **Ecuadorean** or **Mexican white,** which may be wild or farmed. Both the Gulf white and pink are now being farmed on a broad scale, too, mostly in Louisiana. These are plump, sweet-meated shrimp, sometimes such jumbos that you get only fifteen to the pound.

Cold-water shrimp, on the other hand (notably those from the Pacific Northwest and Baltic), are truly "shrimps," so tiny that it may take two hundred of them to make a pound. Far more popular, more common and more reasonably priced are the average-size, all-purpose shrimp that number between twenty and forty to the pound. And what about **prawns** (*scampi,* to give them their Italian name)? These are another species altogether, a European relative not often seen in the United States beyond posh restaurants and fancy fish markets. What are usually pawned off here as prawns are nothing more than jumbo shrimp.

It's best to buy shrimp in the shell and to shuck them yourself. Like other shellfish, shrimp are extremely perishable and should be cooked and served within two days of purchase. Frozen shrimp, even frozen cooked shrimp, are widely available. But these are poor substitutes for the fresh. Shrimp are low in fat and calories, yet good sources of iron, potassium and niacin. Alas, they are also high in sodium and cholesterol (although doctors now believe that the cholesterol in food affects cholesterol blood levels less than do saturated fats).

NUTRIENT CONTENT OF 3 OUNCES (85 GRAMS) STEAMED SHRIMP (SHELLED)	
84 calories	191 mg sodium
18 g protein	155 mg potassium
1 g fat, 0 saturated	0 g dietary fiber
166 mg cholesterol	56 RE vitamin A
0 g carbohydrate	0.03 mg thiamin
33 mg calcium	0.03 mg riboflavin
117 mg phosphorus	2.2 mg niacin
2.6 mg iron	2 mg vitamin C

Sieving, Straining: These methods filter out fiber but affect nutritive values in no way other than that they may accelerate vitamin C loss (the more food is cut, pureed or mashed, the faster vitamin C oxidizes). Those with delicate stomachs or gastrointestinal problems must sometimes eat pureed foods until their digestive problems are corrected. And of course babies graduate to purees before moving up to solid food.

Silica Gel (additive): An anticaking agent used in confectioners' sugar. GRAS.

Silicon: This ubiquitous nonmetallic element, known to be necessary to animals, has only recently been added to the list of trace elements possibly needed by the body. Its particular functions are to aid in the synthesis of healthy collagen (connective tissue) and the development of strong, calcium-rich bones. Silicon exists in blood plasma but its concentrations are greatest in the skin and connective tissue. Some researchers believe that silicon reduces the risk of atherosclerosis and may in some way also retard aging and help prevent or lessen arthritis and osteoporosis. Silicates (silicon salts) are present in much of our drinking water. Silicon is also present in good measure in beer, chicken skin, whole grains and root vegetables. Silicon research continues.

Silicon Dioxide (additive): This compound occurs naturally in 95 percent of the earth's crust—quartz, flint, even such gems as amethyst and agate. Crushed to a clear, flavorless, insoluble powder, silicon dioxide is indispensable to food and beverage manufacturers. Brewers use it to defoam beers and ales; food processors as an anticaking agent for salts and salt substitutes. Silicon dioxide is also an ingredient in some scouring powders. GRAS.

Silicone Coatings: The FDA presently gives these release agents (resinous and polymeric coatings) a clean bill of health. They're used in the manufacture of nonstick parchments and to date have shown no toxicity, no tendency to migrate into food.

Silverstone: The trade name of a new generation of plastic baked on pots and pans to give them a slick, nonstick surface. Silverstone is tougher and longer lasting than some of the earlier plastic coatings; still, it is not indestructible. See also TEFLON.

Simmering: Another word for POACHING.

Simplesse: The people who brought us ASPARTAME (NutraSweet or Equal) have now buzzed up a promising low-calorie "fake fat" out of egg and/or milk protein. For specifics, see FAT SUBSTITUTES.

Simple Sugar: A MONOSACCHARIDE and one of the three basic groups of CARBOHYDRATES. Blood sugar (GLUCOSE), the one that fuels our bodies, is a simple sugar. So are FRUCTOSE and GALACTOSE.

Sippy Diet: A high milk-and-cream diet that was once the classic treatment for gastric ulcers. Stage two of the Sippy Diet (after days of hourly doses of milk and cream) was a bland regimen from which all fresh fruits and vegetables, whole grains and spicy foods were banned. It consisted of six small meals a day plus many glasses of milk. Startingly high in saturated fat and cholesterol, the Sippy Diet has long since been abandoned in favor of more wholesome, more effective treatments. See also PEPTIC ULCERS.

Sirloin: "The King of Steaks," "the King of Roasts," both of which are cut from the sirloin, the chunky cut separating the loin and rump of a steer. Sirloin owes its tenderness to the fact that it comes from a little-exercised part of the animal (it corresponds to our waist). Its succulence, however, is due to the high proportion of fat to lean. For per-serving nutrient counts, see BEEF.

Skate, Ray: Only the wings of the skate are eaten. In Europe they rate as a great delicacy, particularly when sautéed in brown butter. In the United States, however, they are rarely seen beyond sophisticated big-city restaurants. Still, many Americans have unknowingly eaten skate. In years past, unscrupulous fish markets counterfeited sea scallops out of skate wings; their textures and flavors are so similar no one was the wiser.

Skim Milk: See MILK.

Skimming: An effective way to defat stocks, soups, sauces and gravies. Time permitting, chill the liquids until the layer of fat hardens, then lift it right off. When dealing with hot liquids, spoon off as much fat as possible, then blot up any recalcitrant bits with paper toweling. Skimming reduces not only the amount of fat in a recipe but also the calories and cholesterol.

Skin: Skin texture and color reflect both health and nutritional state. Pallor, for example, suggests anemia (which may or may not be brought on by a lack of iron, vitamin B_{12} and folic acid). Yellowness, on the other hand, signals jaundice (or perhaps overdoing the beta-carotene). Frequent bruises indicate a vitamin C deficiency; horny plugs or growths about the hair follicles may mean a lack of vitamin A. Major dermatitis accompanies pellagra, a disease caused by an acute niacin deficiency. Of course, any number of food sensitivities and allergies are manifested in skin rashes, which only a skilled allergist can identify.

Skinfold Tests: Because 50 percent of the body's fat is believed to lie directly under the skin, skinfold or "pinch" tests are used as a quick way to determine total body fat. Using special calipers, technicians measure the thickness of the fat layers over the biceps (called the **biceps skinfold measurement**); over the triceps, the muscle at the back of the upper arm (called the **triceps skinfold measurement**); below the scapula (just under the "wings" of the back); on the upper thigh and elsewhere. The most accurate skinfold measurements are the triceps and subscapular, although even these become less reliable in the grossly obese.

Slow Cookers: When these first appeared in the 1970s, everyone had to have one. Imagine loading in all the makings of a stew first thing in the morning, then coming home after work to find it perfectly cooked. Pretty terrific. Although they've lost some ground to newer gadgets (microwaves and convection ovens), slow cookers remain popular. The newest models boast high and low heat settings and offer greater versatility than their predecessors.

NUTRIENT CONTENT OF 3 OUNCES (85 GRAMS) BROILED/GRILLED SKATE

100 calories	89 mg sodium
21 g protein	293 mg potassium
1 g fat, 0 saturated	0 g dietary fiber
58 mg cholesterol	9 RE vitamin A
0 g carbohydrate	0.07 mg thiamin
15 mg calcium	0.09 mg riboflavin
246 mg phosphorus	1.9 mg niacin
0.3 mg iron	0 mg vitamin C

Still, they aren't without risk. First, many people balk at the thought of leaving an electric appliance *on* all day in an empty house. Chances are slim, but a slow cooker could malfunction and start a fire. A more real concern is the danger of food poisoning. Leaving perishables to languish at low temperatures for hours does shoot the bacterial count up. Here's a bacteriologist's recommendation: Make sure that all food inside a slow cooker reaches a uniform temperature of 125°F. within three hours, that it climbs to 140°F. within four and that it remains at a constant 145°F. for at least one hour—the time and temperature needed to kill harmful microorganisms. Toward that end, thaw all frozen foods before they go into the slow cooker and keep other perishables in the fridge. Finally, don't overload the cooker. If you do, you'll increase, maybe even double the time foods stay in the "bacterial danger zone." And what about nutrient loss? Anytime food cooks long and slow in substantial amounts of liquid, some of the heat-sensitive, water-soluble vitamins (mostly the Bs and C) will be sacrificed.

Small Intestine: See INTESTINE, SMALL.

"Smart Drugs," "Smart Drinks": They're supposed to boost energy, improve memory and satisfy the appetite, but do they? And what *are* they? One of them is PHENYLALANINE, an amino acid, one of the constituents, in fact, of the artificial sweetener ASPARTAME. MIT researchers once believed that phenylalanine increased the brain's output of norepinephrine. It now appears that it actually depresses production of this adrenalinelike hormone. Researchers are now focusing on choline, one of the B vitamins, which seems to sharpen memory (the body converts it to acetylcholine, a neurotransmitter that is indeed involved with memory). Lecithin contains choline, which is why many health-food stores hype it as a way "to increase brain function." To date, however, there's no reliable evidence that lecithin—or for that matter, any of the other so-called smart drugs or drinks—increase brain function in either normal persons or those afflicted with Alzheimer's disease.

Smelt: A family of small, silvery, oily fish that swim nearly all the world's seas. Like salmon, they swim upstream to spawn and like them, too, they may be landlocked in lakes. Among the most popular smelts are the widely distributed **rainbow,** the Pacific **whitebait,** the **surf smelt** and Co-

lumbia River **eulachon** (called **candlefish** by Native Americans because, when dried, these oily fish could be burned like candles). Despite their oiliness, smelts are delicate, their flavor as clean as a cucumber's. Because of their small size (6 to 8 inches is average), smelts fare best fried or crisply deep-fat fried. Smelts are high in potassium and phosphorus and also contain enough riboflavin and niacin to matter.

NUTRIENT CONTENT OF 3 OUNCES (85 GRAMS) BAKED/BROILED SMELT	
105 calories	66 mg sodium
19 g protein	317 mg potassium
3 g fat, 0 saturated	0 g dietary fiber
77 mg cholesterol	25 RE vitamin A
0 g carbohydrate	0.05 mg thiamin
66 mg calcium	0.18 mg riboflavin
251 mg phosphorus	1.8 mg niacin
1.0 mg iron	0 mg vitamin C

Smoke Point: All fats will smoke when overheated, but some fats can take considerably more heat than others. Smoke points are rarely reached when foods are sautéed, but they often are during deep-fat frying. When fats begin to smoke, they also begin to decompose, emitting noxious fumes of ACROLEIN. The highest temperature needed for deep-fat frying is in the 390°F.–400°F. range; still, it's important that the fat's smoke point be at least 20°F. higher. As a general rule, vegetable oils have the highest smoke points (except for olive oil and Asian roasted sesame oil),

Oil or Fat	Smoke Point
Vegetable oils (except olive oil and Asian roasted sesame oil)	441°F.–450°F.
Vegetable/animal shortening blends (without emulsifiers)	448°F.
Lard	361°F.–401°F.
Vegetable shortenings (with emulsifiers)	356°F.–370°F.
Vegetable/animal shortening blends (with emulsifiers)	351°F.–363°F.

Note: The more deep-frying fats and oils are recycled, the lower their smoke points become. Butter and margarine smoke at temperatures well below those needed for deep-fat frying.

then come vegetable shortenings without emulsifiers. The table below opposite shows how well the various deep-frying fats and oils take the heat.

Smoking (in preserving and flavoring food):
Before freezing, before canning, there was smoking. For centuries smoking has been used to preserve meats and fish. Successfully. Here's why: Smoking dries and heats food; both processes discourage microbial growth. Then, too, many of the compounds present in smoke are bactericidal. Unfortunately, some of these are also powerful carcinogens, notably **polycyclic aromatic hydrocarbons** (see PAHs). Some sixteen different PAHs have been found in smoked foods, the most dangerous of which is benzopyrene. Smoked foods also contain **formaldehyde,** which is not only carcinogenic but also makes certain amino acids less available to the body. Does smoking also affect **vitamin content**? Unfortunately, yes. In meats that have first been cured, then smoked, as much as 20 percent of the thiamin (B_1) may be sacrificed together with smaller amounts of riboflavin and niacin. However, the only smoked fish that appears to be similarly affected is salmon.

When it comes to smoking pork, there's the added danger of **trichinosis,** a serious, sometimes fatal disease caused by microscopic parasites occasionally present in raw pork. If the smoked pork is of the cook-before-eating type, federal meat-inspection laws mandate that the internal temperature of the pork must reach 125°F. during the smoking process. For ready-to-eat smoked pork, the internal temperature must be even higher—140°F. or more—because only then will the trichinae be destroyed. Eaten with moderation, smoked foods should present no problems. But they should never become a steady diet. According to more than one study, people eating large amounts of smoked fish suffer high rates of gastrointestinal cancer, as do those who work in smokehouses.

Smoking (of tobacco): See CIGARETTE SMOKING.

Snacks:
Any small between-meals bites qualify as snacks. And very nutritious some of them are—carrots, apples, oranges, a wedge of cabbage, a handful of prunes or salt-free pretzels, a bowl of fresh berries drifted with low-fat yogurt, a couple of graham crackers plus a glass of skim milk, a slice of whole-grain bread thinly spread with peanut butter, even air-popped corn. The trouble is, these are not the snacks most Americans dote upon. Too many of us prefer to junk out on the calorie-, fat-, and sugar- or salt-laden munchies that fill supermarket aisles. We love cheese puffs, tortilla and potato chips, coconut oil-drenched popcorn, doughnuts, muffins and Danish, not to mention a huge variety of cakes, coffeecakes, cookies and candies. Don't be fooled by the new nonfat cakes and cookies (they're plenty caloric). Or by fruit-juice-sweetened cookies (when juices are reduced to syrup, what's left is sugar). Unless children are taught young to appreciate wholesome snacks, they will probably opt for junk. And once they develop an appetite for these highly refined, nonnutritious snacks, they're unlikely to settle for something more nutritious but, in their view, "less delicious."

Snails, Escargots:
From the Romans onward, snails have been eaten with great relish, especially in France, where the classic treatment is to slosh them in garlic butter. Few Americans have acquired a taste for snails, perhaps because they are rarely available here—except in the can. They are very low in fat, low in calories, too—just as well since most people like their snails swimming in garlic butter.

NUTRIENT CONTENT OF 3 OUNCES (85 GRAMS) STEAMED/POACHED SNAILS

153 calories	101 mg sodium
28 g protein	455 mg potassium
2 g fat, 1 saturated	0 g dietary fiber
85 mg cholesterol	46 RE vitamin A
3 g carbohydrate	0.02 mg thiamin
16 mg calcium	0.15 mg riboflavin
324 mg phosphorus	1.8 mg niacin
5.4 mg iron	0 mg vitamin C

Snap Beans: See BEANS, FRESH.

Snow Peas: See PEAS.

Soda, Baking:
Sodium bicarbonate, to give its chemical name. Teamed with an acid food (buttermilk or molasses, for example), it fizzes and foams, releasing carbon dioxide gas, a powerful leavening. See LEAVENING AGENTS.

Soda Crackers:
Also called **common crackers,** these thin, pale wafers, popular since the mid-eighteenth century, are made of stiff yeast doughs neutralized with baking

soda. Commercial bakers roll the dough tissue thin, fold it back on itself, roll again and prick at regular intervals to control surface blistering. Many years ago when Nabisco sprinkled its soda crackers with coarse salt, it called them **saltines**. Today soda crackers are available with or without buttery finishes, with or without sprinklings of salt.

NUTRIENT CONTENT OF 4 SODA CRACKERS (SALTINES)
(about ½ ounce; 12 grams)

52 calories	156 mg sodium
1 g protein	15 mg potassium
1 g fat, 0 saturated	0 g dietary fiber
0 mg cholesterol	0 RE vitamin A
9 g carbohydrate	0.07 mg thiamin
14 mg calcium	0.06 mg riboflavin
13 mg phosphorus	0.6 mg niacin
0.6 mg iron	0 mg vitamin C

Soda Water: See SELTZER.

Sodium: Sodium catches so much flak few of us realize that without it we would die. In a sort of yin-yang relationship with potassium, it regulates fluid balance in our bodies by controlling the flow of liquids in and out of individual cells. Classified as an electrolyte, sodium is also integral to the sparking of nerve impulses, the metabolism of proteins and carbohydrates, the maintenance of the body's acid/alkali balance. Major tasks, all. Yet conventional wisdom tells us to "hold the salt" lest our blood pressure soar. Biomedical researchers believe that this happens mainly in sodium-sensitive persons, that healthy individuals with normal BLOOD PRESSSURES (120/80) are unlikely to become hypertensive if they don't cut down on salt.

Still, those who have high blood pressure (and fifty million Americans do), even those with marginally high blood pressure (140/90), should curb their sodium intake. That means putting the salt shaker away (both at stove and table) and scrutinizing food labels for additives containing sodium as well as for salt (sodium chloride). It also means choosing reduced- or low-sodium canned foods and passing on most cured meats and cheeses, all of which brim with sodium. Finally, it may mean using one of the many SALT SUBSTITUTES.

Although there are no RDAs for sodium, the Committee on Dietary Allowances of the National Academy of Sciences (NAS) has established the Estimated Minimum Requirement at 500 milligrams per day. Further, the NAS's Committee on Diet and Health, in its 1989 report, recommended limiting the daily intake of salt to 6 grams (2,400 milligrams sodium), including that in prepared foods. Table salt is 39 percent sodium and 1 teaspoon of it contains about 2,000 milligrams sodium. Though instances are rare, it is possible to be deficient in sodium. The likeliest candidates? Marathoners, who lose a load of sodium as they sweat, and habitual users of laxatives and/or diuretics. See also "SALT-FREE."

Sodium Acetate (additive): A flavoring and pH controller used in hard candies, breakfast cereals, jams and jellies, plus a huge array of processed meats, soups, sauces and snacks. GRAS when used within FDA guidelines.

Sodium Acid Pyrophosphate (SAP) (additive): A buffer and slow-acting leavener used in a variety of cake, bread and muffin mixes and in self-rising flours, as well as in many commercial baked goods. SAP is also added to franks and cold cuts to heighten and accelerate the development of their rosy color. GRAS.

Sodium Acid Sulfate (additive): An acidifier and a preservative used in dried fruits and bottled lemon juice, also on fresh fruits and vegetables that are to be processed. GRAS; however, sodium acid sulfate may not be used on foods high in thiamin (vitamin B_1), on fruits and vegetables to be sold or served raw or, for that matter, on fruits or vegetables labeled "fresh."

Sodium Alginate (additive): A mucilaginous kelp derivative used as an emulsifier/stabilizer in frozen desserts, baked goods, aerosol whipped cream, cheese dips and spreads. GRAS when used within FDA guidelines.

Sodium Aluminum Phosphate (additive): A leavening added to self-rising flour, cake, muffin and pancake mixes. GRAS when used within FDA guidelines.

Sodium Aluminum Sulfate (SAS) (additive): The principal ingredient of double-acting baking powders, SAS is also used to bleach flours. Not known to be toxic.

Sodium Ascorbate (additive): With all the hysteria about nitrates and nitrites, meat packers began using this form of vitamin C, a powerful antioxidant and preservative, as a way to cut down on the nitrates they added to hams, bacons, hot dogs, corned beef and cold cuts. Sodium ascorbate is also the vitamin C component of many vitamin supplements. GRAS.

Sodium Benzoate (additive): This preservative/antimicrobial is widely used in margarines, soft drinks, bottled fruit juices, pickles, preserves, jams and jellies, mincemeats, maraschino cherries and toothpastes. GRAS when used within FDA guidelines.

Sodium Bicarbonate: Baking soda. See SODA, BAKING; also LEAVENING AGENTS.

Sodium Bisulfite (additive): See SULFITES.

Sodium Carbonate (additive): An alkaline antioxidant and flavoring used in everything from hog butchering to the manufacture of margarines, baked goods, gelatin desserts and assorted instants (puddings, soups and sauces). GRAS when used within FDA guidelines.

Sodium Carboxymethyl Cellulose (additive): A binder/stabilizer/thickener/extender used in commercial pies and poultry products. GRAS when used within FDA guidelines.

Sodium Caseinate (additive): A multitalented binder/stabilizer/texturizer/extender/clarifier used in a long list of processed foods: breads, cereals, cheese products, vegetable sausages, cold cuts, soups and stews, aerosol whipped cream, even wines. GRAS when used within FDA guidelines.

Sodium Chloride (additive): Table SALT. GRAS when used within FDA guidelines.

Sodium Citrate (additive): An acidifier/emulsifier used in commercial ice creams, processed cheeses, evaporated milks, carbonated drinks, frozen fruit-drink concentrates, candies, jams and jellies. GRAS.

Sodium Cyclamate (additive): A nonnutritive, artificial sweetener banned by the FDA in 1969 after it was found to cause cancer in laboratory animals.

Sodium Erythorbate (additive): A salt of ERYTHORBIC ACID, this antioxidant and preservative is widely used in processing meats and poultry, also in the manufacture of soft drinks. GRAS when used within FDA guidelines.

Sodium Fluoride (additive): One of the chemicals used to fluoridate water. Although sodium fluoride can be added to drinking water, the FDA no longer allows its use in food. Its use as a treatment for osteoporosis remains highly controversial.

Sodium Hydroxide (additive): Caustic soda or lye. This strong alkali is added to the water used to scald hogs at butchering time. But that's not all. It's integral to the processing of black olives, lard and tallow, margarines, meat and poultry products containing phosphates. GRAS when used within FDA guidelines.

Sodium Iodide (additive): One of the two most frequently used chemicals to iodize salt. The other is potassium iodide. A third, less used, is cuprous iodide.

Sodium Metabisulfite (additive): See SULFITES.

Sodium Nitrate, Sodium Nitrite (additives): See NITRATES, NITRITES.

Sodium Phosphate (additive): See PHOSPHATES.

Sodium Propionate (additive): A mold inhibitor widely used in commercial breads, cakes, coffee cakes and cookies, also in cheese products, frozen or refrigerated doughs (including heat-and-eat pizzas), fillings, frostings, gelatins, jams and jellies, processed meats, pudding and pie fillings. GRAS when used within FDA guidelines.

Sodium Silico Aluminate (additive): An anticaking agent added to powdered egg yolks, salt and some sugars. Not known to be toxic.

Sodium Sorbate (additive): This preservative is used in a variety of baked goods, cheeses and margarines. GRAS when used within FDA guidelines.

Sodium Stearyl Fumarate, Sodium Stearoyl Lactylate (additives): Compounds used by commercial bakers to condition dough. These two additives are also used as whipping agents for nondairy toppings and powdered eggs. Use regulated by the FDA.

Sodium Sulfite (additive): See SULFITES.

Sodium Tripolyphosphate (additive): A versatile chemical. It's added to processed meats and bakery meringues to minimize juice loss. Food companies also find it a valuable texturizer for a variety of mixes—everything from angel food cake to puddings and gelatins. GRAS when used within FDA guidelines.

Soft Drinks: These bubbly thirst quenchers have been growing in popularity ever since British scientist Joseph Priestley learned how to carbonate water. That was in 1767. In those days sparkling waters were considered medicinal. Indeed, many of them were advertised as cures for this and that right up to the late nineteenth century and the arrival of Coca-Cola, which originally contained both cocaine and caffeine (down South many old-timers still call Cokes dopes; the caffeine remains but the cocaine is long gone).

With huge profits on every can or bottle sold, making soda pop is a multibillion-dollar business. Soft drinks are largely (often 92 percent) water, sweetened either naturally (with corn sugars or syrups) or artificially (with ASPARTAME). In addition to having carbon dioxide gas pumped in to make them bubbly, most soft drinks are further acidified with citric, fumaric, malic, phosphoric or tartaric acid. Their flavors are usually (though not always) synthetic. The same holds for their colorings. Most of the colas contain small amounts of caffeine, which make them poor choices for children.

The main trouble with soft drinks is that they provide little more than empty calories. Children, alas, invariably prefer them to milk, fruit juice or even homemade lemonade or limeade. A steady diet of pop can be harmful. Their sugars and acids can, over time, erode teeth, increasing the risk of decay. More important, soft drinks can dull the appetite so that come mealtime, children have little interest in the nutritious foods put before them.

Solanine: A toxic alkaloid found in high concentrations in the green "sun struck" patches on and just under potato skin and to a lesser degree in the eyes. These should be trimmed away not only because they are bitter but also because the body converts solanine into a poison called solanidine, which has caused spontaneous abortions in lab animals. Pregnant women (also those hoping to become pregnant) should be especially careful about removing all green splotches on potatoes. Indeed, no one should be cavalier about solanine. It has made more than a few people seriously sick and, in rare instances, killed. Can this be why for centuries potatoes were considered poisonous?

Sole: America contains no true sole and must import its supply from Britain or France. The fish passed off on the East Coast as lemon or gray sole and along the Pacific as rex or Petrale sole are all species of FLOUNDER. Sole and flounder *are* related: Both are flatfish and both are lean and white. But, oh, how superior **Dover** or **English sole** is. Firm but tender and as nut-sweet as a Georgia pecan. Many think there is no finer fish, no more versatile fish than the Dover sole. The French twirl it into paupiettes, line molds with it, poach it and sauce it, or sauté it simply in browned butter. Sole are small—plate-size, if you will—and wonderful cooked whole or filleted. For approximate nutrient counts, see FISH, LEAN WHITE.

Soluble Fiber: See FIBER, DIETARY.

Somatotropin, Bovine Growth Hormone: See BOVINE SOMATOTROPIN.

Sorbets: See ICES, GRANITÉS, SORBETS.

Sorbic Acid (additive): A bacteria and mold inhibitor added to dozens of foods and beverages, among them baked goods, cheeses, dried fruits, smoked fish, syrups and salad dressings, soft drinks and wines. GRAS.

Sorbitan Monostearate, SKU700 G, Sorbitan C (additive): An emulsifier. This waxy compound is used as a foaming agent and stabilizer in cake mixes, fillings and frostings; coffee creamers; whipped toppings; and active dry yeast. It is very mildly toxic and the FDA strictly limits its use.

Sorbitol (additive): A sugar substitute (actually it's a sugar alcohol) used in commercially prepared diabetic foods (canned fruits and juices, jams and preserves, chocolates and chewing gums). As a humectant, it helps keep marshmallows and shredded coconut moist and fresh. Sorbitol is only about half as sweet as sugar, and in some people even small amounts of it can cause gas and diarrhea.

Sorghum: A group of Asian and African grains and grasses that grow well in arid areas and nourish millions living below the poverty line. In the United States, sorghums, particularly milo, are grown as livestock fodder. There is an exception—sweet sorghum, which Southerners crush like sugarcane and boil into a dark, thick syrup. Sorghum molasses it's called. **NOTE:** Nutrient counts are unavailable for sorghum molasses, but it's fair to say they would approximate those of molasses.

Sorrel, Sour Grass, Sour Dock: A soft, lemon-flavored green treasured by the French but not much appreciated in the United States. Like rhubarb, to which it is related, sorrel brims with oxalic acid. This accounts for its mouth-puckering astringency and may bind much of the calcium it contains, making it unavailable to the body. Too tart to eat alone, the bright, triangular leaves of sorrel are best mixed about 1:3 or 1:4 with other salad greens and turned in a mellow dressing. Or steamed, in about the same proportion, with spinach (to temper the tartness). Or pureed into *potage germiny*, the classic French sorrel soup. Sorrel is very good, too, mashed with potatoes (2 parts potatoes, 1 part sorrel) or transformed, the British way, into a biting green sauce for meats and poultry. Sorrel is an excellent source of vitamins A and C and a good one of iron and potassium. **NOTE:** Because of the oxalic acid it contains, sorrel should always be cooked in a nonreactive pan—flameproof glass, enameled metal—although stainless steel will do in a pinch. **SEASON:** Year-round because most of the sorrel coming to market is hothouse grown. Homegrown supplies peak in spring and summer.

NUTRIENT CONTENT OF 1 CUP STEAMED SORREL	
(about 3½ ounces; 100 grams)	
20 calories	3 mg sodium
2 g protein	321 mg potassium
1 g fat, 0 saturated	1 g dietary fiber
0 mg cholesterol	347 RE vitamin A
3 g carbohydrate	0.03 mg thiamin
38 mg calcium	0.09 mg riboflavin
52 mg phosphorus	0.4 mg niacin
2.1 mg iron	26 mg vitamin C

Soups: The way to recycle trimmings and leftovers, the way to get a meal on the table fast and, if you choose the soup carefully, the way to put a nutritious meal in a single

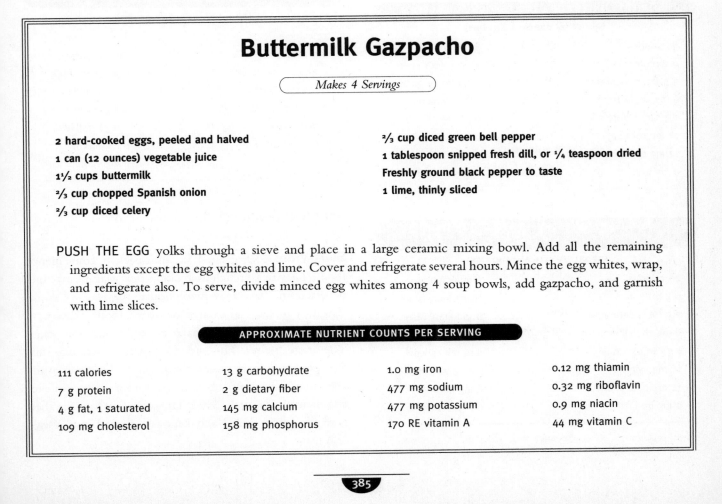

Buttermilk Gazpacho

Makes 4 Servings

2 hard-cooked eggs, peeled and halved
1 can (12 ounces) vegetable juice
1½ cups buttermilk
⅔ cup chopped Spanish onion
⅔ cup diced celery

⅔ cup diced green bell pepper
1 tablespoon snipped fresh dill, or ¼ teaspoon dried
Freshly ground black pepper to taste
1 lime, thinly sliced

PUSH THE EGG yolks through a sieve and place in a large ceramic mixing bowl. Add all the remaining ingredients except the egg whites and lime. Cover and refrigerate several hours. Mince the egg whites, wrap, and refrigerate also. To serve, divide minced egg whites among 4 soup bowls, add gazpacho, and garnish with lime slices.

APPROXIMATE NUTRIENT COUNTS PER SERVING			
111 calories	13 g carbohydrate	1.0 mg iron	0.12 mg thiamin
7 g protein	2 g dietary fiber	477 mg sodium	0.32 mg riboflavin
4 g fat, 1 saturated	145 mg calcium	477 mg potassium	0.9 mg niacin
109 mg cholesterol	158 mg phosphorus	170 RE vitamin A	44 mg vitamin C

bowl. Usually all that's needed to accompany soup is a glass of milk, a slice of whole-grain bread and a piece of fruit for dessert. Homemade soups are best because you can control what goes into them. Commercial soups tend to be glutted with sodium (some of them contain nearly 1,900 milligrams of sodium per 8-ounce cup, nearly the day's suggested total). Some are on fat and calorie overload, too. But big food companies are making every effort to load supermarket shelves with more healthful soups. Look for them, then read labels carefully.

Sour Cream: Light cream soured with lactic-acid-producing bacteria, then homogenized until uniformly smooth and pasteurized. Some **light sour creams** (reduced-fat sour creams) are made with half-and-half; others contain the new fat substitute Simplesse. In either case, light sour cream contains less fat and fewer calories than standard sour cream. **Nonfat sour cream,** an emulsion of skim-milk solids, thickeners and stabilizers, trims the figures even further.

NUTRIENT CONTENT OF 1 TABLESPOON SOUR CREAM
(about ½ ounce; 14 grams)

31 calories	7 mg sodium
0 g protein	21 mg potassium
3 g fat, 2 saturated	0 g dietary fiber
6 mg cholesterol	28 RE vitamin A
1 g carbohydrate	0.01 mg thiamin
17 mg calcium	0.02 mg riboflavin
12 mg phosphorus	0 mg niacin
0 mg iron	0 mg vitamin C

NUTRIENT CONTENT OF 1 TABLESPOON LIGHT SOUR CREAM
(about ½ ounce; 14 grams)

20 calories	6 mg sodium
0 g protein	19 mg potassium
2 g fat, 1 saturated	0 g dietary fiber
6 mg cholesterol	17 RE vitamin A
1 g carbohydrate	0.01 mg thiamin
16 mg calcium	0.02 mg riboflavin
14 mg phosphorus	0 mg niacin
0 mg iron	0 mg vitamin C

NUTRIENT CONTENT OF 1 TABLESPOON NONFAT SOUR CREAM
(about ½ ounce; 14 grams)

9 calories	10 mg sodium
1 g protein	NA mg potassium
0 g fat, 0 saturated	0 g dietary fiber
0 mg cholesterol	20 RE vitamin A
2 g carbohydrate	NA mg thiamin
0 mg calcium	0.03 mg riboflavin
0 mg phosphorus	NA mg niacin
NA mg iron	0 mg vitamin C

Sour Cream Substitutes: Smooth, snowy blends of corn or soybean oil and skim-milk solids plus assorted emulsifiers and stabilizers. These "sour creams" are cholesterol free and average 1 gram of saturated fat and 15 calories per tablespoon. Some are also low in sodium. Study labels.

NUTRIENT CONTENT OF 1 TABLESPOON SOUR CREAM SUBSTITUTE
(about ¼ ounce; 7 grams)

15 calories	7 mg sodium
0 g protein	12 mg potassium
2 g fat, 1 saturated	0 g dietary fiber
0 mg cholesterol	0 RE vitamin A
0 g carbohydrate	0 mg thiamin
0 mg calcium	0 mg riboflavin
3 mg phosphorus	0 mg niacin
0 mg iron	0 mg vitamin C

Sour Salt (additive): See CITRIC ACID.

Sous-Vide: Refrigerated vacuum-packed convenience foods. They're a French innovation (*sous-vide* means "under vacuum") that may revolutionize the way we cook. As quick to serve as canned or frozen foods, these new generation heat-and-eats have an additional advantage. They taste fresher. The *sous-vide* process works like this: Recipes are prepared using the freshest ingredients available, they're put into air- and waterproof plastic pouches and then all air is sucked out. The packets of food are then cooked, quick chilled and kept refrigerated until mealtime. All you have to do is open and eat (if the food is to be served cold) or heat the pouch in boiling water. Although *sous-vide* foods are available to the home cook, restaurant chefs are the ones who've been using them to best advantage and to the hilt. Are they safe? FDA scientists caution that the plastic pouches provide perfect breeding grounds for bacteria that thrive in the absence of air (anaerobes). In particular, they worry about three bugs that can kill—*Clostridium botulinum* (the culprit in botulism), *Listeria monocytogenes* and *Yersinia enterocolitica,* which give no clue to their presence. Still, the FDA admits that if *sous-vide* foods are kept properly refrigerated, there should be no problems. Indeed, there have been none in Europe. Meanwhile, U.S. scientists are researching techniques to make *sous-vide* foods fail-safe, ways to show food handlers and consumers at a glance—or a sniff—whether a packet has spoiled. See also BACTERIA.

Soybean Curd: See TOFU.

Soybean Oil: A pale, bland oil high in unsaturated fats. Soybean oil is a good, all-purpose cooking oil, as Asians have long known and as Americans are now discovering (60 percent of the vegetable oil now used in the United States is soybean oil). In addition to being bottled and sold as is, quantities of soybean oil are blended with other vegetable oils or used in the manufacture of margarines and shortenings. Only 15 percent of the fatty acids in soybean oil are saturated, 24 percent are monounsaturated and the rest polyunsaturated. Because of its high smoke point (441°F.–450°F.), soybean oil is a good choice for deep-fat frying. Like all oils, soybean oil contains 14 grams fat and 120 calories per tablespoon. For a table showing how the fatty acid content of soybean oil compares with that of other fats, see OILS.

Soybeans: One of earth's oldest crops and undeniably one of the most valuable. These high-protein legumes are native to Southeast Asia, where more than a thousand different varieties are grown. The seeds (beans) are the richest plant food known to man, and when teamed in one form or another with rice, as they are throughout Asia, they have sustained millions of people for thousands of years. Early Chinese documents have awarded soybeans a place of honor as one of the "five ancient grains." No part of the soybean plant is ever wasted. The leaves and stems generally become fodder; the sprouts are eaten fresh. The fresh beans may be boiled and eaten, or pressed into cooking oils, or pureed, soaked and cooked down to "milk," which is in turn curded into TOFU. Fresh soybeans are also fermented into soy sauce and TEMPE. Or they may be dried and ground into a high-protein flour. Finally, soybeans are the principal ingredient in TEXTURED VEGETABLE PROTEINS now being used here in meatless burgers and sausages, among other things. See other SOY entries; also PHYTOESTROGENS.

NUTRIENT CONTENT OF 1 CUP COOKED FRESH SOYBEANS
(about 6½ ounces; 180 grams)

254 calories	25 mg sodium
22 g protein	970 mg potassium
12 g fat, 1 saturated	4 g dietary fiber
0 mg cholesterol	29 RE vitamin A
20 g carbohydrate	0.47 mg thiamin
262 mg calcium	0.28 mg riboflavin
284 mg phosphorus	2.3 mg niacin
4.5 mg iron	31 mg vitamin C

Soybean Sprouts: See BEAN SPROUTS.

Soy Flour: A high-protein, low-carbohydrate flour milled from dried soybeans that may or may not have been defatted. There are three types of soy flour: **full-fat** (about 20 percent fat and 35 percent protein), **low-fat** (6 percent fat, 45 percent protein) and **defatted** (less than 1 percent fat, 50 percent protein). Asians use soy flours to make noodles, plus a variety of buns and confections, and know in-

NUTRIENT CONTENT OF 1 CUP DEFATTED SOY FLOUR
(about 3 ounces; 88 grams)

290 calories	18 mg sodium
41 g protein	2,097 mg potassium
1 g fat, 0 saturated	2 g dietary fiber
0 mg cholesterol	4 RE vitamin A
34 g carbohydrate	0.61 mg thiamin
212 mg calcium	0.22 mg riboflavin
593 mg phosphorus	2.3 mg niacin
8.1 mg iron	0 mg vitamin C

stinctively just which flour to use. In the United States, soybean flour is the province of the vegetarian. Or of the big food companies that use tons of it in fabricating meat substitutes. In addition to containing impressive amounts of protein, soy flour is a stellar source of niacin, calcium, iron, phosphorus and potassium.

Soy Milk: This milky substance extracted from pureed fresh soybeans is used in place of animal milk throughout much of Asia. Boiled, filtered and lightly sweetened, it's high in protein, yet easily digested. For all its nutrients, soy milk lacks some of the vitamins and minerals present in cow's milk. For example, it has only a fourth as much calcium. For this reason, commercial processors of soy milk frequently fortify it with vitamins and minerals. A good idea. But read labels to make sure. Soy milk is sold in pasteboard cartons, like those used for fruit juices. It is sterile until opened, then must be stored in the refrigerator.

NUTRIENT CONTENT OF 1 CUP SOY MILK
(8 fluid ounces; 240 grams)

79 calories	29 mg sodium
7 g protein	338 mg potassium
5 g fat, 1 saturated	3 g dietary fiber
0 mg cholesterol	7 RE vitamin A
4 g carbohydrate	0.39 mg thiamin
10 mg calcium	0.17 mg riboflavin
117 mg phosphorus	0.4 mg niacin
1.4 mg iron	0 mg vitamin C

Soy Sauce: A dark, salty liquid seasoning made by fermenting soy beans, which was developed by the Chinese more than three thousand years ago. Today's soy sauces are often made from a soybean/roasted wheat (or rice or barley) mash that's fed yeast starters and left to ferment and age in huge vats for several months. Soy sauces vary in thickness (the Japanese **tamari** is especially dark and dense), in saltiness and in sweetness. As a rule, the Japanese soy sauces are sweeter and mellower than the Chinese. **CAUTION:** If you're on a strict low-sodium diet, consider soy sauce off-limits. A single tablespoon contains 1,027 milligrams sodium, half the day's quota for a healthy person. **NOTE:** There are now lower-sodium soy sauces. These contain about half the sodium of regular soy sauce, but at 500 milligrams per tablespoon they are hardly *low* sodium.

NUTRIENT CONTENT OF 1 TABLESPOON SOY SAUCE (MADE WITH WHEAT)
(about ²/₃ ounce; 18 grams)

10 calories	1,027 mg sodium
1 g protein	32 mg potassium
0 g fat, 0 saturated	0 g dietary fiber
0 mg cholesterol	0 RE vitamin A
2 g carbohydrate	0.01 mg thiamin
3 mg calcium	0.02 mg riboflavin
20 mg phosphorus	0.6 mg niacin
0.4 mg iron	0 mg vitamin C

Spaghetti: See PASTA.

Spaghetti Squash: See SQUASH.

Spanish Mackerel: See MACKEREL.

Special Milk Program for Children: Another of the USDA Food and Nutrition Service's efforts to upgrade child nutrition, this one by making more liquid milk available to them. Simply put, the U.S. government shares the tab for milk drunk by children in nonprofit nursery schools, child-care centers, settlement houses, summer camps, primary and secondary grades, etc., that receive no other federal funds.

Specific Dynamic Action (SDA): Whenever you eat, your metabolic rate increases; this is called specific dynamic action. On average, your metabolism rises about 10 percent each day over that of the fasting level. Some foods have significantly higher SDAs than others. Protein, for example, has an SDA of 30 percent, meaning it will speed your metabolism by about a third. Carbohydrates, on the other hand, have an SDA of only 6 and fats a piddling 4. Is this why fats go straight to the hips?

Spinach: Spinach is believed to have come from Persia and to have been carried long ago by Arab caravans into China, where it quickly became (and remains) a great delicacy. It was the Moors who introduced spinach to Europe—via Spain. The early Dutch always thought of spinach as a Spanish vegetable. So did John Parkinson, the seventeenth-century English herbalist who noted that the Dutch "doe stew the herbe in a pot or pipkin without any other moisture than its owne." Good advice. Although it contains considerable calcium, the oxalates in spinach bind it and make it useless to the body. Fortunately, its impressive stores of iron, potassium and vitamins (A, B$_2$ and C) are not affected. **SEASON:** Year-round, with supplies peaking between January and June. Needless to add, frozen spinach, both the leaf and the chopped, are plentiful right around the calendar. The chopped, in particular, is one frozen vegetable that remains remarkably "fresh."

NUTRIENT CONTENT OF 1 CUP STEAMED SPINACH	
(about 6½ ounces; 180 grams)	
41 calories	126 mg sodium
5 g protein	839 mg potassium
0 g fat, 0 saturated	4 g dietary fiber
0 mg cholesterol	1,474 RE vitamin A
7 g carbohydrate	0.17 mg thiamin
245 mg calcium	0.43 mg riboflavin
100 mg phosphorus	0.9 mg niacin
6.4 mg iron	18 mg vitamin C

Spirulina: These dried ALGAE tablets are, if you believe the claims, a "naturally digestible food that contains concentrations of nutrients unlike any other single grain, herb or plant." Spirulina is said to bolster the immune system, lower blood levels of cholesterol, cleanse and heal the body, stabilize blood sugar and boost mineral absorption. All of this while curbing appetite. But none of these claims has ever been proved.

Split Peas: See PEAS.

Spores: Dormant, encapsulated bacterial cells, some of which are extremely hardy. Spores are a major problem for commercial and home canners because if canned foods are to be safe, all spores must be destroyed. The spore of greatest concern is that of *Clostridium botulinum*. It's present in the air, in soil and proliferates in low-acid canned foods—meats, fish and fowl, vegetables (except tomatoes), soups, sauces, pastas and the like. If its spores are not killed during processing (which takes ten minutes or more at 10 to 15 pounds pressure), they will germinate in the can when stored at room temperature, producing a toxin that can kill. Honey presents special problems. It sometimes contains *C. botulinum* spores and is never heated to tem-

peratures that would do them in. Although the number of spores in honey aren't sufficient to bring adults to grief, there are enough of them to harm a baby. These spores can germinate in the infant's digestive tract, producing a deadly toxin. For this reason, never give infants of one year or less anything containing honey. And never rub honey on baby's pacifier. See also BACTERIA; PRESSURE CANNING.

Sports Anemia, Runner's Anemia: Low blood hemoglobin, which plagues some women athletes, usually at the start of intensive training. Doctors have yet to nail the cause, but they have theories. Sports anemia may be caused by an increase in blood volume and proportionately lower hemoglobin. Menstruation may be responsible, or low iron intake/absorption, or accelerated iron and red blood cell loss or insufficient dietary protein. Usually all that's needed to cure sports anemia is a diet rich in iron and protein— meats (especially liver), poultry and fish. If this transient form of anemia persists, iron supplements may be prescribed.

Sports Drinks: What are these elixirs, these drinks that power athletes to play longer, harder? To win? Most of them are nothing more than blends of water, sugar and two electrolytes (sodium and potassium) plus assorted flavors and colors. Some are carbonated and now that mainstreamers are being targeted as well as professional athletes, artificially sweetened low-cal versions are also available. Do sports drinks work? Are they better thirst quenchers than tap water? For the average person, no. For those who exercise no more than thirty minutes at a time, no. For children, no. None of these people sweats enough, loses enough water, muscle fuel or electrolytes to justify special restorative formulas. When it comes to hard-core athletes, however, to marathoners, to footballers struggling under a downpouring sun, many researchers agree that sports drinks, if not rehydrating their bodies and restoring electrolyte balance and lost calories faster than H$_2$O, do at least reduce fluid loss and keep athletes "pumped." (According to some studies, the only way that sports drinks replace bodily fluids faster than water is by being injected straight into the small intestine.) The kick off of the multibillion-dollar sports drink industry occurred in 1965. That year the University of Florida football team, the Gators, served as guinea pigs for a new power drink. They were seen swilling Gatorade every time they left the field. And they did seem energized. Indeed, 1965 was a championship season for the Gators, and team members were only too happy to attribute their good fortune to Gatorade. See also SWEATING.

Sports Nutrition: Athletes, like everyone else, should eat a well-balanced diet every day, one based on the new FOOD GUIDE PYRAMID. They should also make every effort to maintain optimum weight. This does not mean bone-thin. For most sports, the ideal amount of body fat for men is 15 percent, and for women 20 percent. Runners need to be slightly thinner, swimmers a bit plumper. Seasonal sports—football, baseball, etc.—often mean that athletes gain weight off-season, then must slim down once training begins. Like other dieters, they should settle for a 1½- to 2-pound drop a week instead of going on starvation diets, which may mean lost muscle as well as fat. In periods of active training or competition, the athlete's goal is to increase energy, to improve performance and endurance. This may mean upping the daily calories (mostly through complex CARBOHYDRATES) and eating five or six meals a day instead of three. With B vitamins intricately involved in metabolism (some of them regulate energy expenditure), an athlete who burns 4,000 calories a day will need twice the B-complex of a more sedentary person who burns only 2,000. IRON is essential to oxygenating the blood (and fighting fatigue). Finally, vitamins A, C, E, plus several different minerals, all play roles in the production of red blood cells and hemoglobin. Women athletes, in particular, may suffer from iron-deficiency ANEMIA or SPORTS ANEMIA. And those who are too thin may stop menstruating, which may in turn lead to osteoporosis. And what about bulking up on carbs before the big race, the big game? Does it help? Yes, if done correctly, because it increases body stores of glycogen, the form of carbohydrate that's stored in the liver and muscles as "instant" energy. See also ENERGY BOOSTERS.

Sprouts: These are nothing more than sprouted seeds. BEAN SPROUTS are what we know best. But silvery, filament-thin ALFALFA SPROUTS and peppery RADISH SPROUTS are now staples in many supermarkets, too. Both are delicious sprinkled into sandwiches and salads. For details, see individual entries.

Sprue, Celiac: See GLUTEN INTOLERANCE.

Squabs: These are pigeons, specially raised pigeons that never have seen the sidewalks of New York (or any other city). The squabs that come to market are no more than a month old and weigh about a pound apiece. They are plump of breast, dark of flesh and juicier than white-meated birds.

NUTRIENT CONTENT OF 3 OUNCES (85 GRAMS) ROAST SQUAB	
181 calories	85 mg sodium
27 g protein	349 mg potassium
8 g fat, 3 saturated	0 g dietary fiber
75 mg cholesterol	45 RE vitamin A
0 g carbohydrate	0.03 mg thiamin
42 mg calcium	0.13 mg riboflavin
264 mg phosphorus	5.2 mg niacin
7.1 mg iron	2 mg vitamin C

Squash: Squashes, or "vegetables of the vines," as Native Americans call them, belong to the big five of New World foods (the other four are beans, tomatoes, potatoes and corn). Some botanists believe squashes may have been the

NUTRIENT CONTENT OF 1 CUP BOILED/STEAMED YELLOW SQUASH (about 6½ ounces; 180 grams)	
36 calories	2 mg sodium
2 g protein	346 mg potassium
1 g fat, 0 saturated	3 g dietary fiber
0 mg cholesterol	52 RE vitamin A
8 g carbohydrate	0.09 mg thiamin
49 mg calcium	0.09 mg riboflavin
70 mg phosphorus	0.9 mg niacin
0.6 mg iron	10 mg vitamin C

NUTRIENT CONTENT OF 1 CUP BOILED/STEAMED PATTYPAN SQUASH (about 6½ ounces; 180 grams)	
29 calories	2 mg sodium
2 g protein	252 mg potassium
0 g fat, 0 saturated	3 g dietary fiber
0 mg cholesterol	16 RE vitamin A
6 g carbohydrate	0.09 mg thiamin
27 mg calcium	0.05 mg riboflavin
50 mg phosphorus	0.8 mg niacin
0.6 mg iron	19 mg vitamin C

first food cultivated in the Americas because seeds found in Mexican caves have been carbon-dated at 9000 B.C. Wherever European explorers traveled the New World, they spoke of the squashes they saw growing, often mistaking them for melons or gourds. Vespucci mentioned them, Columbus, de Soto, Cabeza de Vaca, Cartier and, of course, the English colonists. Even then there were too many different squashes to record. And the number of varieties available today is surely tenfold. Fortunately, they can be divided into two categories:

Summer Squash: The most common are **yellow squash** (both crookneck and straight), **zucchini** and the pale green **pattypan** or **cymbling**. SEASON: Year-round for

NUTRIENT CONTENT OF 1 CUP BOILED/STEAMED ZUCCHINI

(about 6½ ounces; 180 grams)

29 calories	5 mg sodium
1 g protein	455 mg potassium
0 g fat, 0 saturated	2 g dietary fiber
0 mg cholesterol	43 RE vitamin A
7 g carbohydrate	0.07 mg thiamin
23 mg calcium	0.07 mg riboflavin
72 mg phosphorus	0.8 mg niacin
0.6 mg iron	8 mg vitamin C

NUTRIENT CONTENT OF 1 CUP MASHED BAKED ACORN SQUASH

(about 8¾ ounces; 245 grams)

136 calories	10 mg sodium
3 g protein	1,070 mg potassium
0 g fat, 0 saturated	11 g dietary fiber
0 mg cholesterol	105 RE vitamin A
36 g carbohydrate	0.41 mg thiamin
108 mg calcium	0.03 mg riboflavin
110 mg phosphorus	2.2 mg niacin
2.3 mg iron	27 mg vitamin C

Casserole of Two Summer Squashes and Tomatoes

Makes 4 Servings

- 1 medium zucchini, washed and thinly sliced
- 1 medium yellow squash, washed and thinly sliced
- 2 medium vine-ripened tomatoes, peeled, cored, and thinly sliced
- ½ teaspoon dried basil
- ½ teaspoon dried marjoram
- ¾ teaspoon salt
- ¼ teaspoon freshly ground black pepper
- 1 cup low-sodium beef or chicken broth
- ¼ cup dry bread crumbs
- 3 tablespoons freshly grated Parmesan cheese
- 1 tablespoon fruity olive oil

PREHEAT OVEN TO 350°F. Layer the zucchini, squash, and tomatoes in a shallow 6-cup casserole coated with nonstick vegetable cooking spray, sprinkling each layer with basil, marjoram, salt, and pepper. Pour the broth over all. In a bowl, combine the crumbs, Parmesan, and oil, tossing well until crumbly. Sprinkle evenly over the casserole and bake, uncovered, for 45 minutes or until bubbling and tipped with brown.

APPROXIMATE NUTRIENT COUNTS PER SERVING

110 calories	11 g carbohydrate	1.2 mg iron	0.11 mg thiamin
5 g protein	2 g dietary fiber	566 mg sodium	0.12 mg riboflavin
6 g fat, 2 saturated	102 mg calcium	351 mg potassium	2.0 mg niacin
4 mg cholesterol	105 mg phosphorus	65 RE vitamin A	19 mg vitamin C

zucchini and yellow squash; July and August for patty-pans.

Winter Squash: Just the short list must include **acorn, banana, buttercup, butternut, delicata, Hubbard, spaghetti, sweet dumpling** and **turban squash,** as well as PUMPKIN, a not too distant relative. **SEASON:** September through March, although acorn and spaghetti squash both are available right around the calendar.

The winter squashes, at least those with dazzling orange flesh, are incomparable sources of beta-carotene, and most

NUTRIENT CONTENT OF 1 CUP MASHED BAKED BUTTERNUT SQUASH
(about 8¾ ounces; 245 grams)

98 calories	10 mg sodium
2 g protein	696 mg potassium
0 g fat, 0 saturated	7 g dietary fiber
0 mg cholesterol	1,715 RE vitamin A
26 g carbohydrate	0.18 mg thiamin
100 mg calcium	0.04 mg riboflavin
66 mg phosphorus	2.4 mg niacin
1.5 mg iron	37 mg vitamin C

Butternut Squash and Snow Pea Salad with Sesame Dressing

Makes 8 Servings

An unusual salad that's as nutritious as it is colorful.

1 small butternut squash (about 12 ounces)
½ pound fresh snow peas, strings removed, cut lengthwise into ¼-inch-wide matchsticks
3 large Belgian endives, halved crosswise, then cut lengthwise into ¼-inch-wide matchsticks
6 large red radishes, trimmed and cut into ¼-inch-wide matchsticks
¼ teaspoon salt
⅛ teaspoon freshly ground black pepper

SESAME DRESSING:
1 small garlic clove, crushed
1½ teaspoons crushed peeled fresh ginger
¼ teaspoon finely grated orange zest
1 tablespoon honey
2 tablespoons soy sauce
3 tablespoons Asian sesame oil
1 tablespoon vegetable oil
2 tablespoons fresh lemon juice

HALVE THE SQUASH lengthwise, scoop out all seeds, then halve crosswise, peel, and cut into matchsticks about 1½ inches long and ¼ inch thick. Place the squash in a large sieve and dip the sieve into a large kettle of boiling lightly salted water for 15 seconds. Rinse in cold water and drain well. In the same water, blanch the snow peas for 5 seconds. Rinse in cold water and drain well. Place squash, snow peas, endives, and radishes in a large bowl and sprinkle with salt and pepper. Combine all the dressing ingredients except the lemon juice, let stand 20 minutes, then whisk well. Drizzle the dressing over the salad, toss lightly, and let stand 10 minutes. Sprinkle lemon juice over the salad, toss well, and serve.

APPROXIMATE NUTRIENT COUNTS PER SERVING

100 calories	9 g carbohydrate	1.0 mg iron	0.08 mg thiamin
2 g protein	2 g dietary fiber	336 mg sodium	0.06 mg riboflavin
7 g fat, 1 saturated	46 mg calcium	241 mg potassium	0.7 mg niacin
0 mg cholesterol	38 mg phosphorus	269 RE vitamin A	28 mg vitamin C

are also rich in iron and potassium. The summer squashes are low in calories, contain traces of vitamins A and C, calcium, iron and phosphorus but their potassium count soars.

(about 8³/₄ ounces; 245 grams)

71 calories	12 mg sodium
3 g protein	505 mg potassium
1 g fat, 0 saturated	7 g dietary fiber
0 mg cholesterol	946 RE vitamin A
15 g carbohydrate	0.10 mg thiamin
24 mg calcium	0.07 mg riboflavin
33 mg phosphorus	0.8 mg niacin
0.7 mg iron	15 mg vitamin C

NUTRIENT CONTENT OF 1 CUP COOKED SPAGHETTI SQUASH

(about 8²/₃ ounces; 243 grams)

45 calories	28 mg sodium
1 g protein	181 mg potassium
0 g fat, 0 saturated	4 g dietary fiber
0 mg cholesterol	17 RE vitamin A
10 g carbohydrate	0.06 mg thiamin
33 mg calcium	0.03 mg riboflavin
22 mg phosphorus	1.3 mg niacin
0.5 mg iron	5 mg vitamin C

Squid, Calamari: A delicacy throughout much of the world, squid are only now winning an appreciative audience in the United States, albeit mainly in large metropolitan areas. Squid are cephalopods, tentacled mollusks that carry their shells inside (the cuttlebone). They are night feeders, devouring fish large and small as they jet-propel themselves through the water. Squid vary widely in size, some being no bigger than one finger joint, others—the giant squid—reaching 60 feet or more. Their flesh is naturally tender, sweet and white. There is little waste with squid. The sac or body is edible (wonderful when stuffed), the tentacles, even the ink, which the Italians sometimes add to seafood muddles or use to color pasta black. Tiny squid can be deep-fried whole and popped into the mouth like shrimp. Squid are high in protein, phosphorus, potassium, riboflavin and niacin. They are also high in sodium and cholesterol.

NUTRIENT CONTENT OF 3 OUNCES (85 GRAMS) BOILED SQUID

117 calories	315 mg sodium
16 g protein	253 mg potassium
4 g fat, 1 saturated	0 g dietary fiber
239 mg cholesterol	45 RE vitamin A
3 g carbohydrate	0.02 mg thiamin
34 mg calcium	0.40 mg riboflavin
227 mg phosphorus	2.1 mg niacin
0.7 mg iron	4 mg vitamin C

Stabilizers, Thickeners: Without them commercial ice creams would be gritty, puddings lumpy, chocolate milk two-tone. The stabilizers most often used by food processors are PECTIN, GELATIN and gelatinous seaweed extracts such as CARRAGEENAN.

Stainless-Steel Cooking Utensils: Stainless-steel pots and pans don't rust, rarely discolor, are quick to clean and react only minimally with acid or alkaline foods (cast iron and aluminum are far more reactive). So when recipes specify a nonreactive pan, a stainless-steel or stainless-steel-lined pan can be used if you have nothing porcelain clad or made of flameproof glass. Stainless steel's biggest shortcoming is that it's a poor conductor of heat, given to "hot spots." The bottoms of better aluminum cookware are now several ply, with copper or aluminum (superconductors both) sandwiched inside so that burner heat is more quickly and uniformly distributed.

Standard of Identity: Over the years, fake foods have been falsely labeled. For example, "peach jam" might be nothing more than water, pectin, sugar, artificial colors and flavors. To stop such fraudulence, the FDA adopted the Standard of Identity program, which monitors and spot-checks several hundred processed foods to ensure that they are what they claim. Manufacturers must meet minimum quality standards determined by the FDA, use required ingredients in the amounts specified, use only permitted ingredients and comply with standards set for color, form and packaging.

Staphyloccus aureus, Staphylococcal Food Poisoning: See BACTERIA.

Starch: See CARBOHYDRATES.

Starch, Modified: See MODIFIED STARCH.

Starch Blockers: See DIET PILLS.

Star Fruit: See CARAMBOLAS.

Starvation: Drought and poverty (the conditions so prevalent in parts of the Third World) cause people to starve. But so do self-induced fasts and extreme low-calorie diets. It's not a pretty picture and the damage done to the body may be permanent. To simplify, here's the scenario: First the body exhausts its stores of glycogen (the form of glucose stored in the liver and muscles). Next it begins to feed upon muscle protein. Then fat stores are depleted and emaciation begins. The body metabolism slows, as if to ration what energy sources remain. "Starved to death" is no joke, because death will surely come unless the starving person begins not only to eat but to eat nutritious food. Dietary rehabilitation, often fortified by vitamin/mineral supplements, should proceed slowly under strict medical supervision so that the starving body has time to readjust. See also DIETS, especially the section on very low-calorie diets.

Steak: See BEEF.

Steak Sauce: A thick, salty/vinegary brown sauce that can be sprinkled on burgers, steaks and chops at table or used as a kitchen seasoner. Recipes differ from brand to brand, but most steak sauces are compounded of water, tomato paste, corn syrup, salt, herbs and spices, caramel, dehydrated onions and garlic. Most are long on sodium.

NUTRIENT CONTENT OF 1 TABLESPOON STEAK SAUCE (A.1.)

(about ½ ounce; 16 grams)

10 calories	227 mg sodium
0 g protein	63 mg potassium
0 g fat, 0 saturated	0 g dietary fiber
0 mg cholesterol	15 RE vitamin A
2 g carbohydrate	0.01 mg thiamin
3 mg calcium	0.01 mg riboflavin
6 mg phosphorus	0.2 mg niacin
0.2 mg iron	3 mg vitamin C

Steaming: A quick way to cook vegetables that requires no fat and preserves most of the vitamins and minerals as well as the color and crunch. Because vegetables cook *over* boiling water, not in it, there's little loss of the water-soluble Bs and C. And because they steam quickly, the heat-sensitive vitamins are also less readily destroyed. Fish and chicken breasts take to steaming, too, remaining succulent. Moreover, some of their fat drips off.

Stearic Acid (additive): A waxy, saturated fatty acid present in many animal fats and vegetable oils. To food manufacturers, it's useful as a flavor enhancer for a variety of baked goods, candies and soft drinks and also as a chewing-gum softener. GRAS when used within FDA guidelines.

Sterilization: Killing microorganisms by heating food or drink to high temperatures for specific periods of time. Times and temperatures vary according to the food being preserved. For high-acid fruits, pickles and relishes, 10 to 15 minutes in a boiling water bath are sufficient, but for low-acid meats, fish, poultry and vegetables, only pressure canning will bring temperatures high enough to destroy disease-causing microorganisms and their spores. See CANNING under FOOD PRESERVATION.

Steroids: A large group of naturally occurring fatty compounds that includes cholesterol, vitamin D, bile salts and a number of body hormones (including the sex hormones). Mention "steroid" to the average person, however, and the immediate association is **anabolic steroids** (synthetic male sex hormones), the drugs athletes use to "power up." Derived from testosterone, these steroids build lean body mass (read *muscles*). But their list of known side effects is both long and frightening. For starters, there are the increased risks of cancer, coronary artery disease, liver disease, edema, even death. And that's the short list. **Corticosteroids,** on the other hand, are valuable medications prescribed for a variety of illnesses, among them asthma, arthritis, cancer, dermatitis and Addison's disease.

Stewing: The way to simmer tough old birds and sinewy cuts of meat into submission. The long, moist heating converts collagen (the tough stuff) to gelatin. It also renders out much of the fat, which can be skimmed from the broth or, better yet, chilled and lifted right off. Vegetables simmered along with the meat will lose some of their heat-sensitive vitamins (mainly C). And some of the water solubles will leach out. But if the stew liquid is served, the leached nutrients are saved.

Stillman Diet: A popular 1970s weight-loss diet developed by Dr. Irwin Stillman. "Eat all you want" was the premise, "as long as it isn't carbohydrate." Stillman's diet banned breads, fruits, vegetables and milk. It was low on carbohydrates, long on protein and fat and required you to drink eight glasses of water a day (small wonder it was dubbed "the water diet"). Consisting mostly of lean meat, fish, poultry, eggs and low-fat cheeses, the Stillman Diet was deficient in calcium, fiber and vitamins A and C. See also DIETS.

Stilton: England's superlative blue cheese. Made from cow's milk, Stilton is buttery with veins of blue-green mold radiating from the center outward. The best Stiltons are aged about six months. They are creamier than Roquefort, somewhat mellower, too. More like Gorgonzola. **NOTE:** Nutrient counts are unavailable for Stilton, but it's safe to say it's long on calories, fat and cholesterol.

Stir-frying: It's a Chinese technique of sautéing performed in a wok, but clumsy chefs often slosh in the oil and heat it to the smoke point before tossing in the food. If done with a minimum of oil in a sizzling-hot skillet, stir-frying is an excellent way to cook diced, shredded or thinly sliced meats, chicken and vegetables because it preserves the lion's share of vitamins and minerals.

Stomach: A muscular pouch located between the esophagus and duodenum that's an important part of the digestive process. The stomach consists of three parts, each with a specific duty. The upper part (or **cardia**) receives the food and delivers it into the middle portion (**fundus**) to be stored briefly and mixed with digestive juices. From here food moves into the lower part of the stomach (**antrum**), which churns it with hydrochloric acid and four vital secretions (intrinsic factor, lipase, pepsin and rennin). The combination of acid, enzymes and vigorous mixing partially breaks down carbohydrates, fats and proteins before dispatching them to the small intestine to finish the job.

Stone Crabs: See CRABS.

Stout: A hoppy, dark, sometimes bitter brew popular in Ireland. See ALCOHOL, ALCOHOLIC BEVERAGES.

Strawberries: "Doubtless God could have made a better berry, but doubtless God never did." Thus wrote Englishman William Butler along about 1600. Unlike many fruits, whose geographic origins can be pinpointed, strawberries seem to have grown wild in both the Old World and New. But only in temperate or northern climes. The Bible doesn't mention strawberries. They don't show up in Egyptian art. The Greeks seemed to have confused strawberries with the strawberry tree, a different species altogether. And the Romans paid them little mind. But strawberry seeds have surfaced in Stone Age sites in Switzerland and Denmark. Wild strawberries grew so abundantly over half the world they've only recently been cultivated and, alas, bred more for endurance than for succulence or savor. There's a lesson here: Buy homegrown strawberries when they are red straight through, plump and heady with their own perfume. Strawberries are a major source of vitamin C and potassium, yet they are extremely low in calories and sodium. **SEASON:** Late April through August.

NUTRIENT CONTENT OF 1 CUP FRESH STRAWBERRIES
(about 6 ounces; 166 grams)

50 calories	2 mg sodium
1 g protein	276 mg potassium
1 g fat, 0 saturated	4 g dietary fiber
0 mg cholesterol	5 RE vitamin A
12 g carbohydrate	0.03 mg thiamin
23 mg calcium	0.11 mg riboflavin
32 mg phosphorus	0.4 mg niacin
0.6 mg iron	94 mg vitamin C

Streptococcus lactis, S. thermophilus: Two benign strains of bacteria used in souring milk and cream, in making butter, buttermilk, yogurt and a variety of cheeses (Cheddar, cottage cheese and Emmentaler, to name three).

Stress (diet and): Is the hyping of vitamin and mineral supplements for the stressed-out a ploy to make money? Or do those under stress really need nutritional boosters? It depends on what you mean by stress. Physicians and nutritionists acknowledge that four types of stress can change your nutrient requirements: (1) **physiological**—pregnancy, breast feeding or just plain growing up; (2) **pathological**—disease, fever, infection, alcoholism; (3) **physical**—hard labor, heavy-duty exercise, environmental extremes; (4) **psychological**—bulimia, anorexia nervosa, compulsive overeating. And what about the pressures of daily life, job stresses, family crises? Emotional tension can put you at greater risk of high blood pressure, cardiac and gastrointestinal disease. It can also weaken your immune system. But solving these problems isn't as easy as popping vitamin pills. It requires medical attention, often with internists, psychiatrists and nutritionists working in concert. Often it means retooling the diet because poor eating habits may be partly responsible for the psychological distress.

String Beans: See GREEN BEANS under BEANS, FRESH.

Striped Bass: "The Basse is an excellent Fish, both fresh and salte . . . and for daintinesse of diet they excell the Marybones [marrowbones] of Beefe. There are such multitudes that I have seene stopped close in the river adjoining to my house with a sande at one tyde so many as will loade a ship of 100 tonnes. I myselfe, at the turning of the tyde have seene such multitudes pass out of a pounde that it seemed to me that one might go over their backs drishod." That was what Captain John Smith of the Jamestown colony had to say about striped bass in 1607. The *Mayflower* Pilgrims were no less enthusiastic and baited "stripers" with lobsters. In those days, stripers of 80 or 100 pounds were not uncommon. Today, a sportfisherman considers himself lucky to land a 20-pounder. Striped bass swim the entire Atlantic coast, mostly in inshore waters because they move up the great rivers to spawn. They have also been introduced into the Pacific. Striper flesh is whitish, firm and sweet, especially when the fish are young (6 to 8 pounds); these are the ones Japanese chefs choose for sushi. The larger the striped bass, the coarser its meat. Striped bass also tend to take on the taste of what they've eaten. Down South, striped bass (**rock** or **rockfish,** as they're known locally) feed upon shrimp and their flesh is supremely sweet. Chesapeake stripers are gamier because they gobble oily menhaden. And those swimming the waters off Long Island—"powerboat heaven"—sometimes taste of diesel. For approximate nutrient counts, see FISH, LEAN WHITE.

Strontium: Like other minerals, strontium exists naturally in food, plants and seawater. It's present, too, in our bodies although no one's determined that we need it. Indeed, there's a danger because strontium can replace calcium in bones. The strontium that had everyone on red alert in the 1950s, however, was radioactive **strontium 90,** which aboveground nuclear explosions rained down upon us. It showed up in grass, silage, in cow's milk and ultimately those who drank that milk. Once absorbed into the bones, strontium 90, with a half-life of twenty-eight years, continues to assault the body with internal radiation. Even small doses of it can cause leukemia and bone cancer, particularly in children less than ten years old. The Federal Radiation Council quickly set acceptable levels of strontium 90. As a result, estimates suggest that internal radiation (by strontium 90 and other radioactive substances in food or drink) now accounts for only 0.3 percent of the fatal cancers in the United States.

Struvite: Harmless glassy crystals often found in canned seafood, principally shrimp and tuna. These form during the canning process from the minerals the fish have absorbed from seawater. The chemical name for struvite is a tongue twister—**magnesium ammonium phosphate hexahydrate.** These crystals are usually soft enough to crush with your fingers. Failing that, you can pick them out and discard.

Stuffings: The best part of the Thanksgiving turkey, most people would agree, is the stuffing. Unfortunately, it's a bacteria factory and, unless handled with care, can cause serious food poisoning. Indeed, the USDA now urges erring on the side of caution; that is, roasting the turkey unstuffed and baking the stuffing separately. Stuffings inside a bird—especially a whopper—remain in the bacterial danger zone too long, giving potentially harmful bugs a chance to proliferate. Small birds—of 10 pounds or less—pose less risk, especially when stuffed just before they go into the oven. Mixing the stuffing at the last minute helps, too. It's safe to chop everything ahead of time as long as you refrigerate the ingredients in separate bowls. **ANOTHER CAUTION:** If you do stuff a bird, scoop out all stuffing at meal's end, spread in a shallow casserole, cover and refrigerate immediately to reduce the risk of food poisoning. Certain stuffings are more likely to cause grief than others—those containing egg, for example; those with oysters or giblets. The safest stuffings are merely minces of fruits and vegetables. So much for tradition.

Sturgeon: A snouted, plated prehistoric fish that's the source of CAVIAR. But sturgeon is also uncommonly meaty, its firm ivory-pink flesh as bland, as tender as veal. Although sturgeon, a saltwater fish, once ascended America's mighty rivers by the thousands to spawn—the Potomac, the Delaware, Hudson and Columbia—most of that on the market today is farm raised in California and sold as steaks or fillets. Like veal, it costs the earth. Like salmon and swordfish, sturgeon is an oily fish. But delicately so.

NUTRIENT CONTENT OF 3 OUNCES (85 GRAMS) BROILED/BAKED STURGEON	
114 calories	59 mg sodium
18 g protein	309 mg potassium
4 g fat, 1 saturated	0 g dietary fiber
66 mg cholesterol	206 RE vitamin A
0 g carbohydrate	0.07 mg thiamin
15 mg calcium	0.08 mg riboflavin
231 mg phosphorus	8.6 mg niacin
0.7 mg iron	0 mg vitamin C

Styrofoam: Styrofoam is a trademarked product name. The millions upon millions of fast-food cups and trays we use are popularly called Styrofoam, but real Styrofoam is not used for food and beverage containers. What is used is an extruded featherweight plastic foam. Until the early 1980s (when environmentalists' cries rang around the world), ozone-zapping chlorofluorocarbons were used to pump bubbles into polystyrene. Today more environmentally correct compounds are employed and most plastic foam containers, if not biodegradable, can at least be recycled. Indeed, some schools and fast-food chains are going all out by stationing special recycling bins beside their trash cans. Still, McDonald's, for one, has sworn off foam containers. Apart from endangering the environment, plastic foam may also be hazardous to your health. Styrene, from which polystyrene comes, is toxic, perhaps carcinogenic, although that remains to be seen. What is certain is that plastic foam should never be used in the microwave. It will melt.

Subcutaneous Fat: The layer of fat just beneath the skin. Its thickness is one way physicians and nutritionists can determine degree of obesity. See SKINFOLD TESTS.

Sucralose: A new artificial sweetener still awaiting FDA approval. It's 600 times sweeter than sugar, yet contains zero calories. Called Splenda by its manufacturer, Johnson & Johnson, sucralose is more stable than aspartame, meaning its sweetness does not fade over time or during cooking. Stay tuned.

Sucrose: Table sugar. See SUGARS.

Sucrose Polyesters: Lab-synthesized fat substitutes that look like fat, taste like fat, have the same rich "mouth feel" but lack the carload of calories. See OLESTRA.

Suet: Beef fat, the finest of which encases the kidneys. Although cooks made puddings, stuffings, even mincemeats using suet, its high percentage of saturated fats puts modern cooks off.

Sugar Alcohols: These are being used in place of sugar in many dietetic foods. See MANNITOL; SORBITOL; XYLITOL.

Sugar Labeling: With the new labeling laws in force, the following terms have been redefined:

"Low Sugar": Cannot be used.

"No Added Sugar": Just what it says. This means not only no table sugar but also no alternative sweeteners like honey, corn syrup, molasses, etc. Further, there can be no jams or jellies or concentrated fruit juices, all of which contain sugar. There's more: The standard version of the product must be one that normally does contain added sugars. Finally, the label must state that the food neither is low in calories nor has had its calories reduced. Unless such is the case (as defined by the new labeling laws). Acceptable synonyms: "without added sugar," "no sugar added."

"Reduced Sugar": At least 25 percent less sugar per Reference Amount (standard serving size as set forth in the Nutirion Labeling and Education Act of 1990). Packaged main dishes (these must weigh at least 6 ounces per serving and feature two or more different foods) and meal products (TV dinners—or lunches or breakfasts—weighing at least 10 ounces and including at least three items from two or more food groups) must contain at least 25 percent less sugar per 100 grams (3½ ounces). Acceptable synonyms: "reduced in sugar," "sugar-reduced," "less sugar," "lower sugar," "lower in sugar."

"Sugar-Free": Contains less than ½ gram of sugar per Reference Amount (standard serving size) or, for that matter, of any ingredient generally understood to contain sugar unless asterisked and accompanied by a qualifying statement such as "Adds a trivial [or "negligible" or "dietarily insignificant"] amount of sugar." Further, the label must state that the product is "not a reduced- or low-calorie food," or that it is "not for weight control" unless it also meets those requirements. Acceptable synonyms: "free of sugar," "no sugar," "zero sugar," "without sugar," "sugarless," "trivial source of sugar," "negligible source of sugar," "dietarily insignificant source of sugar."

Sugars:

This is not a chemical discussion of sugars (for that, see CARBOHYDRATES). It's a quick survey of the sugars carried by every supermarket. Most of our sugar comes from sugarcane, fleshy bamboolike stalks that are about 80 percent sweet juice. No one knows where sugarcane originated. Some believe the East Indies; some Southeast Asia. At any rate, sugar was a major crop in India as early as 327 B.C. (etymologists trace our word *sugar* to the Sanskrit *sárkarā*). The Portuguese and Spaniards brought sugar to the New World at the turn of the sixteenth century and within one hundred years it was flourishing all over the Caribbean. But sugarcane is not the only source of sugar. We also get plenty of it from sugar beets. These plump, white

tubers thrive in cold climates where summer temperatures rarely exceed 70°F. Refined beet sugar and cane sugar look and taste the same and indeed are chemically identical. Two specialty sugars—JAGGARY and MAPLE SUGAR—are covered in individual entries.

Brown Sugar: Sugar crystals suspended in molasses syrup. Dark brown sugar has more molasses; light brown less. Brown sugars are equally good for sweets (gingerbread, butterscotch cookies, etc.) and savories (ham glazes, baked beans). Their only shortcoming is that they harden into bricks. No problem. **TO SOFTEN BROWN SUGAR:** Place sugar in a large, wide-mouth preserving jar, drape with a piece of plastic food wrap, then a moist paper towel and screw the lid down tight. In twelve hours the sugar will be soft. Or, even quicker, place sugar and a peeled apple slice in a microwave-safe bowl, cover with plastic food wrap, rolling back a corner to vent. Microwave on high power, allowing 30 seconds for each 1 cup sugar and crumbling with a fork every 30 seconds. **CALORIES:** 50 per tablespoon (firmly packed). Brown sugar also contains tiny amounts of calcium, iron, phosphorus and potassium.

Confectioners' Sugar: Pulverized granulated sugar that's had something added to keep it from caking. That something might be cornstarch, silica gel or tricalcium phosphate (all GRAS additives). Although confectioners' sugar is supposed to be available in different grinds, the only one known to supermarket shelves is 10× (ultra-fine). Bakers and confectioners are familiar with very fine (6×), fine (4×), medium and coarse. Confectioners' sugar is a specialist, the sugar for dredging, dusting and butter frostings. **CALORIES:** 25 per tablespoon.

Granulated Sugar: Fine sucrose crystals. Table sugar, the kitchen staple. **CALORIES:** 46 per tablespoon.

Raw Sugar: The FDA forbids the sale of raw sugar in the United States because this dark first crystallization is contaminated with yeasts, molds, waxes and bits of soil and fiber. What health-food stores sell as raw sugar is actually **turbinado,** meaning it has been centrifuged and steam washed to cleanse it of all impurities. It loses some of its molasses in the process yet is 99 percent pure. Turbinado can be used interchangeably with brown sugar, with granulated sugar, too—except for baking. **CALORIES:** 50 per tablespoon (firmly packed).

Superfine Sugar: Semipulverized granulated sugar that dissolves the instant it's moistened. This is the sugar to use for cocktails, meringues, boiled icings, sherbets and ice cream. **CALORIES:** 46 per tablespoon.

Sugar Snaps: See PEAS.

Sugar Substitutes: See ARTIFICIAL SWEETENERS.

Sulfa Drugs (residuals in food): To control disease and boost feed efficiency, pork producers, chicken farmers and cattle raisers have been adding a triple-threat chlortetracycline/penicillin/sulfamethazine formula to feed—with FDA approval. Indeed, 80 percent of American poultry, 75 percent of pork and dairy calves and 60 percent of beef have been raised on this antibiotic cocktail. The doses are supposed to be small—**subtherapeutic.** But many animals have been fed larger, **therapeutic** doses (with 10 percent of the swine affected), which can put humans at risk. Violations among poultry growers and cattle raisers were far less (less than 0.2 percent). The greatest hazard, it turns out, has been the residuals of sulfamethazine in milk. It is carcinogenic and as such has not been approved for use in dairy cows. Cooking depowers these antibiotics, but usually milk is poured and drunk cold. After the discovery in 1989 of sulfamethazine in milk, the government has cracked down on dairies and pumped up its monitoring of milk. See also ANTIBIOTICS.

Sulfide Spoilage: Unlike its deadly cousin *Clostridium botulinum, Clostridium nigrificans* lets you know right away that it has spoiled a can of food. There are splotches of black (ferrous sulfide, the same compound that causes that ugly dark layer between hard-cooked egg yolks and whites) plus a sickening smell of rotten eggs. Not for nothing are these contaminated cans called sulfur stinkers. The foods most susceptible to sulfide spoilage are low-acid vegetables like peas and corn. The cause? Underprocessing—too little time in the pressure canner and/or insufficient pressure. Needless to say, any sulfide-spoiled food should be disposed of where neither people nor animals will find it.

Sulfites (additives): Antioxidants widely used by food processors to keep foods from turning brown and to preserve certain nutrients, among them vitamin C. The trouble is, some people are so sensitive to sulfites that they may, within minutes, have trouble breathing, break out in hives, become dizzy, suffer violent headaches or abdominal pain. A few have even died. When reports of sulfite problems began funneling into the FDA, the agency set up the Adverse Reaction Monitoring System. That was in 1985, and since then, more than a thousand allergic reactions to sulfites have been logged.

A year later, the FDA ruled that any food containing sulfites must list them on its label. That same year it also banned the use of sulfites on salad-bar fruits and vegetables; indeed, on any that were to be eaten raw (restaurateurs and grocers routinely gave them a sulfite dip to keep them fresh and pretty). In 1990, FDA regulations were broadened to require listings on standardized foods (foods that meet the FDA's STANDARD OF IDENTITY).

There were, of course, glitches. In 1990, a sulfite ban on peeled fresh potatoes sold unmarked and in bulk to restaurants for french fries and hash browns was overturned. The FDA aims to repropose the ban and expects it to stick. Sulfite use is forbidden on meats (it keeps them bright red, possibly masking signs of spoilage) and also in such high-thiamin foods as enriched flours because it destroys this important B vitamin.

At present, the FDA allows food processors to add six different sulfiting agents to packaged foods: **sodium sulfite, sodium bisulfite** and **sodium metabisulfite, sulfur dioxide, potassium bisulfite** and **potassium metabisulfite.** It also strictly limits amounts that can be used. What foods and beverages are likely to contain them? The list is long and includes everything from beer and baked goods to dried candied fruits to soup mixes, processed seafoods and syrups to vinegars and wines. Scrutinize labels.

Sulforaphane: A sulfurous compound recently isolated from broccoli and shown to block tumor growth in rats (sulforaphane is also present in other members of the cabbage family). According to a Johns Hopkins study, sulforaphane appears to stimulate the body's production of cancer-fighting enzymes, particularly those involved with

breast cancer. Although the lab rat tests hold promise for treating and/or thwarting cancer in people, there's no proof that sulforaphane will be equally effective other than the fact that those who eat plenty of broccoli, brussels sprouts, cabbage, cauliflower, collards, kale and mustard greens do seem more resistant to cancer.

Sulfur: Although the body doesn't use this mineral as a nutrient, it's present in thiamin (vitamin B$_1$); in methionine, an essential amino acid; and in cysteine, a nonessential one. Sulfur appears to contour and stabilize protein molecules in the body, particularly those in the hair, nails and skin. There are no recommended intakes for sulfur and deficiencies are unheard of.

Sulfur Dioxide (additive): One of the sulfiting agents used to keep fruits and vegetables from turning brown and wines from spoiling. In addition to triggering violent reactions in sulfite-sensitive people, it destroys some vitamin B$_1$ (thiamin). See SULFITES.

Sultanas: See RAISINS.

Summer Food Service Program for Children: Yet another of the USDA's programs designed to nourish children. It consists of grants that enable states to provide nutritionally balanced meals to needy preschoolers and schoolchildren attending nonprofit summer schools and residential camps.

Sunchokes: See ARTICHOKES, JERUSALEM.

Sun-Dried Tomatoes: See TOMATOES, DRIED.

Sunette: See ACESULFAME-K; ARTIFICIAL SWEETENERS.

Sunfish: America's most popular freshwater fish. Correction, fishes, for the family includes **bluegills, crappies, redears** and **rock bass,** among others. These are the fish teens and old-timers hook in ponds and lakes, most of them perfect frying size, meaning small enough to fit in a skillet. As a group, they have lean, sweet and white flesh. But mind the bones! For approximate nutrient counts, see FISH, LEAN WHITE.

Sunflower-Seed Oil: On Portugal's Alentejo plains, groves of olive are being axed to make way for sunflowers. These are grown not for their blossoms but for their oil,

which is less labor intensive than olive oil and thus much cheaper to produce. So much so that sunflower oil is becoming a staple in the Portuguese kitchen, the all-purpose cooking oil, with olive oil being added at the last minute for flavor. Sunflower-seed oil is bland, nearly colorless, too. But it is high in polyunsaturates (only safflower oil is higher). In the United States, sunflower-seed oil is a component of many all-purpose vegetable-oil blends, and because of its semidrying properties, it's added to paints, soaps and varnishes, too. Like most oils, it's a nutritional cipher, offering nothing other than fat and calories: 1 tablespoon = 120 calories, 14 grams total fat (1.4 grams saturated). Because of its high smoke point (441°F.–450°F.), it's a good choice for deep-fat frying. To compare the composition of sunflower oil with that of other cooking oils, see OILS.

Sunflower Seeds: Once considered "hippie food," sunflower seeds have gone so mainstream they're bagged and sold like peanuts in many supermarkets. You can buy them whole or husked, raw or roasted, salted or unsalted. Sunflower seeds are a superior source of iron, phosphorus and potassium. And if unsalted, they contain almost no sodium.

NUTRIENT CONTENT OF 1 OUNCE (28 GRAMS) RAW, HUSKED SUNFLOWER SEEDS (UNSALTED)	
161 calories	1 mg sodium
6 g protein	195 mg potassium
14 g fat, 1 saturated	2 g dietary fiber
0 mg cholesterol	1 RE vitamin A
5 g carbohydrate	0.65 mg thiamin
33 mg calcium	0.07 mg riboflavin
199 mg phosphorus	1.3 mg niacin
1.9 mg iron	0 mg vitamin C

NUTRIENT CONTENT OF 1 OUNCE (28 GRAMS) OIL-ROASTED, HUSKED SUNFLOWER SEEDS (UNSALTED)	
174 calories	1 mg sodium
6 g protein	137 mg potassium
16 g fat, 2 saturated	2 g dietary fiber
0 mg cholesterol	1 RE vitamin A
4 g carbohydrate	0.09 mg thiamin
16 mg calcium	0.08 mg riboflavin
323 mg phosphorus	1.2 mg niacin
1.9 mg iron	0 mg vitamin C

Sunlight (effect on nutrients): Though sunlight is essential to life, it wreaks havoc on many food nutrients. Riboflavin (vitamin B_2), for example, is so light sensitive that when glass bottles of milk were left on sunny doorsteps, half the milk's riboflavin was lost within two hours. Even vitamin D becomes unstable when subjected to light, despite the fact that the sun's ultraviolet rays actually form vitamin D on the skin. Eight other vitamins are also partially destabilized and/or destroyed by light: A (and its beta-carotene precursor or forerunner), C, four of the B-complex besides riboflavin (thiamin, B_{12}, folic acid and pyridoxine or B_6), E and K. All essential fatty acids are similarly affected by light, as is at least one essential amino acid, tryptophan. **THE LESSONS HERE:** Those farmer's stand fruits and vegetables that look so country-fresh under the downstreaming sun will certainly have lost some of their nutrients within a few hours, especially if they've been cut open. And cooking oils, though pretty in glass bottles, should be stored in opaque bottles on a dark, cool shelf.

Supplements, Dietary: These may be vitamin/mineral pills, brewer's yeast, herbs, botanicals, wheat germ, cod-liver oil, in short any concentrated source of nutrients taken in addition to food. The big question, of course, is are they necessary? If you're healthy, if you eat a well-balanced diet based on the FOOD GUIDE PYRAMID, most nutritionists agree that supplements are unnecessary. A well-balanced diet, they explain, supplies not only the RDAs of all the necessary nutrients but also important nonnutrients that vitamin pills lack. Fiber, for one. Disease-fighting phytochemicals, for another. Nutritionists also believe that taking supplements perpetuates bad eating habits by making you think everything will be okay as long as you get your "vities."

They worry, in particular, about the misinformation being spread about the disease-preventing—or curing—merits of this pill or that potion.

A compromise version of the Nutrition Labeling and Education Act, which had the supplement industry in a tizzy for several years, was passed by the House and Senate in 1994. Nicknamed the pill bill, it empowers the FDA to bar health claims on the labels of nutritional supplements and herbal products unless there is "significant scientific agreement" to substantiate them. For example, until the cancer-fighting powers of vitamin C are established, no label can claim that it fights cancer.

On the other hand, the new ruling does permit supplement manufacturers to state on labels how their products "affect a structure or function of the body"—the role of vitamin A, for example, in promoting good eyesight. The distinction between health claims and function claims is already murky, and critics of the pill bill expect it to get murkier.

The Nutrition Labeling and Education Act also authorizes the FDA to establish safety standards for supplements and herbals. Seventy-five days before any new product goes on sale, the manufacturer must, with convincing evidence, show the FDA that it poses no "significant or unreasonable risk of illness or injury." Beginning January 1, 1997, label health claims must also be accompanied by this caveat: "This statement has not been evaluated by the Food and Drug Administration. This product is not intended to diagnose, treat, cure or prevent any disease."

As for products already on the market, they can be withdrawn only if the FDA can prove that they "present significant or unreasonable risks."

Some herbs and botanicals can be downright dangerous: CHAPARRAL (after causing acute toxic hepatitis, it's been voluntarily withdrawn from the market), COMFREY (liver disease, death), GERANIUM (irreversible kidney damage, death), JIN BU HUAN (it sent three Colorado preschoolers to the hospital with breathing problems, depressed central nervous systems, life-threateningly slow heartbeats), MA HUANG (high blood pressure, runaway heartbeat, stroke, nerve damage) and YOHIMBE (kidney failure, seizures, death).

Even megadoses of certain vitamins and minerals can be harmful: **vitamin A** (liver and bone damage, birth defects), **vitamin B_6** (numbness, muscle weakness, bone pain), **niacin** (liver damage, severe gastrointestinal distress), **vitamin C** (inflamed urinary tract, diarrhea), **vitamin D** (deformed bones, kidney damage), **folic acid** (masks B_{12} deficiency, allowing pernicious anemia to progress undiagnosed), **L-tryptophan** (an often fatal connective-tissue disorder called eosinophilia-myalgia syndrome, or EMS).

While physicians and nutritionists admit that balanced vitamin/mineral supplements are harmless when taken as directed, most disapprove of bulking up on individual nutrients. *Except* when they are prescribed by a doctor for certain conditions. Babies of six months or more, for example, may need extra iron; pregnant women four vitamins (folic acid, B_6, C and D) plus four minerals (calcium, copper, iron, zinc), and nursing mothers those same four vitamins plus three minerals (calcium, magnesium and zinc). In addition, milk haters should take calcium carbonate or swill calcium-fortified OJ, vegans will need vitamins B_{12} and D plus three minerals (calcium, iron, zinc) and smokers double the RDA for vitamin C. Finally, the fifty-plus crowd may require more antioxidants (beta-carotene, vitamins C and E), more vitamin D, more of three B-complexers (folic acid, B_6 and B_{12}) and, finally, more calcium—just what a well-balanced multivitamin/mineral pill delivers.

Surgery (diet and): For elective surgery, the obese are often put on reducing diets before they go under the knife. And the malnourished are built up. Just before surgery and until the patient is fully awake, no food is given orally to reduce the risk of vomiting and aspiration (sucking partially digested food into the lungs). Initially, postop patients are put on IVs of glucose, then, depending on the type of surgery, may be given clear liquids by mouth, then full liquids, then soft, bland foods. Finally, they are phased back on to a normal diet. How fast the sequence progresses depends on the speed of recovery. It's not unusual, however, for a postop patient to be on soft foods within a few hours of emerging from anesthesia and on solids within a few days.

Surimi: Salty, sweet, low-fat pastes made out of pollack or other cheap white-fleshed fish that can be flavored, colored and shaped into convincing counterfeits of Alaska king crab, shrimp, scallops or other pricey seafood. The process was developed by the Japanese and is now widely used in the United States. United States labeling laws require that *surimi* not be identified as real Alaska king crab, shrimp, scallops or whatever else it apes.

NUTRIENT CONTENT OF 3 OUNCES (85 GRAMS) SURIMI	
84 calories	122 mg sodium
13 g protein	95 mg potassium
1 g fat, 0 saturated	0 g dietary fiber
26 mg cholesterol	17 RE vitamin A
6 g carbohydrate	0.02 mg thiamin
8 mg calcium	0.02 mg riboflavin
240 mg phosphorus	0.2 mg niacin
0.2 mg iron	0 mg vitamin C

Susceptors: Metalized plastic films bonded to microwave cartons that draw the lion's share of the microwaves and get hot enough to crisp and brown pizza, also the metalized strips embedded in bags of popcorn that become searingly hot within minutes. The possibility of these materials' breaking down under such intense heat and releasing possibly noxious chemicals into food has been a matter of ongoing concern. See also PLASTIC.

Sushi: See SASHIMI, SUSHI.

Sustainable Agriculture: Farming that's both profitable and environmentally correct. The aim is to develop pest-resistant plants of high yield that produce top-quality food *and* protect the environment.

Sweating (nutrient loss and): You might call sweating nature's own air-conditioning; it's the way our bodies keep cool whenever temperatures soar or whenever we exercise long and hard. But like mechanical cooling systems, our own can fail. For example, if you lose more than 2 percent of your body weight through sweating, your temperature rises, your heart is stressed and your performance ebbs. In steamy weather, it's possible to lose a quart of sweat in half an hour. A fact all marathon runners know. They also know that if they're to have any shot at winning the race, they must continually replenish the fluid lost via perspiration, which is why you always see marathoners drinking on the run. Enter SPORTS DRINKS. These carefully formulated solutions of water, sodium, potassium and glucose plus other simple sugars may not rehydrate the body any faster than tap water, but they do appear to fight fatigue and reduce fluid loss.

Sweetbreads: The thymus gland and pancreas of calves (or lambs)—white, tender and as rich as all get out. Sweetbreads are loaded with cholesterol (3 ounces more than the day's quota). But they are also good sources of iron, phosphorus and potassium.

NUTRIENT CONTENT OF 3 OUNCES (85 GRAMS) BRAISED CALF SWEETBREADS

148 calories	56 mg sodium
27 g protein	291 mg potassium
4 g fat, 1 saturated	0 g dietary fiber
399 mg cholesterol	0 RE vitamin A
0 g carbohydrate	0.05 mg thiamin
3 mg calcium	0.14 mg riboflavin
583 mg phosphorus	1.7 mg niacin
1.7 mg iron	63 mg vitamin C

NUTRIENT CONTENT OF 3 OUNCES (85 GRAMS) BRAISED LAMB SWEETBREADS

199 calories	44 mg sodium
19 g protein	247 mg potassium
13 g fat, 6 saturated	0 g dietary fiber
340 mg cholesterol	0 RE vitamin A
0 g carbohydrate	0.02 mg thiamin
10 mg calcium	0.18 mg riboflavin
367 mg phosphorus	2.2 mg niacin
1.8 mg iron	17 mg vitamin C

Sweet Corn: See CORN.

Sweet Dumpling Squash: See SQUASH.

Sweetened Condensed Milk: See MILK.

Sweeteners: See ARTIFICIAL SWEETENERS; HONEY; MOLASSES; SUGARS.

Sweet'n Low: A popular brand of saccharin. See SACCHARIN; also ARTIFICIAL SWEETENERS.

Sweet One: A brand name for ACESULFAME-K, an artificial sweetener also known as **Sunette**.

Sweet Potatoes, Yams: Compared to the belated acceptance of that other New World potato, sweet potatoes landed on world tables with the speed of light. Columbus brought them back to Spain after his first voyage to the West Indies. And not many years later, the Portuguese ferried them from Brazil to Africa to Asia, where they remain staples to this day. The Spaniards planted sweet potatoes within a year of Columbus's homecoming, indeed were exporting them to England. History tells us that the English called them Spanish potatoes and that they were a particular favorite of Henry VIII, who loved them mashed and spiced and baked into pies. Even the French fancied sweet potatoes, for a time at least. First, Louis XV had them planted at the Trianon, but they plummeted from favor after he died. Then some thirty years later, Empress Josephine, who hailed from Martinique and longed for the sweet potatoes of her childhood, reintroduced them at Malmaison. Once again they became the rage, with Paris restaurants paying *beaucoup* for them. And once again they passed out of fashion, this time never to return.

It's a different story in the American South, where passions for sweet potatoes have never cooled. That's understandable. This is sweet-potato country, with miles of sandy flats in North Carolina, Georgia and Louisiana devoted to growing these fleshy tubers. Tabor City, North Carolina, has dubbed itself the Yam Capital of the World. Which brings up another point. What we call yams are no such thing. They are the moister, sweeter, orangier varieties of sweet potato beloved by Southerners. The rest of America prefers the drier, mealier, yellower, less sugary species called simply sweet potatoes. True yams (*Dioscorea alata*), which grow in the tropics and subtropics right around the globe, are as pale as ivory. They are plenty starchy but not very sweet. Sweet potatoes, especially the intensely orange ones, are bonanzas of beta-carotene. They

NUTRIENT CONTENT OF 1 MEDIUM-SIZED BAKED SWEET POTATO (WITHOUT SKIN)
(about 4 ounces; 114 grams)

117 calories	11 mg sodium
2 g protein	396 mg potassium
0 g fat, 0 saturated	3 g dietary fiber
0 mg cholesterol	2,486 RE vitamin A
28 g carbohydrate	0.08 mg thiamin
32 mg calcium	0.15 mg riboflavin
63 mg phosphorus	0.7 mg niacin
0.5 mg iron	28 mg vitamin C

Honeyed Sweets and Beets with Orange

Makes 6 Servings

1 pound medium beets, scrubbed well and trimmed of
    all but 1 inch of tops
1 pound small sweet potatoes, scrubbed but not peeled
¼ cup honey
2 tablespoons unsalted margarine, melted
½ teaspoon finely grated orange zest

¼ teaspoon ground ginger
⅛ teaspoon mace or grated nutmeg
¼ teaspoon salt
⅛ teaspoon freshly ground black pepper

PREHEAT OVEN TO 400°F. Parboil the beets and sweet potatoes in separate pans until firm-tender; the beets will take about 30 minutes, the sweets 20. Drain, cool, peel, and cut both into 1-inch cubes. Arrange the beets and sweet potatoes in a 9-inch pie pan lightly coated with nonstick vegetable spray, tossing lightly to mix. In a bowl, combine the honey, margarine, orange zest, ginger, mace or nutmeg, salt, and pepper and drizzle evenly over vegetables. Bake, uncovered, 20 to 25 minutes, basting occasionally with pan juices, until richly glazed.

APPROXIMATE NUTRIENT COUNTS PER SERVING

188 calories	31 g carbohydrate	1.1 mg iron	0.06 mg thiamin
3 g protein	3 g dietary fiber	153 mg sodium	0.14 mg riboflavin
4 g fat, 1 saturated	30 mg calcium	364 mg potassium	0.7 mg niacin
0 mg cholesterol	49 mg phosphorus	1,351 RE vitamin A	16 mg vitamin C

are also excellent sources of potassium and vitamin C and moderate ones of dietary fiber. Despite their sweetness, they are not very caloric. **SEASON:** Year-round.

Sweet Tooth: This craving for sweets not only exists but may well be inherited. Certainly, you are born with it. When researchers tested babies' reactions to different tastes, here's what happened. A drop of water on the tongue elicited no response. A drop of something sour made them screw up their faces; a drop of salt set them wailing. And a drop of sugar? Smiles all around.

Swiss Chard: See CHARD.

Swiss Cheese: A generic term applied to GRUYÈRE and Gruyère-type cheeses such as EMMENTALER—firm, pale yellow, nut-sweet and shot through with holes.

Swordfish: These deep-sea giants, which occasionally weigh 1,000 pounds or more, swim temperate and tropical waters around the world. They are feisty, often running their swords through a boat's hull, but they are elusive,

NUTRIENT CONTENT OF 3 OUNCES (85 GRAMS) BROILED/BAKED SWORDFISH

132 calories	98 mg sodium
22 g protein	314 mg potassium
4 g fat, 1 saturated	0 g dietary fiber
43 mg cholesterol	35 RE vitamin A
0 g carbohydrate	0.04 mg thiamin
5 mg calcium	0.10 mg riboflavin
286 mg phosphorus	10.0 mg niacin
0.9 mg iron	1 mg vitamin C

too—one reason sportfishermen consider them such a prize. Another is the meatiness of their pink flesh, which can be cooked like steak. Swordfish are classified as oily fish, meaning that their natural fats are evenly dispersed throughout their bodies instead of being concentrated in their livers. Because of their heft, swordfish have no pesky little bones, only big ones that can be lifted out with ease. The most common market forms of swordfish are steaks, either fresh or frozen. They are a powerhouse of niacin and a good source of phosphorus and potassium. Best of all, they're low in calories. **NOTE:** Ever since swordfish were found to have excessively high levels of mercury, a toxic metal, the FDA has been monitoring all catches— both domestic and imported—and banning the sale of those deemed unsafe.

Symphytine: An alkaloid in comfrey tea that is suspected of being a carcinogen.

Synthetic Vitamins and Minerals: Chemically they are identical to "natural" vitamins and minerals and are believed to be equally effective in the body. The principal difference? Price. The synthetics are usually significantly cheaper than the "naturals."

Syrups: See CORN SYRUP; MAPLE SYRUP.

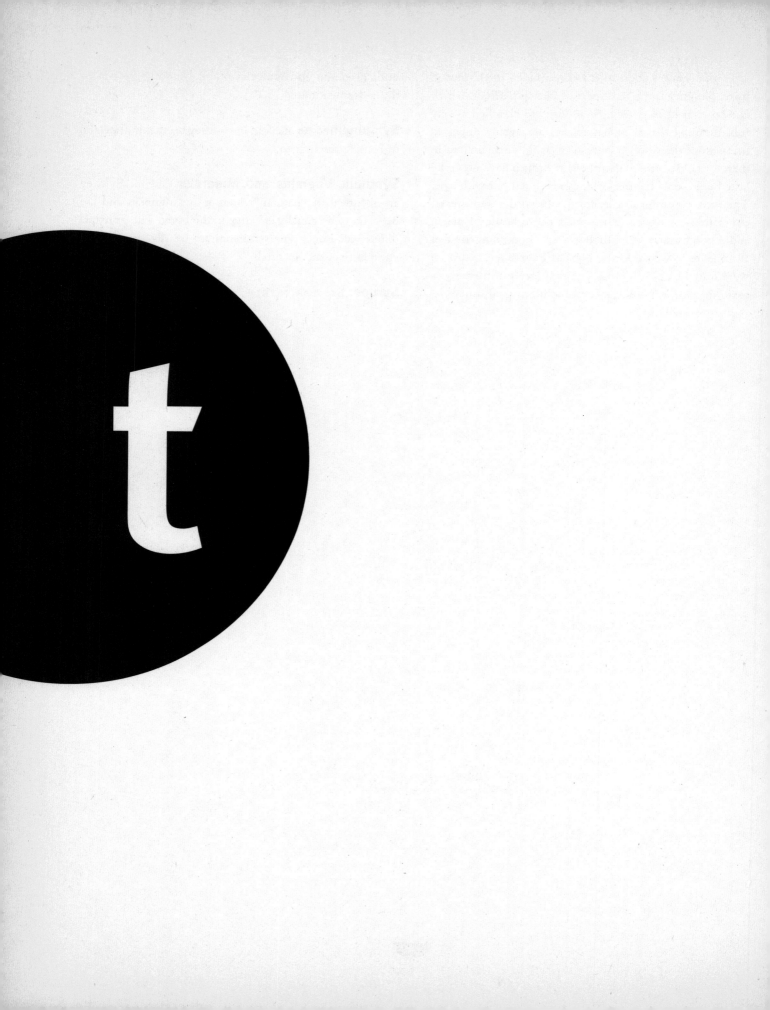

Tabasco Sauce: The trademarked name of a patented aged-in-oak hot red pepper sauce bottled in 1868 by Edmund McIlhenny of Avery Island, Louisiana, and now mass-produced by his descendants. America's first liquid red-pepper seasoning, Tabasco is a blend of vinegar, fermented red peppers and a dash of salt. No artificial colors. No stabilizers. No preservatives. And very little salt, so this is a good choice for those on low-sodium diets. A drop or two are all it takes to jazz up lackluster food.

Tabbouleh: The name by which cracked wheat is known throughout the Middle East, although spellings may vary from country to country. To prepare it, women boil wheat just until it splits, spread it in the sun and parch it for days. Then it's ground—fine, medium or coarse. *Tabbouleh* is also the name of a chopped tomato, mint and BULGUR salad that is popular throughout the countries that rim the eastern Mediterranean.

NUTRIENT CONTENT OF 1 TABLESPOON TABASCO SAUCE	
(about ½ ounce; 16 grams)	
2 calories	103 mg sodium
0 g protein	20 mg potassium
0 g fat, 0 saturated	0 g dietary fiber
0 mg cholesterol	44 RE vitamin A
Trace carbohydrate	0.01 mg thiamin
1 mg calcium	0.01 mg riboflavin
3 mg phosphorus	0.1 mg niacin
0.1 mg iron	0 mg vitamin C

Bulgur, Tomato, Onion, and Mint Salad (Tabbouleh)

Makes 4 Servings

Every Middle Eastern country has its own version of this crunchy cracked-wheat salad. This particular recipe comes from Lebanon, where the proportions of mint, parsley, and lemon are somewhat higher than in more arid countries. In Beirut, tabbouleh is integral to *mezze,* that nonstop procession of appetizers that amounts to a meal in itself. Tabbouleh is equally good with grilled chicken, fish, or lamb. Serve it on a bed of crisp romaine leaves.

⅔ cup bulgur

2 cups boiling water

½ cup coarsely chopped Italian (flat-leaf) parsley

⅓ cup coarsely chopped fresh mint leaves

¾ cup finely chopped yellow onion (about 1 medium onion)

1 cup diced vine-ripened tomato (about 1 medium tomato)

Juice of 1 large lemon

¼ teaspoon salt

¼ teaspoon freshly ground black pepper

3 tablespoons fruity olive oil

SOAK BULGUR IN boiling water for 15 minutes; drain well, bundle in a clean dry towel, and squeeze out as much water as possible. Place the bulgur in a deep mixing bowl, add remaining ingredients, and toss well. Let stand at room temperature 30 minutes, toss again, and serve.

APPROXIMATE NUTRIENT COUNTS PER SERVING			
200 calories	25 g carbohydrate	1.7 mg iron	0.11 mg thiamin
4 g protein	6 g dietary fiber	149 mg sodium	0.07 mg riboflavin
11 g fat, 1 saturated	36 mg calcium	339 mg potassium	1.7 mg niacin
0 mg cholesterol	100 mg phosphorus	93 RE vitamin A	36 mg vitamin C

Tacos: In Mexico, *taco* means a folded and stuffed tortilla, but in the United States it's a crisply fried, U-shaped tortilla. Popularized by fast-food taco stands, tacos are now packaged and sold like potato chips as shells for a variety of stuffings. Most tacos are made with cornmeal.

NUTRIENT CONTENT OF 1 CORN TACO SHELL
(about ½ ounce; 14 grams)

62 calories	24 mg sodium
1 g protein	33 mg potassium
3 g fat, 0 saturated	1 g dietary fiber
0 mg cholesterol	6 RE vitamin A
9 g carbohydrate	0.04 mg thiamin
34 mg calcium	0.02 mg riboflavin
31 mg phosphorus	0.2 mg niacin
0.4 mg iron	0 mg vitamin C

Tagatose, D-Tagatose: Artificial sweeteners now being researched for effectiveness and safety. Stay tuned.

Tahini: Sesame seed paste, which is integral to many Middle Eastern recipes, among them the creamy ivory dip called hummus. Made of pale, unroasted sesame seeds, tahini is slightly thinner than peanut butter and tastes faintly of nuts. Asians make a stronger, browner paste of roasted sesame seeds. Unless refrigerated, tahini quickly turns rancid.

NUTRIENT CONTENT OF 1 TABLESPOON TAHINI
(about ½ ounce; 15 grams)

91 calories	25 mg sodium
3 g protein	1 mg potassium
8 g fat, 1 saturated	1 g dietary fiber
0 mg cholesterol	1 RE vitamin A
3 g carbohydrate	0.24 mg thiamin
21 mg calcium	0.02 mg riboflavin
118 mg phosphorus	0.8 mg niacin
0.9 mg iron	0 mg vitamin C

Take-out Food: The danger is that the perishables may not be kept sufficiently cold—or hot—either on store counters or in transit. If they are left too long in the "danger zone," bacteria may proliferate and cause food poisoning. See BACTERIA; also SALAD BARS.

Taleggio: A supremely creamy Italian cheese also known as **Stracchino.** It has been made for centuries in the Taleggio Valley from the milk of cows that graze Lombardy's Alpine meadows directly above. The age-old recipes and methods haven't changed much—at least on farms where cheese making remains a cottage industry. There are two distinctly different Taleggios: an uncooked, mold-ripened one that's spreadable and "stinky" and a cooked, quickly aged one that's milder and a bit firmer. Both are the color of whipped butter. And almost as rich. **NOTE:** Specific nutrient counts are unavailable for Taleggio, but it's safe to say it's loaded with saturated fat, cholesterol and calories.

Tallow: The fat of lamb, mutton and beef (except that surrounding beef kidneys, which is suet). It's very brittle, very firm and highly saturated. Occasionally tallow is rendered and used as a cooking fat, mostly by fast-food restaurants.

Tallow Flakes (additive): These refined flecks of tallow are used to refine sugar and defoam beer. In tests with lab animals, they have clogged arteries in record time—within about a year. GRAS when used as the FDA directs.

Tamales: Any of a variety of fillings (usually savory), encased in cornmeal dough, then steamed in corn husks or banana leaves. Popular in Mexico since the days of the Aztecs, tamales long ago crossed the border to become staples throughout Texas and the Southwest. Today they are enjoyed from Maine to Monterey, the most common version being a spicy pork or beef/tomato/onion mincemeat wrapped first in cornmeal dough, then dried corn husks. If made with enriched cornmeal, tamales are a good source of thiamin, riboflavin, niacin and iron.

NUTRIENT CONTENT OF 1 MEDIUM-SIZE TAMALE
(about 2½ ounces; 70 grams)

182 calories	229 mg sodium
7 g protein	154 mg potassium
10 g fat, 4 saturated	2 g dietary fiber
24 mg cholesterol	18 RE vitamin A
16 g carbohydrate	0.24 mg thiamin
33 mg calcium	0.18 mg riboflavin
80 mg phosphorus	2.9 mg niacin
1.9 mg iron	4 mg vitamin C

Tamari: A dark, intense soy sauce that is popular in Japan and that is brewed the age-old way without the addition of wheat. See SOY SAUCE.

Tamarillos: Also called **tree tomatoes**—because they taste something like true tomatoes and, when sliced, look a little like them—these egg-shaped South American fruits now grow abundantly in the Caribbean, East Indies, Australia and New Zealand, from which most of our supply comes. Too tart to eat out of hand, tamarillos make splendid chutneys and sherbets. **SEASON:** Summer and fall. **NOTE:** Although nutrient counts are unavailable for tamarillos, their bright orange suggests that they brim with beta-carotene.

Tangelos: Slip-skinned, tart-sweet hybrids—part grapefruit (or pummelo), part tangerine. Tangelos are about the size of navel oranges but have a noticeable knob at the stem end. Like all citrus fruits, they are stellar sources of vitamin C and potassium. They are also low in calories, contain zero fat, cholesterol or sodium. **SEASON:** November to January.

NUTRIENT CONTENT OF 1 MEDIUM-SIZE TANGELO	
(about 3½ ounces; 95 grams)	
45 calories	0 mg sodium
1 g protein	172 mg potassium
0 g fat, 0 saturated	2 g dietary fiber
0 mg cholesterol	20 RE vitamin A
11 g carbohydrate	0.08 mg thiamin
38 mg calcium	0.04 mg riboflavin
13 mg phosphorus	0.3 mg niacin
0.1 mg iron	51 mg vitamin C

Tangerines: Also known as **mandarin oranges** (*mandarin* is an umbrella term applied to a number of loose-skinned citrus fruits), these easy-to-peel, easy-to-eat fruits have been tucked into millions of school lunch boxes, American mothers' stab at getting vitamin C into their kids. Sometimes it works. Would more schoolchildren eat tangerines if they knew how precious they were in ancient China, where they are believed to be native? That they are the treats St. Nikolaus leaves good German children at Christmastime? Or that they were introduced into the United States only in 1882? Probably not. Five varieties of

tangerines are now available: **Dancy** (the most popular), **Fairchild, sunburst, Robinson** and **honey, or Murcott. SEASON:** October through April.

NUTRIENT CONTENT OF 1 MEDIUM-SIZE TANGERINE	
(about 3 ounces; 84 grams)	
37 calories	1 mg sodium
1 g protein	131 mg potassium
0 g fat, 0 saturated	1 g dietary fiber
0 mg cholesterol	77 RE vitamin A
9 g carbohydrate	0.09 mg thiamin
12 mg calcium	0.02 mg riboflavin
8 mg phosphorus	0.1 mg niacin
0.1 mg iron	26 mg vitamin C

Tannic Acid (additive): This bitter commercial form of tannin is not a true acid but an acidlike substance called a polyphenol. It occurs naturally in tea, coffee, oak and sumac bark, and is used to clarify beers and wines, to refine fats, even to impart butter, caramel, maple and fruit flavorings to baked goods, candies, ice creams and liqueurs. GRAS when used as the FDA directs.

Tansy: An old-fashioned herbal remedy, still used in some quarters as a tonic and dewormer, also as a way to bring on the monthly period. Modern botanists consider tansy ineffective at best and unsafe at worst.

Tapeworms: See PARASITES.

Tapioca: Pearly little starch pellets obtained from raw cassava roots that are used to thicken puddings and pie fillings. Extracting cassava starch is fairly complex. Once peeled,

NUTRIENT CONTENT OF 1 CUP HOMEMADE VANILLA TAPIOCA PUDDING (WITH WHOLE MILK)	
(about 6 ounces; 165 grams)	
206 calories	314 mg sodium
8 g protein	234 mg potassium
7 g fat, 4 saturated	0 g dietary fiber
135 mg cholesterol	128 RE vitamin A
28 g carbohydrate	0.06 mg thiamin
172 mg calcium	0.35 mg riboflavin
173 mg phosphorus	0.1 mg niacin
0.5 mg iron	2 mg vitamin C

the roots are shredded to express the milky juices. These are soaked and their starch removed and sieved of impurities. The starch is then kneaded and sun-dried, then slowly heated on iron plates until it beads into tapioca. Today, quick-cooking tapioca has all but phased out the old-fashioned **pearl** or **fish-eye** variety.

Tapioca Starch, Tapioca Flour: Finely ground tapioca sold mostly in Asian groceries. It disperses quickly and completely, thus can be used to thicken sauces and gravies. Its thickening power approximates that of flour, but unlike flour, tapioca-thickened sauces are translucent, not opaque.

Tarama: The salty, cured roe of the gray mullet that is widely used in Greek cookery. Like all preserved roe, tarama is loaded with sodium. The eggs are small, not much bigger than grains of sand, and intensely orange, which gives *taramasalata,* the creamy, bread-thickened dip beloved by Greeks, its lovely salmon color.

Taro: See DASHEENS.

Tartaric Acid (additive): The acid found in grapes. Crystallized tartaric acid is one of the active ingredients in tartrate baking powders, the single-acting leaveners that produce cakes of uncommonly fine crumb. Tartaric acid is also used to acidify, emulsify and/or flavor baked goods, candies, processed cheeses, dehydrated egg whites, preserves and soft drinks. GRAS.

Tartrate Baking Powder: See LEAVENING AGENTS.

Tartrazine (additive): This is **Yellow Dye No. 5,** one of the most widely used artificial food colorings in the United States. A coal tar derivative, tartrazine has been tested for toxicity, carcinogenicity and ability to cause mutations in lab animals, so far with nothing to incriminate it on any of these counts. There's no denying, however, that some people are extremely sensitive to tartrazine—breaking out in hives, having trouble breathing. In addition, those who can't tolerate aspirin are apt to encounter similar problems with tartrazine. The FDA requires that tartrazine be identified on the labels of all the foods in which it is used.

TA Spoilage: *TA* stands for "thermophilic anaerobe." In plain English this means a microorganism with heat-resistant spores that thrive in the airless environment of canned foods. These bugs, unlike those responsible for foul-smelling SULFIDE SPOILAGE, form acids plus carbon dioxide and hydrogen gases as they grow, causing the food to sour. TA spoilage is most apt to occur in canned foods of low to medium acid—tomatoes and tomato pastes, for example, canned apricots, peaches, pears, even pineapple. The usual culprit? A benign cousin of the deadly *Clostridium botulinum* named *C. thermosaccharolyticum,* which splits the sugars in canned foods, building up sufficient heads of gas to bulge the ends of tightly sealed cans and sometimes enough to explode them. Needless to add, any spoiled foods should be disposed of at once where neither people nor animals will find them.

Taste: Acid . . . salt . . . sweet . . . bitter. Four distinctly different flavors and the only ones the taste buds on our tongues can detect. Everything else—flowery . . . spicy . . . grassy . . . musky—is a scent sniffed out by the nose. Our tongues are so highly specialized that certain areas zero in on specific tastes. The back of the tongue picks up sweet, the left or right side acid, the front salt, and the very tip bitter. See also TONGUE (FUNCTION OF).

Taurine: One of the nonessential amino acids. Rich in sulfur, taurine is a constituent of bile and helps, among other things, to regulate heartbeat, develop nerve tissue and stabilize cellular membranes. Meats and fish contain plenty of taurine, the reason VEGANS are apt to lack it. So, too, are infants, especially preemies. To approximate the nutritional value of breast milk, most baby formulas are now fortified with taurine.

TBHQ (additive): This stands for **tertiary butylhydroquinone,** a controversial petroleum-based antioxidant that's mixed into everything from beef patties to dried cereals to margarines to potato chips to pizza toppings. The FDA strictly limits amounts that can be used. Consumer-advocate groups want it off the market and out of our food.

T-bone: One of the choicest steaks. Cut from the loin, it contains nuggets of tenderloin. See BEEF.

Tea: The oldest caffeine drink known to man, a stimulant sipped down the centuries in China, Japan, India, Sri Lanka and the rest of Asia. The champion tea drinkers today, however, are the English, with iced-tea-guzzling Americans not far behind. All tea comes from a resinous evergreen Asian shrub (*Camellia sinensis*), so what determines whether tea will be **green, black** or **semifermented** is the way it's processed.

The most natural is green tea, which accounts for 22 percent of the world production. Once picked, the leaves are quickly steamed, then rolled and dried before they can oxidize (ferment) and change color. The best known green tea is **gunpowder** tea, so called because its tightly furled tiny leaves resemble buckshot. There are two other types of green tea: **young hyson** (medium-size leaves rolled lengthwise) and **imperial** (large leaves rolled, like gunpowder tea, into balls).

Making black tea is more complex. The leaves are first withered under waftings of warm, humid air, then rolled or broken to speed oxidation (fermentation), which converts the tea's colorless flavanols to orangy-brown phenols and mellows aroma and taste. Finally, black tea is fired or belted through a hot-air dryer, a trip of maybe twenty minutes. Black tea contains more caffeine than green tea but both have about half that of coffee.

Semifermented teas are less pure than green teas but less oxidized than the black. **Pouchong**, for example, is only 30 percent oxidized, **oolong** about 70 percent. Semifermented teas are often scented—with jasmine or other perfumy flowers.

Most of the other words in the tea lexicon have to do with the size or shape of the leaves. Or the part of the plant from which they come. For example, **orange pekoe** leaves are the longest and most delicate; **pekoe** and **souchong** second and third longest and strongest, respectively. Most of the teas sold in the United States are blends of teas grown in different parts of Asia—Ceylon (Sri Lanka), Darjeeling, Formosa. Blends, too, of orange pekoe and pekoe. Some are flowery, some citrusy, some smoky.

The buzz these days, however, centers on the cancer-fighting powers of both green tea and black tea. Results of a recent Shanghai study, reported in the *Journal of the National Cancer Institute*, show that nonsmoking, non-alcohol-drinking women who sipped green tea regularly lowered their risk of esophageal cancer by 60 percent (and men by 57 percent). Some American researchers also believe that green tea may help cure—or at least prevent—skin, stomach and lung cancers. And now research with mice at Rutgers State University in New Jersey suggests that black tea is as effective as green tea in preventing skin cancer. Al-

	A QUICK ALPHABET OF POPULAR HERBAL TEAS	
Type of Tea	**Health Claims**	**The Facts**
Alfalfa (leaves, tops)	Eases ulcers and other stomach disorders, lowers blood cholesterol, reduces stiffness and pain of arthritis, eliminates water retention.	It's ineffective and possibly unsafe for some people.
Aloe	Soothes the stomach, cleanses the colon. Applied directly, strong aloe tea speeds healing of superficial burns and wounds.	Can cause severe diarrhea but probably safe for healthy individuals.
Bayberry bark	Cures spongy, bleeding gums. As a gargle it relieves scratchy throat.	Too much of it can cause vomiting.
Burdock root	A diuretic that detoxes the system and soothes the kidneys.	Can blur vision, slur speech, cause hallucinations.
Catnip	Aids digestion; fights insomnia.	Probably safe for healthy individuals but of questionable efficacy.
Chamomile	A mild sedative that relieves stomach spasms and colic.	Can trigger severe reactions in those allergic to asters, chrysanthemums, goldenrod, ragweed, etc.

Type of Tea	Health Claims	The Facts
Comfrey (root, leaves)	Speeds healing of broken bones, wounds, internal irritations.	Unsafe.
Dandelion	Detoxes the body, may prevent anemia.	It's a powerful diuretic.
Devil's claw root	An antiinflammatory agent that reduces pain and swelling of arthritis and rheumatism.	Claims of miscarriage and abortion not verified. This is no miracle drug for arthritis, rheumatism or anything else.
Echinacea	Purges body, boosts immune system. Applied topically, disinfects boils and wounds.	Probably effective and safe for healthy people.
Eyebright	Cures conjunctivitis.	Ineffective, unsafe.
Ginseng	Alleviates impotence, high blood pressure, diabetes, chest colds, congestion, boosts immune system, protects against radiation.	Too much can raise blood pressure, cause nervousness, insomnia.
Goldenseal	Eases gastric distress, helps cure genitourinary disorders.	Ineffective and possibly unsafe yet should cause no problems for healthy persons.
Hops	Soothes nerves, cures insomnia, nervous diarrhea.	Of questionable use but safe.
Horehound (tops, leaves)	An expectorant that relieves bronchial congestion.	Safe and effective.
Hyssop (leaves, flowers)	Another expectorant that relieves chest congestion.	Also safe and effective.
Juniper berry	Aids digestion, eases gastrointestinal inflammation as well as pain of gout and rheumatism.	A powerful diuretic that can irritate digestive tract and cause hallucinations.
Licorice root	Releases a natural cortisone that restores hormonal balance. Also aids in healing of inflamed membranes and tissues.	Large doses can cause swelling, high blood pressure and cardiac arrest.
Lobelia	This tranquilizer makes it easier to stop smoking.	Can cause hallucinations, rapid heartbeat, acute respiratory distress, coma, even death.
Mistletoe (leaves)	Lowers blood pressure, prevents muscle spasms.	Unsafe.
Nettle (leaves)	Stimulates milk flow in nursing mothers. It also aids digestion, relieves neuralgia and kidney problems.	An effective diuretic.
Red raspberry (leaves)	Strengthens the uterus, prevents miscarriage, eases childbirth.	Safe, yes. Effective, no.
Sassafras	Soothes the nerves.	It contains the carcinogen SAFROLE.
Yarrow	Relieves menstrual cramps, aids digestion.	Like ragweed, to which it is related, yarrow can trigger allergic reactions..

Note: The name-brand herbal teas and blends sold in supermarkets are perfectly safe and good choices for those who want caffeine-free beverages. The reason these "teas" are caffeine free is because they contain no true tea.

though studies with humans are only preliminary, scientists are hopeful that black tea drinkers may also lower their chances of getting certain cancers.

What are the magic ingredients in tea? Phytochemists are focusing on a group of bitter polyphenols (tannins), among them catechin, gallocatechin and QUERCITIN. The race is on to isolate these compounds, to combine them with other known anticarcinogens in DESIGNER FOODS that may one day keep us all hale and hearty. See also PHYTOCHEMICALS.

In addition to the true teas, there are dozens of caffeine-free herbal teas drunk for a variety of reasons. Most are soothing, calming even. But health faddists also attribute preposterous healing powers to some of them. Those bottled as soft drinks may average 100 calories or more per 8 ounces. Check the label.

Teeth: See DENTAL HEALTH.

Teff: These dark brown "dust specks"—grains so tiny it takes 150 of them to equal the weight of a single wheat kernel—aren't to be sneezed at. They're nutritional giants. Two ounces of cooked teff supplies 25 percent of the Reference Daily Intake (Daily Value) of iron, 15 percent of the thiamin (vitamin B_1), 10 percent each of the protein and calcium plus moderate amounts of two other B vita-

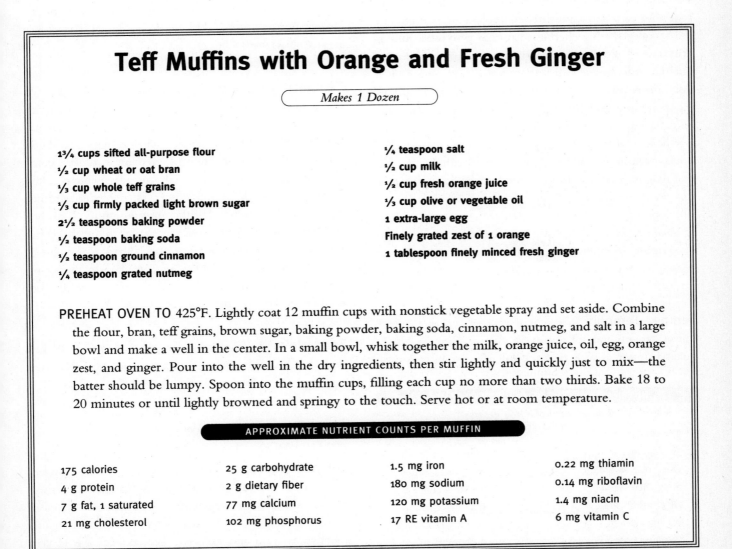

Teff Muffins with Orange and Fresh Ginger

Makes 1 Dozen

1¾ cups sifted all-purpose flour
½ cup wheat or oat bran
⅓ cup whole teff grains
⅓ cup firmly packed light brown sugar
2½ teaspoons baking powder
½ teaspoon baking soda
½ teaspoon ground cinnamon
¼ teaspoon grated nutmeg

¼ teaspoon salt
½ cup milk
½ cup fresh orange juice
⅓ cup olive or vegetable oil
1 extra-large egg
Finely grated zest of 1 orange
1 tablespoon finely minced fresh ginger

PREHEAT OVEN TO 425°F. Lightly coat 12 muffin cups with nonstick vegetable spray and set aside. Combine the flour, bran, teff grains, brown sugar, baking powder, baking soda, cinnamon, nutmeg, and salt in a large bowl and make a well in the center. In a small bowl, whisk together the milk, orange juice, oil, egg, orange zest, and ginger. Pour into the well in the dry ingredients, then stir lightly and quickly just to mix—the batter should be lumpy. Spoon into the muffin cups, filling each cup no more than two thirds. Bake 18 to 20 minutes or until lightly browned and springy to the touch. Serve hot or at room temperature.

APPROXIMATE NUTRIENT COUNTS PER MUFFIN

175 calories	25 g carbohydrate	1.5 mg iron	0.22 mg thiamin
4 g protein	2 g dietary fiber	180 mg sodium	0.14 mg riboflavin
7 g fat, 1 saturated	77 mg calcium	120 mg potassium	1.4 mg niacin
21 mg cholesterol	102 mg phosphorus	17 RE vitamin A	6 mg vitamin C

mins (riboflavin and niacin). And make a note, this same portion contains only 1 gram of fat, 0 cholesterol and, if unsalted, almost no sodium. Small wonder teff has been the "rice and wheat" of Ethiopia for centuries. Raw teff looks like celery salt; cooked teff, wet brown sugar. Either way, teff tastes good. There are hints of nuts, of new-mown hay, even, some say, of molasses or burnt sugar. Although boiled teff is a pleasant enough porridge (especially when cooked with raisins, then tossed with a handful of toasted hazelnuts or pecans), it's even better used to pump up the nutritional value of meat loaves, muffins and such. **NOTE:** Nutrient counts for teff more complete than those described above are unavailable.

Teflon: The commercial word for a slick plastic used to coat pots, pans and some kitchen implements that goes by the tongue-twisting chemical name of **polytetrafluoro-ethylene.** Teflon's plus: It allows you to cook with minimal fat, sometimes with no fat at all. Its minuses? Over time, many plastic coatings discolor, scratch and scuff, losing their nonstick abilities. As a result, they must eventually be replaced. There is concern in some quarters that when overheated, plastic coatings (particularly some of the earlier ones) break down, releasing potentially harmful chemicals that may migrate into food. Some researchers worry, too, that when used again and again to cook high-acid foods (tomato sauces, for example) or when repeatedly washed in alkaline detergents, plastic coatings may also begin to decompose. In other words, they are *reactive* (not so flame-proof glass or porcelain-clad cookware, which remain inert no matter what is put into them). See also SILVERSTONE.

Tempe, Tempeh: Fermented soybean cakes that are "meat" to millions of Southeast Asians. High in good-quality protein as well as chock-full of vitamins and min-

erals, *tempe* is a staple among strict vegetarians. Fairly bland of flavor and firm of texture, it can be diced and slipped into salads, soups, stews and stir-fries. Or it can be "frenched" and deep-fat fried.

Temperature: If perishable foods are to remain edible for days—or months—they must be properly refrigerated or frozen. This means keeping freezer and fridge at safe temperatures. Refrigerators should stay in the 32°F.–40°F. zone and the nearer 32°F. the better. For freezing food and storing frozen foods, freezer temps should never exceed 0°F. If there's a power outage, keep refrigerator and freezer tightly shut. Food will remain safe in the fridge for several hours; in a fully loaded freezer one to two days. Any frozen food containing ice crystals may safely be refrozen, but toss out squishy ones. See also REFREEZING; REFRIGERATION.

Tenderizing Agents: Tropical women have long known that a papaya, pineapple or fig juice rub would tenderize tough cuts of meat. All contain enzymes—PAPAIN for papaya, BROMELIN for pineapple, ficin for figs—that digest muscle and sinew. The active ingredient in today's commercial tenderizers is crystallized papain, which can soften 300 times its weight in lean muscle. These tenderizers must be used with discretion lest the meat go mushy. Usually a light sprinkle plus several jabs with a fork are sufficient. Most of the tenderizing takes place during cooking—at temperatures between 140°F. and 160°F.—so there's no need to marinate the meat at room temperature. Further cooking deactivates the enzymes.

Tenderloin: The long, moderately lean muscle tucked underneath the ribs. Because it receives no exercise, it's the tenderest cut of beef, veal, lamb and pork.

Tequila: See ALCOHOL, ALCOHOLIC BEVERAGES.

Teriyaki Sauce: A sweet but salty soy-based brown sauce used both at table and in the kitchen to season meats, fish, fowl and vegetables. It is a Japanese creation, a bottled version of the sauce put out as an accompaniment to teriyaki and sukiyaki. Teriyaki sauce is low in calories, contains no fat or cholesterol. But watch out for the sodium!

NUTRIENT CONTENT OF 1 CUP DICED TEMPE
(about 6 ounces; 166 grams)

330 calories	10 mg sodium
32 g protein	609 mg potassium
13 g fat, 2 saturated	NA g dietary fiber
0 mg cholesterol	115 RE vitamin A
28 g carbohydrate	0.22 mg thiamin
154 mg calcium	0.18 mg riboflavin
342 mg phosphorus	7.7 mg niacin
3.8 mg iron	0 mg vitamin C

NUTRIENT CONTENT OF 1 TABLESPOON TERIYAKI SAUCE
(about ⅔ ounce; 18 grams)

15 calories	689 mg sodium
1 g protein	41 mg potassium
0 g fat, 0 saturated	0 g dietary fiber
0 mg cholesterol	0 RE vitamin A
3 g carbohydrate	0.01 mg thiamin
5 mg calcium	0.01 mg riboflavin
28 mg phosphorus	0.2 mg niacin
0.3 mg iron	0 mg vitamin C

Tetracycline (in animal feed): See ANTIBIOTICS.

Tetrahydrolipstatin: The chemical name of a new "fat pill," known generically as ORLISTAT.

Textured Vegetable Protein (TVP): Chewy granules or spun fibers made from soy or other vegetable proteins that are used to make meat substitutes, to extend processed meats and fast-food burgers and to pump up the protein in pastas. Dried textured vegetable proteins, artificially colored and flavored and vitamin enriched, are sold by many groceries as ground meat extenders. They're a cheap but nutritious way to stretch meat loaves, burgers, meat sauces and stuffings. The USDA approves the use of TVP in public school lunches, provided it doesn't account for more than 30 percent of the combined meat/vegetable protein total and also meets the nutritional standards set by the department's Food and Nutrition Service.

To prevent fraudulent use of TVP in processed foods, the USDA devised the Ratio Rule. Here's how it works. When raw meat products contain as little as 1 part TVP to 13 parts meat (or cooked meats 1 part TVP to 9 parts meat), package labels need not list TVP except among the ingredients. Lower ratios (but no lower than 10:1 for raw meat products and 7:1 for cooked meat products) must be labeled "with textured vegetable protein added." For example, "beef lasagne with textured vegetable protein added." When the ratio of meat is even less, the label wording changes to indicate a more lavish use of TVP: "lasagne made with beef and textured vegetable protein."

Thawing Methods: No harm done if breads, cakes and cookies thaw at room temperature. Or frozen fruits and juices. But when perishables thaw, the microorganisms dormant inside them stir and, depending on how long the thawing takes and at what temperature, proliferate. The point is to thwart that proliferation.

Some frozen foods—precooked casseroles, lasagne and such—can move directly from freezer to oven. So can frozen raw meat loaves and brown-and-serve breads. Frozen vegetables, soups and sauces, needless to say, can go straight into the pot. But frozen roasts, steaks, chops, fish and fowl fare better if thawed, then cooked. The safest way is in the refrigerator because the cold slows bacterial growth. Small items soften quickly, but big ones—especially turkeys—take forever (about five hours per pound, to be specific). Be patient. *Or* thaw the turkey, still in its original plastic wrapper or sealed inside a plastic bag, submerged in a large kettle of cold water, changing the water every half hour. This trims thawing time to about thirty minutes per pound. Even faster is the microwave, but here you should follow the directions in the user's manual. Consult it, too, for microwave defrosting of everything from frozen juice concentrates to roasts to homemade soups and sauces. See also REFREEZING.

Theobromine: An alkaloid present in chocolate and cocoa. Like caffeine, to which it's related, theobromine is a stimulant, diuretic and vessel dilator.

Thermal Effect of Food: See SPECIFIC DYNAMIC ACTION.

Thermophiles: Literally, "heat-loving organisms," in particular bacteria with heat-resistant spores. If foods are faultily canned, these may survive, causing three different types of spoilage: FLAT-SOUR, SULFIDE SPOILAGE and TA SPOILAGE.

Thiamin, Thiamine: Vitamin B_1 (see B_1, VITAMIN).

Thiaminase: An enzyme that splits and deactivates the thiamin molecule. It's present in raw clams and mussels as well as in a variety of fruits and vegetables. Too much thiaminase can cause a vitamin B_1 deficiency. Fortunately, cooking depowers it.

Thiamin Hydrochloride, Thiamin Mononitrate: The forms of vitamin B_1 used in vitamin pills, enriched flours and cornmeals.

Thickening Agents (additives): Processors use oh, so many to smooth puddings and ice creams, to enrich soups and salad dressings, to improve the "mouth feel" of soft drinks and yogurts. Most are natural carbohydrates: **starches** of one sort or another (arrowroot, cornstarch, potato starch, rice starch), **gelatins, seaweed extracts, pectins, gums.** Of all the additives used, thickeners probably have the cleanest bill of health. See entries for individual thickeners.

Thirst (the elderly and): As people age, their need for water remains the same but their thirst decreases (so, too, may their kidney function). If they're to replace the 2½ quarts of water they lose every day (in urine, perspiration, stools, even by breathing), they must drink plenty of fluids. Otherwise they may become seriously dehydrated and die. Most physicians advise elderly patients to make a habit of drinking water, milk or fruit juices at certain hours every day.

Thompson Seedless: See GRAPES.

Threonine: One of the essential AMINO ACIDS. It's a major player in the synthesis of PURINES, which in turn break down uric acid, itself a by-product of protein digestion. Threonine is also key to bodily processes requiring glycine, a nonessential amino acid. Further, it piggybacks phosphate in phosphoproteins.

Thuringer: A smoky, hard, dry German sausage created in the German state of Thuringia. It may be made of pork or of a combination of pork, beef and/or veal. It is fairly fat and fine of grain. Today domestic varieties are widely available.

Thyme Oil (additive): A flavoring used primarily in sausages and processed meats. Yet thyme oil also shows up in everything from baked goods to candies to ice creams. It's extracted from the leaves and flowers of wild thyme, a creeper that grows abundantly both in the United States and abroad. GRAS.

Thymol (additive): An aromatic preservative obtained from the oils of lavender and sweet marjoram that's mixed into soft drinks, frozen desserts, baked goods, processed meats and soups. Some people may be allergic to thymol.

Thyroid Gland: This vital butterfly-shaped gland in the neck bracketing the larynx regulates body metabolism, speeds the absorption and use of glucose, sets the rate at which fats, carbs, proteins, vitamins, minerals and water are metabolized. Equally important, the thyroid absorbs and concentrates iodine, which in turn governs thyroid function. To do its appointed work, the thyroid secretes a number of hormones, among them thyroxine and triiodothyronine, which work in tandem not only to boost the conversion of glucose to energy but also to protect the body against physical and mental stress. Essential to proper thyroid function is the pituitary gland's thyroid-stimulating hormone (TSH) or thyrotropin, which controls iodine uptake and the synthesis of thyroxine. Major functions, all.

Thyroid-Stimulating Hormone (TSH), Thyrotropin: A pituitary hormone that directly affects two important thyroid functions: the absorption of iodine and the manufacture of THYROXINE.

Thyroxine: A hormone, the major secretion of the THYROID GLAND.

Tilapia: Is this St. Peter's fish? Some say that this Nile perch is indeed the fish of the apostle. It is a lean white-fleshed African fish now being farmed in the United States that shows up on restaurant menus with increasing frequency. But tilapia is not to everyone's taste. Says Mark Bittman in his definitive book, *Fish: The Complete Guide to Buying and Cooking:* "Every farm-raised tilapia I've ever had (and all the tilapia sold here is farm-raised) has had an undesirable, muddy flavor. I avoid this fish when I see it, and recommend that you do also." For approximate nutrient counts, see FISH, LEAN WHITE.

Tilefish: Three species of this deep-sea fish swim the Atlantic, the most abundant of which is the **common tilefish**, which prefers the cold waters of Nova Scotia, New England, New York and New Jersey. The other two Atlantic tilefish (**sand** and **blackline**) roam the warmer waters of the South, Florida and the Gulf. There's a **Pacific tilefish**, too, but its flesh is often bitter. When cooks speak of tilefish, they mean the common northern variety. This yellow, polka-dotted creature feeds on shrimps and crabs and its flesh is as white, as sweet, as firm as lobster. Although tilefish may weigh upward of 50 pounds, most common market sizes are in the 6- to 8-pound range. Tilefish are available whole, filleted and "steaked." Because of their firmness, they can be chunked and tossed into salads. They're also popular sashimi fish. As for nutritive value, tilefish are powerhouses of niacin, phosphorus and potassium. Yet they are low in calories, fat and sodium.

NUTRIENT CONTENT OF 3 OUNCES (85 GRAMS) BAKED/BROILED TILEFISH	
125 calories	50 mg sodium
21 g protein	435 mg potassium
4 g fat, 1 saturated	0 g dietary fiber
54 mg cholesterol	18 RE vitamin A
0 g carbohydrate	0.12 mg thiamin
22 mg calcium	0.16 mg riboflavin
201 mg phosphorus	3.0 mg niacin
0.3 mg iron	0 mg vitamin C

Tilsit, Tilsiter: This ivory cow's-milk cheese strewn with tiny holes is made in Germany, Switzerland and the United States. It's semisoft, loaf-shaped, a good all-purpose cheese that ranges from mild to robust, depending on age. There are plain tilsits, also tilsits studded with caraway seeds or peppercorns. Depending on the richness of the milk used, tilsit butterfat percentages range from 10 to 30 with some premium German varieties running as high as 60.

NUTRIENT CONTENT OF 1 OUNCE (28 GRAMS) TILSIT CHEESE (MADE WITH WHOLE MILK)	
96 calories	213 mg sodium
7 g protein	18 mg potassium
7 g fat, 5 saturated	0 g dietary fiber
29 mg cholesterol	83 RE vitamin A
1 g carbohydrate	0.02 mg thiamin
198 mg calcium	0.10 mg riboflavin
142 mg phosphorus	0.1 mg niacin
0.1 mg iron	0 mg vitamin C

Tin: Certain crimson/blue/purple foods (beets, red cabbage, blueberries, strawberries, raspberries and anything else containing anthocyanin pigments) turn blue-green when cooked or canned in tin. For that reason, tin-lined cans are lacquered. And for that reason, these fruits and vegetables should not be cooked in tin-lined copper pans, tin pie pans or other tin vessels. The chemical reaction doesn't make them unsafe to eat. But who can work up an appetite for blue beets?

Tin is one of the trace elements needed by the body. Concentrated in the liver and spleen, it appears to enhance growth. People eating a balanced diet get 3 to 4 milligrams of tin a day and deficiencies are unknown. Scientists worry about overdoses, however, which have upset iron and zinc metabolism in lab animals, lowering both their blood hemoglobin and serum iron. Apart from industrial contamination, the greatest potential tin hazards are unlacquered tin cans and cookware.

Tobacco: See CIGARETTE SMOKING.

Tocopherol: See E, VITAMIN.

Tofu: The Japanese word for **soybean curd** and the one by which it's generally known. Although the Chinese learned to curd soybean milk with seawater extracts before the time of Christ (and the Japanese, some thousand years later), tofu became a household word in the United States only in the 1960s. Most people thought of it as "hippie food," bland, boring stuff vegetarians ate instead of meat. Today millions of buttoned-down Americans have taken to tofu and supermarkets stock the two basic types—**soft** and **firm.** A few high-end markets sell fresh tofu, snowy blocks submerged in tubs of water. Most, however, sell mass-produced versions (curded, for the most part, with calcium sulfate or magnesium chloride) that are precut and packaged in plastic. Whole cookbooks have been devoted to tofu in recent years, and anyone interested in learning how to prepare it should ferret these out. There is every reason to explore tofu's potential. Not only is it a source

NUTRIENT CONTENT OF ½ CUP SOFT TOFU (about 4½ ounces; 124 grams)	
94 calories	9 mg sodium
10 g protein	150 mg potassium
6 g fat, 1 saturated	1 g dietary fiber
0 mg cholesterol	11 RE vitamin A
2 g carbohydrate	0.10 mg thiamin
130 mg calcium	0.06 mg riboflavin
120 mg phosphorus	0.2 mg niacin
6.7 mg iron	0 mg vitamin C

of high-quality protein, but it's also loaded with iron, phosphorus and potassium, and if curded with calcium salts (calcium sulfate, for example), it will also contain an impressive amount of calcium (the label should tell). Yet tofu is fairly low in calories and saturated fat, contains zero cholesterol and has almost no sodium. The newest development? "Lite" tofu with 75 percent less fat and only 35 calories per 3-ounce serving. See also PHYTOESTROGENS.

Tofutti: The brand name of a cholesterol-free ice cream made with TOFU. Several flavors are available and, depending upon recipe, may or may not be lower in fat than some of the new low-fat ice creams. Read labels carefully.

Tokay: Red table grapes. Several table wines, not necessarily made from this grape, are also called Tokay. See GRAPES.

Tomatillos: Some call them **Mexican green tomatoes;** others **Chinese lanterns.** In Spanish, they go by half a dozen different names. These tart, top-shaped, little green fruits with slip-off parchment husks are widely used throughout Mexico and the rest of Latin America to sharpen the flavor of sauces both raw and cooked. Though husked tomatillos resemble green cherry tomatoes, the two are only distantly related (both are in the nightshade family). Only recently have tomatillos begun to find their way into American supermarkets. They're bitingly tart, lemony, too, with musky hints of coriander—an acquired taste. Although tomatillos can be used raw (try them in salsa), cooking tames their tartness. **SEASON:** Spasmodically year-round.

NUTRIENT CONTENT OF 1 MEDIUM-SIZE TOMATILLO	
(about 1¼ ounces; 34 grams)	
11 calories	0 mg sodium
0 g protein	91 mg potassium
0 g fat, 0 saturated	NA g dietary fiber
0 mg cholesterol	4 RE vitamin A
2 g carbohydrate	0.02 mg thiamin
2 mg calcium	0.01 mg riboflavin
13 mg phosphorus	0.6 mg niacin
0.2 mg iron	4 mg vitamin C

Tomatoes, Canned: Not so long ago there were two choices—whole, peeled tomatoes and broken tomatoes. Today there are whole, peeled tomatoes packed in juice or tomato puree with or without basil, there are crushed tomatoes, broken tomatoes and sometimes tomatoes mixed with celery and assorted seasonings. For the health conscious, there are also canned tomatoes with considerably less sodium.

NUTRIENT CONTENT OF 1 CUP CANNED TOMATOES (PACKED IN JUICE)	
(about 8½ ounces; 240 grams)	
48 calories	391* mg sodium
2 g protein	530 mg potassium
1 g fat, 0 saturated	3 g dietary fiber
0 mg cholesterol	144 RE vitamin A
10 g carbohydrate	0.11 mg thiamin
62 mg calcium	0.07 mg riboflavin
46 mg phosphorus	1.8 mg niacin
1.5 mg iron	36 mg vitamin C

*In low-sodium brands, there are 31 milligrams sodium per cup.

NUTRIENT CONTENT OF 1 CUP CANNED CRUSHED TOMATOES (PACKED IN PUREE)	
(about 8½ ounces; 240 grams)	
60 calories	700 mg sodium
2 g protein	700 mg potassium
1 g fat, 0 saturated	NA g dietary fiber
0 mg cholesterol	100 RE vitamin A
12 g carbohydrate	0.06 mg thiamin
92 mg calcium	0.10 mg riboflavin
60 mg phosphorus	2.2 mg niacin
2.2 mg iron	12 mg vitamin C

Tomatoes, Dried: The oldest form of preserved tomatoes yet the newest to American cooks. Originally tomatoes were dried under the downpouring sun, but today they are air dried in ovens at low temperature. Most of our supply comes from California and can be bought as dried halves, dried bits or marinated in oil (the most expensive). All that's needed to plump dried tomatoes is two minutes in boiling water (3 ounces dried tomatoes will plump up

Spaghetti with Low-Fat Marinara Sauce

Makes 4 Servings

The sauce is so rich you'd never guess it contains just 2 teaspoons olive oil.

- **2 teaspoons fruity olive oil**
- **1 medium yellow onion, minced**
- **2 garlic cloves, minced**
- **1 small carrot, peeled and finely chopped**
- **2½ cups low-sodium canned tomatoes, chopped with their juice**
- **½ teaspoon finely grated orange zest**

- **2 tablespoons fresh orange juice**
- **¼ teaspoon salt**
- **⅛ teaspoon freshly ground black pepper**
- **⅛ teaspoon cayenne pepper**
- **2 tablespoons chopped fresh basil, or 2 teaspoons dried**
- **8 ounces fettuccine, cooked according to package directions and drained**

HEAT THE OIL for 1 minute in a large heavy nonstick skillet over moderate heat. Add the onion and garlic, and cook, stirring frequently, until golden brown and soft, about 10 minutes. Add the carrot and cook, stirring often, until carrot is tender, about 7 minutes. Add tomatoes, orange zest and juice, salt, pepper, and cayenne, and cook until sauce thickens and flavors marry, about 7 minutes longer. Stir in basil and toss with the hot pasta. Serve, if you like, with freshly grated Parmesan cheese.

APPROXIMATE NUTRIENT COUNTS PER SERVING

296 calories	57 g carbohydrate	3.4 mg iron	0.42 mg thiamin
10 g protein	6 g dietary fiber	166 mg sodium	0.22 mg riboflavin
4 g fat, 1 saturated	67 mg calcium	487 mg potassium	3.9 mg niacin
0 mg cholesterol	132 mg phosphorus	506 RE vitamin A	29 mg vitamin C

to 2 cups). What cooks love about dried tomatoes is their intense roasted tomato flavor. Also the fact that stored airtight in a cool, dry spot, they'll keep for about a year. Dried

NUTRIENT CONTENT OF 1 OUNCE (28 GRAMS) DRIED TOMATOES (NOT RECONSTITUTED)

73 calories	594 mg sodium
4 g protein	971 mg potassium
1 g fat, 0 saturated	4 g dietary fiber
0 mg cholesterol	25 RE vitamin A
16 g carbohydrate	0.15 mg thiamin
31 mg calcium	0.14 mg riboflavin
101 mg phosphorus	2.6 mg niacin
2.6 mg iron	11 mg vitamin C

tomatoes are endlessly versatile. Use them to enrich stews or pasta sauces, to enliven salads, risottos and scalloped potatoes. Mince them and mix into meatballs or loaves, sliver and scatter over pizza, or puree with garlic, dry mustard, freshly ground pepper and mayonnaise for a stellar cocktail dip or spread. The biggest disadvantage of dried tomatoes is the amount of sodium they contain (salt is added to help preserve them). Newer methods developed in California have now made it possible to dry tomatoes with minimal sodium.

Tomatoes, Fresh: Tomatoes didn't go mainstream America until World War I and then only because the government considered them highly nutritious and urged farmers to plant them. Given the popularity of tomatoes today, it's hard to imagine that just eighty years ago many Americans considered them poisonous. They were, after all, a member of the deadly nightshade family. Never mind that Mexicans and South Americans had been happily eating them for thousands of years, beginning with the cranberry-size wild tomato of Ecuador and Peru.

The juicy *tomatl* the conquistadores found in Mexico was a plumper, sweeter yellow variety developed by the Aztecs and Toltecs. These were the tomatoes carried back to Spain in the sixteenth century, the tomatoes the Spaniards grew mostly for show until an enterprising court chef simmered them into sauce with garlic, onions and olive oil. From that day forward, tomatoes changed the way Spaniards cooked. Italians, too, for they accepted the *pomi d'oro* (golden apple) at once. Still, the rest of Europe didn't trust tomatoes.

"In Spaine and those hot Regions," wrote the sixteenth-century English herbalist Gerard, "they used to eat the Apples of Love prepared and boiled with pepper, salt and oyle; but they yeeld very little nourishment to the body and the same naught and corrupt."

Today, tomatoes overflow supermarket bins. Red tomatoes, pink ones, orange, yellow, ivory and several shades of green. There are giant, meaty beefsteaks, common salad tomatoes, plum- and pear-shaped tomatoes, juicy little cherries and tart cranberries. But the tomato that's got everyone talking—and many *worried*—is the new genetically engineered **Flavr Savr** developed by Calgene, a biotech company in Davis, California. Ten years and twenty-five million dollars have gone into creating this summer-flavored winter tomato, which is tough enough to take cross-country shipping. Scientists did it by identifying the "softening" gene in tomatoes, reversing its structure to slow the ripening process, then injecting the backward gene into tomatoes. Their seeds contained the new genetic code, as did all the tomatoes descended from them.

The FDA spent four years testing the Flavr Savr for safety, reviewed the research with its food advisory committee composed of academics, nutritionists and scientists. All gave this new "test-tube tomato" a clean bill of health. Higher marks, too, than the "Styrofoam"-texture winter tomatoes that have been our lot. No one's ready to abandon homegrown, sun-ripened summer tomatoes, however. The Flavr Savr is on the market now, yet many Americans are loath to try it and consider it unsafe and possibly dangerous. The tomato, it seems, has come full circle. **SEASON:** Year-round with homegrown supplies peaking between mid-June and mid-September.

NUTRIENT CONTENT OF 1 MEDIUM-SIZE TOMATO
(about 4½ ounces; 123 grams)

26 calories	11 mg sodium
1 g protein	273 mg potassium
0 g fat, 0 saturated	2 g dietary fiber
0 mg cholesterol	76 RE vitamin A
6 g carbohydrate	0.07 mg thiamin
6 mg calcium	0.06 mg riboflavin
30 mg phosphorus	0.8 mg niacin
0.6 mg iron	24 mg vitamin C

NUTRIENT CONTENT OF 5 CHERRY TOMATOES
(about 3 ounces; 85 grams)

18 calories	8 mg sodium
1 g protein	189 mg potassium
0 g fat, 0 saturated	1 g dietary fiber
0 mg cholesterol	53 RE vitamin A
4 g carbohydrate	0.05 mg thiamin
4 mg calcium	0.04 mg riboflavin
20 mg phosphorus	0.5 mg niacin
0.4 mg iron	16 mg vitamin C

NUTRIENT CONTENT OF 1 MEDIUM-SIZE PLUM TOMATO
(about 2¼ ounces; 62 grams)

13 calories	6 mg sodium
1 g protein	138 mg potassium
0 g fat, 0 saturated	1 g dietary fiber
0 mg cholesterol	38 RE vitamin A
3 g carbohydrate	0.04 mg thiamin
3 mg calcium	0.03 mg riboflavin
15 mg phosphorus	0.4 mg niacin
0.3 mg iron	12 mg vitamin C

Tomato Juice: Canned or bottled tomato juices often contain a measure of tomato pulp as well as juice and some are slightly concentrated. The good news is that tomato juice is a surprisingly good source of beta-carotene, iron and vitamin C. Unfortunately, many brands are heavily salted. Scrutinize labels.

NUTRIENT CONTENT OF 1 CUP CANNED TOMATO JUICE
(8 fluid ounces; 244 grams)

42 calories	881 mg sodium
2 g protein	537 mg potassium
0 g fat, 0 saturated	2 g dietary fiber
0 mg cholesterol	137 RE vitamin A
10 g carbohydrate	0.12 mg thiamin
22 mg calcium	0.08 mg riboflavin
46 mg phosphorus	1.6 mg niacin
1.4 mg iron	45 mg vitamin C

Tomato Ketchup: That this was called a vegetable back in the Nixon years is laughable. When the president caught a lot of flak for lunching on ketchup-doused cottage cheese, his aides, in a silly stab at damage control, upgraded ketchup to "vegetable" lest Americans think their leader was junking out. For calorie counts and additional info, see KETCHUP.

Tomato Paste: A highly concentrated, often intensely salty tomato puree now sold in handy squeeze tubes as well as in cans. (Those on low-sodium diets please note: Low-sodium brands are now available.) Most tomato pastes are blended with spices and citric acid (an antioxidant that keeps the sauce bright red). Just a tablespoon or two enriches the flavor of tomato soups and sauces as well as a huge assortment of stews, meat loaves and meatballs.

NUTRIENT CONTENT OF 1 TABLESPOON TOMATO PASTE
(about ½ ounce; 16 grams)

14 calories	129* mg sodium
1 g protein	153 mg potassium
0 g fat, 0 saturated	1 g dietary fiber
0 mg cholesterol	40 RE vitamin A
3 g carbohydrate	0.03 mg thiamin
6 mg calcium	0.03 mg riboflavin
13 mg phosphorus	0.5 mg niacin
0.5 mg iron	7 mg vitamin C

*In low-sodium brands of tomato paste, there are 11 milligrams sodium per tablespoon.

Tomato Sauce: Canned tomato purees cooked with herbs and spices according to the manufacturers' well-guarded recipes. Many mass-produced tomato sauces are good enough to ladle over hot pasta—and they're significantly cheaper than the boutique tomato and marinara sauces sold in supermarket refrigerator sections. Canned tomato sauces do much to boost the color and flavor of soups, stews, chilis, meatballs and meat loaves. The nutritional value, too, for they supply hefty doses of beta-carotene, vitamin C and potassium—but, alas, equally hefty shots of sodium. Low-sodium tomato sauces are available.

NUTRIENT CONTENT OF ½ CUP CANNED TOMATO SAUCE
(about 4½ ounces; 123 grams)

37 calories	741 mg sodium
2 g protein	455 mg potassium
0 g fat, 0 saturated	2 g dietary fiber
0 mg cholesterol	120 RE vitamin A
9 g carbohydrate	0.08 mg thiamin
17 mg calcium	0.07 mg riboflavin
39 mg phosphorus	1.4 mg niacin
0.9 mg iron	16 mg vitamin C

Tongue (as food): Beef, veal, lamb and pork tongues are all highly nutritious, supplying impressive amounts of top-quality protein and iron plus moderate amounts of niacin and riboflavin. They are extremely tough, however, and must be simmered long and slow if they're to lose their rubberiness (not to mention some of their fat and salt). Beef tongue is available fresh, corned, canned, pickled and smoked, also chopped, jellied, sliced into cold cuts. Veal tongue is usually sold fresh; pork and lamb tongues precooked and ready to eat.

NUTRIENT CONTENT OF 3 OUNCES (85 GRAMS) COOKED BEEF TONGUE

240 calories	51 mg sodium
19 g protein	153 mg potassium
18 g fat, 8 saturated	0 g dietary fiber
91 mg cholesterol	0 RE vitamin A
0 g carbohydrate	0.03 mg thiamin
6 mg calcium	0.30 mg riboflavin
120 mg phosphorus	1.8 mg niacin
2.9 mg iron	0 mg vitamin C

NUTRIENT CONTENT OF 3 OUNCES (85 GRAMS) CURED BEEF TONGUE

235 calories	874 mg sodium
18 g protein	149 mg potassium
17 g fat, 7 saturated	0 g dietary fiber
89 mg cholesterol	0 RE vitamin A
0 g carbohydrate	0.02 mg thiamin
7 mg calcium	0.29 mg riboflavin
118 mg phosphorus	1.8 mg niacin
2.8 mg iron	0 mg vitamin C

NUTRIENT CONTENT OF 3 OUNCES (85 GRAMS) COOKED VEAL TONGUE

172 calories	54 mg sodium
22 g protein	138 mg potassium
9 g fat, 4 saturated	0 g dietary fiber
202 mg cholesterol	0 RE vitamin A
0 g carbohydrate	0.06 mg thiamin
8 mg calcium	0.30 mg riboflavin
141 mg phosphorus	1.3 mg niacin
1.8 mg iron	5 mg vitamin C

Tongue (function of): We taste with our tongues, but that's only one of the jobs of this muscular organ. Without a tongue it's difficult to chew and impossible to swallow. Once food is chewed, the tongue rolls it into small balls and pushes them down the throat toward the esophagus. The condition of the tongue is an indication of health in general and nutritional health in particular. Normal tongues are slightly rough, plump and pink. A sore tongue may be an indication of riboflavin deficiency; a swollen, mottled tongue a lack of niacin; a smooth tongue insufficient vitamin B_6; and a tongue that's both smooth and swollen a folic acid shortfall.

Tonic Water: See QUININE WATER.

Tonka Beans: These tropical pods are the source of artificial vanilla flavorings. The trouble is, they contain COUMARIN, which thins the blood and makes it slow to clot.

Tortillas: Unleavened Mexican "pancakes," paper thin and pliable enough to roll. Tortillas are usually made with a flour called MASA HARINA, which is milled from whole corn kernels that have been steeped in lime, dried and cured. But there are wheat tortillas, too. When tortillas are rolled and stuffed, they become TACOS. Tortilla chips are simply tortilla triangles or rounds crisped in deep fat. Popular for dipping guacamole and salsa, they're now almost as popular north of the border as potato chips.

NUTRIENT CONTENT OF 1 (8-INCH) CORN TORTILLA
(about 1 ounce; 30 grams)

67 calories	48 mg sodium
2 g protein	46 mg potassium
1 g fat, 0 saturated	2 g dietary fiber
0 mg cholesterol	8 RE vitamin A
14 g carbohydrate	0.03 mg thiamin
53 mg calcium	0.02 mg riboflavin
94 mg phosphorus	0.5 mg niacin
0.4 mg iron	0 mg vitamin C

NUTRIENT CONTENT OF 1 (8-INCH) WHEAT FLOUR TORTILLA
(about 1¼ ounces; 35 grams)

115 calories	169 mg sodium
3 g protein	46 mg potassium
3 g fat, 0 saturated	1 g dietary fiber
0 mg cholesterol	0 RE vitamin A
20 g carbohydrate	0.19 mg thiamin
44 mg calcium	0.10 mg riboflavin
44 mg phosphorus	1.3 mg niacin
1.2 mg iron	0 mg vitamin C

NUTRIENT CONTENT OF 1 OUNCE (28 GRAMS) CORN TORTILLA CHIPS

142 calories	150 mg sodium
2 g protein	56 mg potassium
7 g fat, 1 saturated	2 g dietary fiber
0 mg cholesterol	6 RE vitamin A
18 g carbohydrate	0.02 mg thiamin
44 mg calcium	0.05 mg riboflavin
58 mg phosphorus	0.4 mg niacin
0.4 mg iron	0 mg vitamin C

Total Parenteral Nutrition (TPN): Tube feeding, usually directly into the superior vena cava, completely bypassing the gastrointestinal tract. TPN is given to those who can't take food by mouth. The superior vena cava is a major vein, the one that carries blood from the head, chest, arms and hands directly to the heart.

Toxemia: See ECLAMPSIA.

Toxicity: The extent or degree to which something is poisonous.

Toxins: Poisons, some of them deadly, manufactured by plants or microorganisms that can contaminate food. See BACTERIA; FLOWERS AND PLANTS, POISONOUS; MOLDS.

Toxoplasmosis: An infection caused by a microscopic protozoan that's present in meats and poultry (also cats) that can be transmitted to humans. Toxoplasmosis has caused women to miscarry, also to deliver stillborn babies. See also PARASITES.

TPN: See TOTAL PARENTERAL NUTRITION.

Trace Elements, Trace Minerals: Minerals the body needs in minute amounts. The trace elements now generally recognized as necessary for good health are ARSENIC, BORON, CHROMIUM, COBALT, COPPER, FLUORINE, IODINE, IRON, MANGANESE, MOLYBDENUM, NICKEL, SELENIUM, SILICON, TIN, VANADIUM and ZINC. These utilitarian elements perform four basic functions: (1) They help the body burn (oxidize) fuel; (2) they help shuttle oxygen to red blood cells; (3) they are a component of proteins and nucleic acids; (4) they serve as coenzymes.

Trans Fatty Acids: Though these exist in small amounts in nature, the current concern today is that they are created when vegetable oils are hydrogenated to give margarines the consistency of butter or to create fluffy shortenings. American researchers have been aware of, indeed wary of, trans fatty acids (or trans fats) since the 1950s. But only in 1990, when two Dutch scientists, after studying fifty-nine men and women, reported that margarine actually increases the risk of coronary heart disease, did trans fatty acids take center stage. The anomaly is that trans fats are unsaturated yet substantially raise blood levels of "bad" cholesterol (LDL), which in turn accelerates the formation of fatty, artery-clogging plaques. At the same time, they reduce levels of HDL, the so-called "good" cholesterol, which flushes plaques away.

A more recent Harvard report estimates that trans fatty acids may be responsible for thirty thousand deaths from heart disease in the United States. *Each year!* That statistic has consumer action groups scrambling, demanding that food labels now include trans fatty acid content as well as total fat, saturated fat and cholesterol. Or, better yet, hazardous-to-your-health warnings.

Until then, you can often calculate the trans fat content of many food items. For example, if a label states that there are 15 grams total fat per serving (2 of them saturated, 3 monounsaturated and 5 polyunsaturated), the missing 5 grams are probably trans fats. You can also significantly cut down on trans fatty acids by (1) cooking with olive, canola or other largely unsaturated vegetable oils instead of margarine or shortening; (2) using soft tub margarine only and as little of that as possible; (3) shunning fast-food burgers, fries and hash browns, which may have been cooked in hydrogenated fats; (4) eating as few commercially baked cakes, cookies, muffins and pastries as possible; (5) cutting down on fat, period.

Transferrin: A globulin that binds and transports IRON in blood plasma. Synthesized by the liver, transferrin can be decreased by a number of conditions, among them kidney disease, uremia and chronic infections. During pregnancy, estrogen therapy, acute hepatitis and iron deficiency, transferrin levels rise. To test for transferrin (and whether there's too much or too little stored iron), doctors analyze a blood sample.

Transgenics: Genetically altered crops. See GENETIC ENGINEERING.

Travel (eating safely and): No one wants to get *turista*—or worse—while traveling. Although it isn't always preventable, you can reduce the risk if you know what to eat. Or, more important, what *not* to eat or drink. Most problems occur abroad because in the United States the FDA sets and enforces standards of sanitation for airline caterers, Amtrak, all forms of interstate public transportation. Still, it pays to be careful.

Veteran travelers don't drink the water, insisting instead on carbonated mineral waters with plenty of fizz (these are less likely to have been tampered with than nonsparkling waters) and they take their drinks neat, never with ice. They eat simply, sticking with well-done meat, fish or fowl (and avoiding these in much of the Third World). They refuse fussy foods, overhandled dishes such as salads (especially those containing meat, poultry or fish), meatballs and meat loaves, casseroles, aspics and gelatins. They pass on cream sauces and gravies, raw vegetables, raw fish or shellfish and eat only thick-skinned fruits they can peel themselves. They insist that hot foods be steaming and all dairy foods pasteurized, packaged in tightly sealed serving-size containers and properly cold. They shun buffets, especially those that have languished on sunny decks or patios, confining themselves to breads, crackers, well-aged hard cheeses and the safe fruits just mentioned. Finally, they brush their teeth with mouthwash.

Such measures may seem extreme. And they are unnecessary throughout Western Europe (except maybe the boonies). But in Asia, the Middle East, Africa, Latin and South America they have kept many travelers on their feet while their more careless companions were flattened for days. See also AIRPLANE FOOD; BACTERIA; PARASITES.

Tree Tomatoes: See TAMARILLOS.

Tribasic Calcium Phosphate: See PHOSPHATES.

Triceps Skinfold Measurement: See SKINFOLD TESTS.

Trichinosis: A serious, sometimes fatal parasitic infection caused by eating raw or rare pork. In the old days when pigs were slopped (thrown buckets of kitchen garbage), trichinosis was more common than it is in these days of pampered, ration-fed hogs. Still, it pays to cook pork to an internal temperature of at least 140°F. or, better yet 150°F., because not all meat thermometers are on the mark. And many people—old-time Southerners mostly—won't touch pork unless it's well done (170°F.). **NOTE:** Freezing also kills trichinae, the microscopic parasites that cause trichinosis. See also PARASITES.

Triglycerides: See GLYCERIDES.

Tripe: The muscular lining of the stomach of steers, calves, lambs or hogs. The most delicate, **honeycomb tripe,** comes from the second stomach of beef. The next best is **pocket tripe** from lower down in the stomach, and the cheapest (and strongest) is **smooth** or **plain tripe.** Much of the tripe available today is frozen, pickled or canned although big-city markets also sell it fresh (this has been parboiled but needs further cooking, indeed *long* simmering, to make it tender). Tripe is riddled with fat, but these chunks are easily separated from the lean and discarded. Most Europeans like tripe but the French and Portuguese take top honors, if only for two classic recipes—Tripes à la Mode de Caen and Tripas à Moda de Porto. Unfortunately, few Americans have acquired a taste for tripe.

NUTRIENT CONTENT OF 3 OUNCES (85 GRAMS) BOILED HONEYCOMB TRIPE	
85 calories	62 mg sodium
13 g protein	85 mg potassium
4 g fat, 2 saturated	0 g dietary fiber
58 mg cholesterol	0 RE vitamin A
0 g carbohydrate	0 mg thiamin
128 mg calcium	0.07 mg riboflavin
77 mg phosphorus	0 mg niacin
0.6 mg iron	3 mg vitamin C

Trisodium Phosphate (TSP) (additive): Long employed as a preservative/stabilizer in evaporated milk and processed cheeses, TSP, an intensely alkaline compound, is now being used by poultry producers to reduce salmonella contamination in chickens. According to the USDA's Food Safety and Inspection Service, the incidence of salmonella among untreated birds is about 25 percent. But when inspected birds are dipped in a TSP solution (which alters neither taste nor texture), that rate plummets to less than 5 percent. The USDA has given TSP dips its blessing but points out that they do not kill all bacteria and that unless birds are carefully handled, they can be recontaminated once they leave the processing plant. GRAS.

Triterpenoids: Natural compounds present in citrus fruits, licorice root extracts and other foods that may reduce the risk of breast cancer. See also PHYTOCHEMICALS.

Triticale, Triticale Flour: Triticale (pronounced *trit-uh-KAY-lee*) is a man-made, high-protein rye-wheat hybrid with impressive amounts of lysine (an essential amino acid) and a pleasant nutty flavor. Although triticale is rolled into flakes and toasted like oatmeal, the bulk of the U.S. crop is milled into flour. Triticale flour contains more gluten than rye but less than wheat, thus it makes heavy bread unless combined with wheat flour (2 parts wheat to 1 part triticale is a good ratio).

NUTRIENT CONTENT OF 1 CUP TRITICALE FLOUR
(about 4²/₃ ounces; 130 grams)

439 calories	3 mg sodium
17 g protein	605 mg potassium
2 g fat, 0 saturated	19 g dietary fiber
0 mg cholesterol	0 RE vitamin A
95 g carbohydrate	0.49 mg thiamin
46 mg calcium	0.17 mg riboflavin
417 mg phosphorus	3.7 mg niacin
3.4 mg iron	0 mg vitamin C

Trout: Unless you go after your own or have anglers in the family, the trout you eat will be farm raised. And pallid compared to the **rainbow, golden, brook** and **brown trout** that swim America's cold, rushing rivers. Wild trout feed upon crayfish when they're available and a steady diet of these yields superbly sweet, salmon-pink flesh. Farm-raised trout are paler and disappointingly bland. Like salmon, trout are oily fish, meaning their fat is evenly distributed throughout the lean. They come to market both fresh and frozen, whole (averaging 6 to 12 inches in length), gutted, split or filleted. See also SALMON TROUT.

NUTRIENT CONTENT OF 3 OUNCES (85 GRAMS) BROILED/BAKED RAINBOW TROUT

128 calories	48 mg sodium
20 g protein	381 mg potassium
5 g fat, 1 saturated	0 g dietary fiber
59 mg cholesterol	13 RE vitamin A
0 g carbohydrate	0.13 mg thiamin
73 mg calcium	0.08 mg riboflavin
229 mg phosphorus	4.9 mg niacin
0.3 mg iron	2 mg vitamin C

NUTRIENT CONTENT OF 3 OUNCES (85 GRAMS) PANFRIED RAINBOW TROUT

151 calories	68 mg sodium
20 g protein	472 mg potassium
7 g fat, 3 saturated	0 g dietary fiber
67 mg cholesterol	43 RE vitamin A
0 g carbohydrate	0.11 mg thiamin
12 mg calcium	0.18 mg riboflavin
231 mg phosphorus	4.3 mg niacin
0.6 mg iron	1 mg vitamin C

Truffles: Edible fungi that mature underground and cost (you'll excuse it) the earth. They have neither roots nor stems, look like lumps of coal or clay and grow best in porous limestone soil among the roots of scrub oaks, beeches and birches. The world's finest truffles, by most accounts, are the black truffles of the Périgord in southwest France (most of us must settle for the canned, no match for the fresh). Some liken the flavor of black truffles to oysters, others to meaty porcini mushrooms, still others to roasted hazelnuts. Perhaps a bit of all three is more on target. There are white truffles, too, gnarled lumps of beige or brown, that grow best in the north of Italy. Both species elude man, so the French use pigs to root them out and the Italians, specially trained dogs. For centuries man has tried to cultivate truffles—so far with little success. Even today only the rich can afford them, which has given truffles considerable snob appeal. Apparently it was ever thus. Pliny urged wealthy Romans to prepare truffles with their own hands; they were too precious to entrust to servants. Centuries later (in 1825) Brillat-Savarin wrote, "Nobody dares admit that he has been present at a meal where there was not at least one dish of truffles." And seventy-five or one hundred years after that, when asked by a social-climbing Paris hostess how he liked his truffles, the celebrated gourmet Curnonsky replied, "In great quantity, madame. In great quantity." **NOTE:** Nutrient counts unavailable for truffles.

Trypsin: An enzyme integral to the digestion of protein foods. The pancreas manufactures its precursor, trypsinogen, which is activated in the small intestine.

Trypsin Inhibitor: A substance found in raw egg white, soybeans and other legumes that inhibits the body's ability to digest and use protein. Fortunately, cooking destroys the trypsin inhibitor.

Tryptophan: One of the nine essential AMINO ACIDS. Tryptophan is also a precursor of NIACIN (a B vitamin) and of SEROTONIN, a brain neurotransmitter that regulates appetite, pain, mood and sleep. Because of tryptophan's mood-elevating, sleep-inducing capabilities, it is prescribed in Canada, Germany and other European countries as both a sleeping pill and an antidepressant. Until recently, the United States considered this amino acid a food supplement and as such it was exempt from the rules governing drugs. This meant megabucks for health-food stores and supplement manufacturers who touted their L-tryptophan supplements as "nature's own sleeping pills." Insomniacs began popping L-tryptophan pills, powders and potions as if there were no tomorrow. For some, alas, there *was* none. In 1989, an outbreak of eosinophilia-myalgia syndrome (EMS), a rare and incurable blood disease, felled more than fifteen hundred people and killed nearly forty (the FDA now puts the total number affected at five thousand). While tracking the source of the illness, biomedical researchers discovered that all victims had one thing in common. They'd been taking high doses of L-tryptophan supplements manufactured in Japan, supplements, it turns out, that were contaminated. Were the contaminants responsible? Or was tryptophan itself dangerous? The FDA wasted no time ordering recalls of all tryptophan supplements. It now aims to study tryptophan carefully to determine its efficacy and safety and to make it available only by prescription.

Tuna: Few fish are more fabled than tuna. In his endlessly fascinating *Encyclopedia of Fish Cookery*, A. J. McClane writes that Aristotle believed "tuna grew to a weight of 15 talents [1,200 pounds] . . . and lived for two years, becoming fat to the point of exploding." Later Greeks believed tuna fed on the acorns of submarine Mediterranean oaks, which accounted for their rich, sweet flesh. Not for nothing did they call tuna *porco marino* ("sea pig"). Even today, some of the lighter, fatter tunas taste like pork. And the leaner, redder ones like beef. Unfortunately, few Americans living beyond the megalopolises of the East Coast and West have tasted fresh tuna. Sadly, only about 1 percent of the supply, most of it caught in the Pacific, comes to market fresh or frozen. The rest goes into cans. From a commercial standpoint, the most important tunas, all members of the mackerel family, are **albacore** (white meat), **bluefin** (dark to light meat), **bonito** (so dark and strong it cannot legally be labeled "tuna"), **skipjack** (light meat, a sashimi favorite) and **yellowfin** (light). Tuna is categorized as an oily fish, meaning its oils are distributed throughout its flesh instead of being concentrated in the liver, as they are in halibut and cod. Nearly all fresh and frozen tuna is sold as steak. With canned tuna there's more variety. It may be flaked or chunked, all white meat, all light or a mixture of light and dark. Finally, it may be packed in water or in oil with or without added salt.

In recent years there's been noisy media hysteria about the presence of cockroach legs in canned tuna—all brands,

---

NUTRIENT CONTENT OF 3 OUNCES (85 GRAMS) CANNED ALBACORE TUNA (PACKED IN WATER)

116 calories	333 mg sodium
23 g protein	241 mg potassium
2 g fat, 1 saturated	0 g dietary fiber
36 mg cholesterol	20 RE vitamin A
0 g carbohydrate	0 mg thiamin
3 mg calcium	0.04 mg riboflavin
227 mg phosphorus	4.9 mg niacin
0.5 mg iron	0 mg vitamin C

NUTRIENT CONTENT OF 3 OUNCES (85 GRAMS) CANNED ALBACORE TUNA (PACKED IN OIL)

158 calories	337 mg sodium
23 g protein	283 mg potassium
7 g fat, 1 saturated	0 g dietary fiber
26 mg cholesterol	20 RE vitamin A
0 g carbohydrate	0.01 mg thiamin
3 mg calcium	0.07 mg riboflavin
227 mg phosphorus	9.9 mg niacin
0.6 mg iron	0 mg vitamin C

NUTRIENT CONTENT OF 3 OUNCES (85 GRAMS) CANNED LIGHT TUNA (PACKED IN WATER)

99 calories	288 mg sodium
22 g protein	202 mg potassium
1 g fat, 0 saturated	0 g dietary fiber
26 mg cholesterol	14 RE vitamin A
0 g carbohydrate	0.03 mg thiamin
9 mg calcium	0.06 mg riboflavin
138 mg phosphorus	11.3 mg niacin
1.3 mg iron	0 mg vitamin C

NUTRIENT CONTENT OF 3 OUNCES (85 GRAMS) CANNED LIGHT TUNA (PACKED IN OIL)

169 calories	301 mg sodium
25 g protein	175 mg potassium
7 g fat, 1 saturated	0 g dietary fiber
15 mg cholesterol	20 RE vitamin A
0 g carbohydrate	0.03 mg thiamin
11 mg calcium	0.10 mg riboflavin
265 mg phosphorus	10.6 mg niacin
1.2 mg iron	0 mg vitamin C

all grades. Not to worry. The FDA sets action levels, meaning allowable amounts (always minute) of foreign bodies in food. These (hairs, insect parts, etc.) occur in everything we eat, not just in cans of tuna. For manufacturers to ensure that every box, every can, every container of food is purer than God made it would be prohibitive. Moreover, the canning, processing and/or pasteurization of food make these foreign bodies completely harmless. **AND HERE'S AN IRONY:** Water-packed tuna contains more of the cholesterol-lowering omega-3 fatty acids than the oil packed,

NUTRIENT CONTENT OF 3 OUNCES (85 GRAMS) GRILLED/BROILED FRESH ALBACORE TUNA	
128 calories	60 mg sodium
21 g protein	390 mg potassium
4 g fat, 1 saturated	0 g dietary fiber
54 mg cholesterol	34 RE vitamin A
0 g carbohydrate	0.09 mg thiamin
26 mg calcium	0.09 mg riboflavin
208 mg phosphorus	5.4 mg niacin
1.2 mg iron	1 mg vitamin C

NUTRIENT CONTENT OF 3 OUNCES (85 GRAMS) GRILLED/BROILED FRESH BLUEFIN TUNA	
156 calories	43 mg sodium
26 g protein	275 mg potassium
5 g fat, 1 saturated	0 g dietary fiber
42 mg cholesterol	644 RE vitamin A
0 g carbohydrate	0.24 mg thiamin
9 mg calcium	0.26 mg riboflavin
278 mg phosphorus	8.9 mg niacin
1.1 mg iron	0 mg vitamin C

Hi-Vi Tuna Salad

Makes 8 Servings

If you chop the onion in a food processor, you can add all remaining dressing ingredients and pulse quickly to combine. Pour over salad and toss well to mix.

- **1 cup finely diced carrots (about 2 medium carrots)**
- **¾ cup finely diced celery (about 2 small to medium ribs)**
- **2 cans (12¼ ounces each) water-packed solid white tuna, well drained and flaked**
- **2 tablespoons well-drained small capers**
- **¾ cup coarsely chopped yellow onion (about 1 medium onion)**
- **¾ cup nonfat mayonnaise**
- **⅓ cup plain nonfat yogurt**
- **1 tablespoon Dijon mustard**
- **1 teaspoon ketchup**
- **1 teaspoon dried marjoram**
- **½ teaspoon dried dill**
- **½ teaspoon finely grated lemon zest**
- **¼ teaspoon freshly ground black pepper**
- **¼ teaspoon hot red pepper sauce**

PARBOIL THE CARROTS in a small pan of boiling water for 4 minutes. Add the celery and boil 1 minute longer. Drain well, spread between clean dish towels, and cool. Meanwhile, place the tuna, capers, and onion in a large mixing bowl. In a small bowl, combine all remaining ingredients and add to tuna mixture along with the carrot mixture. Toss well, cover, and refrigerate at least 1 hour before serving.

APPROXIMATE NUTRIENT COUNTS PER SERVING

165 calories	9 g carbohydrate	1.2 mg iron	0.04 mg thiamin
25 g protein	1 g dietary fiber	676 mg sodium	0.11 mg riboflavin
3 g fat, 1 saturated	43 mg calcium	421 mg potassium	5.4 mg niacin
45 mg cholesterol	276 mg phosphorus	531 RE vitamin A	4 mg vitamin C

mostly because these fatty acids dissolve in the vegetable oils used to pack the tuna, which are drained off. See also FISH OILS.

Turban Squash: See SQUASH.

Turbinado: See SUGARS.

Turbot: There is turbot (Pacific flounder) and there is turbot (a fine European flatfish of the sole family). The European is far superior, firmer of flesh, sweeter, too. All turbot are lean and white and can be cooked in any way

that suits sole or flounder. They are available both fresh and frozen, usually as fillets. For approximate nutrient counts, see FISH, LEAN WHITE.

Turkey: "I wish the Bald Eagle had not been chosen as the Representative of our country! The turkey is a much more respectable Bird, and withall a true original native of America." Thus wrote Benjamin Franklin. No doubt many Americans would agree with him today, not least the turkey growers, who raise some three hundred million of these birds every year. Today's white-feathered turkeys are a far cry from what the Pilgrims ate. They are broad-

Forty-Minute Hot-as-You-Like-It Turkey Chili

Makes 6 Servings

Old-timey beef chili brims with fat, cholesterol, and calories. But not this healthful variation made with ground turkey.

- 1 tablespoon olive oil
- 1 large yellow onion, chopped
- 3 garlic cloves, minced
- 1 large green bell pepper, cored, seeded, and diced
- 1¾ teaspoons chile powder
- 1¼ teaspoons dried oregano
- ¾ teaspoon ground cumin
- 1 can (14½ ounces) no-salt-added stewed tomatoes, chopped with their juices

- 2 tablespoons no-salt-added tomato paste
- ¾ cup water
- 1 pound ground turkey
- 3 cups cooked or canned red kidney beans, rinsed and drained
- ½ teaspoon salt, or to taste
- 1 tablespoon fresh lime juice
- 6 drops hot red pepper sauce, or to taste

HEAT THE OIL for 1 minute in a large heavy kettle over moderate heat. Add the onion and garlic, and cook, stirring occasionally, until onion is limp and glassy, about 7 minutes. Stir in the green pepper, and cook, stirring occasionally, until softened, about 5 minutes. Blend in the chile powder, oregano, and cumin and cook, stirring, 1 minute. Add the tomatoes, tomato paste, and water, and bring to a boil. Adjust heat so mixture bubbles gently, cover, and cook 4 to 5 minutes to blend flavors. Mix in the turkey, breaking up clumps, and then add beans and salt. Simmer, uncovered, until turkey is cooked through and chili is lightly thickened, about 20 minutes. Stir in lime juice and hot pepper sauce and serve.

APPROXIMATE NUTRIENT COUNTS PER SERVING

301 calories	30 g carbohydrate	4.8 mg iron	0.23 mg thiamin
24 g protein	9 g dietary fiber	260 mg sodium	0.19 mg riboflavin
10 g fat, 2 saturated	80 mg calcium	801 mg potassium	4.0 mg niacin
55 mg cholesterol	265 mg phosphorus	87 RE vitamin A	25 mg vitamin C

breasted, tender and succulent thanks to rations of soy, corn and vitamins (but no hormones, which the government forbids). Nearly all farm-raised turkeys coming to market are infants or adolescents and all are available either fresh or frozen. The National Turkey Federation classifies them thus:

Fryer-Roasters: Males or females less than sixteen weeks old weighing between 6 and 9 pounds.

Young Hens: Sixteen-week-old females averaging 16 to 18 pounds.

Young Toms: Nineteen-week-old males averaging 28 to 30 pounds.

Young Turkeys: Males or females weighing 10 to 15 pounds.

There are also **self-basting turkeys,** birds that have been injected with mixes of partially hydrogenated soybean oil, water, salt, sodium phosphate and emulsifiers made to taste like butter. Because these birds all but cook themselves, they land on 20 percent of America's Thanksgiving tables. The once-popular **prestuffed turkeys** have fallen from favor because of the danger of salmonella food poisoning. For absolute safety, these prestuffed birds must be kept solidly frozen throughout their long journey from processing plant to supermarket to oven.

Today's newly popular "**wild turkeys**" are nothing more than the old **Bronze,** a small, dark-feathered breed averaging 7 to 10 pounds that was phased out in the fifties and sixties in favor of the plump white "super turkey." Many farmers let their Bronzes run free, scratching about for berries, seeds, acorns and insects, which, they say, give them gamier flavor. But make no mistake. These "wild" turkeys are farm raised. The only way to enjoy honest to God wild turkey is to shoot it yourself.

Ninety-five percent of America's turkeys are inspected for wholesomeness by the USDA and bear round inspection stamps on their packages. Many are also graded for quality (look for a shield-shaped emblem). Most turkeys are Grade A, meaning they're well shaped, meaty, free of nicks, tears, bruises, broken bones and almost all pinfeathers.

Turnip Cabbage: See KOHLRABI.

Turnip Greens, Turnip Salad: "Mess o' greens" is what they call these down South. And Southerners are among the few Americans who enjoy these bitter, beta-carotene-rich leaves. If young and tender, turnip greens can be steamed like spinach, drizzled with oil and vinegar or tossed with a little butter. But the Southern way is to boil them an hour or more with a piece of side meat (pork). The greens are then served with plenty of pot likker and chunks of corn bread for sopping up every drop. Turnip greens are a first-rate nondairy source of calcium. **SEASON:** Year-round with supplies at their best in autumn.

NUTRIENT CONTENT OF 3 OUNCES (85 GRAMS) ROAST TURKEY (LIGHT MEAT, NO SKIN)	
119 calories	48 mg sodium
26 g protein	234 mg potassium
1 g fat, 0 saturated	0 g dietary fiber
73 mg cholesterol	0 RE vitamin A
0 g carbohydrate	0.04 mg thiamin
13 mg calcium	0.12 mg riboflavin
183 mg phosphorus	5.9 mg niacin
1.3 mg iron	0 mg vitamin C

NUTRIENT CONTENT OF 3 OUNCES (85 GRAMS) ROAST TURKEY (DARK MEAT, NO SKIN)	
158 calories	67 mg sodium
24 g protein	247 mg potassium
6 g fat, 2 saturated	0 g dietary fiber
72 mg cholesterol	0 RE vitamin A
0 g carbohydrate	0.05 mg thiamin
27 mg calcium	0.21 mg riboflavin
174 mg phosphorus	3.1 mg niacin
2.0 mg iron	0 mg vitamin C

NUTRIENT CONTENT OF 1 CUP STEAMED/BOILED TURNIP GREENS (about 5 ounces; 144 grams)	
29 calories	42 mg sodium
2 g protein	292 mg potassium
0 g fat, 0 saturated	5 g dietary fiber
0 mg cholesterol	792 RE vitamin A
6 g carbohydrate	0.07 mg thiamin
197 mg calcium	0.10 mg riboflavin
42 mg phosphorus	0.6 mg niacin
1.2 mg iron	40 mg vitamin C

Turnips: It's written that Henry VIII liked turnips roasted in ashes and the tender young tops served raw as salad, but there's no record that the court shared his passion. In truth, this most ancient of vegetables (it's about four thousand years old) has come down the ages as a lowly root, eaten in lean times by the poor and in fat times by the cattle of the poor. The best turnips are about the size of crab apples, firm, ivory skinned with blushes of purple about the stem. Larger turnips tend to be fibrous, watery and biting. **SEA-SON:** Year-round with supplies peaking in October and November.

NUTRIENT CONTENT OF 1 CUP STEAMED/BOILED DICED TURNIPS
(about 5½ ounces; 156 grams)

28 calories	78 mg sodium
1 g protein	210 mg potassium
0 g fat, 0 saturated	3 g dietary fiber
0 mg cholesterol	0 RE vitamin A
8 g carbohydrate	0.04 mg thiamin
34 mg calcium	0.04 mg riboflavin
30 mg phosphorus	0.5 mg niacin
0.3 mg iron	18 mg vitamin C

TV (obesity and): This should come as no surprise. Researchers studying a group of adolescents have found a direct correlation between degree of obesity and hours spent watching television. Lack of exercise is only partly to blame. Coculprits are the high-fat, high-calorie snacks teenagers wolf down while couched out. Studies haven't zeroed in on older people, but you don't have to be a rocket scientist to know that the same principles apply.

TV Dinners: Not so long ago what TV dinners lacked in taste and texture were more than made up for in fat, calories, salt and cholesterol. Today low-fat, low-calorie frozen dinners and side dishes are pushing the less healthful choices out of supermarket freezer bins. Between 1985 and 1992 sales of "lean" TV dinners have doubled, with more than a dozen different companies dreaming up appetizing new combos. Still, it pays to scrutinize the nutrient labels to see just how "healthy" a particular frozen dinner or side dish actually is. Does fat account for more than 30 percent of its calories? That's the cutoff point recommended not only by the surgeon general but also by the American Heart Association and National Cancer Institute. Many so-called healthy TV dinners don't meet that criterion. What about sodium? To qualify as healthy, there should be no more than 600 milligrams per serving. Finally, how much food are you getting? A proper frozen meal should weigh at least 9 ounces. Calorie limits, nutritionists say, are harder to define because all manner of people eat TV dinners—hunks who may need 500 calories just to keep going and picky dieters who want something in the 250-calorie range. The new food labels plainly state number of calories per serving, so choices are easy. No frozen dinner by itself is a complete meal. To supply missing vitamins and minerals, it should be accompanied by a salad or fresh vegetable, a glass of milk or yogurt dessert. Those who have benefited most from TV dinners are not fat and calorie counters. They are the elderly, the ill and the handicapped who might otherwise nibble crackers, popcorn and chips. With TV dinners so available, so quick to fix, they can enjoy a variety of relatively healthful meals.

Twinkies: For years these spongy, cream-filled little cakes have been the butt of jokes. They were even indicted not so long ago by lawyers representing Dan White, the man who shot Mayor George Moscone of San Francisco. In what has come to be known as the "Twinkies defense," defense attorneys maintained that the assassin was a Twinkies junkie and that his high blood sugar levels "made him do it." They based their case on a theory advanced in the 1970s by Dr. Benjamin Feingold, a California physician, which blamed sugar, among other things, for aggressive behavior in children (see FEINGOLD DIET). The truth about Twinkies is somewhat different. Made with enriched flour, they are very modest sources of thiamin, riboflavin, niacin and iron. The main problem with Twinkies is that for many people, one is never enough. Thus the fat, calories and sodium quickly escalate.

NUTRIENT CONTENT OF 1 TWINKIES
(about 1½ ounces; 42 grams)

153 calories	153 mg sodium
1 g protein	38 mg potassium
5 g fat, 1 saturated	0 g dietary fiber
7 mg cholesterol	2 RE vitamin A
27 g carbohydrate	0.06 mg thiamin
19 mg calcium	0.06 mg riboflavin
32 mg phosphorus	0.5 mg niacin
0.5 mg iron	0 mg vitamin C

Tylenol: See ACETAMINOPHEN.

Type I Diabetes: See DIABETES.

Type II Diabetes: See DIABETES.

Tyramine: After eating foods high in tyramine, a powerful adrenalinelike substance, people on certain antidepressants (phenelzine sulfate and isocarboxazide) sometimes experience serious reactions—dangerously high blood pressure, headaches, nausea. For that reason physicians and/or pharmacists should caution them that as long as they are taking these medications they should keep their tyramine intake to less than 5 milligrams a day. This means avoiding well-aged cheeses such as Brie, Camembert, Cheddar, Emmentaler and Gruyère, all of which are loaded with tyramine. It also means skipping beer, red wine, port, sherry, liver (especially beef and chicken), pickled herring, dead-ripe bananas and avocados, coffee and yeast extracts. Finally, it means cutting down on chocolate, peanuts, soy sauce, raspberries, yogurt and all whiskey. What's safe? Fresh fish, cucumbers, sweet corn, mushrooms, beets, tomato juice, cottage cheese, cream cheese, boiled eggs, raisins. Tyramine counts are highest in aged, pickled or fermented foods or those that have ripened beyond the point of no return.

Tyrosine: Originally classified as a nonessential amino acid (see AMINO ACIDS), tyrosine is now considered semiessential by most nutritionists, because if the body gets enough of it, it can be used in place of phenylalanine to make protein. Milk, meat, fish and legumes are good sources of tyrosine. The brain uses tyrosine to manufacture NOREPINEPHRINE, an upper that boosts mental alertness. Army researchers, aware that fatigue and psychological stress deplete norepinephrine, have been testing tyrosine pills on volunteers to learn if they can improve mental and physical performance. Results look promising. Taking tyrosine tablets remains highly controversial, however—especially after supplements of another amino acid, TRYPTOPHAN, recently crippled and killed so many people. To prevent such incidents in future, the FDA wants amino acids reclassified as medicines so that they cannot be sold over the counter as food supplements and possibly cause serious harm. See also MOOD FLUCTUATIONS.

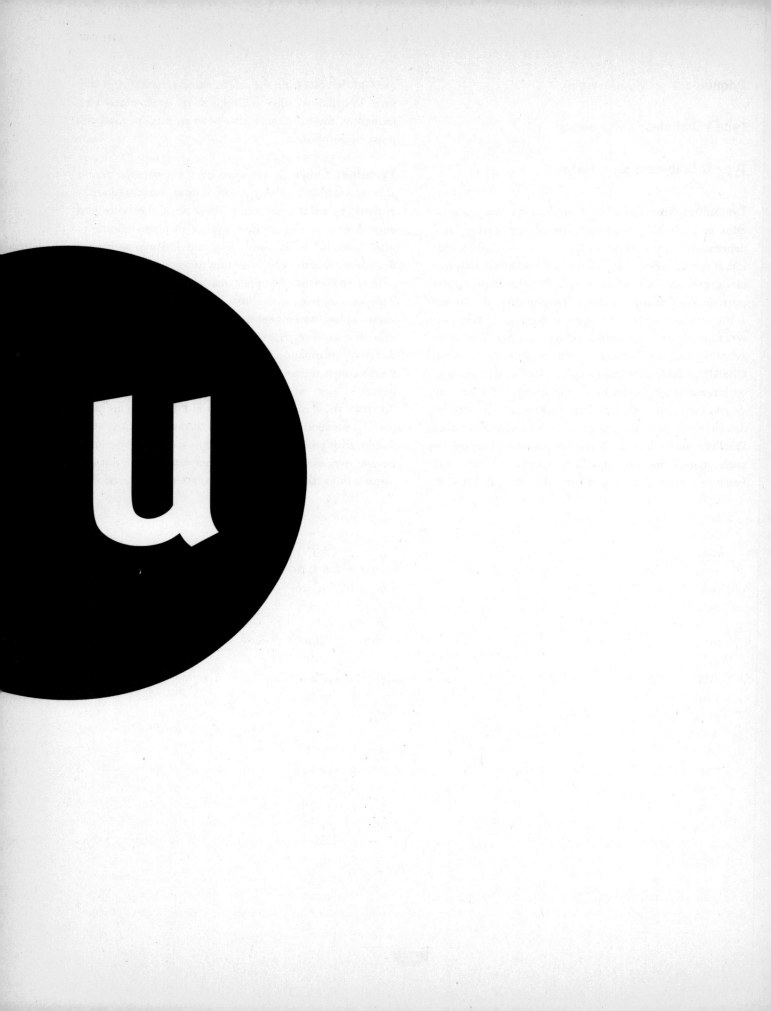

Ubiquinone: See COENZYME Q.

Ugli Fruit: A grapefruit/tangerine hybrid that's believed to be native to Jamaica and is now grown in Florida. Ugli fruit is wrapped in a thick, flabby, furrowed rind that strips off easily. Its flesh is pinkish, sweeter than grapefruit, tarter than tangerine. Like tangerines, uglis segment easily and their juices fairly spurt. They may be as small as navel oranges or as big as grapefruits (use interchangeably with grapefruit). Although no nutrient counts are available for ugli, it is, like all citrus fruits, a good source of vitamin C. And the pinker the flesh, the greater the dose of beta-carotene. **SEASON:** Erratic, year-round.

UHT: See ULTRAHIGH TEMPERATURE TREATMENT.

Ulcerative Colitis (diet and): Chronic inflammation of the large intestine (colon) and rectum. Usually brief but intermittent, bouts of ulcerative colitis mean abdominal cramps, fever, diarrhea and often weight loss and anemia, too. During attacks, a low-fiber diet is prescribed to minimize irritation of the lower digestive tract. Or perhaps the patient is put on a commercial fiber-free formula. In stubborn cases, IVs may be necessary. Once the inflammation subsides, the proper protocol is a high-protein, high-carb, low-fat diet with vitamin and mineral supplements high in chromium, copper, selenium and zinc. Though the amount of fiber the patient can safely eat varies from person to person, dietary fiber should be increased gradually. See also CROHN'S DISEASE.

Ulcers: See PEPTIC ULCERS.

Ultrahigh Temperature Treatment (UHT): A method of sterilizing milk and other perishables at extremely high temperatures so they can be stored at room temperature for six to eight weeks (once opened, of course, these "long-life" foods must be refrigerated). UHT, a variation on ultrapasteurization, works like this: First milk (or other food) is heated to 280°F., held there for two seconds, then quick chilled to 45°F. and sealed inside sterile cartons— usually waxed pasteboard much like milk cartons. Much of the UHT milk and tomatoes now on supermarket shelves are produced by an Italian firm that's established itself in the United States. UHT tomatoes and tomato sauces taste bright, rich and fresh but the milk has a cooked flavor. Still, it's handy to have on hand.

Ultrapasteurization: Heating dairy products (usually half-and-half, heavy cream and eggnog) to between 275°F. and 300°F. for 1 to 4 seconds to extend refrigerator shelf life. Ultrapasteurized cream is much slower to whip than ordinary pasteurized heavy cream. But if icy cold (the bowl and beaters, too), it will whip well.

Ultraviolet Light: See LIGHT; also SUNLIGHT.

Umami: A Japanese word for the rounding and enriching of flavor contributed by a number of natural substances in food, notably glutamate. The *umami* effect was identified more than twelve hundred years ago by Asian cooks and acknowledged by U.S. scientists at the turn of this century. Some say *umami* is a "fifth taste" that should be added to the basic four (salt, sour, sweet and bitter). Others maintain that *umami* is merely a knack for intensifying bouquets and aromas—the brand of magic performed by MONOSODIUM GLUTAMATE.

Unbleached Flour: See FLOUR.

(Gamma)-Undecalactone (additive): An artificial peach flavoring used in a variety of candies, gelatins, ice creams and soft drinks. The FDA limits amounts that can be used.

Undecanals 1, 10 (additives): Flowery flavorings used in a variety of processed foods. The FDA limits amounts of each that can be used.

Undernutrition: A form of MALNUTRITION.

Underweight: Being at least 10 percent below the norm for persons of the same age, height and sex. Mild underweight isn't dangerous unless accompanied by malnutrition (the case with anorexics, bulimics and many of the terminally ill). For a pound-per-week gain, nutritionists recommend a 750- to 800-calorie-a-day overload spread across six to eight high-protein, high-carb meals plus, sometimes, a multivitamin/mineral supplement. At least at first, then perhaps 500 excess calories per day. Like the obese, the underweight must adopt healthful eating habits that will bring their weight within the normal range and keep it there. What causes underweight? Sometimes it's in the genes. Sometimes it's poor eating habits. Sometimes a combination of intense, ongoing exercise and insufficient calories. In the case of anorexia nervosa and bulimia, there may be serious psychological problems that require both mental and physical treatment.

Unit Pricing: Cost per ounce, pound, quart or count as opposed to per package. Its purpose is to make it easier to compare prices, but it fails to consider quality. Thus three small splotchy lemons at eighty cents may not be a better bargain than three perfect ones at ninety.

Universal Product Code (UPC): The bar code used to identify every supermarket item. At the bottom of each code are ten numbers. The first five identify the manufacturer; the last five the product. Bar codes speed checkouts because all the checker has to do is run the bar code over a laser scanner, which rings up prices on the register. The biggest shortcoming of UPCs (apart from faulty scanners) is that shoppers can't keep track of prices unless these are also stamped on each and every item.

Unsaturated Fatty Acid: A fatty acid containing reduced amounts of hydrogen. Among the better known fatty acids present in food are LINOLEIC ACID (polyunsaturated), OLEIC ACID (monounsaturated) and ARACHIDONIC ACID (polyunsaturated). From the standpoint of health, unsaturated fatty acids (and the fats composed of them) are easier on the cardiovascular system because they reduce the risk of plaque buildup. See also FAT; OILS.

Urea: The nitrogen-rich end product of protein metabolism, which is excreted in the urine. Purified urea crystals are also used as yeast food by wine makers and bakers to accelerate fermentation.

Uremia, Uremic Poisoning: Progressive kidney disease marked by impaired function, a buildup of urea and other toxic substances in the blood. Uremia upsets blood chemistry (specifically the acid/alkali balance) and also disrupts fluid and electrolyte metabolism. Unless reversed (or stabilized), it can kill. Because the kidneys' ability to handle protein is diminished, patients are allowed only 15 to 20 grams of it a day—usually 1 egg and 4 to 6 ounces of milk. Nothing more in the way of protein. To prevent body tissue breakdown, there must be sufficient nonprotein calories—from fats, sugars, fruits and vegetables. In acute cases of uremia, special commercial high-calorie, low-protein formulas may be prescribed.

Urethane, Ethyl Carbamate: This compound, known to cause cancer in animals, forms during the fermentation of wine and whiskey. If these beverages are also heated while fermenting—the case with Madeira, sherry and bourbon—the level of urethane is even higher. There are also traces of urethane in yogurt, bread, olives, some fermented cheeses and soy sauce. The federal government is now actively researching the hazards of urethane for humans. Stay tuned.

Uric Acid: A nitrogenous acid found in small amounts in the urine. Uric acid is a by-product of the metabolism of purines, themselves by-products of protein digestion. When blood levels of uric acid rise, it may crystallize out, causing stones in the urinary tract. Or there may be GOUT. Patients with either condition are often told to avoid meats or other protein foods high in purines.

Urinary Tract Infections: For years, folk medicine prescribed cranberry juice as a cure for urinary infections, the idea being that it made urine so acidic bacteria could not grow. Until recently, most researchers pooh-poohed the "cranberry cure." Now come two studies, one from Boston, the other from Israel, suggesting that there may be something to it after all. In Boston, two groups of elderly women were tested, one being given 10 ounces of cranberry juice cocktail a day, the second a look- and taste-alike placebo. Six weeks into the six-month study, the cranberry drinkers had fewer bacteria and white blood cells in their urine and continued to improve throughout the study. The placebo group showed no improvement. The Israeli study suggests that it's not the acid in cranberry juice that fights infection, but rather an as-yet-unidentified substance (also present in blueberries) that thwarts bacteria's ability to cling to urinary tract walls. Whether they subscribe to the cranberry juice cure or not, many physicians and nutritionists do believe that a well-balanced diet accompanied by plenty of fluids (water and/or fruit juices) reduces the incidence of urinary tract infections.

Urine: A liquid filtered out of the blood by the kidneys, the medium by which wastes are excreted. Healthy kidneys filter more than a quart of blood per minute and, depending on the quantity of liquids drunk, produce between 1 and 2 quarts of urine every twenty-four hours. Urine is slightly acidic and its chemical composition resembles that of blood plasma except that in normal individuals it contains no sugar, no protein or large colloidal bits. For physicians and nutritionists, urinalysis is a valuable diagnostic test because it's a measure of nutritional health and health overall.

Urticaria: The medical term for HIVES.

U.S. Department of Agriculture (USDA): An important federal agency whose aims include developing new markets to boost farm income; eradicating hunger, malnutrition and poverty; conducting nutritional research; inspecting and grading meats, eggs, poultry, dairy products plus some fruits and vegetables. In addition, the USDA oversees several national programs: Food Stamps, School Breakfast and School Lunch, Child Care Food, Special Milk for Children and the Commodity Supplemental Food Program. Also under the aegis of the USDA are the Agricultural Extensive Service (including 4-H), the Human Nutrition Center, Food and Nutrition Service (FNS), Food Safety and Inspection Service, Agricultural Research, Cooperative Research and the Technical Information Service.

U.S. Department of Commerce: Under the Fish and Wildlife Act of 1956, this federal agency, through its National Marine Fisheries Service, sets standards and urges voluntary grading of fish and shellfish. With many waters now contaminated by industrial fallout or toxin-producing organisms, the department's powers are expected to be increased. And stiff standards of seafood inspection made mandatory. Meanwhile, the Marine Fisheries Service, cooperating with the Food Marketing Institute (an arm of the supermarket industry), has established a Standard of Excellence Award. Its purpose is to ensure the safety and quality of seafood. First, by urging the seafood industry to continue careful inspection and, second, by encouraging groceries to maintain high standards of sanitation. It's a voluntary program, but the Standard of Excellence Seal displayed at fish counters and printed in ads should be an incentive.

U.S. Department of Health and Human Services (USDHHS): Originally called the U.S. Department of Health, Education, and Welfare, this vast government agency was renamed in late 1979, when the Department of Education was established. Among its many divisions is the FOOD AND DRUG ADMINISTRATION. For more information about USDHHS, see HEALTH AND HUMAN SERVICES, U.S. DEPARTMENT OF.

U.S. Recommended Daily Allowances (USRDAs): Based on the 1968 recommendations of the Food and Nutrition Board, these nutritional guidelines were developed by the Food and Drug Administration for use in labeling foods. Obsolete since the implementation in 1994 of the Nutrition Labeling and Education Act of 1990, USRDAs have been replaced by Reference Daily Intakes (see RDIs). For now, the numerical values of the two are identical. But in future, they will no doubt change. See also FOOD LABELING; NLEA.

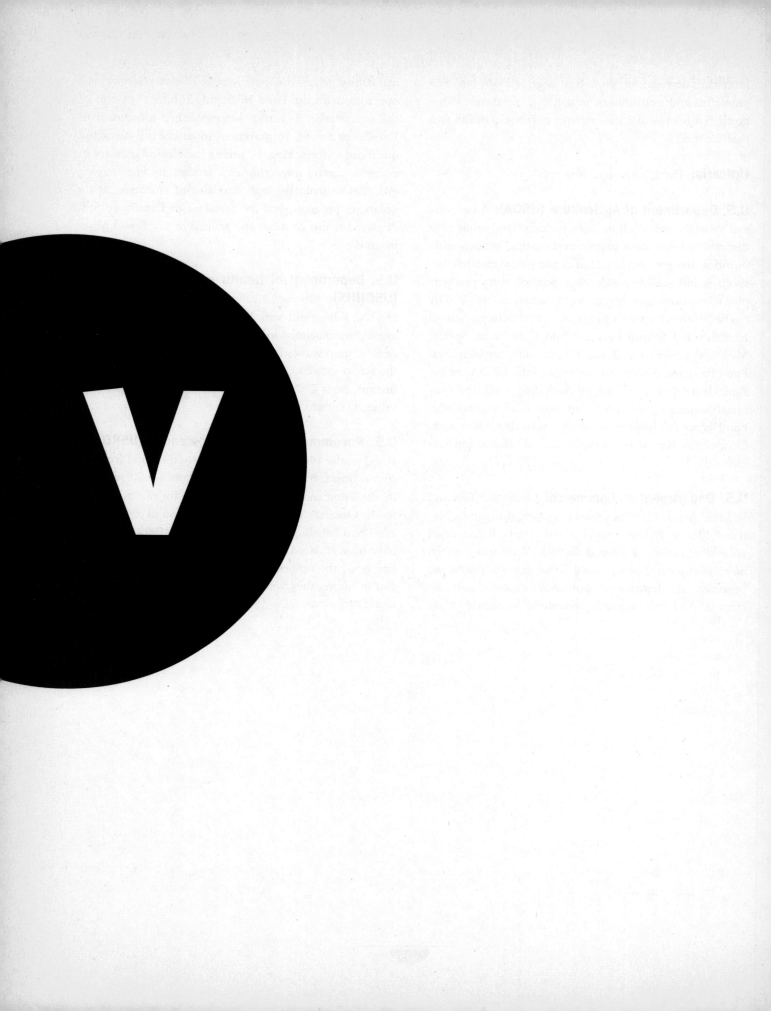

Vacuum-Packed Foods: A method of keeping food safe and fresh by sealing containers from which all (or almost all) air is withdrawn. Sometimes another gas—usually nitrogen or carbon dioxide—is pumped in to replace the air. Sometimes the food is also heat treated—canned meats, for example. The idea is to prevent oxidation, which hastens staling and discoloring. Also to thwart the growth of harmful microorganisms like *Escherichia coli,* salmonella, *Staphylococcus aureus* and *Yersinia enterocolitica.* Vacuum packing does a good job of stopping these bugs. But it has little or no effect on *Clostridium botulinum,* the culprit behind the deadly form of food poisoning known as botulism. Because *C. botulinum* gives no clue to its presence, food researchers are developing biosensors for vacuum packs and other processed foods that will turn color whenever there is a risk of botulism. The vacuum-packed and canned foods most familiar to us are coffees, nuts and meats, but more are on the way.

Valerian, Valeric Acid (additive): Although present in apples, cocoa, coffee, peaches and strawberries, most of what's used to flavor baked goods, candies, ice creams and soft drinks is extracted from valerian root. The FDA considers valeric acid safe when used within reason to achieve the desired butter, butterscotch or rum flavors. Health-food stores push valerian root as a cure for everything from insomnia to tension to hysteria and epileptic fits. The truth? It does seem to be something of a tranquilizer and it's considered safe for healthy individuals.

Valine: An essential amino acid that's a major player in the growth and maintenance of body tissues (it's found primarily in fibrous animal proteins). Shortfalls of valine have produced loss of muscular coordination in lab rats as well as hypersensitivity to pain, heat and cold. Like isoleucine and leucine, valine is an amino acid some infants can't metabolize. This metabolic disorder produces a condition called maple syrup urine disease (see ISOLEUCINE). See also AMINO ACIDS.

Vanadium: A trace element named for the Scandinavian goddess of youth and beauty that's essential to animals and probably to humans as well. Its main function is to activate enzymes involved in fat metabolism and nerve hormone production. Taken in pharmacological doses, vanadium not only blocks cholesterol production by the liver but also lowers blood levels of cholesterol and triglycerides. Because vanadium is present in a wide variety of foods (seafood, soybeans and grains are especially good sources), deficiencies are unknown. Overdoses, on the other hand, are fairly common due to industrial pollution (vanadium can be inhaled, even absorbed by the skin) and it doesn't take much to cause trouble. **SYMPTOMS OF VANADIUM TOXICITY:** Dermatitis, sore eyes, diarrhea, loss of appetite, high blood levels of vanadium and, in rare instances, death.

Vanilla, Vanilla Extract (additives): It took hundreds of years for vanilla to make the global leap from Mexico, where Cortés found the Aztecs drinking vanilla-spiked hot chocolate, to the royal tables of Europe to the kitchens of everyday America. Thomas Jefferson first tasted vanilla in France and missed it so, after returning to America, that he wrote a friend "to send me a packet of 50 pods which may come very well in the middle of a packet of newspapers." Jefferson's yearning for vanilla is understandable. Who today could cook without it? Purists use only vanilla beans, the pods of a wild climbing orchid native to the rain forests of southern Mexico, which have been ripened, cured and fermented to bring out their perfumy flavor. Vanilla extract, a solution that's at least 35 percent alcohol, is harsher. It may also contain sugar or corn syrup, glycerin and/or propylene glycol. GRAS.

Vanillin (additive): Although this compound exists naturally in wood pulp, potato parings, even vanilla extract, it's classified as a synthetic flavoring. Vanillin packs more punch than vanilla beans or extract; it's cheaper, too, which is why food manufacturers like to use it to flavor baked goods, candies, puddings, ice creams, liqueurs and soft drinks. Though mildly toxic, vanillin is considered safe by the FDA because such small amounts of it are needed to impart vanilla flavor.

Variety Meats: A portmanteau term that includes not only organ meats (heart, liver, kidneys, sweetbreads, etc.) but also a nearly endless list of sausages and cold cuts. Many are discussed in individual entries.

Veal: Twenty-five years ago, it was virtually impossible to buy a decent piece of veal in America except in a few pricey metropolitan markets. Indeed, few Americans had ever eaten good veal, let alone knew what it looked like.

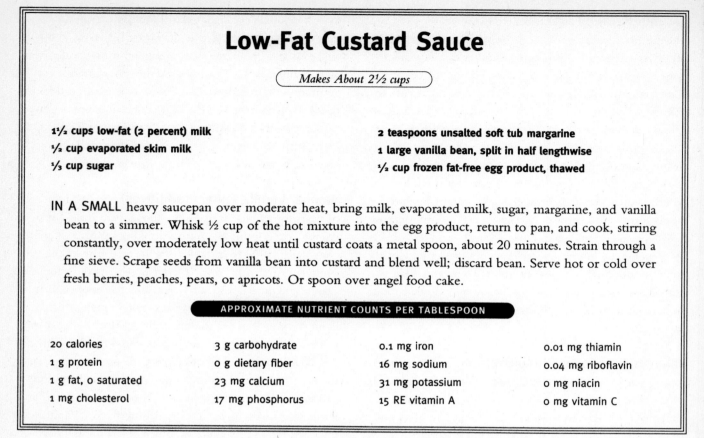

Low-Fat Custard Sauce

Makes About 2½ cups

1½ cups low-fat (2 percent) milk

½ cup evaporated skim milk

⅓ cup sugar

2 teaspoons unsalted soft tub margarine

1 large vanilla bean, split in half lengthwise

½ cup frozen fat-free egg product, thawed

IN A SMALL heavy saucepan over moderate heat, bring milk, evaporated milk, sugar, margarine, and vanilla bean to a simmer. Whisk ½ cup of the hot mixture into the egg product, return to pan, and cook, stirring constantly, over moderately low heat until custard coats a metal spoon, about 20 minutes. Strain through a fine sieve. Scrape seeds from vanilla bean into custard and blend well; discard bean. Serve hot or cold over fresh berries, peaches, pears, or apricots. Or spoon over angel food cake.

APPROXIMATE NUTRIENT COUNTS PER TABLESPOON

20 calories	3 g carbohydrate	0.1 mg iron	0.01 mg thiamin
1 g protein	0 g dietary fiber	16 mg sodium	0.04 mg riboflavin
1 g fat, 0 saturated	23 mg calcium	31 mg potassium	0 mg niacin
1 mg cholesterol	17 mg phosphorus	15 RE vitamin A	0 mg vitamin C

Then mass America began traveling abroad and tasting such classics as the French *blanquette de veau,* the Austrian *Wiener schnitzel,* the Italian *vitello tonnato,* all made with a delicate white meat wholly unlike the chewy, reddish cuts palmed off as veal back home.

Today, fine European-style veal is available across most of America—and not just in fancy French restaurants or gold-plated butcher shops. It has come to the supermarket. This is true veal, mind you—"nature," "special-fed," "fancy quality"—meat from bull Holstein calves no more than sixteen weeks old that have been penned since the day they were born and fattened on a ration of milk solids, vitamins and minerals and sometimes HORMONES as well.

Wisconsin produces the bulk of America's milk-fed veal, not surprising considering that it is our leading dairy state and that veal is a by-product of the dairy industry (not of the beef industry). Holsteins, from which the best American veal comes, are dairy animals, abundant milk producers, provided the cows freshen (calve) each year. The female calves usually grow up into the dairy herd. The males become lean, fine-fleshed veal.

Several types of veal are available today: **bob veal** (the meat of newborns which is too young to have developed much flavor or character); **grain-fed veal** (really "baby beef" eight to twelve months old with reddish, not very flavorful meat); and **special-fed, nature** or **fancy-quality veal** (European-style veal from suckling calves so fine it's often sold by brand name—usually Plume de Veau or Provimi Delft Blue. This veal costs plenty). All three types of veal may be federally graded for quality. The two top

NUTRIENT CONTENT OF 3 OUNCES (85 GRAMS) SAUTÉED VEAL CUTLET

156 calories	65 mg sodium
18 g protein	376 mg potassium
4 g fat, 1 saturated	0 g dietary fiber
91 mg cholesterol	30 RE vitamin A
0 g carbohydrate	0.06 mg thiamin
6 mg calcium	0.27 mg riboflavin
247 mg phosphorus	10.7 mg niacin
0.7 mg iron	0 mg vitamin C

grades of veal, as with beef, are USDA Prime and USDA Choice. Frankly, there's no point in settling for less.

Compared to beef, lamb or pork, veal is low in fat, but it is high in cholesterol. Yet, it is a stellar source of niacin (one of the B-complex) and a good source of riboflavin, phosphorus and potassium.

NUTRIENT CONTENT OF 3 OUNCES (85 GRAMS) BRAISED VEAL LOIN CHOP	
192 calories	71 mg sodium
29 g protein	253 mg potassium
8 g fat, 6 saturated	0 g dietary fiber
106 mg cholesterol	0 RE vitamin A
0 g carbohydrate	0.04 mg thiamin
27 mg calcium	0.29 mg riboflavin
202 mg phosphorus	8.6 mg niacin
0.9 mg iron	0 mg vitamin C

NUTRIENT CONTENT OF 3 OUNCES (85 GRAMS) ROAST LEG OF VEAL	
136 calories	58 mg sodium
23 g protein	330 mg potassium
4 g fat, 2 saturated	0 g dietary fiber
88 mg cholesterol	0 RE vitamin A
0 g carbohydrate	0.05 mg thiamin
5 mg calcium	0.27 mg riboflavin
198 mg phosphorus	8.4 mg niacin
0.8 mg iron	0 mg vitamin C

NUTRIENT CONTENT OF 3 OUNCES (85 GRAMS) BRAISED, TRIMMED VEAL ARM STEAK	
170 calories	77 mg sodium
31 g protein	294 mg potassium
5 g fat, 1 saturated	0 g dietary fiber
131 mg cholesterol	0 RE vitamin A
0 g carbohydrate	0.05 mg thiamin
26 mg calcium	0.28 mg riboflavin
234 mg phosphorus	9.1 mg niacin
1.2 mg iron	0 mg vitamin C

Vegans: "Pure" or "total" vegetarians who won't touch animal food—milk or milk products, eggs, meat, fish or fowl. Vegans (pronounced *VEE-ganz,* with a hard *g*) must plan their diet carefully if they're to get all the essential amino acids (protein building blocks), iron, calcium and zinc they need. They also need supplementary vitamin B_{12}, either from fortified soy milk or in tablet form.

Vegetable Gums: Assorted mucilaginous plant extracts used by food processors to thicken, smooth and stabilize puddings, frozen desserts, salad dressings, etc. See GUMS, VEGETABLE; also GUM ARABIC; GUM GHATTI; GUM GUAIAC; GUM KARAYA; GUM TRAGACANTH.

Vegetable Oils: See OILS. See also individual oils: CANOLA OIL; CORN OIL; OLIVE OIL; SAFFLOWER OIL; SUNFLOWER-SEED OIL; etc.

Vegetable Oil Sprays: See NONSTICK VEGETABLE COOKING SPRAYS.

Vegetables: The closer the vegetable is to the farm, the better it will be from every standpoint—color, texture, flavor and nutritive value. Those shipped cross-country suffer on all four counts, as do canned vegetables, dried vegetables and some frozen vegetables. Most good cooks admit that the only frozen vegetables they keep on hand are whole-kernel corn, chopped spinach and kale, pureed winter squash, artichoke hearts and maybe green peas or black-eyed peas. Still, resorting to the canned, dried and frozen is better than forgoing out-of-season vegetables. According to the recommendations set forth by the new FOOD GUIDE PYRAMID, we should all get three to five servings of vegetables every day. And the greater the variety, the better. Vegetables are low in fat and calories, contain no cholesterol, yet many of them are packed with fiber, vitamins and minerals. All major vegetables are discussed—in some detail—in individual entries. To learn what nutrients are most likely to be sacrificed when foods are canned, dried or frozen, see FOOD PRESERVATION.

Vegetable Shortening: Vegetable oils pumped up with hydrogen to stiffen them and make them fluffy. Shortenings produce cakes of tender crumb, wispy pastries and cookies of incomparable crispness. Unfortunately, hydrogenating vegetable oils not only saturates them but also creates trans fatty acids, which biomedical researchers now believe significantly raise blood cholesterol levels and increase the risk of heart disease. **THE LESSON HERE:** Use unsaturated vegetable oils everywhere possible in cooking and reserve shortenings for those cakes, cookies and pastries whose success depends upon them. See also TRANS FATTY ACIDS.

Vegetable Steamers:
Perforated metal stands, steel mesh or woven bamboo baskets in which vegetables can be steamed without touching the water boiling directly underneath, meaning minimal water-soluble nutrient loss. Steaming is also quick, thus few heat-sensitive vitamins are lost. Not every vegetable, however, is a candidate for steaming. Potatoes and sweet potatoes are better when baked or boiled, as are hard winter squashes.

Vegetarians:
People who eat mostly plant foods for one reason or another (religious, philosophical, cultural, health). There are several degrees of vegetarianism. **Ovo-lacto-vegetarians,** for example, will eat eggs and dairy products but no meat, fish or fowl. **Lactovegetarians** include milk and other dairy products in their diet but avoid eggs, meat, poultry and seafood. **Ovovegetarians** permit themselves eggs but no milk, meat or other animal products. **Fruitarians** limit themselves to fruits and nuts. And then there are VEGANS, the strictest vegetarians of all. One nutritional challenge facing strict vegetarians is getting enough top-quality protein because much of it comes from animal sources. For that reason, nutritionists stress the importance of eating plenty of soybean products, dried beans, peas, lentils and brown rice, which supply not only many of the important amino acids but also hefty shots of B vitamins, iron and fiber. Even so, there is a risk of iron-deficiency anemia among vegetarians, particularly among babies, children and pregnant women, so iron supplements may be necessary (zinc and calcium are likely to be missing, too). In addition, a supplementary source of vitamin B_{12} is essential for vegans. The good news is that vegetarians have lower blood cholesterol levels than nonvegetarians. They also consume greater amounts of fiber and vitamins A and C, plus minerals other than iron, calcium and zinc. Balancing a vegetarian diet, though not difficult, does take dedication and experience. As with nonvegetarians, the wisest course is to go for variety.

Vending Machine Food:
Long given a bad rap as purveyors of instant junk food, vending machine companies are going all out to offer healthful choices for America's more nutritionally aware public: fat-free, cooked-to-order french fries; low-fat/low-salt pizzas; skim milk; low-fat yogurt; lean, white-meat turkey sandwiches; even fresh fruit and fruit juice. Chips and candy bars still abound, to be sure, and will disappear only when there's no longer a demand for them. Meanwhile, nutritionists urge those with high blood pressure, high cholesterol or excess pounds to avoid such old-time vending machine staples as salt-, fat- and cholesterol-laden hot dogs, cheese puffs, tortilla and potato chips, cakes, cookies and pastries and to settle, instead, for yogurt, unsalted pretzels, sugar-free soft drinks and, when their sweet tooth demands a sugar fix, lower-fat, higher-fiber Fig Newtons.

Venison:
The meat of deer. It is leaner than beef, gamier and tougher, too, if the animal was wild. Venison sold by fancy butchers will be top quality, federally inspected for wholesomeness, and possibly ranch-raised. Raising venison has become big business because it's one way to produce the top-quality venison restaurants and knowledgeable cooks demand. In the wild, there's no quality control, and how good a specific animal is is determined by several factors: age (the younger, the tenderer), diet (animals that have fed on resinous needles and juniper berries, etc., will have strong flavor) and the care the kill was given in the field. Sloppy handling can ruin perfectly good meat and only painstaking, experienced hunters should be trusted to bring home venison that's edible. As with any animal, the tenderest cuts of venison—the ''roastables'' and ''broilables''—will come from the least exercised portions—the rib, loin and tenderloin. Shoulder and rump are candidates for stews, pot roasts and burgers. Shanks can be braised like osso buco. For red-meat lovers, venison is a good substitute for beef. It is a

NUTRIENT CONTENT OF 3 OUNCES (85 GRAMS) ROASTED VENISON	
134 calories	46 mg sodium
26 g protein	284 mg potassium
3 g fat, 1 saturated	0 g dietary fiber
95 mg cholesterol	0 RE vitamin A
0 g carbohydrate	0.15 mg thiamin
6 mg calcium	0.51 mg riboflavin
192 mg phosphorus	5.7 mg niacin
3.8 mg iron	0 mg vitamin C

superior source of top-quality protein, riboflavin, niacin, iron, phosphorus and potassium yet is lower in fat (especially saturated fat).

Vermouth: Fortified aperitif wines infused with secret blends of herbs and spices that are, by volume, 16 to 18 percent alcohol. The quintessential **French vermouth** is dry and white, and the **Italian** sweet and brown. As for calories, dry vermouth contains 27 calories per ounce, sweet vermouth 43. See also ALCOHOL, ALCOHOLIC BEVERAGES.

Very Low-Density Lipoprotein (VLDL): The least dense of all the body's lipoproteins, VLDL is about 10 percent protein, with the remainder being lipid (fat) and lipidlike compounds, among them cholesterol. VLDL is specially synthesized by the liver to shuttle triglycerides, which it also synthesizes, through the bloodstream to areas where they're needed. Or where they can be stored, then released in future. Along with LDL (the so-called "bad" cholesterol), VLDL is considered undesirable. Comparatively high levels may indicate atherosclerosis and coronary artery disease.

Veterinary Drugs (residuals in food): See ANTIBIOTICS; also HORMONES; SULFA DRUGS.

Vibrio vulnificus: A bacterium that thrives in warm oceans and saltwater seas. It's widespread in the Gulf of Mexico between April and October and can contaminate any mollusks living there—clams, conchs, mussels, oysters and scallops. These shellfish feed by filtering salt water through their bodies and if *V. vulnificus* is present, high levels of it can build up in their flesh. If you eat contaminated clams, conchs, mussels, oysters or scallops raw, you can become very sick and, depending on your state of health, may die (50 percent of those in run-down condition or with weakened immune systems do die from *V. vulnificus* infections). The best preventive: Eat no shellfish that hasn't been thoroughly cooked.

Vidalia Onions: See ONIONS.

Vienna Sausage: Fine-textured finger-size frankfurters most often sold by the can. They are fatty, salty and not particularly nutritious.

NUTRIENT CONTENT OF 1 OUNCE (28 GRAMS) CANNED VIENNA SAUSAGE	
79 calories	269 mg sodium
3 g protein	29 mg potassium
7 g fat, 3 saturated	0 g dietary fiber
15 mg cholesterol	0 RE vitamin A
1 g carbohydrate	0.03 mg thiamin
3 mg calcium	0.03 mg riboflavin
14 mg phosphorus	0.5 mg niacin
0.3 mg iron	0 mg vitamin C

Villi, Microvilli: Small (or very small) "fingers" lining the small intestine that maximize the absorption of nutrients and excretion of mucus.

Vinegar: As long as there's been wine, there's been vinegar. And that means since Old Testament times. The French word for vinegar—*vinaigre,* originally *vin aigre*—means "soured wine." Precisely what vinegar is, a wine (or ale or beer or other lightly fermented liquid) made sour by bacteria turning the alcohol to acetic acid. Most vinegars sold today average 4 to 6 percent acetic acid. In the major wine-producing countries—France, Italy and Spain—vinegar is made from wine. Red wine, white wine, sherry. The specialty of Modena in northern Italy is a warm, brown wine vinegar called *aceto balsamico* (**balsamic vinegar**), which is aged ten, fifty, sometimes even one hundred years in oaken barrels. Some of these, the so-called **artesanal vinegars,** are so rich, so syrupy they're sprinkled over fruit and served as dessert. Beer-drinking countries like Great Britain prefer **malt vinegars** to grape; Asians prefer delicate **rice wine vinegars.** In the United States, **cider** (or apple) **vinegar** is the staple, with **white** (distilled) **vinegar** first choice for pickling. Boutique **flavored vinegars** abound, too—garlic, shallot, herbal, raspberry, you name it.

Since ancient times, vinegar has been used as a disinfectant and medicine. Even today, champions of folk medicine (with no hard evidence to back their claims) swear that vinegar banishes headaches faster than aspirin, stops hiccups cold, cools the fire of sunburn and bee stings, cures dandruff, eases the pain of arthritis and varicose veins, soothes the stomach and helps prevent food poisoning. Most people, however, simply use vinegar for cooking, pickling and preserving. And, needless to add, for dressing salads. The classic is vinaigrette, roughly 3 parts olive oil to 1 part vinegar plus seasonings (for a lovely mellow variation, see HONEY).

NUTRIENT CONTENT OF 1 TABLESPOON CIDER VINEGAR	
(about ½ ounce; 15 grams)	
2 calories	0 mg sodium
0 g protein	15 mg potassium
0 g fat, 0 saturated	0 g dietary fiber
0 mg cholesterol	0 RE vitamin A
1 g carbohydrate	0.03 mg thiamin
1 mg calcium	0.03 mg riboflavin
1 mg phosphorus	0.5 mg niacin
0.1 mg iron	0 mg vitamin C

Violets: Yes, they are edible. Pluck them and sprinkle into green salads and fruit salads. Or use candied violets to decorate fancy desserts. Although specific nutrient counts are unavailable for violets, they are said to be fair sources of beta-carotene and vitamin C. See also FLOWERS, EDIBLE.

Viruses: Disease-causing microorganisms smaller than bacteria (some are so tiny they can't be seen with an ordinary microscope). Viruses are responsible for many illnesses, but the ones of particular interest here are the food-borne viruses. The most prevalent and troublesome are these:

Acute Hepatitis A: A serious liver infection transmitted, for the most part, via contaminated food or water. And not just in developing countries. Over one recent two-year period, more than six thousand cases of acute hepatitis A in the United States were traced to raw or insufficiently cooked shellfish. **VIRAL SOURCE:** Any food or water contaminated with fecal matter or sewage, also infected food handlers (a North Carolina outbreak was traced to iced tea prepared by an asymptomatic restaurant worker), flies, cockroaches and rodents. In the Third World, drinking water is especially chancy; also eating raw fruits and vegetables, which might have been irrigated with contaminated water, or improperly cooked fish and shellfish. Clams, oysters, mussels and other mollusks pose the greatest risk. On two counts. First, they concentrate viruses as they filter seawater through their bodies. Second, they're often eaten on the half shell. **SYMPTOMS OF ACUTE HEPATITIS A:** Tender, enlarged liver; fever; severe vomiting. **HOW SOON SYMPTOMS OCCUR:** Within fifteen to fifty days. **PREVENTIVES:** Avoid raw or rare cooked fish and shellfish everywhere. When traveling, stay out of greasy spoons or eateries that look unclean, especially in developing countries. Don't drink the water; in fact, don't even brush your teeth with it (mouthwash works well) and take all drinks without ice. Pass on raw salads and vegetables and on fussy, overhandled dishes (sandwiches, rice, pasta, meat or fish salads, fruit cocktails, etc.); eat only thick-skinned fruits that you peel yourself. Drink only bottled fizzy mineral water (less apt to have been adulterated than still water), only pasteurized milk from sealed containers, well-boiled coffee or tea. Veteran travelers pack jars of peanut butter and packs of soda crackers, even nutritionally balanced diet bars to snack on whenever the going gets rough. Good thinking. Many also take preventive shots before they travel.

Astrovirus: It hasn't been identified in the United States yet, but it's made many people sick in England. **VIRAL SOURCE:** Polluted water and contaminated shellfish. **SYMPTOMS:** Diarrhea and sometimes fever, too. **HOW SOON SYMPTOMS OCCUR:** One to four days. **PREVENTIVES:** Drink fizzy bottled water and eat only well-cooked seafood.

Calcivirus: Another food-borne virus that is confined so far to England. **VIRAL SOURCE:** Contaminated water and shellfish. **SYMPTOMS:** Diarrhea, vomiting, low-grade fever. **HOW SOON SYMPTOMS OCCUR:** One to three days. **PREVENTIVES:** Drink fizzy bottled water and insist that all fish and shellfish be cooked well done.

Human Rotavirus: A common cause of gastrointestinal problems, especially among young children and the elderly, whose immune systems are weak. **VIRAL SOURCE:** Less than fastidious food handlers. **SYMPTOMS:** Vomiting, fever, diarrhea and dehydration. **HOW SOON SYMPTOMS OCCUR:** One to three days. **PREVENTIVES:** Personal cleanliness.

Norwalk-Type Viruses: These bugs, which surfaced only in 1982 in Norwalk, Ohio, have caused more than 150 large outbreaks of gastroenteritis and are spreading rapidly. The 1982 outbreak was attributed to butter-cream frosting, mixed by an infected commercial bakery worker. It made three thousand people sick. Though mild and mercifully short-lived, Norwalk virus infections are severe enough to flatten you for several days. **VIRAL SOURCE:** Two outbreaks have occurred on Caribbean cruise ships; several have been traced to large public banquets and some to eating raw or insufficiently cooked clams and oysters. The problem? Unsanitary conditions, infected but symptomless food handlers, sloppy food handling. **SYMPTOMS:** Intestinal cramps, vomiting, diarrhea, low-grade fever. **HOW SOON SYMPTOMS OCCUR:** Within one to two days. **PREVENTIVES:** Be choosy about what you take from buffets that have been spread in sunny spots, declining all fancy salads (especially those containing meat, fish or fowl), all creamed dishes (even dessert). Insist that all fish and shellfish be thoroughly cooked. And while traveling in areas of poor sanitation, drink fizzy bottled water and take all beverages neat—without ice.

Visible and Invisible Fat in Foods:
Everyone trying to cut down on fat trims the fat off steaks and chops; holds the butter, margarine and oil; swears off bacon and fat-studded cold cuts; tries, too, to avoid fried foods and to opt for sherbet over superpremium ice cream. The trouble is, many foods that look lean are filled with fat. Take cream of mushroom soup. Even when prepared with water, 66 percent of its calories come from fat. Salad bars are minefields of hidden fat. Those shreds of Swiss or Cheddar cheese, those gloppy dressings, those croutons, those slivers of avocado can send the fat in a tossed salad soaring (82 percent of an avocado's calories come from fat). Then there

are coleslaws and potato salads, to say nothing of macaroni, tuna, chicken, ham and turkey salads, all of which are heavily freighted with fat. So are doughnuts and Danish, pizzas and many tortellini, ravioli, lasagne and other beloved pasta recipes. In fact, invisible fat riddles the American diet. Small wonder so many Americans—even youngsters—are overweight. And small wonder cardiovascular disease is the number-one killer in the United States.

Visual Purple: See RHODOPSIN; also RETINA.

Vitamins:
Essential to life, these thirteen organic compounds perform dozens of vital jobs in the body. Yet *vitamin* entered our vocabulary only in 1912, when the first one—thiamin or B_1—was isolated. We now know that some of the devastating diseases of the past—beriberi, rickets, scurvy—were nothing more than acute vitamin deficiencies. To prevent future deficiencies, the Food and Nutrition Board of the National Academy of Sciences devised Recommended Dietary Allowances (see RDAs), the daily amounts of the different food nutrients considered adequate for healthy individuals. These figures are updated every five to ten years, the last update being 1989. The book on vitamins is far from complete. Research continues and few scientists doubt that new vitamins, even new roles for existing vitamins, will surface. Meanwhile, below is a quick summary of the thirteen vitamins now known. (All, by the way, are discussed in detail in individual entries.)

CHARTING THE VITAMINS

Vitamin	Good Sources	Functions	Solubility/Stability
A	Dark leafy greens, yellow/orange fruits and vegetables; liver, margarine, milk (whole, fortified skim)	Aids in formation and upkeep of skin, mucous membranes; promotes eye health, building of sturdy bones, teeth.	Fat soluble. Stable in cooking; gradually destroyed by oxygen, heat, drying.

Additional notes: Carotenes, notably beta-carotene, are vitamin A precursors. ODing on vitamin A (not beta-carotene) can blur vision, slow growth, increase skull pressure and cause hair loss.

THE B-COMPLEX

Vitamin	Good Sources	Functions	Solubility/Stability
B_1 (thiamin)	Pork, liver, other meats, whole grains, legumes, nuts	Assists in carbohydrate metabolism, promotes normal appetite and nerve function.	Water soluble. Destroyed by heat; lost in milling of grains; restored via enrichment.

Additional notes: Deficiency causes nerve dysfunction, beriberi.

Vitamin	Good Sources	Functions	Solubility/Stability
THE B-COMPLEX			
B₂ (riboflavin)	Milk, yogurt, cheese, liver, meat, whole and enriched grains, eggs, leafy vegetables	Helps release food energy; promotes good vision, healthy skin.	Water soluble. Destroyed by sunlight, ultraviolet light, milling of grains; restored via enrichment.

Additional notes: Deficiency inflames mouth, dries and scales facial skin.

....

Niacin	Meat, poultry, fish, liver, peanuts, whole and enriched grains, legumes	Assists in carbohydrate metabolism and release of energy. Promotes skin health, nerve and digestive tract function.	Water soluble. Heat and light stable; lost in milling of grains; restored via enrichment.

Additional notes: Body can convert tryptophan, an essential amino acid, into niacin. Acute deficiency causes pellagra.

....

B₆ (pyridoxine)	Poultry, fish, meat, potatoes, sweet potatoes, avocados, bananas	Aids protein, fat and carbohydrate metabolism.	Water soluble. Destroyed by heat, light, processing and refinement.

Additional notes: Large quantities toxic; may cause nerve damage.

....

B₁₂ (cobalamin)	Meats (especially organs), poultry, eggs, fish, milk	Promotes development of healthy red blood cells and maintenance of nerve tissue.	Water soluble. Fairly stable. Some loss in pasteurization.

Additional notes: Exists in animal foods only. Cannot be absorbed without INTRINSIC FACTOR. Deficiency results in pernicious anemia.

....

Folic acid (folacin)	Leafy green vegetables, legumes, whole grains, nuts, liver, oranges	Promotes formation of healthy red blood cells.	Water soluble. Heat sensitive; can be destroyed in cooking; some lost in processing of food.

Additional notes: Pregnant women (even those planning to become pregnant) urged to take folic acid supplements to reduce risk of birth defects. Folic acid now also thought to help prevent heart disease. Overdoses can mask symptoms of pernicious anemia.

....

Pantothenic acid	Meats, organ meats, fish, whole grains, legumes, egg yolks	Integral to metabolism of fat, carbohydrate and proteins. Fosters growth and maintenance of body tissues.	Water soluble. Sensitive to heat, acids and alkalis. Some lost in processing/milling.

Additional notes: Dietary deficiencies unknown.

....

Vitamin	Good Sources	Functions	Solubility/Stability
THE B-COMPLEX			
Biotin	Eggs, milk, meats, nuts, legumes, whole grains	Integral to protein, carbohydrate and fat metabolism.	Water soluble. *Raw* egg white contains AVIDIN, which blocks biotin absorption.

Additional notes: Deficiencies occur only when raw egg whites are eaten too much and too often. But in this age of salmonella, few people are likely to be eating raw egg whites.

C (ascorbic acid)	Citrus fruits, peppers sweet and hot, dark leafy greens, broccoli, cabbage, brussels sprouts, tomatoes, potatoes, strawberries	Forms "glue" that holds body cells together; strengthens blood vessels; assists in iron absorption; speeds healing; boosts immune system.	Water soluble. Destroyed by heat, air (oxygen). Can be lost in cooking water.

Additional notes: Megadoses cause dependency; when doses are cut, deficiency symptoms may develop.

D	Sunlight, vitamin D-enriched dairy foods and margarine, egg yolks, fish oils	Helps bones and teeth harden; increases calcium and phosphorus absorption and utilization.	Fat soluble. Not easily destroyed by cooking or food processing.

Additional notes: Overdoses toxic; can stunt growth, cause weight loss and calcification of soft tissues.

E	Vegetable oils, margarines, butter, eggs, whole grains, wheat germ, liver, leafy greens	Works as antioxidant preventing destruction of vitamins A, C, fatty acids and cell membranes.	Fat soluble. Destroyed by high heat, freezing and long storage and, to lesser degree, by milling of grains and refining of vegetable oils.

Additional notes: Researchers studying E's cancer-fighting potential.

K	Leafy green vegetables, milk, soybean oil, egg yolks (intestinal bacteria synthesize most of the vitamin K the body needs)	Helps blood clot.	Fat soluble. Antibiotics kill intestinal bacteria that produce vitamin K, so those on these drugs may be deficient.

Additional notes: Newborns are given a single hefty dose of K because their sterile digestive tracts can't synthesize it.

Vitamin Supplements: See SUPPLEMENTS, DIETARY.

Vodka: See ALCOHOL, ALCOHOLIC BEVERAGES.

Vomiting: "Throwing up," "tossing your cookies," "barfing." Whatever you call it, this means forcing stomach contents up through the esophagus and out the mouth. It's dangerous only when it's violent and can't be stopped. Prolonged vomiting leads to dehydration and nutritional deficiencies. The physician's first move is to determine the cause, stop the vomiting, then prescribe easily digested carbohydrates such as rice or toast. If vomiting persists, IVs (or other tube feeding) may be needed until the stomach settles.

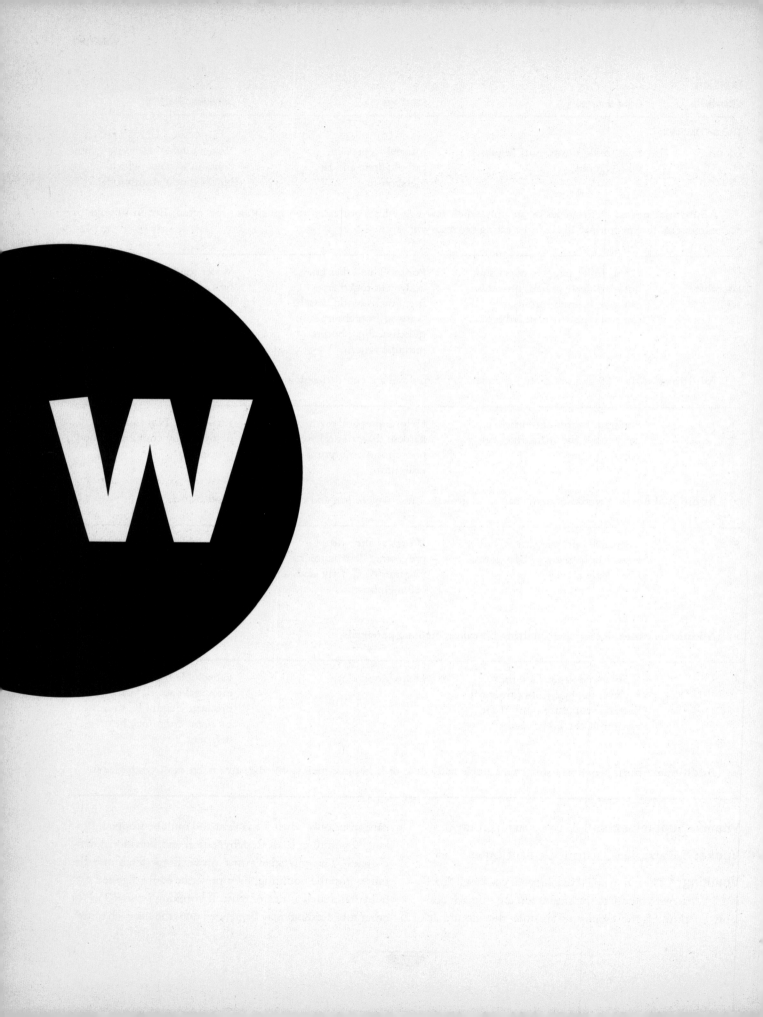

Waffles: Quick batter breads cooked and crisped in special gridded irons. Long a breakfast favorite in this country, waffles originated in Holland (the word comes from the Dutch *wafel*). According to John Mariani in his ever-fascinating *Dictionary of American Food and Drink,* waffles were "known to the Pilgrims, who had spent time in Holland before sailing to America in 1620." Mariani also writes that Thomas Jefferson lugged a long-handled waffle iron home from France. Although the classic way to serve waffles is topped with butter and maple syrup, they are very good, too, smothered with creamed chicken, shellfish or chipped beef. After the Belgian pavilion at the 1964 New York World's Fair served yeast-raised waffles, they became the rage, and they remain a staple at many fast-food restaurants. Waffles are a splendid way to recycle leftovers: Simply mix ½ cup of cooked rice or wild rice, finely cut cooked vegetables, chicken, fish or shellfish into the batter.

NUTRIENT CONTENT OF 1 TOASTED FROZEN WAFFLE	
(about 1⅓ ounces; 35 grams)	
92 calories	275 mg sodium
2 g protein	45 mg potassium
3 g fat, 1 saturated	1 g dietary fiber
8 mg cholesterol	127 RE vitamin A
14 g carbohydrate	0.14 mg thiamin
81 mg calcium	0.17 mg riboflavin
147 mg phosphorus	1.6 mg niacin
1.6 mg iron	0 mg vitamin C

Waist-Hip Ratio (WHR): An index used to determine body shape and healthy weight. The waist is measured at the narrowest point, the hips at the widest, then the larger number (hips) is divided into the smaller (waist) to determine the ratio. Women with a ratio higher than 0.8 and men with one above 0.95 are more likely to develop such obesity-related illnesses as diabetes and heart disease.

Walla Walla Onions: See ONIONS.

Walleye, Walleyed Pike: See PIKE.

Walnut Oil: A mellow, amber oil pressed from English walnuts. It stales very fast, so should be bought in small amounts and stored in a cool, dark, dry spot. Mixed about 2:1 or 50-50 with a bland vegetable oil, walnut oil is terrific for sautéing and imparts a lovely nut flavor (but its smoke point is too low to use for deep-frying). Full strength, walnut oil makes gorgeous vinaigrette (until the price of it touched the sky, it was as essential to the French kitchen as olive oil). As for nutritive value, walnut oils offer nothing other than fat and calories: 1 tablespoon walnut oil = 120 calories, 14 grams total fat (1 gram saturated). But like other vegetable oils, it's cholesterol free.

Walnuts: Black walnuts are all-American, a food the Native Americans relished and relied upon to help bring them through lean times. Their flavor is sweet and woodsy, but being tough nuts to crack, black walnuts have lost ground to English walnuts. "English" is a misnomer because these nuts originated in Iran (or so botanists believe). Their biggest producer today is France, with California not far behind. The English do fancy "English" walnuts, however, especially the soft green ones of late June that can be made into pickles, ketchup and jam. In this country we prefer mature walnuts, which every supermarket sells both in the shell and out. Because of their high fat content, walnuts quickly go rancid (the best way to keep them sweet and fresh is to buy them in the shell [or vacuum-packed tin] and store in the freezer). In addition to being high in polyunsaturated fat and containing some monounsaturates, too, walnuts are a good source of potassium. They may even lower blood cholesterol—or so a just-completed six-year California study now suggests. At least they did among those in the study (healthy men) who ate walnuts frequently—but in moderation.

NUTRIENT CONTENT OF 1 OUNCE (28 GRAMS) SHELLED ENGLISH WALNUTS	
182 calories	3 mg sodium
4 g protein	142 mg potassium
18 g fat, 2 saturated	1 g dietary fiber
0 mg cholesterol	4 RE vitamin A
5 g carbohydrate	0.11 mg thiamin
27 mg calcium	0.04 mg riboflavin
90 mg phosphorus	0.3 mg niacin
0.7 mg iron	1 mg vitamin C

Water: We can live without food for a few weeks. But denied water, we would die within days. Our bodies are 50 to 70 percent water. Blood is mostly water; so are brains and muscle. Even bones are about 20 percent water. Just to keep things running smoothly, adults need 2 quarts (8 cups) of water (milk, fruit juice or other liquid) a day and children 4 to 8 cups (depending on age and size). It's the regulator of body temperature and waste disposal, joint lubricant, cell shaper and fetal cushion. Moreover, water is crucial to the thousands of biochemical processes constantly taking place in the body.

Fresh, pure tap water is something Americans take for granted until disaster—natural or man-made—shuts off the supply. Truth to tell, not all of our water is as safe as it should be. By some estimates, nearly a million Americans sicken each year from waterborne diseases and nearly ten thousand die, mostly because hundreds of thousands of violations of the Safe Drinking Water Act go undetected or uncorrected. At present, state and federal officials take action against only about 1 percent of such violations as failing to test water for contamination, failing to report contamination to the EPA (or the public), using improper water treatment techniques.

One of the major water contaminants today is RADON. It makes water radioactive and, together with radium, the EPA estimates, accounts for more than one hundred to eighteen hundred cancer cases a year. Other troublesome chemical pollutants include lead (from old pipes or soldered joints), nitrates and pesticides (agricultural fallout that seeps into groundwater), industrial waste such as trichloroethylene and trihalomethanes, by-products of chlorination, and chloroform, which is formed when chlorine bonds with some of the organic matter dissolved in water.

Then there are biological hazards. In the Saranac Lake area of upstate New York, there are ongoing outbreaks of giardiasis, a disease caused by microscopic parasites, which chlorination alone won't control (see PARASITES). Although cholera and typhoid fever have virtually been eliminated in the United States, they remain threats whenever sewage plants are flooded and water systems polluted, as has happened repeatedly in various parts of the country.

If you're concerned about your drinking water, contact your nearest EPA office. The staff can tell you how to get it tested. See also BACTERIA; VIRUSES.

Water, Bottled: See MINERAL WATER.

Water Chestnuts: The ivory-fleshed, chestnut-skinned tubers of an aquatic sedge that flourishes throughout China and is a kitchen staple there. Though freshwater chestnuts can be bought in the Chinatowns of America and at some specialty groceries, the masses must be content with the canned. These lack the subtle sweetness of freshwater chestnuts but have lost none of the crunch. Although they supply some iron, potassium and fiber together with a modicum of B vitamins, water chestnuts are the cook's best friend because they are extremely low in calories and sodium and contain zero fat or cholesterol. Yet they add "weight" and interest to stir-fries, salads and casseroles.

NUTRIENT CONTENT OF ½ CUP CANNED SLICED WATER CHESTNUTS	
(about 2½ ounces; 70 grams)	
35 calories	6 mg sodium
1 g protein	83 mg potassium
0 g fat, 0 saturated	2 g dietary fiber
0 mg cholesterol	0 RE vitamin A
9 g carbohydrate	0.01 mg thiamin
3 mg calcium	0.02 mg riboflavin
13 mg phosphorus	0.3 mg niacin
0.6 mg iron	1 mg vitamin C

Watercress: A peppery aquatic perennial that grows wild over much of Europe but nowhere more lushly than along the *levadas* (irrigation ditches) of the Portuguese island of Madeira. Watercress grows wild in American streams, too, although what comes to market is cultivated. Watercress is equally good in soups and salads and can be steamed, half and half, with spinach. It's a moderate source of beta-carotene and vitamin C.

NUTRIENT CONTENT OF ½ CUP RAW WATERCRESS	
(about ½ ounce; 17 grams)	
2 calories	7 mg sodium
Trace protein	56 mg potassium
0 g fat, 0 saturated	0 g dietary fiber
0 mg cholesterol	80 RE vitamin A
Trace carbohydrate	0.02 mg thiamin
20 mg calcium	0.02 mg riboflavin
10 mg phosphorus	0 mg niacin
0 mg iron	7 mg vitamin C

Watercress Sprouts: The new darling of chefs, who scatter them into salads and use them to trim plates. Watercress sprouts are silvery except for a pair of tiny green

Bowl of Jade Watercress Soup

Makes 6 Servings

The texture shouts "cream," yet this nutritious soup contains very little fat or calories.

1 quart reduced-sodium chicken broth
1 large yellow onion, chopped
1 tablespoon unsalted butter
1 large Idaho potato (about 8 ounces), peeled, halved, and thinly sliced
⅓ cup water
1 large egg yolk
1 cup evaporated skim milk

⅛ to ¼ teaspoon cayenne pepper
⅛ teaspoon white pepper
¼ teaspoon salt
3 bunches (6 ounces each) watercress, trimmed of tough stems, washed, and patted dry on paper toweling (6 cups)
3 tablespoons fresh lemon juice
⅓ cup light sour cream

SIMMER THE BROTH, uncovered, in a large heavy nonreactive pan for 30 minutes or until reduced to 3 cups. Meanwhile, in a very large heavy nonstick skillet over moderate heat, stir-fry the onion in the butter until limp, about 5 minutes. Add the potato and water, stir to combine, turn heat to low, cover, and cook until the onion and potato are soft, about 10 minutes. Whisk egg yolk and evaporated milk together. Blend in a little hot broth, stir back into pan, and season with cayenne, white pepper, and salt. Heat and stir over low heat for about 5 minutes or until slightly thickened and smooth (do not boil). Remove from heat. Pile the watercress into the skillet, cover, and wilt 2 minutes; stir well, cover again, and wilt about 1 minute longer or until limp. Place the watercress mixture in a food processor fitted with the metal chopping blade and churn 30 seconds. Scrape down bowl and churn 60 seconds longer, until smooth. Stir into soup along with lemon juice and bring just to serving temperature, stirring occasionally. Remove from heat and stir in sour cream. Serve hot or chill well and serve cold.

APPROXIMATE NUTRIENT COUNTS PER SERVING

147 calories	16 g carbohydrate	0.8 mg iron	0.10 mg thiamin
9 g protein	1 g dietary fiber	213 mg sodium	0.27 mg riboflavin
6 g fat, 3 saturated	196 mg calcium	577 mg potassium	2.8 mg niacin
47 mg cholesterol	201 mg phosphorus	260 RE vitamin A	24 mg vitamin C

leaves at the tip of the hairlike stem. Despite their small size, they are blessed with plenty of bite. Nutrient counts are unavailable.

Water Filters: Three basic types exist: **carbon filters** full of activated charcoal, **reverse-osmosis systems** and **distillation units.** Each is a specialist, but none will remove bacteria or viruses. Heavy-duty carbon filters (forget small countertop or faucet-mounted models) remove chlorine, also organic chemicals like pesticides and chloroform, plus bad smells and tastes, plus some sediment. But they don't get the lead (or other heavy metals) out, or, for that matter, nitrates, fluorides, calcium, magnesium or sodium. Reverse-osmosis systems remove organic and inorganic pollutants but are extremely wasteful of water, sending 13 gallons a day (or more) down the drain. Distillers, which operate something like giant coffeepots, raise heads of steam, which then condense, leaving the impurities behind. The trouble is, some impurities are also volatile—benzene, chlorine, chloroform and so on. So these vaporize and condense, too, landing back in the "purified" water.

Water Ices: See ICES, GRANITÉS, SORBETS.

Water Intoxication: When there's an excess of water, fluid builds up in body tissues. If the kidneys are unable to function effectively, brain cells swell, causing headache, twitching, nausea, vomiting, stupor and, unless corrected, death. There may also be blurred vision and blindness. Water intoxication occurs mainly in postop or trauma patients although it can afflict infants given highly diluted formulas or if water is fed to the exclusion of milk.

Watermelons: Native to Africa, these sugary members of the gourd family spread eastward to Egypt and India thousands of years before they landed in the New World. They grow best in sandy soil—and in warm climates—which explains their popularity throughout the Mediterranean and the American South. Their varieties are nearly endless—green-and-white-striped blimps with shocking pink flesh; smooth green globes with crimson meat; chartreuse-fleshed ovals; even watermelons as orange as pumpkins. There are seeded varieties and seedless, thick skinned and thin. Babies weighing 5 to 8 pounds, and 50-pound behemoths. But only the sweet and juicy will do. The best way to eat watermelon? Cut into wedges and nibbled like ears of corn. Only moderately caloric, watermelons brim with beta-carotene, thiamin, vitamin C and potassium.

NUTRIENT CONTENT OF 1 WEDGE/SLICE WATERMELON
(about 17 ounces; 482 grams)

154 calories	10 mg sodium
3 g protein	559 mg potassium
2 g fat, 0 saturated	2 g dietary fiber
0 mg cholesterol	178 RE vitamin A
35 g carbohydrate	0.39 mg thiamin
39 mg calcium	0.10 mg riboflavin
43 mg phosphorus	1.0 mg niacin
0.8 mg iron	46 mg vitamin C

Water Pills: See DIURETIC.

Water Retention: See EDEMA.

Water Softeners: These do nothing to purify water. They merely remove the calcium and/or magnesium, which make soap scum. Many softeners, now billed as water conditioners, mislead unknowing consumers into thinking they both cleanse and soften water. They don't.

Water-Soluble Vitamins: All the Bs and C are water soluble. What this means is that if food (mainly vegetables) is cut into small pieces and cooked in lots of boiling water, much of the Bs and C will be sacrificed. The best way to preserve them? Steam vegetables. Or boil whole, preferably in the skin, using a small amount of water and cooking only until crisp-tender. See also VITAMINS.

Wax Beans: See BEANS, FRESH.

Waxing of Fruits and Vegetables: It's been going on since the 1920s and its function is not just cosmetic. Waxing is a way to keep many fruits and vegetables from drying and shriveling during their long trek from farm to kitchen. Several different waxes are used, some animal (**beeswax; lac–resin,** a food-grade shellac extracted from an East Indian insect), some vegetable (**carnauba wax,** from the fronds of the Brazilian wax palm; **candelilla wax,** the resinous exudate of a Latin American shrub) and some mineral (**paraffin**). Usually applied as a thin spray, these waxes, all of which must have FDA approval, reduce moisture loss in fruits and vegetables by nearly half. But that's not all. Artificial colors and fungicides may be added to the wax spray. Or the fruits and vegetables may be treated with fungicides before they're sprayed (it's a way to prolong shelf life and prevent the growth of molds, which may themselves produce deadly toxins). Either way, the wax seals in the fungicides.

According to the National Academy of Sciences, 90 percent of these fungicides are potentially carcinogenic. A distinct violation of the Delaney Clause of the Food, Drug, and Cosmetic Act, which bans the use of all cancer-causing agents with food. But here's the kicker: Under the very same law, the EPA can allow significant fungicide and pesticide residues on food. And only now are researchers reviewing their aggregate effect and their possible harm, especially to young children. Meanwhile, the law allows farmers and food processors to use a variety of pesticides and fungicides, some of which—benomyl, captan and folpet—are known to increase the risk of cancer.

Although the FDA now requires that all waxed fruits and vegetables be identified at point of purchase, they seldom are (and the FDA hasn't the manpower to enforce every facet of the new labeling laws). So consumer advocates cry foul. And assorted public and private agencies (the FDA, the EPA, the Natural Resources Defense Council [NRDC], the National Academy of Sciences, the United Fresh Fruit and Vegetable Association) continue to debate the merits and dangers of waxing. Until the verdict is in, here are some ways to beat "the whole ball of wax":

- Buy produce from local farms as soon as it comes into season. Better yet, grow your own.

- Peel fruits and vegetables whenever possible.

- When waxed produce can't be peeled, wash in warm soapy water, then rinse well.

- Buy "organic," concentrating on those fruits and vegetables *certified* as being organically grown. Remember, too, that even these may contain some pesticide residues.

- Reject any produce imported from Mexico or Chile. These countries permit higher pesticide residues than the United States, yet the United States allows them to be sold here.

- Educate yourself. Learn which fruits and vegetables are most likely to be waxed. The short list includes apples, avocados, beets, bell peppers, cucumbers, eggplants, lemons, limes, melons, papayas, parsnips, peaches, pineapples, potatoes, rutabagas, summer and winter squash, sweet potatoes, tangerines, tomatoes, turnips, and watermelons.

Waxy Cornstarch, Waxy Rice Flour (additives):
Obtained from waxy corn and waxy rice, respectively, these high-amylopectin starches form clear, smooth, stable gels when blended with liquid and heated. They're widely used in prepared puddings and sauces. GRAS.

Weakfish: A smallish, delicate white fish whose cousins include at least three sea trout. There are several different species, some of which swim the North Atlantic, some the Caribbean and South Atlantic and others the Pacific. In the United States they're more commonly known as **corvinas.** Weakfish flake beautifully when cooked; indeed, they're so fragile they're difficult to flip in skillet or broiler, especially if you're dealing with fillets instead of whole fish. For approximate nutrient counts, see FISH, LEAN WHITE.

Weaning: Gradually phasing babies off breast milk and on to infant formulas or other food appropriate to their age. For babies up to the age of one year, the American Academy of Pediatrics recommends that the formulas be fortified with iron to ensure that babies don't lack this essential mineral.

Weight Control, Weight Loss: For most Americans, the problem is keeping trim, and it seems there's a new diet every year that promises the impossible: quick, permanent weight loss. If a diet is to be successful, it must, according to the American Dietetic Association (ADA), incorporate these six steps:

1. Supply all the necessary nutrients but with fewer calories. Women should get at least 1,200 calories a day, men 1,500, which will mean slow but steady weight loss.

2. Consider your tastes and eating habits.

3. Keep your energy up and appetite down.

4. Let you dine out with ease and without embarrassment.

5. Readjust your eating habits so you can keep the weight off.

6. Improve your health overall.

The most successful reducing diets are built around the new FOOD GUIDE PYRAMID and include a sane program of exercise. For more details, see DIETS; OBESITY, OVERWEIGHT. See also LEPTIN.

Weisswurst: A bland white veal sausage created in Munich nearly a century and a half ago. Quite by accident. It seems that a Munich butcher, lacking the necessary ingredients for bratwurst, began improvising with some leftover sausage meat and boiled veal, adding minced parsley, grated onion and lemon rind for oomph. Today *weisswurst* is what every Municher eats when it's too late for coffee but too early for lunch. The secret of cooking *weisswurst* is that it should never be boiled, only coddled in simmering water until steaming hot. The traditional accompaniments? Sweet Bavarian mustard, *Weissbier* (a light beer made with wheat) and soft pretzels. **NOTE:** Specific nutrient counts are unavailable for *weisswurst*, but it is surely high in saturated fat, cholesterol and sodium.

Wheat: Known to all the nations of antiquity, wheat is so old no one can say where it originated. The best evidence points to the highlands of Syria. Wheat was grown early on in the Fertile Crescent; indeed it was the foundation of the Babylonian civilization. The Chinese were cultivating wheat nearly three thousand years before Christ, and it was a staple among the Stone Age Lake Dwellers of Switzerland. Wheat was introduced repeatedly to the New World. In 1529 the Spaniards carried it to Mexico. In 1602 an English explorer named Gosnold planted it in New England and by 1611 the Virginia colonists were harvesting wheat.

Strangely, wheat came to America's breadbasket late. Only in 1845 did it reach Minnesota, nearly one hundred years after its arrival in California. Today more world acreage is devoted to wheat than to any other grain, and throughout the temperate zone it is king. As might be expected of a cereal of such ancient lineage, there are hundreds of varieties of wheat: the primitive, fragile-headed **einkorn, emmer** and **spelt** still grown in parts of Europe and the Middle East; the **club wheats** of Central Europe; the **durum** of arid Mediterranean regions (its high-gluten flour goes into pasta and semolina); **common wheats** (the principal source of bread and cake flour). Among the most important wheats grown in the United States are **hard red winter** (the Great Plains staple that accounts for nearly half of our total crop), **hard red spring, soft red winter** (the Southern favorite because its flour, being lower in gluten, produces supremely flaky biscuits and tender-crumbed cakes) and **durum**. These wheats are made into various types of CEREALS, PASTA and FLOUR, both whole-grain and refined.

The ripe wheat grain consists largely of starchy endo-

sperm (it accounts for some 82 percent of the kernel). The rest is comprised of bran or husk (8 to 9 percent), embryo or germ (6 percent) and a nitrogen-rich aleurone layer (3 to 4 percent).

Wheat Berries: Only the name is new. When great grandmother bought these kernels to grind into flour, they were known as **whole wheat.** Though she'd probably snicker at their being called wheat berries, she'd be impressed by the many ways today's cooks are using them. Both **soft** and **hard** wheat berries are available, mostly at health-food stores and specialty groceries. "Soft" and "hard" don't refer to the kernel's tenderness—both types are as hard as BBs—but to the amount of gluten (protein) in the wheat. Soft wheat is low gluten, what millers grind into cake and pastry flours. Hard wheat is milled into sturdy bread flours (**all-purpose** is a blend of the two). Cooks buying wheat berries today aren't likely to mill them into flour as their grandmothers did. They're more interested in parboiling and folding them into multigrain breads. Or in cooking them like rice and serving as a nutritious alternative. Wheat berries are a go-everywhere ingredient. If soaked and boiled or parboiled, they can be slipped into a variety of casseroles in place of rice or pasta, into chilis and curries, soups and stews. They can be teamed 50-50 with rice or wild rice, lentils or other legumes. Wheat berries can also be added to meat and vegetable salads, even to poultry stuffings. See also BULGUR.

NUTRIENT CONTENT OF 1 CUP COOKED WHEAT BERRIES	
(about 5½ ounces; 150 grams)	
84 calories	1 mg sodium
4 g protein	99 mg potassium
0* g fat, 0 saturated	3 g dietary fiber
0 mg cholesterol	0 RE vitamin A
20 g carbohydrate	0.12 mg thiamin
9 mg calcium	0.03 mg riboflavin
78 mg phosphorus	1.5 mg niacin
0.9 mg iron	0 mg vitamin C

*Although they contain the germ, wheat berries are virtually fat free—just 0.426 grams per cup of cooked berries. Since our style is to round off grams to the nearest whole number, it appears above as 0 grams fat.

Wheat Bran: The fibrous husk of the wheat grain. It's mixed into cereals and whole-grain breads and is also packaged and sold by health-food stores to be used as an ingredient. It looks a little like sawdust and is just about as flavorful. Fortunately, it's much more nutritious.

NUTRIENT CONTENT OF 1 CUP WHEAT BRAN
(about 2 ounces; 60 grams)

130 calories	1 mg sodium
9 g protein	708 mg potassium
3 g fat, 0 saturated	25 g dietary fiber
0 mg cholesterol	0 RE vitamin A
39 g carbohydrate	0.31 mg thiamin
44 mg calcium	0.35 mg riboflavin
606 mg phosphorus	8.2 mg niacin
6.4 mg iron	0 mg vitamin C

Wheatena: The brand name of a hot, nourishing whole-wheat cereal that cooks up much like oatmeal.

NUTRIENT CONTENT OF 1 CUP COOKED WHEATENA
(about 8¾ ounces; 243 grams)

136 calories	5 mg sodium
5 g protein	187 mg potassium
1 g fat, 0 saturated	3 g dietary fiber
0 mg cholesterol	0 RE vitamin A
29 g carbohydrate	0.02 mg thiamin
10 mg calcium	0.05 mg riboflavin
145 mg phosphorus	1.3 mg niacin
1.4 mg iron	0 mg vitamin C

Wheat Germ: The oily embryo of the wheat grain, the part that sprouts. It contains two thirds of the grain's thiamin, a fourth of its riboflavin and a fifth of its pyridoxine. It can be bought by the bottle, sprinkled over cereals, mixed into meat loaves and burgers, or baked into a variety of breads and cookies. There's no denying it will boost their nutritive value, adding hefty shots of iron, niacin, thiamin, phosphorus and potassium. Health faddists attribute magical powers to wheat-germ oil because of its high vitamin E content. Unfortunately, wheat germ and wheat-germ oil both turn rancid very quickly and should be kept refrigerated.

NUTRIENT CONTENT OF 1 CUP RAW WHEAT GERM
(about 3½ ounces; 100 grams)

360 calories	12 mg sodium
23 g protein	892 mg potassium
10 g fat, 2 saturated	13 g dietary fiber
0 mg cholesterol	0 RE vitamin A
52 g carbohydrate	1.88 mg thiamin
39 mg calcium	0.50 mg riboflavin
842 mg phosphorus	6.8 mg niacin
6.3 mg iron	0 mg vitamin C

Wheat Gluten: A complex protein present in great quantities in durum and other hard wheats, to a lesser extent in soft wheats. It forms the framework of breads, cakes and pastries. For sturdy breads, high-gluten hard-wheat bread flours are the baker's choice; for feathery cakes and pastry, low-gluten soft-wheat cake or pastry flours.

Wheat Sprouts: Sprouted wheat berries, crunchy, nutty and delicious in stir-fries, salads, pancakes and frittatas.

NUTRIENT CONTENT OF 1 CUP WHEAT SPROUTS
(about 4 ounces; 108 grams)

213 calories	17 mg sodium
8 g protein	183 mg potassium
1 g fat, 0 saturated	9 g dietary fiber
0 mg cholesterol	6 RE vitamin A
46 g carbohydrate	0.24 mg thiamin
30 mg calcium	0.17 mg riboflavin
216 mg phosphorus	3.3 mg niacin
2.3 mg iron	3 mg vitamin C

Whey: The milky liquid left after milk or cream has clotted (curded). There are **sweet wheys** (those produced when rennet is used to curd milk for Cheddars and Swiss cheeses) and **sour** or **acid wheys,** a by-product of cottage-cheese manufacturing. Wheys are a good source of milk sugar and proteins and shouldn't be thrown away. Add them to ranch-style salad dressings; mix 50-50 with sour milk or buttermilk when baking; use to heighten the tartness of certain soups and sauces just as you would lemon juice.

Whipping Cream, Heavy Cream: See CREAM.

Whiskeys: See ALCOHOL, ALCOHOLIC BEVERAGES.

Whitebait: A portmanteau term used for a variety of just-hatched fish—herring, eel, silverside, etc. No more than an inch or two long, these hatchlings are eaten whole—head, spine, tail. The most popular way to cook whitebait is to crisp them in hot fat like shoestring potatoes. **NOTE:** No nutrient counts are available for whitebait, but this much can be said: They are oily fish.

White Chocolate: Cocoa butter blended with sugar and milk solids. It's a poor keeper, tricky to work with, as every confectioner knows, because it "seizes" (clumps) easily. With more than half of its fat saturated, white chocolate is a poor choice for anyone with cardiovascular disease—or anyone wishing to avoid it.

NUTRIENT CONTENT OF 1 OUNCE (28 GRAMS) WHITE CHOCOLATE CHIPS

151 calories	25 mg sodium
2 g protein	87 mg potassium
9 g fat, 5 saturated	0 g dietary fiber
6 mg cholesterol	18 RE vitamin A
17 g carbohydrate	0.01 mg thiamin
58 mg calcium	0.08 mg riboflavin
54 mg phosphorus	0 mg niacin
0 mg iron	0 mg vitamin C

Whitefish: A group of fish of the salmon and trout family that swim the world's icy inlets, lakes and rivers. Among them are the **ciscos** (often sold in the United States as

NUTRIENT CONTENT OF 3 OUNCES (85 GRAMS) BAKED/BROILED WHITEFISH

146 calories	55 mg sodium
21 g protein	345 mg potassium
6 g fat, 1 saturated	0 g dietary fiber
66 mg cholesterol	33 RE vitamin A
0 g carbohydrate	0.15 mg thiamin
28 mg calcium	0.13 mg riboflavin
294 mg phosphorus	3.3 mg niacin
0.4 mg iron	0 mg vitamin C

chub) with sweet, snowy flesh that flakes easily. Because their fat is distributed evenly throughout their flesh, whitefish are classified as oily fish. Like trout and salmon, they're best when baked, broiled or sautéed.

White Perch: See PERCH.

White Sauces: The "mother" of flour-thickened sauces, the formula from which dozens of other sauces descend. As for nutrient value, 1 tablespoon medium white sauce (2 tablespoons each butter and flour, 1 cup whole milk, ¼ teaspoon salt) contains 26 calories, 2 grams fat (1 gram saturated) and 6 milligrams cholesterol, plus small amounts of vitamins and minerals. Thinner white sauces contain slightly fewer calories, slightly less fat and cholesterol; thicker sauces slightly more of each. **NOTE:** To lower saturated fat and cholesterol, substitute soft margarine for butter and low-fat or skim milk for whole milk.

White Wines: Light, dry to sweet table wines, the most popular of which include **Chablis, Chardonnay, Gewürztraminer, Pinot Grigio, Riesling, Sauternes, Sauvignon Blanc,** even the crisp and prickly Portuguese **Vinho Verde.** See WINES; also ALCOHOL, ALCOHOLIC BEVERAGES.

Whiting: Another name for HAKE.

Whole Milk: See MILK.

Whole-Wheat Flour: See GRAHAM FLOUR; also FLOUR.

WIC Program: WIC stands for Supplemental Food Program for Women, Infants and Children. The purpose of this program, underwritten by the federal government and administered by state health departments, is to provide nutrition education as well as vouchers for supplemental food. To qualify for the program, women must be pregnant, or breast-feeding or have children less than five years old. They must also meet income requirements, be at nutritional risk and live in a WIC service area.

Wieners: See FRANKFURTERS.

Wild Leeks: See RAMPS.

Wild Mushrooms: Mushrooming is risky business because there are dozens of deadly look-alikes and only an expert can tell the difference. See also MUSHROOMS.

Wild Rice: In the old days, the Chippewa would travel with little pouches of wild rice. It was as good as gold. The seed of a swamp grass that thrives in Wisconsin and Minnesota, wild rice botanically isn't rice. Although wild rice is still gathered in the wild, much of it is also now cultivated. Still, its delicate woodsy flavor hasn't been tamed any more than its crackle and crunch. Wild rice not only is blessed with significant amounts of iron and protein but is also a first-class source of niacin and dietary fiber.

NUTRIENT CONTENT OF 1 CUP COOKED WILD RICE	
(about 5¾ ounces; 164 grams)	
166 calories	5 mg sodium
7 g protein	166 mg potassium
1 g fat, 0 saturated	4 g dietary fiber
0 mg cholesterol	0 RE vitamin A
35 g carbohydrate	0.09 mg thiamin
5 mg calcium	0.14 mg riboflavin
134 mg phosphorus	2.1 mg niacin
2.0 mg iron	0 mg vitamin C

Wilson's Disease: An inability to metabolize copper that's both rare and inherited. Unless corrected (usually through a low-copper diet plus drugs that either block absorption of this metal or boost urinary excretion of it), copper accumulates in the brain, cornea, kidneys and liver. The result? Permanent liver damage and progressive neurological dysfunction.

Wines: "The nectar of the grape," wine is a beverage that has soothed and sustained man down the ages. With so many thousands of different wines being produced, the subject is encyclopedic. What concerns us here is the nutritional value of wine. Although wines in general contain small amounts of potassium and red wines tiny shots of iron, none of them lacks for calories. **Table wines** and **sparkling wines** (whether red, white or rosé) are, by volume, 9 to 14 percent alcohol, and **fortified wines** (sherry, port, Madeira, Malaga and Marsala) 14 to 24 percent. In each category there are sweet wines, semisweet, dry and semidry. What most determines the calorie count is the alcohol content, although sugar plays a role, too. Thus if two wines are both 12 percent alcohol, the sweeter wine will be higher in calories. Here's a quick calorie table. (See also VERMOUTH, the most popular of the aromatized wines; see, too, FRENCH PARADOX.)

1 oz table wine = 17 to 29 calories
(depending on sweetness and alcoholic content)
1 oz sparkling wine = 21 to 42 calories
(depending on sweetness and alcoholic content)
1 oz dessert (fortified) wine = 35 to 52 calories
(depending on sweetness and alcoholic content)

Winged Beans, Wing Beans: See BEANS, FRESH.

Wintergreen, Oil of Wintergreen: See METHYL SALICYLATE.

Wok Cooking: A wok is the bowl-shaped metal container the Chinese use for STIR-FRYING. Its advantage is that it heats quickly and cooks food fast. But unless the cook is deft, fat will puddle in the bottom of the wok and saturate the food. It may also heat to the smoke point, giving off noxious fumes.

Wolffish: Also called **ocean catfish,** perhaps because of their large heads and fearsome incisors, wolffish swim the North Atlantic. They are so highly prized in Scandinavia that Norwegians are beginning to raise them for the table lest supplies run short. The meat of wolffish is as snowy, firm and sea-sweet as lobster and can be sautéed, grilled, baked or steamed with equal success. Although wolffish sometimes attain weights of 40 pounds, those making it to American markets are in the 5- to 10-pound range. Wolffish can be bought whole or filleted. For approximate nutrient counts, see FISH, LEAN WHITE.

Wood Alcohol: See METHANOL.

Wooden Cutting Boards: After condemning hardwood cutting boards as breeding grounds for bacteria, bacteriologists have reversed themselves and now believe them safer than PLASTIC CUTTING BOARDS. Wood, it seems, discourages microbial growth. Not so plastic. Needless to say, wooden cutting boards should be kept scrupulously clean and washed in hot sudsy water immediately after they've been used to cut raw meat, fish or fowl so the next item to go on the board doesn't pick up their bacteria.

Woodruff: This herb, which blooms in May in German meadows and woodlands, is what gives *Maiebowle*, a wine punch, its distinctive flavor. In the United States, woodruff is grown mostly for show. Just as well, because woodruff can thin the blood and make it slow to clot.

Worcestershire Sauce: Two British chemists, one named Lea, the other Perrins, developed this spicy brown sauce at the time of Queen Victoria. For obvious reasons, the recipe remains secret. But the label lists these ingredients in descending order: "water, vinegar, molasses, corn syrup, anchovies, hydrolyzed soy and corn protein, fresh onions, tamarinds, salt, fresh garlic, cloves, chili peppers, natural flavorings and fresh eschalots." Worcestershire sauce doesn't require refrigeration, lasts almost indefinitely, but its flavors will gather strength over time. The surprise of Worcestershire sauce is that it's a good source of potassium and a modest one of iron.

Wormwood: A licorice-flavor herb (*Artemisia absinthium*) that was used to flavor absinthe, a green French liqueur, which, when mixed with water, turned milky white. Wormwood is hallucinogenic, and its oil, thujone, so toxic it can eat away at the brain. In Edwardian days, absinthe was as trendy among artists, writers and swingers as cocaine is today. Many became addicted and destroyed their health. As a result, absinthe was banned in 1915 throughout most of Western Europe and in the United States, too.

Wrist Circumference: A quick and easy way to determine whether you're small boned, big boned or somewhere in between. And thus a factor to be considered in determining proper weight. To determine wrist circumference, a health professional places a measuring tape around the right wrist just above the wrist bone on the hand side of the wrist, then uses this value to calculate frame size.

NUTRIENT CONTENT OF 1 TABLESPOON WORCESTERSHIRE SAUCE

(about ½ ounce; 17 grams)

11 calories	167 mg sodium
0 g protein	136 mg potassium
0 g fat, 0 saturated	0 g dietary fiber
0 mg cholesterol	2 RE vitamin A
3 g carbohydrate	0.01 mg thiamin
18 mg calcium	0.02 mg riboflavin
10 mg phosphorus	0.1 mg niacin
0.9 mg iron	2 mg vitamin C

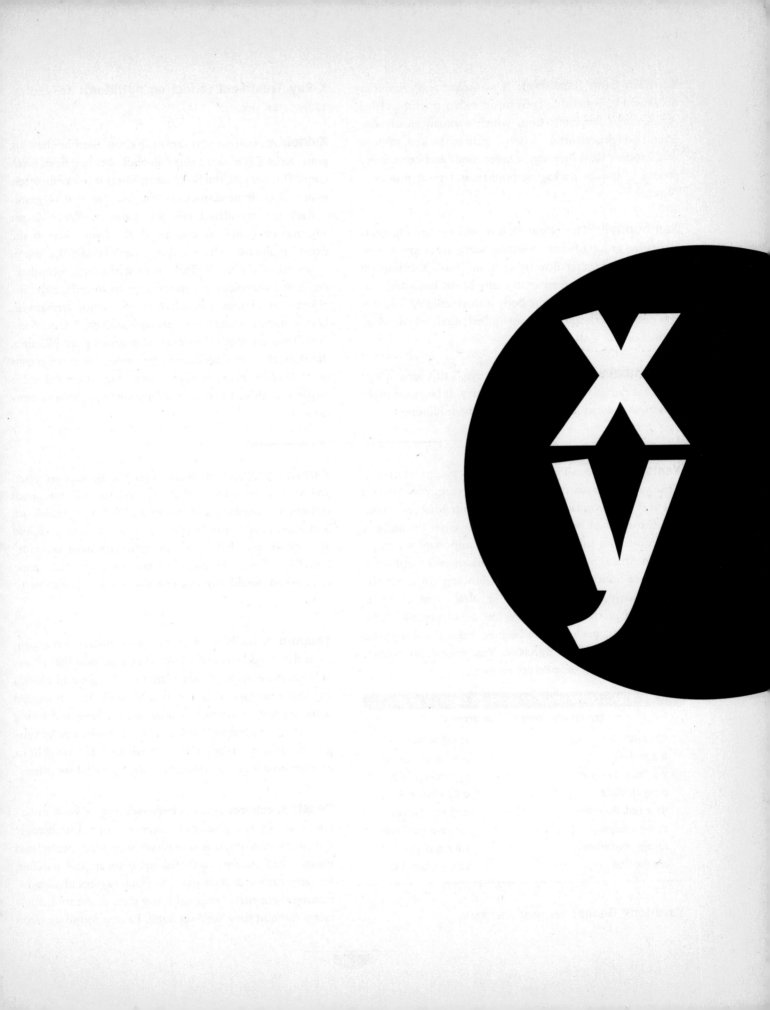

Xanthan Gum (additive): A plasticizer and emulsifier obtained by fermenting corn sugar with a microbe called *Xanthomonas campestris,* from which xanthan clearly derives. Food processors use xanthan gum to thicken, smooth and stabilize salad dressings, cheese foods and other dairy products, also in packaging poultry and meat products. Nontoxic.

Xanthophyll: The bright yellow and orange pigments (actually a group of carotenoids) in oranges, autumn leaves, marigolds and other flowers of sunny hue. Xanthophyll coexists with beta-carotene in many plants but, unlike it, cannot be converted by the body into vitamin A. There is also some xanthophyll in just-milled unbleached white flour. See also CAROTENE.

Xerophthalmia: Greek for "dry eye," this serious eye disease is caused by vitamin A deficiency. It begins as night blindness and can lead to total, permanent blindness.

X-Ray Treatment (effect on nutrition): See RADIATION THERAPY.

Xylitol: A controversial sugar substitute used in chewing gum. Xylitol is in fact a sugar alcohol obtained from birch chips. But because the body metabolizes it less completely than sucrose, limited amounts of it (no more than 60 grams a day) are considered safe for diabetics. When larger amounts of xylitol are consumed, the liver converts the excess to glucose, which diabetics can't handle because of a shortfall of insulin. Xylitol has created a buzz recently in the dental profession because it appears to reduce the incidence of cavities—mouth bacteria cannot ferment it. Unfortunately, some researchers question the safety of xylitol. Too much of it can cause abdominal pain, bloating, diarrhea, excessive calcium in the urine, calcium deposits in the bladder, even, perhaps, cancer (high doses fed to lab rats in one British test did produce tumors). Studies continue.

Yams: What we call yams are actually SWEET POTATOES. True yams are ivory fleshed, brown and shaggy of skin and not very sweet. In fact, they're nearer Irish potatoes in taste and texture than sweet potatoes. Yams grow throughout the tropics and subtropics and are an important source of food in Africa, Indonesia, parts of Asia and the Caribbean. There are hundreds of species, all climbing vines, but the most widely grown is *Dioscorea alata,* whose tubers sometimes reach awesome size (30 or 40 pounds). Like Irish potatoes, yams take to boiling, baking and deep-fat frying with equal ease. **SEASON:** Year-round, but mainly in Latin American or specialty groceries.

NUTRIENT CONTENT OF 1 CUP DICED COOKED YAMS	
(about 4¾ ounces; 136 grams)	
156 calories	11 mg sodium
2 g protein	911 mg potassium
0 g fat, 0 saturated	4 g dietary fiber
0 mg cholesterol	0 RE vitamin A
38 g carbohydrate	0.13 mg thiamin
19 mg calcium	0.04 mg riboflavin
67 mg phosphorus	0.8 mg niacin
0.7 mg iron	17 mg vitamin C

Yard-long Beans: See BEANS, FRESH.

Yarrow: A relative of chamomile. The flowers are dried and sold as herbal teas that are said to ease menstrual cramps, aid digestion and relieve assorted skin conditions. Some few people may be allergic to yarrow, however, and as a result may break out in rashes or have difficulty breathing. Those allergic to asters, chrysanthemums and/or ragweed should avoid yarrow tea. See also CHAMOMILE TEA.

Yaupon: A tea brewed by Southern Native Americans from the dried leaves of a holly (*Ilex vomitoria*) that grows wild on the Atlantic coastal plain from Virginia to Florida and along the Gulf as far south as Mexico. As its botanical name suggests, yaupon was used as an emetic and spring "purifier." On North Carolina's Outer Banks, smoky yaupon tea is a specialty. It's too weak to cause trouble or embarrassment and is, Bankers insist, "pow'ful soothing."

Yeast: Saccharomyces cerevisiae, to give yeast its scientific name, is a powerful leavener. These microscopic organisms (not fungi, as some have suggested, but related plants called ascomycetes) feed upon sugars and starches, releasing carbon dioxide gas. This bubbles through doughs, making them rise. Yeasts exist so widely in nature the ancients thought they lived on dung. Pasteur found them on ripe grapes (but didn't know where they lived the rest of the year). His contemporary, Danish botanist E. C. Hansen, then discovered that rain washed vineyard yeasts into the soil, where they wintered over.

Come summer, they would be blown about by dust and disseminated by insects. Man learned early on to catch these free-floating yeasts in starchy pastes and turn them into frothy fermented drinks and sourdough starters. Today every supermarket sells ¼-ounce packets containing 2¼ teaspoons of **active dry** or **quick-rising yeast** (the two are interchangeable); some also stock 4-ounce jars of dry yeast. **Cake yeast,** which pros consider livelier, can be bought at specialty food stores and baker's supply houses. Cake yeasts are more perishable than the dry and must be used quickly. But even dry yeasts have a life expectancy—clearly printed on each label. The point to remember when working with yeast is that heat kills it; for rapid growth, 105°F. to 115°F. is considered optimum.

Does yeast affect the nutritional content of food? One (¼-ounce) packet of yeast granules (either active dry or quick rising) contains 21 calories, 3 grams each of protein and carbohydrate, 1.2 milligrams of iron, 4 milligrams of sodium and 140 of potassium. But only a trace of fat and 0 cholesterol. As for compressed yeast, a 6-ounce cake (the size bakers use) contains 179 calories, 14 grams protein, 2 grams fat, 31 grams carbohydrate, 16 grams fiber, 5.6 milligrams iron, 32 of calcium, 51 of sodium, 1,022 of potassium. But again, no cholesterol. See also BREWER'S YEAST.

Yeast Breads: Breads leavened with yeast as opposed to quick breads that are leavened with baking powder or soda. Yeast breads take longer to prepare because they must rise once, twice, sometimes three times before they're shaped and baked. As a rule, they're spongier, sturdier, chewier than quick breads. See also BREAD.

Yeast Infections (diet and): *Candida albicans,* a normally benign yeast, lives in the bodies of healthy people, especially in such warm, moist places as the vagina and mouth (the "thrush" that plagues some babies is caused by *C. albicans*). But occasionally *C. albicans* multiplies on fast forward, infecting almost every tissue. Those most prone to yeast infections are diabetics, pregnant women and those on birth control pills, all of which raise blood sugar levels. Also prime candidates for **candidiasis,** the medical term for yeast infection, are those taking antibiotics over a period of time. Antibiotics kill the body's beneficial bacteria, which check yeast growth.

Proponents of the yeast syndrome theory advanced in the early 1980s by William G. Crook, M.D., in his book *The Yeast Connection,* believe that yeast infections generate a toxin that depowers the immune system, triggers headaches, irritability, depression, menstrual problems, respiratory and digestive disorders, not to mention aches and pains. Crook's cure consists of prolonged antifungal medication plus herbs and vitamin/mineral supplements plus a diet devoid of sugar, mold-ripened cheeses, mushrooms, vinegar and anything containing yeast, be it bread, beer or wine. Crook also recommends garlic capsules, acidophilus milk or pills and caprylic acid, a saturated fatty acid found in butter and coconut oil that's also a GRAS-rated antimicrobial/defoamer/synthetic flavoring used in baked goods, candies, gelatins and ice creams. Much of his regimen makes sense—*for everyone,* not just those with yeast infections—avoiding junk foods and sugar; eating more green vegetables, complex carbohydrates, fish and chicken; swearing off tobacco and getting plenty of exercise. Does the cure work? There's no solid clinical evidence that it does and most doctors consider it of questionable value.

What does seem to help vaginal yeast infections, however, is yogurt containing active *Lactobacillus acidophilus* cultures. In studies conducted recently among chronic yeast infection sufferers at Long Island Jewish Medical Center, women who ate a cup of *L. acidophilus*-cultured yogurt every day for six months were three times less likely to suffer from vaginitis as those in the control group. Unfortunately, some major brands of yogurt are not made with *L. acidophilus* although more and more manufacturers are beginning to add it. Read labels carefully or call the manufacturer to learn what bacterial cultures are used. Better yet, make your own yogurt using acidophilus milk as a starter.

Yeast Syndrome: See YEAST INFECTIONS.

Yellow Bell Peppers: See SWEET PEPPERS under PEPPERS, CAPSICUMS.

Yellowfin: A light-meat TUNA.

Yellow Perch: See PERCH.

Yellow Squash: See SQUASH.

Yellowtail: A Pacific fish that is a member of the jack family and one that's particularly abundant around San Diego. Some yellowtail are giants weighing 100 pounds or more, but, to the sportsman's despair, the usual catch is much smaller. Yellowtail seldom come to market fresh, and when they do, it's usually as steaks or fillets. But they do appear with increasing frequency on restaurant menus. Unfortunately, yellowtail is one of the saltwater fish likely to cause CIGUATERA POISONING.

NUTRIENT CONTENT OF 3 OUNCES (85 GRAMS) BAKED/BROILED YELLOWTAIL	
159 calories	43 mg sodium
25 g protein	457 mg potassium
6 g fat, NA saturated	0 g dietary fiber
61 mg cholesterol	26 RE vitamin A
0 g carbohydrate	0.15 mg thiamin
25 mg calcium	0.04 mg riboflavin
171 mg phosphorus	7.4 mg niacin
0.5 mg iron	2 mg vitamin C

Yersinia enterocolitica: One of the sources of food poisoning. See BACTERIA.

Yin-Yang Foods: The Chinese believe that to achieve bodily harmony, you must balance your intake of yin (cool, bland) foods with yang (the rich and hot). They further believe that winter is yang season (the time for spicy, heavy food) and summer yin; that new mothers should eat yang foods, as should the chronically fatigued. Yin foods, on the other hand, are recommended for the irritable. The Chinese classify ailments as yin (cold) or yang (hot) and believe that as the body ages, it becomes increasingly yin. Such yin diseases as anemia are treated with yang foods, and assorted yang infections (sore throats, measles, etc.) with yin foods. Not all Chinese agree on which foods are yin or yang, but as a general rule, they break down as follows:

Yin Foods: Bean curd and sprouts, all bland or boiled foods, the cabbage family, carrots and celery, cucumber, duck, some fish and fruits, American ginseng, most greens, honey, melons, milk, pears, pork, potatoes, seaweed and soybean products, white turnips, water and watercress, winter squash, most white foods.

Yang Foods: Bamboo, beef, broiled meats, catfish, chicken and chicken soup, eggs and eggplant, fatty meats and fried foods, garlic and ginger, Korean ginseng, glutinous rice, green peppers, hot and spicy foods, leeks and onions, liquor, mushrooms, peanuts, persimmons, pig's knuckles and pork liver, red foods (beans, peppers, tomatoes, etc.), sesame oil, shellfish, sour foods, tangerines, vinegar and wine.

Yogurt: In ancient times, as early as two thousand years before Christ, women found that if they let milk ferment into curds and whey, the tart and creamy curd could be kept much longer than fresh milk. We now know that curd as yogurt. It first surfaced in the United States in the 1940s as "health food," gained recognition in the sixties as "hippie food" and now at long last has gone mainstream, as a cruise down any supermarket dairy aisle quickly proves. Still, health claims for yogurt persist: It strengthens the immune system, lowers blood cholesterol, reduces the risk of cancer, fights yeast infections, aids digestion and is, in fact, a sort of fountain of youth. Microbiologists, physicians and nutritionists discount nearly all of these claims (except perhaps that yogurts containing active *Lactobacillus acidophilus* cultures may lower the incidence of vaginal yeast infections). They do agree, however, that yogurt is a good source of calcium and top-quality protein.

Clearly, not all yogurts are created equal. Although required by the U.S. government to be fermented with *Lactobacillus bulgaricus* and *Streptococcus thermophilus,* some yogurts may have additional cultures of *L. acidophilus* and/or *Bifido bacterium*. The curative powers of yogurt are attributed to these last two "good" bacteria, which fight the "bad" bugs in the body. Unfortunately, many yogurts are heat treated after they've been cultured, meaning they contain no live cultures (if so, the label must clearly state that fact). And **frozen yogurts,** to which bacterial cultures are added just before freezing, are never fermented. Worse, "yogurt-dipped" candies and raisins contain no cultures at all and are merely given a sour taste that masquerades as yogurt.

Today's yogurt terminology is both vast and confusing. To help set things straight, here's a quick dictionary, arranged in order of fat content.

DEFINING FAT CONTENT

Nonfat Yogurt: Often labeled "fat-free," "light" or "lite," these yogurts are made from skim milk containing less than 0.5 percent fat. Still, they do contain some fat (it supplies about 6 percent of the calories in plain yogurt and 3 percent in the flavored). Nonfat does not necessarily mean low calorie, however. Some nonfat yogurts contain as few as 90 calories per 8-ounce cup, but in others the calorie count zooms to 200 per cup. Once again, sugar is the culprit (with some flavored nonfat yogurts containing nearly ¼ cup). Truly low-calorie nonfat yogurts (in the 90- to 100-calorie bracket) are artificially sweetened, usually with aspartame.

Low-Fat Yogurt: Made from low-fat or part-skim milk containing 0.5 to 2 percent milk fat, these yogurts are about half as fat as whole-milk yogurts (in the unflavored, fat supplies 23 percent of the calories; in the flavored, a mere 10 percent). The downside is that the flavored yogurts may contain more than 3 tablespoons sugar. As for calories, low-fat yogurts weigh in at from 140 to 270 calories per 8-ounce cup (with added sugar contributing the lion's share).

Whole-Milk Yogurt: Yogurt made from whole milk (with at least 3.25 percent milk fat). It contains anywhere from 150 to 250 calories per 8-ounce cup depending upon whether it's sweetened with sugar, fruit jam or an artificial sweetener. Plain yogurts get about 40 percent of their calories from fat, flavored yogurts 22 percent (but these may contain as much as 3 tablespoons of sugar).

OTHER YOGURT-SPEAK

Chiffon: A light and creamy yogurt custard.

"Contains Active Yogurt Cultures": The yogurt has not been heat treated after culturing and thus does contain active bacterial cultures. The one that is supposed to be the most beneficial is *Lactobacillus acidophilus* and the label may or may not state whether it is present. This may be written a number of different ways. On one popular brand, it's "Meets National Yogurt Association criteria for live and active culture yogurt."

Custard Style, Swiss Style: Completely homogenous yogurt with fruit or other flavors pureed in. To keep them from separating, many manufacturers add stabilizers or gelatin.

Frozen Yogurt: To date, the federal government has failed to define frozen yogurt and, until it does, almost anything goes. Some frozen yogurts, for example, are nothing more than ice milk or ice cream to which yogurt cultures have been added. Others are just what they say—frozen yogurt with significant amounts of active bacterial cultures. Look for "LAC" on the label. It stands for "live, active cultures" and is a designation dreamed up by the National Yogurt Association. The nutritional profile of many frozen yogurts approximates that of ice cream; indeed, some ice creams are lower in fat and calories than some frozen yogurts. A number of the fancier frozen yogurts have been clocked at 9 grams of fat and 220 calories per half cup (4 ounces). Hardly health food! Read labels carefully and avoid tricked-out flavors made with cookie chunks, syrup swirls and candies.

Heat Treated After Culturing: Yogurt that's been heated to prolong shelf life. It contains none of the live or active bacterial cultures that are supposed to be so beneficial.

Liquid: A yogurt thin enough to drink. Usually it's a blend of yogurt and pureed fruit.

Made with Active Cultures: An entirely deceptive description that implies that the yogurt contains active cultures. If it's been heat treated after culturing, it does not. Scrutinize labels.

Sundae: An umbrella term that includes all the stir-up, fruit-on-the-bottom yogurts.

Yogurt Cheese: Called **labna** in the Middle East, this is nothing more than plain yogurt from which every last drop of whey has been drained. Yogurt cheese is thicker, sweeter than yogurt, a dandy substitute for whipped cream or cream cheese. It couldn't be easier to make. Simply line a fine sieve with cheesecloth or coffee filters, set it over a 1-quart glass measure, pour in 1 pint plain nonfat yogurt, score top crisscross fashion with a sharp knife, cover, refrigerate and let drain for 24 hours. **YIELD:** About ¾ cup.

NUTRIENT CONTENT OF 1 TABLESPOON YOGURT CHEESE

15 calories	0 mg iron
1 g protein	13 mg sodium
0 g fat, 0 saturated	46 mg potassium
1 mg cholesterol	4 RE vitamin A
1 g carbohydrate	0.01 mg thiamin
0 g dietary fiber	0.04 mg riboflavin
49 mg calcium	0 mg niacin
37 mg phosphorus	0 mg vitamin C

NUTRIENT CONTENT OF 1 CUP PLAIN WHOLE-MILK YOGURT
(about 8¾ ounces; 245 grams)

150 calories	113 mg sodium
9 g protein	377 mg potassium
8 g fat, 5 saturated	0 g dietary fiber
31 mg cholesterol	74 RE vitamin A
11 g carbohydrate	0.07 mg thiamin
294 mg calcium	0.35 mg riboflavin
232 mg phosphorus	0.2 mg niacin
0.1 mg iron	1 mg vitamin C

NUTRIENT CONTENT OF 1 CUP WHOLE-MILK FRUIT YOGURT
(about 8¾ ounces; 245 grams)

292 calories	292 mg sodium
11 g protein	466 mg potassium
8 g fat, 5 saturated	0 g dietary fiber
24 mg cholesterol	67 RE vitamin A
46 g carbohydrate	0.10 mg thiamin
365 mg calcium	0.42 mg riboflavin
287 mg phosphorus	0.22 mg niacin
0.2 mg iron	2 mg vitamin C

NUTRIENT CONTENT OF 1 CUP PLAIN LOW-FAT YOGURT
(about 8¾ ounces; 245 grams)

154* calories	172 mg sodium
13* g protein	571 mg potassium
4 g fat, 2 saturated	0 g dietary fiber
15 mg cholesterol	39 RE vitamin A
17 g carbohydrate	0.11 mg thiamin
446* mg calcium	0.52 mg riboflavin
350 mg phosphorus	0.3 mg niacin
0.2 mg iron	2 mg vitamin C

NUTRIENT CONTENT OF 1 CUP LOW-FAT FRUIT YOGURT
(about 8¾ ounces; 245 grams)

250 calories	142 mg sodium
11 g protein	475 mg potassium
3 g fat, 2 saturated	0 g dietary fiber
10 mg cholesterol	27 RE vitamin A
47 g carbohydrate	0.09 mg thiamin
372 mg calcium	0.44 mg riboflavin
292 mg phosphorus	0.2 mg niacin
0.2 mg iron	2 mg vitamin C

*The reason calories, protein and calcium are higher in low-fat
 yogurt than in whole-milk yogurt is that nonfat dry milk solids
 are added for body and creaminess.

NUTRIENT CONTENT OF 1 CUP PLAIN NONFAT YOGURT
(about 8¾ ounces; 245 grams)

136 calories	187 mg sodium
14 g protein	625 mg potassium
0 g fat, 0 saturated	0 g dietary fiber
4 mg cholesterol	5 RE vitamin A
19 g carbohydrate	0.12 mg thiamin
488 mg calcium	0.57 mg riboflavin
382 mg phosphorus	0.3 mg niacin
0.2 mg iron	2 mg vitamin C

NUTRIENT CONTENT OF 1 CUP NONFAT FRUIT YOGURT (WITH ARTIFICIAL SWEETENER)
(about 8⅔ ounces; 241 grams)

122 calories	139 mg sodium
11 g protein	550 mg potassium
0 g fat, 0 saturated	1 g dietary fiber
3 mg cholesterol	6 RE vitamin A
19 g carbohydrate	0.10 mg thiamin
369 mg calcium	0.45 mg riboflavin
291 mg phosphorus	0.5 mg niacin
0.6 mg iron	2 mg vitamin C

Yohimbe: Health-food stores claim this tree bark boosts potency and builds muscles. The truth? It's caused serious side effects: kidney failure, seizures and death. The FDA is scrutinizing health aids containing yohimbe.

Yokan: See BEANS, DRIED.

Yolk: The yellow part of the egg, the more nutritious half. But make a note, the yolk also contains all the fat and cholesterol. Indeed, one large egg yolk supplies more than two thirds of the daily quota for cholesterol suggested by the American Heart Association. For nutrient counts see EGGS.

Yo-yo Dieting: See DIETING, YO-YO OR SEESAW.

Yucca Extract (additive): Obtained from the spiky subtropical yucca plant, this dark brown, bittersweet foaming agent is used in a variety of cocktail mixers, root beers, also some ices and ice creams. Not known to be toxic.

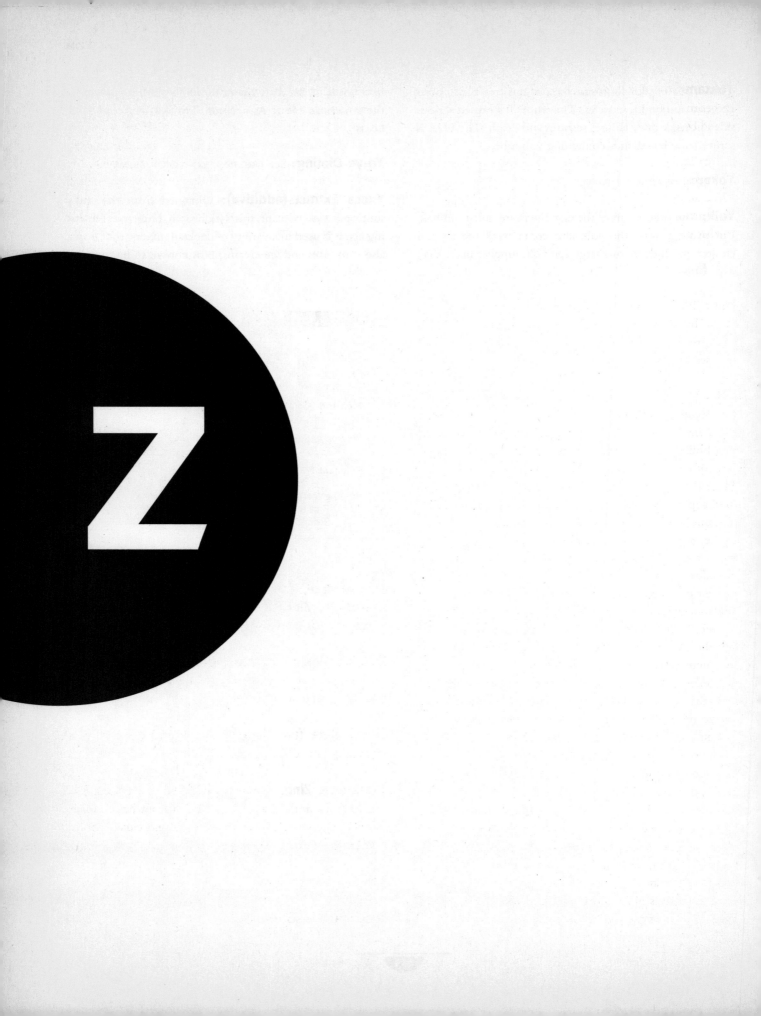

Zeaxanthin: One of the yellow pigments in egg yolks and corn. Though a carotene, zeaxanthin cannot be converted by the body into vitamin A.

Zein: The principal protein in corn, but an incomplete one because it is very low in two essential amino acids—lysine and tryptophan. Zein is not soluble in water, a trait food manufacturers put to good advantage by using zein to coat candies and nuts.

Zen Macrobiotic Diet: See MACROBIOTIC DIET.

Zest: The colored part of citrus rind that's rich in flavonoids, biflavonoids and limonoids. These PHYTOCHEMICALS, researchers now believe, reduce the risk of certain diseases, among them cancer.

Zinc: The body cannot function without this heavy metal. It's essential to the synthesis of DNA and RNA, of proteins, insulin and sperm. The body needs zinc, too, to metabolize carbohydrates, fats, protein and alcohol; to dispose of carbon dioxide; to make good use of vitamin A. More than seventy different enzymes require zinc to do their appointed work. And that's not all. Zinc bolsters the immune system and makes wounds heal faster. It's integral to the growth and maintenance of body tissues; it plays a major role in the development of fetuses and the growth of children. It even hones the palate. Does zinc stop colds in their tracks, as folk practitioners have claimed for years? Well, maybe. When zinc lozenges are dissolved on the tongue, Dartmouth researchers say, the runny nose dries and the cold virus fails to multiply. But only if the zinc treatment starts at first sneeze. Swallowing zinc pills has little effect although some nutritionists and physicians believe that if you've been getting your daily dose of zinc, you're more likely to resist colds. **DEFICIENCY SYMPTOMS:** Stunted growth, loss of appetite and ability to taste food, slowness to heal. Substantial amounts of zinc are lost in milling and processing, also in the soaking water of dried peas and beans unless that water is recycled. In addition, the fiber and PHYTATES in food bind zinc, making some of it unavailable to the body. **GOOD SOURCES OF ZINC:** High-protein foods like meat, poultry (especially dark meat), shellfish, legumes and whole grains. **PRECAUTIONS:** Only those on zinc supplements risk ODing. The first symptom is likely to be vomiting, the body's way of purging itself of the excess. The zinc in galvanized containers can combine with acid fruit drinks, producing a toxin that apes the symptoms of food poisoning—a fact a group of Southern picnickers learned the hard way after drinking lemonade carried to the picnic site in a tin bucket. A more common problem is that zinc interferes with the body's ability to use copper, another reason to avoid high doses. Now comes word from a new Massachusetts study that links zinc with Alzheimer's. Researchers suggest that zinc may trigger the formation of the destructive plaque that shows up so prominently in the brains of Alzheimer's patients (all the more reason not to scarf down zinc tablets). See also ALZHEIMER'S DISEASE.

RDA FOR ZINC	
Babies:	
Birth to 1 year	5 mg per day
Children:	
1 to 10 years	10 mg per day
Men and Boys:	
11 to 51+ years	15 mg per day
Women and Girls:	
11 to 51+ years	12 mg per day
Pregnant Women:	15 mg per day
Nursing Mothers:	
First 6 months	19 mg per day
Second 6 months	16 mg per day

Zinc Acetate, Zinc Carbonate, Zinc Chloride, Zinc Gluconate, Zinc Oxide (additives): Different forms of zinc used as dietary supplements. GRAS.

Zinc Methionine Sulfate (additive): The form of zinc commonly used in vitamin/mineral pills. The FDA regulates amounts that can be used.

Zinc Sulfate (additive): A zinc salt used in some frozen egg products and substitutes. GRAS.

Zingerone, Zingiberone (additive): A flavoring extracted from fresh ginger that's used in root beer, ginger ale, chewing gum, candies, ice creams and baked goods. Not known to be toxic.

Ziti: See PASTA.

Zucchini: See SQUASH.

Zucchini Blossoms: See FLOWERS, EDIBLE.

Zungenwurst: Blood sausage strewn with cubes of cooked tongue. A German specialty. **NOTE:** Specific nutrient counts are unavailable for *zungenwurst* but it's safe to say that it doesn't short-shrift fat, cholesterol or sodium.

Zwieback: To translate from the German, this means "twice baked." And that's precisely what these crisp, dry crackers are. Baked rusks that are sliced thin, then rebaked until hard and dry.

NUTRIENT CONTENT OF 1 PIECE ZWIEBACK
(about ¼ ounce; 7 grams)

30 calories	18 mg sodium
1 g protein	11 mg potassium
1 g fat, 0 saturated	NA g dietary fiber
0 mg cholesterol	0 RE vitamin A
5 g carbohydrate	0 mg thiamin
1 mg calcium	0 mg riboflavin
5 mg phosphorus	0.1 mg niacin
0 mg iron	0 mg vitamin C

Bibliography

The American Heritage Cookbook and Illustrated History of American Eating & Drinking. New York: American Heritage Publishing, 1964.

American Home Economics Association. *Handbook of Food Preparation,* 9th edition. Dubuque, Ia: Kendall/Hunt Publishing, 1993.

Anderson, Kenneth. *The Pocket Guide to Coffees & Teas.* New York: Perigee, 1982.

Aresty, Esther B. *The Delectable Past.* New York: Simon & Schuster, 1964.

Battistotti, Bruno, Vittorio Bottazzi, Antonio Piccinardi and Giancarlo Volpato. *Cheese: A Guide to the World of Cheese and Cheesemaking.* Translated by Sara Harris. New York: Facts on File, 1984.

Bennion, Marion. *Introductory Foods,* 10th edition. Englewood Cliffs, N.J.: Prentice Hall, 1995.

Better Homes and Gardens Staff, eds. *Complete Guide to Food and Cooking.* Des Moines, Ia.: Meredith, 1991.

Bittman, Mark. *Fish: The Complete Guide to Buying and Cooking.* New York: Macmillan, 1994.

Black, Jacquelyn G. *Microbiology Principles and Applications,* 2d edition. Englewood Cliffs, N.J.: Prentice Hall, 1992.

Boston Children's Hospital with Susan Baker and Roberta R. Henry. *Parents' Guide to Nutrition.* Reading, Mass.: Addison-Wesley, 1986.

Brennan, Georgeanne, Isaac Cronin and Charlotte Glenn. *The New American Vegetable Cookbook: The Definitive Guide to America's Exotic & Traditional Vegetables.* Berkeley, Calif.: Aris Books, 1985.

Brillat-Savarin, J. A. *The Physiology of Taste.* Translated by M.F.K. Fisher. New York: Harcourt Brace Jovanovich, 1978.

Brody, Jane. *Jane Brody's Nutrition Book.* New York: Bantam, 1982.

———. *Jane Brody's Good Food Book: Living the High-Carbohydrate Way.* New York: Norton, 1985.

Bryant, Carol A., Anita Courtney, Barbara A. Markesbery and Kathleen M. DeWalt. *The Cultural Feast.* St. Paul, Minn.: West Publishing, 1985.

Campbell, Ada Marie, Marjorie P. Penfield and Ruth M. Griswold. *The Experimental Study of Food,* 2d edition. Boston: Houghton Mifflin, 1979.

Christian, Janet L., and Janet L. Greger. *Nutrition for Living,* 3d edition. Redwood City, Calif.: Benjamin/Cummings Publishing, 1991.

Clarke, Ethne. *The Art of the Kitchen Garden.* New York: Knopf, 1987.

Claudio, Virginia S., and Rosalinda T. Lagua. *Nutrition and Diet Therapy Dictionary,* 3d edition. New York: Van Nostrand Reinhold, 1991.

Cody, Mildred M., and Mary Keith. *Food Safety for Professionals.* Chicago: The American Dietetic Association, 1991.

Cook's and Diner's Dictionary. Introduction by M.F.K. Fisher. New York: Funk & Wagnalls, 1968.

Cost, Bruce. *Bruce Cost's Asian Ingredients.* Foreword by Alice Waters. New York: Morrow, 1988.

Creasy, Rosalind. *Cooking from the Garden.* San Francisco: Sierra Club Books, 1988.

Davidson, Alan. *North Atlantic Seafood.* New York: Viking, 1979.

———. *Seafood: A Connoisseur's Guide and Cookbook.* New York: Simon & Schuster, 1989.

————. *Fruit: A Connoisseur's Guide and Cookbook*. New York: Simon & Schuster, 1991.

Deskins, Barbara B. *Everyone's Guide to Better Food and Nutrition*. Middle Village, N.Y.: Jonathan David Publishers, 1975.

DeWitt, Dave, and Nancy Gerlach. *The Whole Chile Pepper Book*. Boston: Little, Brown, 1990.

Dowell, Philip, and Adrian Bailey. *Cooks' Ingredients*. New York: Morrow, 1980.

Duff, Gail. *A Book of Herbs & Spices: Recipes, Remedies, and Lore*. Topsfield, Mass.: Salem House Publishers, 1987.

Eckstein, Eleanor F. *Menu Planning,* 3d edition. Westport, Conn.: Avi Publishing, 1983.

Ensminger, Audrey H., M. E. Ensminger, James E. Kolande and John R. K. Robson. *Foods & Nutrition Encyclopedia,* 2d edition. Boca Raton, Fla.: CRC Press, 1994.

Eskin, N. A. Michael. *Biochemistry of Foods,* 2d edition. San Diego: Academic Press, 1990.

Fletcher, Anne M. *Eat Fish, Live Better*. New York: Harper & Row, 1989.

Food and Nutrition Board, National Research Council. *Recommended Dietary Allowances,* 10th edition. Washington, D.C.: National Academy Press, 1989.

Frankle, Reva T., and Anita L. Owen. *Nutrition in the Community,* 3d edition. St. Louis: Mosby, 1993.

Frazier, W. C., and D. C. Westhoff. *Food Microbiology,* 4th edition. New York: McGraw-Hill, 1988.

Freeland-Graves, Jeanne H., and Gladys C. Peckham. *Foundations of Food Preparation,* 5th edition. New York: Macmillan, 1987.

Gastronomic Routes of France. Paris: Sopexa, 1991.

Gershoff, Stanley, with Catherine Whitney and the Editorial Advisory Board of the *Tufts University Diet & Nutrition Letter. The Tufts University Guide to Total Nutrition.* New York: Harper & Row, 1990.

Grieve, M. *Culinary Herbs and Condiments*. New York: Dover Publications, 1971.

Guthrie, Helen A. *Introductory Nutrition,* 7th edition. St. Louis: Times Mirror, Mosby College Publishing, 1989.

Hale, William Harlan, and the Editors of *Horizon Magazine. The Horizon Cookbook and Illustrated History of Eating and Drinking Through the Ages*. Wendy Buehr, ed.; Tatiana McKenna, recipes ed.; Mimi Sheraton, historical foods consultant. New York: American Heritage Publishing Co., 1968.

Harris, Robert S., and Endel Karmas. *Nutritional Evaluation of Food Processing,* 2d edition. Westport, Conn.: Avi Publishing, 1975.

Hedrick, U. P., ed. *Sturtevant's Notes on Edible Plants*. Albany, N.Y.: J. B. Lyon Co., 1919.

Hill, Albert F. *Economic Botany*. New York: McGraw-Hill, 1952.

Holmberg, Rita. *Meal Management Today*. Prospect Heights, Ill.: Waveland Press, 1983.

Igoe, Robert S. *Dictionary of Food Ingredients,* 2d edition. New York: Van Nostrand Reinhold, 1989.

Institute of Medicine. *Nutrition During Pregnancy*. Washington, D.C.: National Academy Press, 1990.

Jackson, Michael. *Pocket Guide to Beer*. New York: Simon & Schuster, 1991.

Jacobson, Michael F. *The Consumer's Factbook of Food Additives,* updated. New York: Doubleday, 1976.

Jacobson, Michael F., Lisa Y. Lefferts and Anne Witte Garland. *Safe Food: Eating Wisely in a Risky World*. Los Angeles: Living Planet Press, 1991.

Jenkins, Nancy Harmon. *The Mediterranean Diet Cookbook*. New York: Bantam, 1994.

Johnson, G. Timothy, and Stephen E. Goldfinger, eds. *The Harvard Medical School Health Letter Book*. Cambridge, Mass.: Harvard University Press, 1981.

Johnson, Hugh. *Hugh Johnson's Modern Encyclopedia of Wine,* 3d edition, revised and updated. New York: Simon & Schuster, 1991.

Jones, Julie Miller. *Food Safety*. St. Paul, Minn.: Eagan Press, 1992.

Kinder, Faye, Nancy R. Green and Natholyn Harris. *Meal Management,* 6th edition. New York: Macmillan, 1984.

Kittler, Pamela G., and Kathryn Sucher. *Food and Culture in America*. New York: Van Nostrand Reinhold, 1989.

Kunz, Jeffrey R. M., M.D., and Asher J. Finkel, M.D., eds. *The American Medical Association Family Medical Guide,* revised and updated. New York: Random House, 1987.

Layton, T. A. *The Wine and Food Society's Guide to Cheese and Cheese Cookery*. Cleveland, Ohio: World Publishing, 1967.

leRiche, W. Harding. *A Chemical Feast*. New York: Facts on File, 1982.

Lewis, Richard J., Sr. *Food Additives Handbook*. New York: Van Nostrand Reinhold, 1989.

Lichine, Alexis. *Alexis Lichine's Encyclopedia of Wines & Spirits*. New York: Knopf, 1967.

Linder, Maria, ed. *Nutritional Biochemistry and Metabolism,* 2d edition. New York: Elsevier, 1991.

Loewenfeld, Claire, and Philippa Back. *The Complete Book of Herbs & Spices,* new edition. London and North Pomfret, Vt.: David & Charles, 1985.

McClane, A. J. *The Encyclopedia of Fish Cookery*. Photography by Arie de Zanger. New York: Holt, Rinehart and Winston, 1977.

McGee, Harold. *On Food and Cooking: The Science and Lore of the Kitchen*. New York: Scribners, 1984.

Mahan, L. Kathleen, and Marian Arlin. *Krause's Food, Nutrition and Diet Therapy,* 8th edition. Philadelphia: W. B. Saunders, 1992.

Margen, Sheldon, and the Editors of the University of California at Berkeley *Wellness Letter*. *The Wellness Encyclopedia of Food and Nutrition*. New York: Rebus, 1992.

Mariani, John F. *The Dictionary of American Food and Drink,* completely revised and updated. New York: Hearst Books, 1994.

Marquis, Vivienne, and Patricia Haskell. *The Cheese Book*. New York: Simon & Schuster, 1965.

Masefield, G. B., M. Wallis, S. G. Harrison and B. E. Nicholson. *The Oxford Book of Food Plants*. London: Oxford University Press, 1969.

Mayer, Jean, and Jeanne P. Goldberg. *Dr. Jean Mayer's Diet & Nutrition Guide*. New York: Pharos, 1990.

Miller, Mark, with John Harrisson. *The Great Chile Book*. Photography by Lois Ellen Frank. Berkeley, Calif.: Ten Speed Press, 1991.

Obert, Jessie Craig. *Community Nutrition,* 2d edition. New York: Wiley, 1986.

Ody, Penelope. *The Complete Medicinal Herbal*. London: Dorling Kindersley, 1993.

Owen, Sri. *The Rice Book*. New York: St. Martin's Press, 1993.

Passmore, Jacki. *The Encyclopedia of Asian Food and Cooking*. New York: Morrow, 1991.

Peterson, Lee Allen. *A Field Guide to Edible Wild Plants*. Boston: Houghton Mifflin, 1977.

Pike, Ruth L., and Myrtle L. Brown. *Nutrition: An Integrated Approach,* 3d edition. New York: Wiley, 1984.

Potter, Norman. *Food Science,* 5th edition. New York: Chapman & Hall, 1995.

Pronsky, Zaneta M. *Food Medication Interactions,* 8th edition. Pottstown, Pa.: Food-Medication Interactions, 1993.

Revel, Jean-François. *Culture and Cuisine: A Journey Through the History of Food*. Translated by Helen R. Lane. New York: Doubleday, 1982.

Robbins, Chandler S., Bertel Bruun and Herbert S. Zim. *Birds of North America*. New York: Golden Press, 1966.

Roe, Daphne A. *A Handbook on Drug and Nutrient Interactions,* 4th edition. Chicago: The American Dietetic Association, 1989.

Rogers, Sheridan. *The Cook's Garden*. Illustrations by Skye Rogers. New York: Viking, 1992.

Rolfes, Sharon R., Linda K. DeBruyne, and Eleanor N. Whitney, eds. *Life Span Nutrition*. St. Paul, Minn.: West Publishing, 1990.

Root, Waverley. *Food*. New York: Simon & Schuster, 1980.

————, and Richard de Rochemont. *Eating in America*. New York: Morrow, 1976.

Saltman, Paul, Joel Gurin and Ira Mothner. *The University of California San Diego Nutrition Book*. Boston: Little, Brown, 1993.

Schneider, Elizabeth. *Uncommon Fruits & Vegetables: A Commonsense Guide*. New York: Harper & Row, 1986.

Shibamoto, Takayuki, and Leonard F. Bjeldanes. *Introduction to Food Toxicology*. San Diego: Academic Press, 1993.

Shils, Maurice E., ed. *Modern Nutrition in Health and Disease,* 8th edition. Philadelphia: Lea & Febiger, 1993.

Silverman, Harold M., and Gilbert I. Simon. *The Pill Book*. New York: Bantam Books, 1980.

Simmons, Marie. *Rice, the Amazing Grain*. New York: Henry Holt, 1991.

Simon, André L., and Robin Howe. *Dictionary of Gastronomy*. New York: McGraw-Hill, 1970.

Spears, Marian C. *Foodservice Organizations,* 2d edition. Englewood Cliffs, N.J.: Prentice-Hall, 1991.

Steinman, David. *Diet for a Poisoned Planet: How to Choose Safe Foods for You and Your Family*. New York: Harmony Books, 1990.

Stobart, Tom. *The Cook's Encyclopedia: Ingredients & Processes*. Millie Owen, ed. New York: Harper & Row, 1980.

————. *Herbs, Spices and Flavorings*. Woodstock, N.Y.: Overlook Press, 1982.

Tannahill, Reay. *Food in History,* new, fully revised and updated edition. New York: Crown, 1988.

Taylor, Clara Mae, and Orrea Florence Pye. *Foundations of Nutrition,* 6th edition. New York: Macmillan, 1966.

Thomas, Clayton L., ed. *Taber's Cyclopedic Medical Dictionary,* 16th edition. Philadelphia: F. A. Davis, 1985.

Trager, James. *Foodbook.* New York: Grossman, 1970.

Turgeon, Charlotte, American ed. *The New Larousse Gastronomique.* New York: Crown, 1977.

Tver, David F., and Percy Russell. *The Nutrition and Health Encyclopedia,* 2d edition. New York: Van Nostrand Reinhold, 1989.

Tyler, Varro E. *The Honest Herbal.* Binghamton, N.Y.: Pharmaceutical Products Press, 1993.

United States Pharmacopeial Convention. *The Physicians' and Pharmacists' Guide to Your Medicines.* New York: Ballantine.

von Welanetz, Diana and Paul. *The von Welanetz Guide to Ethnic Ingredients.* Los Angeles: J. P. Tarcher, 1982.

Ward, Artemus. *The Encyclopedia of Food.* New York: Artemus Ward, 1923.

Wardlaw, Gordon M., and Paul M. Insel. *Perspectives in Nutrition,* 2d edition. St. Louis: Mosby, 1993.

Wason, Betty. *Cooks, Gluttons, and Gourmets.* Garden City, N.Y.: Doubleday, 1962.

Whitney, Eleanor N., Corrine B. Cataldo and Sharon R. Rolfes. *Understanding Normal and Clinical Nutrition,* 3rd edition. St. Paul, Minn.: West Publishing, 1991.

Williams, Sue Rodwell, and Bonnie S. Worthington-Roberts. *Nutrition Throughout the Life Cycle,* 2d edition. St. Louis: Mosby, 1992.

Winter, Ruth. *A Consumer's Dictionary of Food Additives,* 3d revised edition. New York: Crown, 1989.

Wood, Rebecca. *Quinoa, the Supergrain.* New York: Japan Publications, Kodansha International, 1989.

The World Atlas of Food. Jane Grigson, contributing ed. London: Mitchell Beazley Publishers; New York: Simon & Schuster, 1974.

Younger, William. *Gods, Men, and Wine.* The Wine and Food Society. Cleveland: World, 1966.

Newspapers, Magazines and Periodicals

Consumer Reports on Health
Eating Well
Environmental Nutrition
FDA Consumer
Food Review
Food Safety Notebook
Food Technology
Harvard Medical School Health Letter
Johns Hopkins Medical Letter Health After 50
Journal of the American Dietetic Association
Natural History
The New England Journal of Medicine
New York Newsday
The New York Times
Nutrition Action
Nutrition Week (Community Nutrition Institute)
Priorities
Scientific American
Smithsonian
Tufts University Diet & Nutrition Letter
University of California at Berkeley Wellness Letter

Databases for Nutrient Values

Books

Ensminger, Audrey H., M. E. Ensminger, James E. Kolande and John R. K. Robson. *Foods & Nutrition Encyclopedia,* 2d edition. Boca Raton, Fla.: CRC Press, 1994.

Pennington, Jean A. T. *Bowes & Church's Food Values of Portions Commonly Used,* 16th edition. Philadelphia: Lippincott, 1994.

United States Department of Agriculture. *Composition of Foods: Raw, Processed, Prepared,* Parts 1 through 21.★ Washington, D.C.: USDA, 1976–1993.

Software

The Food Processor.★ ESHA Research. Salem, Oreg.
Nutrition Data System. Minneapolis, Minn.
Nutritionist IV. N-Squared Computing. San Bruno, Calif.

★Principal sources.